Selected Topics in Food Science and Nutrition

Selected Topics in Food Science and Nutrition

Editor: Dephne Rowland

Callisto Reference
www.callistoreference.com

Callisto Reference,
118-35 Queens Blvd., Suite 400,
Forest Hills, NY 11375, USA

Visit us on the World Wide Web at:
www.callistoreference.com

ISBN: 978-1-64116-250-0 (Hardback)

Printed in China.

Cataloging-in-Publication Data

Selected topics in food science and nutrition / edited by Dephne Rowland.
p. cm.
Includes bibliographical references and index.
ISBN 978-1-64116-250-0
1. Food science. 2. Nutrition. 3. Cooking. 4. Diet. 5. Dietetics. I. Rowland, Dephne.
TP370.8 .S45 2020
641.3--dc23

Table of Contents

Preface

Over the recent decade, advancements and applications have progressed exponentially. This has led to the increased interest in this field and projects are being conducted to enhance knowledge. The main objective of this book is to present some of the critical challenges and provide insights into possible solutions. This book will answer the varied questions that arise in the field and also provide an increased scope for furthering studies.

Nutrition is the science concerned with the study of nutrients in food and their action in promoting growth, reproduction and health. An unhealthy diet can lead to diseases like anemia, scurvy, blindness, cretinism, obesity, cardiovascular disease, osteoporosis, etc. Nutrients are of two types-macronutrients and micronutrients. Macronutrients such as fiber, fats, carbohydrates, proteins and water are needed in large amounts, while micronutrients like minerals and vitamins are needed in smaller quantities. The nature of foods, the causes of food deterioration and the principles of food processing are studied under the domain of food science. The development of new food products, choice of packaging materials, shelf-life studies, and microbiological and chemical testing fall under the scope of food science. Most of the topics introduced herein cover new techniques and applications of food science and nutrition. Food science and nutrition are closely linked as one directly affects the other. The book presents researches and studies performed by experts across the globe. It is an essential guide for both academicians and those who wish to pursue these disciplines further.

I hope that this book, with its visionary approach, will be a valuable addition and will promote interest among readers. Each of the authors has provided their extraordinary competence in their specific fields by providing different perspectives as they come from diverse nations and regions. I thank them for their contributions.

Editor

Effect of Sodium Chloride (NaCl) on the Growth of *Pediococcus acidilactici* used for the Improvement of Nutritional and Microbial Quality of Tsire

Aina AT*

Department of Microbiology, University of Ibadan, Ibadan, Nigeria

***Corresponding author:** Aina AT, Department of Microbiology, University of Ibadan, Ibadan, Nigeria, E-mail: ainaadetinuke@gmail.com

Abstract

This finding was aimed at investigating the effect of varying sodium chloride concentration on the growth of *Pediococcus acidilactici* used for improving the nutritional and microbial quality of Nigerian grilled meat product; tsire. *P. acidilactici* used in the study was isolated from raw beef. *P. acidilactici* was cultured in 5.5, 6.5, 7.5, 8.5 and 9.5% NaCl concentration and incubation time. Tsire was prepared using traditional method and *P. acidilactici* was inoculated on the product and stored for 5 days at 28 ± 2°C. The samples were analysed for microbial and nutritional content after 5 days. *P. acidilactici* and *Lactobacillus confusus* (23%) each, *Lactobacillus kandleri, Lactobacillus plantarum* and *Lactobacillus fermentum* (12% each) and *Lactobacillus rhamnosus, Lactobacillus viridiscences* and *Lactobacillus vaccinostercus* (6% each) were isolated from raw beef samples. Growth of *P. acidilactici* decreased with increase in NaCl concentration and steady growth was observed with 5.5-7.5% NaCl concentration. LAB counts were high in tsire treated with *P. acidilactici* cultured in 6.5 and 7.5% NaCl (10.75 and 10.10 log cfu/g respectively) and corresponding low coliform counts was also observed (1.17 and 1.05 log cfu/g). Crude protein content was higher in tsire treated with *P. acidilactici* cultured in 5.5, 6.5 and 7.5% NaCl (24.49, 21.17 and 22.54% respectively) with corresponding low FFA values (18.39, 16.13 and 17.00% respectively). Data obtained in this research is being applied in harmonized in further research to obtain tsire of acceptable quality in terms of microbial content, nutritional value and sensory attributes.

Keywords: Tsire; *Pediococcus acidilactici*; Lactic acid bacteria; Sodium chloride; Crude protein; Free fatty acid

Introduction

Lactic Acid Bacteria (LAB) have been implicated in various studies on meat and meat products [1-3]. Lactic acid bacteria plays a very important role in food fermentation as products obtained through them are characterized by hygienic safety, storage stability and attractive sensory properties [4]. Their microbial antagonism results from the lone or combined production of organic acids, ethanol, diacetyl, hydrogen peroxide, and carbon dioxide [5]. Lactic acid bacteria that have been reportedly used in meat production include Pediococcus species *(P. cerevisae* and *P. acidilactici)* and *Lactobacillus* species (*L. plantarum, L. brevis* and *L. buchneri)* and *Lactococcus* species [1,6,7].

Meat is a major source of protein and vitamins for most people in many parts of the world, thus they are essential for the growth repair and maintenance of body cells and necessary for our everyday activities [8]. Meats are highly perishable foods due to their chemical and physiological composition thus they support the growth of a wide range of microorganisms [9]. Several methods have been used to preserve meat including cooking, fermenting, salting, smoking and drying. **Salting** meat is an ancient preservation technique in which the salt draws out moisture and creates an environment inhospitable to bacteria [10]. Other functions of salts include microbial growth suppression, water reduction, salt-soluble protein release, and pro-oxidant effects [11]. NaCl and $NaNO_2$ are the common curing salts used in meat production with NaCl making the bulk of the mixture.

Tsire is a Nigerian grilled meat product consumed as evening delicacies. Tsire is synonymous to suya. Tsire vendors often have left over from their daily sales thus the chances of contamination as storage facilities are often unavailable or inadequate. Tsire is prepared using de-boned meat (often beef) spiced with ingredients such as common salt (NaCl), garlic, pepper, groundnut cake etc. Studies by Onilude et al. [12], established that lactic cultures influence the quality attributes of tsire and Olaoye [13] also found that organisms such as *P. acidilactici* could be used as starter cultures for extending the shelf-life of the product. This research is thus aimed at investigating the effect of NaCl on the growth of *P. acidilactici* used for the improvement of nutritional and microbial quality of tsire.

This study is aimed at studying the effect of varying sodium chloride concentration on the growth of *P. acidilactici* used for improving the nutritional and microbial quality of Nigerian grilled meat product; tsire.

Materials and Methods

Raw meat samples were purchased from local vendors at retail outlets in Ibadan, Oyo State. The samples were incubated at 37C for 24 h to allow bacterial colonization. Ten grams of the meat samples was homogenized in 90 mL sterile normal saline solution, pour-plated on de Mann Rogosa and Sharpe (MRS) agar and incubated at 37C for 48 h in an anaerobic jar. [14]. Isolates were identified using API 50CH and CHL medium (API system, Montalieu, Vericeu, France).

Effect of sodium chloride concentration on the growth of the isolate

P. acidilactici was aseptically inoculated into 15 mL peptone water in test tubes and incubated at 32 ± 5°C for 18 h. 1 mL aliquot of *P. acidilactici* was inoculated into sterile MRS broth with sodium chloride concentration of the media was supplemented with 5.5, 6.5, 7.5, 8.5 and 9.5% sodium chloride. The bottles were incubated at 32 ± 5C for 12, 24, 36 and 48 h. Growth measurement was determined as Optical density (OD) at 620 nm using Spectronic 20 D.

Tsire sample preparation

Tsire was produced from beef using a traditional method described by Onilude et al. [12].

Fresh beef and tsire spices including onion, ginger and garlic were purchased from a local market in Lagos, Nigeria.

The meat(fat-free) was washed in 5% sterile saline water and sliced into layers to about 10 × 6 × 0.5 cm^3, not exceeding a weight of 20 g each. The meat pieces cured with ground pepper and all other spices were hung on stick and allowed to marinate for 10-15 min after which they were grilled on hot coals at a temperature of 130-150°C for 15-20 min with intermittent sprinkling of groundnut oil to stimulate the traditional processing method and to prevent burning of the stick meat samples.

The samples were allowed to cool to ambient temperature and inoculated *P. acidilactici* cultured at different NaCl concentration. Inoculated tsire samples were incubated in a sterile environment at 29 ± 2°C for 48 h before further analysis. Un-inoculated tsire served as the control.

Proximate analyses of tsire samples inoculated with the stressed isolate

The Protein, Moisture, Ash and Free Fatty Acid (FFA) content of the tsire samples were analysed as described by AOAC [15].

Microbiological analyses of tsire samples inoculated with the stressed isolate

10-15 g of each of tsire samples were cut into small pieces and blended in 90 mL sterile distilled water in a disinfected blender to make the initial dilution. Serial dilutions of the samples were then prepared and 1 mL of the appropriate dilutions was plated out using the pour plate method described by Totora et al. [16]. MRS agar was used to enumerate for Lactic acid bacteria, MacConkey agar for Coliforms and Yeast Extract agar for Yeasts. Samples were incubated for 48 h in Gallenkomp 9052 laboratory incubator.

Results

Figure 1 shows the frequency of occurrence of Lactic Acid Bacteria isolated from raw beef sample.

The result of the isolation shows that the highest occurring microorganisms were *P. acidilactici* and L. confusus (23%) each followed by *L. kandleri, L. plantarum* and *L. fermentum* (12% each) and the least occurring were *L. rhamnosus, L. viridiscences* and *L. vaccinostercus* (6% each).

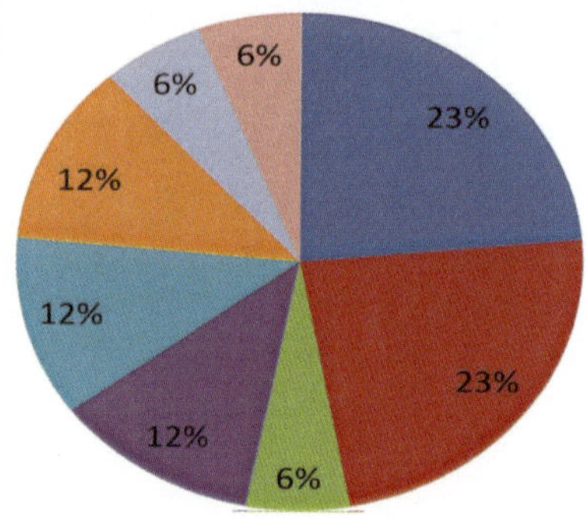

Figure 1: Percentage occurrence of Lactic acid bacteria isolated from raw beef samples.

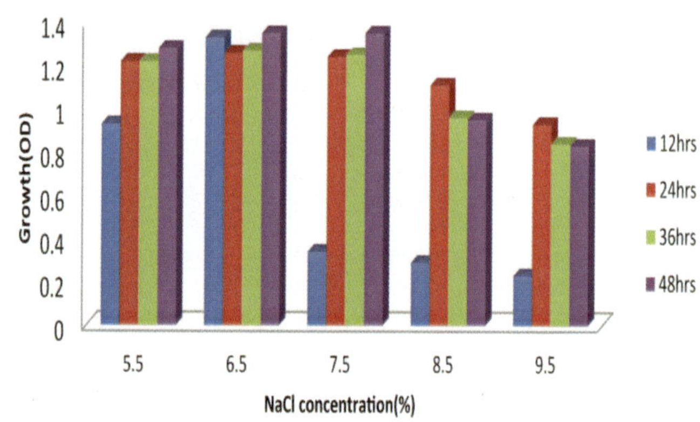

Figure 2: Growth of *Pediococcus acidilactici* at different concentrations of NaCl and incubation time.

NaCl Concentration (%)	LAB	Yeast	Coliforms	Mold
5.5	7.95	2.06	2.53	1.5
6.5	10.75	3.11	1.17	1.71
7.5	10.1	3.5	1.05	2.55
8.5	8.35	2.14	2.02	1.09
9.5	5.15	2.98	3.41	1.12
*Values are mean of three replicates				

Table 1: Microbial load (log cfu/g) of tsire samples inoculated with *Pediococcus acidilactici* (cultured at different NaCl concentration) after storing for 5 days at 28 ± 2°C.

Discussion

Figure 1 shows the percentage occurrence of LAB isolated from raw beef samples and they were identified as *L. confusus, P. acidilactici, L. rhamnosus, L. plantarum, L. fermentum, L. kandleri, L. viridiscences* and *L. vaccinostercus.* Oliveira et al. [17] reported the isolation of *L. plantarum, P. acidilactici* and *L. fermentum* from vacuum packaged beef. Collins et al. [18] reported the isolation of *L. confusus* in meat, *L. viridiscences* was reported to cause greening in meat due to excessive production of hydrogen peroxide [19]. Meat supports the growth of a wide range of micro-organisms because of its nutritious nature.

NaCl Concentration (%)	Ash	Crude Protein	Free Fatty Acid (FFA)	TBA
5.5	9.4	24.49	18.39	1.25
6.5	9.87	21.17	16.13	1.04
7.5	8.92	22.54	17	1.15
8.5	11.27	18.44	20.98	1.05
9.5	10.47	15.2	21.06	1.27
*Values are mean of three replicates				

Table 2: Nutritional analysis (%) of tsire samples inoculated with *P. acidilactici* (cultured at different NaCl concentration) after storing for 5 days at room temperature.

Figure 2 shows the growth of *P. acidilactici* at different NaCl concentration and incubation time. Similar to previous reports by Altuntas et al. [20], growth of *P. acidilactici* decreased with increase in NaCl concentration. *P. acidilactici* was observed to have steady growth with 5.5-7.5% NaCl concentration. It is believed that the organisms are at the exponential phase of growth with favorable growth conditions while at higher NaCl concentration of 8.5-9.5% growth decreased with increased contact time.

Microbial contamination can lower the quality and shorten the shelf life of meat and meat products resulting in economic loss or health hazard [3]. As shown in Table 1, the highest LAB count (10.75%) was observed on tsire sample treated with *P. acidilactici* grown in 6.5% NaCl. LAB count was least (5.15 log cfu/g) on sample treated with *P. acidilactici* grown in 9.5% NaCl. Lower coliform value was observed in tsire sample treated with *P. acidilactici* grown in 6.5% NaCl being 1.17 log cfu/g and 7.5% NaCl being 1.05 log cfu/g. The lower coliform values observed on samples with higher LAB proliferation can be due to the production of antimicrobial compounds such as lactic acid, bacteriocin, hydrogen peroxide and diacetyl [7]. Tsire produced with *P. acidilactici* cultured in 6.5 and 7.5% NaCl can be considered safe for consumption based on the low coliform values as coliform have direct impact on health and within limit of hot smoked meat product specified by the Food Administration Manual. Yeasts and moulds invade and grow on almost all food items at any time resulting in deterioration and decomposition of foods. They may be hazardous to human health because of their ability to produce mycotoxins. Gandi [21] reported the isolation of *A. niger, A. flavs, Penicillum* spp. and *Fusarium* spp. from suya (Table 2).

The ash content of a food sample is synonymous to the mineral content of the sample. Ash content of tsire samples in this study was between 8.92 and 11.27% which agrees with reports by authors such as Olusola et al. [22] reported 10.31% ash on Kilishi which is a dry meat product and Torres et al. [23]; 9.40-11.27% ash content of tsire samples. Ash content of various samples depends on the meat type. The crude protein of tsire samples in this study was within 15.20-24.49%. Proteins are Polymers of Amino acids and it is the only macro nutrient in food that contains nitrogen. Groundnut cake was not used in the production of tsire in this study. Studies by Abdullahi et al. [24]; 31.88% crude protein on tsire and Gandi [21] reported higher crude protein content (31.88 and 40-45% respectively)

Free Fatty Acid (FFA) content of a sample indicates the extent to which the oils in the sample have been decomposed by Lipase action. FFA formation is often accompanied by rancidity and also heat and light accelerate FFA formation. The lower the FFA content of a sample, the better the sample, the better the sample is. The least FFA in this study was observed on tsire samples treated with *P. acidilactici* cultured at 6.5% NaCl concentration. The meat type and part has a direct relationship to the FFA content of meat products. Thiobabituric Acid (TBA) reactive substances are formed as a byproduct of lipid peroxidation measured as the malonaldehyde per weight of the sample. TBA values of tsire samples in this study ranged between 1.04% and 1.27%. Lipids are susceptible to oxidation and enzymatic oxidation under different conditions usually involving free radicals or oxygen species [25].

Conclusion

P. acidilactici can grow in NaCl concentrations up to 9.5%, the effect of culturing *P. acidilactici* in varying NaCl concentration is not significant with respect to the microbial quality of tsire produced using these organisms. However, higher crude protein and lower free fatty acid content was observed in tsire samples treated with *P. acidilactici* cultured in <7.5% NaCl. Data obtained in this study is being applied in further work to obtain tsire of acceptable quality in terms of microbial content, nutritional value and sensory attributes.

References

1. Olaoye OA, Onilude AA (2010) Investigation on the potential use of biological agents in the extension of fresh beef in Nigeria. World J Microbiol Biotechnol 26: 1445-1454.
2. Afolabi RO, Bankole OM, Olaitan JO (2008) Production and characterization of antimicrobial agents by lactic acid bacteria isolated from fermented foods. Int J Microbiol 4: 12-17.
3. Kalalo I, Faid M, Ahami AT (2004) Extending the shelf life of fresh minced camel meat at ambient temperature by *Lactobacillus delbruekii* sub sp *delbruekii.* Elect J Biotechnol 7: 246-251.
4. Savadogo A, Quatarra CAT, Bassole IHN, Traore AS (2004) Antimicrobial activities of lactic acid bacteria strains isolated from *Burkina faso* fermented milk. Pak J of Nutr 3: 174-179.
5. De Vuyst L, Vandamme EJ (1994) Antimicrobial potential of lactic acid bacteria. In: De Vuyst L, Vandamme EJ (Eds.) Bacteriocins of Lactic Acid Bacteria: Microbiology, Genetics and Applications. Blackie Academic and Professional, London, pp: 91-142.
6. Jay JM (2005) Modern Food Microbiology (4th edn.). CBS Publishers and distributors. New Delhi, India pp: 384-385.
7. Cizeikiene D, Juodeikune G, Paskevicius A, Bartkieize E (2013) Antimicrobial activity of Lactic acid bacteria against pathogenic and spoilage microorganism isolated from food and their control in wheat bread. Food Control 31: 539-545.
8. Hassan El-S, Ferage M, Nahla T (2006) Lactic acid and pH as indication for bacterial spoilage of meat and some meat products. J Appl Sci Res 2: 522-528
9. Kim JW, Rajagopal SN (2001) Antimicrobial activities of *Lactobacillus crispatus* ATCC 33820 and *Lactobacillus gasseri* ATCC 33323. J Microbiol 39: 146-148.
10. Alonge DO, Hiko AA (1981) Traditional methods of meat preservation and preparation in Nigeria. West Afr Farm Food Proc pp: 19-21.
11. Fontana C, Cocconcelli P, Vignolo G (2005) Monitoring the bacterial population dynamics during fermentation of artisanal Argentinean sausages. Int J Food Microbiol 103: 131-142.
12. Onilude AA, Sanni AI, Olaoye OA, Ogunbanwo ST (2002) Influence of lactic cultures on the quality attributes of tsire, a West African stick meat. World J Microbiol Biotechnol 18: 615-619.

13. Olaoye (2014) Characteristics of Lactic Acid Bacteria being proposed as starter cultures for extending the shelf life of a Nigerian grilled meat product Tsire. Asian J Sci Technol 5: 639-643.
14. Olaoye AO, Onilude AA, Dodd ER (2008) Identification of *Pediococcus* spp. from beef and evaluation of their lactic acid production in varying concentration of different carbon sources. Adv Nat Appl Sci 2: 197-207.
15. AOAC International (AOAC) (2005) Official methods of analysis of AOAC International (18th edn.).
16. Totora GJ, Funke BR, Case CL (2002) Microbiology: An introduction (7th edn.). Pearson Education Inc. publishing as Benham in Cummings. San Fransisco, USA.
17. Oliveiria RBP, Oliveria AL, Gloria MBA (2008) Screening of lactic acid bacteria from vacuum packaged beef for antimicrobial activity. Braz J Microbiol.
18. Collins MD, Rodriguez V, Ash C, Aguirre M, Farrow JAE (1993) Phylogenetic analysis of the genus Lactobacillus and related lactic acid bacteria as determined by reverse transcriptase sequencing of 16SrRNA. FEMS Microbiol Lett 77: 5-12.
19. Ammor S, Tauveron G, Dufour E, Chevallier I (2006) Antibacterial activity of lactic acid bacteria against spoilage pathogenic bacteria isolated from scale meat facility: Screening and characterization of the antibacterial compounds. Food Control 17: 454-461.
20. Altuntas EG, Cosansu S, Ayhan K (2010) Some growth parameters and antimicrobial activity of bacteriocin-producing strains of *P. acidilactici* GL2213. Int J Food Microbiol 141: 28-31
21. Gandi BR (2014) Quality characteristics and microbial status of beef smoked with different plant materials and suya produced from round muscles. "A thesis to the school of postgraduate studies Ahmadu Bello University, Zaria, Nigeria p: 56.
22. Olusola OO, Okubanjo AO, Omojola AB (2012) Nutritive and organoleptic characteristics of kilishi as affected by meat type and ingredient formulation. J Anim Prod Adv 2: 221-232
23. Torres EEFS, Shimokomaki M, Franco BDGM, Landgrant M (1994) Parameter determining the quality of "charqui" on intermediate moisture meat product. Meat Sci 38: 229-234
24. Abdullahi IO, Umoh VJ, Ameh JB, Galadima M (2010) Environmental impact and hazards analysis critical control point (HACCP) concept in the production of Tsire at Zaria, Nigeria. Anim Prod Res Advs.
25. Fereidon S, Ying Z (2005) Bailey's industrial oil and fat products (6th edn.). John Wiley and sons Inc. pp: 357-367.

2

Magnesium: A Mineral Essential for Health Yet Generally Underestimated or Even Ignored

Adel AA Ismail[1*] **and Nour A Ismail**[2]

[1]*Consultant in Clinical Biochemistry and Chemical Endocrinology (RTD), Pinderfiels and Leeds Teaching Hospitals, West Yorkshire, England*

[2]*Pinderfiels and Leeds Teaching Hospitals, West Yorkshire, England*

[*]**Corresponding author:** Adel AA Ismail, Consultant in Chemical Endocrinology, Pinderfiels and Leeds Teaching Hospitals, West Yorkshire, England
E-mail: adelaaismail@aol.com

Abstract

Magnesium is the fourth most common mineral in the human body after calcium, potassium and sodium. Magnesium must be continuously replenished through foods and water intake because it is not synthesizable. Chronic inadequate intake of magnesium over long period of time can manifest as latent magnesium deficiency with symptoms such as muscle weakness, cramps, fatigue, neurological and cardiovascular dysfunctions, reduced bone mineralization and strength. Reports published by WHO have estimated that ~two thirds of Americans and French have magnesium intake below the recommended amounts but only a small numbers are overtly depleted. The authorities in Finland were concerned of the negative impact of geochemical magnesium deficiency in the eastern region of Finland and its adverse effect on heart health. A program was initiated to increase magnesium intake though supplementation; this has contributed to progressive fall of death rate due to heart-related issues. Restoring and sustaining adequate magnesium store are easy and inexpensive.

Some 40% of total body magnesium is intracellular and ~60% in bone and teeth with less than 1% in circulation. Intracellular magnesium deficiency may or may not be reflected as overt hypomagnesaemia making measurement of plasma/serum magnesium potentially misleading when "normal" plasma/serum concentration is "interpreted" to exclude deficiency.

In this review, the role of magnesium at cellular level, its homeostasis and major clinical conditions associated with magnesium deficiency in adults will be briefly discussed. Assessment of magnesium status and its potential deficiency by examining individual's "modus vivendi" and/or the use of laboratory tests will be highlighted. Finally, various therapeutic modalities and monitoring of treatment will be summarized.

Keywords: Magnesium; Mineral; Human health; Food

Background

The relationship between magnesium and health has been recognized some 400 years ago and well before magnesium was even identified as an element. The English summer in 1618 was exceptionally hot and dry. A farmer by the name of Henry Wicker in Epsom, Surrey dug out few wells in his farm to get water for his herd of cows. He noticed that his thirsty animals refused to drink this water because it had a tarty and bitter taste. However he noted that this water has the ability to rapidly heal scratches, sores and rashes both in animals and humans. Tried by others, the fame of this water was spread by the word of mouth. Londoners flocked to Epsom which became a Spa town, surpassing others more fashionable ones at the time such as Tunbridge wells in Kent for its water and salt. A physician (also a Botanist) with extensive practice in London by the name of Nehemiah Grew noted that the salt in this water had a laxative effect. This "mind-boggling" discovery was patented as a purging salt and a factory in London was established for world-wide marketing. In England this salt was (and still is) known as "Epsom Salt" and in continental Europe as "Salt Anglicum".

Late in the 17th century and thereafter, Epsom salt was one of the most popular medicinal drugs. The people who used it did not know exactly why it was so beneficial, but they did understand that in some way it was good for health and promoted longevity. Even now, it is surprising to know that there is an "Epsom Salt Council" in the UK whose members are wild about the goodness of "Epsom Salt". Currently, 13 wonderful ways have been described for the use of "Epsom Salt" by this council.

Epsom Salt is a magnesium salt (hydrated magnesium sulphate; $MgSO_4.7H_2O$). In 1755, the Scottish Chemist Joseph Black in Edinburgh identified magnesium as an element and the English chemist Sir Humphrey Davy was the first to isolate magnesium by electrolysis in 1808. The 19th century was the age of chemistry of magnesium; its biology however became clearer during the 20th century. The importance of magnesium in health remained overlooked or even ignored in the 21st century. This may be attributed to (a) the amorphous ramifications of magnesium deficiency causing a wide range of clinical manifestations and (b) the common and overuse of plasma/serum magnesium measurement when deficiency is suspected, the lack of understanding of the limitations of this test and it's often misinterpretation by health practitioners [1]. It is not therefore surprising that magnesium deficiency is not uncommon in the general population and even in some people with apparently healthy life style who may be deficient of such important mineral.

Magnesium, a Major But Under-recognized and Underestimated Mineral

Of the 90 naturally occurring elements in the planet earth, ~25 are considered to be essential for health in humans. Four of these 25 namely carbon, oxygen, hydrogen and nitrogen constitute ~97% of body building blocks. The other 21 elements accounting for ~3% of all elements in human's body, of which 8 are "anions" namely phosphorous, sulphur, chlorine, iodine, fluorine, boron, chromium and silicon; and 13 are metals "cations". Based on body contents and recommended daily allowance (RDA), only four metals are regarded as "majors"; these are calcium, potassium, sodium and magnesium; the other 9 are required in relatively much smaller amounts and are designated as "trace-metals"; these are iron, zinc, manganese, copper, selenium, molybdenum, cobalt, tin and vanadium.

Although calcium, potassium and sodium are readily recognizable as major minerals, magnesium is neither commonly known nor perceived as a major one, even by some health professionals despite its relatively high recommended daily allowance (RDA). For example, the RDA of magnesium is ~50% and ~25% that recommended for calcium and sodium respectively and ~26 times greater than that of iron, the top of all trace metals in terms of RDA. Sustaining magnesium balance is not only dependent on RDA but its absorption and retention in the body. Age is an important physiological factor because absorption of magnesium from the gut is reduced and its loss from the body in urine increases with age in both genders. Consequently, magnesium deficiency occurs more often in the elderly than in the young. Furthermore, the incidence is also likely to vary significantly from one area to another because of the large variation in magnesium contents in drinking water which can provide up to 30% of daily requirement.

Brief Note on the Biological Role of Magnesium at Cellular Level

The 19th century was the age of chemistry of magnesium; its biology however became clearer during the 20th century. Approximately 40% of magnesium is intracellular and some 60% in bone and teeth with 1% or less is present in the circulation [1].

It may be important to reiterate that although magnesium intake is in the form of elemental radical, in body fluids magnesium do not function nor operate biologically in this form i.e., "native chemical radicals" but as "hydrated-ions", enclosed within shells of water which confer and exert a profound influence on their electrochemical, biochemical and physiological roles.

Magnesium *in vivo* (Mg^{2+}) exhibits a rather unique or even peculiar characteristic in its ionic hydration form, being distinctly different from the other three major minerals namely Ca^{2+}, K^+ and Na^+. Such difference is important to highlight because it illustrates the physical uniqueness of hydrated Mg^{2+} ion and its recognition at molecular level (Table 1).

Table 1 shows the massive and disproportionate increase in the Mg^{2+} atomic radius upon hydration compared with the other three major ions [2,3]. This is because Mg^{2+} is a highly "charge dense" ion compared not only with Na^+, K^+ or Ca^{2+}, but all other cations, thus holding the waters' shell tightly by a factor of 10^3-10^4, rigidly within hexa-coordinated hydration shell. It was suggested that this unique characteristic makes the hydrated Mg^{2+} ion more recognisable for various molecular actions/transport.

Atomic Wt. radius (Est)	Ionic radius, picometer (Est)	Increase in hydrated
Na^+ 23	102-116 pm ?	X25 fold
K^+ 39	138-152 pm ?	X4 fold
Ca^{2+} 40	100-114 pm ?	X25 fold
Mg^{2+} 24	72-86 pm ?	X400 fold

Table 1: Changes in atomic radius on hydration (estimated).

Biologically, magnesium is regarded with justification as a "chronic regulator" and biochemically as a "forgotten electrolyte". The number of cells in an adult is ~37 trillion [4] and cellular biochemistry/physiology is complex. Biological processes carried out within each cell and between adjacent cells have to be orderly and function harmoniously and in synchrony using highly complex systems of neuroendocrine bio-communication. Individual living cell receives a large number of signals such as stimulation to grow, to divide, to initiate or stop the making of specific bio-components, to trigger an immune response et cetera. Each signal needs to be correctly transmitted, properly read, interpreted and clearly communicated both within individual cell and between adjacent cells in the first place. These processes are regulated by specific intracellular proteins/enzymes each dedicated to a specific biological task which may not be only sequential but require appropriate activation/initiation to start a process followed by deactivation/stoppage signal to terminate such task. Mitochondria within individual cell also generate its own energy utilizing a cascade of proteins/enzymes which drive this process. When a cell dysfunction, repairing processes is attempted and when fails, the dysfunctional cell commits orderly and voluntary suicide (i.e., apoptosis). Central to all these cellular processes is that each cellular component must be at the right place and function at the right time, both within and between cells.

The regulators of all the above examples of cellular functions are catalysed by some 500 enzymes known biochemically as Kinases which essentially coordinate, control and integrate such complex web of orderly processes. Kinases have a vital role in signal transduction and the production and actions of second messengers such as c-AMP, diacylglycerol, calmodulin and c-GMP. Kinases activate or inhibit individual protein/component, route them to a specific cellular location, or block their interaction with others (i.e., establishing an orderly production-line). To transmit their orders, kinases label specific location(s) within a corresponding protein/component with polar phosphate group (PO^{3-}) i.e., phosphorylation. The source of polar phosphate group is ATP and Kinases can only bind "Mg-ATP" complex, allowing it to cleave the γ phosphate group which is subsequently transferred to the recipient molecule. Phosphorylation is an ion-radical, electron-spin selective process [5-7] which transforms (switches on) an inactive molecule into an active or "functional" one which can then perform a specific biological/biochemical task (or vice versa). In addition to the phosphorylation of small organic molecules, up to 30% of functional body proteins are activated by magnesium-dependent kinases.

Physiologically, magnesium plays an important role in electrolyte homeostasis being necessary for the activation of ATP/ATPase pumps such as Na^+/K^+ pump, Na^+/Ca^{++} , Na^+/Mg^{++} and Mg^{++}/Ca^{++} pumps which if deficient causes impairment and reduction in their efficacy and activities. Chronic magnesium deficiency with time may eventually lead to overt pathology and electrolyte disturbances such as "refractory" hypokalaemia and/or hypocalcaemia. Neither the former nor the later can be corrected by potassium or calcium treatment alone and magnesium replacement becomes essential for restitution. It is therefore paramount to note that magnesium itself is an electrolyte which plays a major role in the homeostasis of other major electrolytes, namely Na^+, K^+ and Ca^{++}. Furthermore, magnesium is necessary for bone mineral density and strength, protein, carbohydrate and fat metabolism, energy transfer, storage and use (i.e., bioenergetics, and oxidative energy metabolism). About 150 magnesium-dependent kinases are linked to a wide variety of diseases; it is not therefore surprising that magnesium deficiency can potentially cause/exacerbate a wide range of disorders [8-16].

Magnesium also encourages bone formation [12], directly and indirectly through its effect on bone hormones such as parathyroid and vitamin D. Magnesium plays a role in bone mineralization and its mechanical strength. Several studies have shown a positive relationship between dietary magnesium intake and bone mineral density (BMD). There is evidence to suggest that magnesium supplementation increases BMD over the course of one year but its impact on bone fractures is not yet known.

Finally, the underlying reaction mechanism seems to be the same for all known kinase. Up to 300 different kinases are present within a single cell; each devoted to a particular task, route individual component to a specific cellular location, or blocks their interaction with others (i.e., streamlining an orderly production-line). The dependence of Kinases on magnesium for their function has led to their nomenclature as "magnesium-dependent kinases". Magnesium deficiency if present impairs and if depleted impedes kinase's activity. Kinases are the largest superfamily of all enzymes in the human body to which ~one fifties of the ~24,000 human genes are dedicated to their encoding, highlighting their important role in regulating nearly all intracellular biological processes. The central role of these regulatory mechanisms in biochemistry/physiology is reflected in the worldwide publication of some 200,000 papers on these subjects over a period of only 18 months between March 2012 and July 2014.

Magnesium Homeostasis

Considering the many vital roles of magnesium, there was surprisingly lack of information regarding its homeostasis. Only in the last decade however two ion channels have been suggested as magnesium transporters which appear to play a pivotal role in its homeostasis through the dual processes of its absorption from the gut and reabsorption by the kidneys. Ion channels conduct a particular ion after which it is named while excluding others e.g. Na^+, K^+ and Ca^{++} channels. Ion hydration energy (water shell surrounding each ion) and the charges at the binding sites by the ligand make the internal milieu within each channel favourable for conducting only a specific ion. The two dedicated ion channels specifically aimed at transporting Mg^{++} belong to the Transient receptor potential melastatin (TRPM), a sub-family of the transient receptor potential proteins super-family involved in transporting other cellular cations such as calcium by TPRM 3. Recently, TRPM 6 and TRPM 7 have been suggested as unique transporters for Mg^{++} termed chanzymes because they possess a channel and a kinase domain. These two chanzymes may therefore represent molecular mechanism aimed at regulating magnesium homeostasis at cellular level [2,17-22]. They are differentially expressed, with TRPM6 being found primarily in colon and renal distal tubules. Up-regulation of TRPM 6 occurs in response to reduction in intracellular magnesium; this in turn enhances magnesium absorption from the gut and its reabsorption by the kidneys and can therefore alter whole-body magnesium homeostasis. TRPM7 is ubiquitous, occurring in numerous organs (e.g. lung). These two chanzymes may therefore represent a molecular mechanism specifically aimed at regulating body magnesium balance [2,17-22].

Clinical Conditions Associated with Magnesium Deficiency in Adults

Magnesium deficiency is common in the general population as well as in hospitalized patients and can occur in individuals with an apparently healthy lifestyle. Latent magnesium deficiency is more common in the elderly, probably exacerbated by oestrogen which decline in women and men with age. Oestrogen influence body magnesium balance through its effect on TRPM6 which may help explaining the hypermagnesuria in the elderly in general and postmenopausal in particular. Magnesium deficiency is clinically under-diagnosed condition, yet surprisingly easy to treat [23-27].

We have researched peer reviewed articles on magnesium published in English between 1990 and April 2011 in MEDLINE and EMBASE and updated thereafter till April 2015 using database keywords "magnesium, deficiency, diagnosis, treatment and hypomagnesaemia". Bibliographies of retrieved articles have been searched and followed. We have also carried out a manual search of each individual issue of major clinical and biochemical journals in which most of these reports have appeared.

Clinically magnesium deficiency may present acutely or with chronic latent manifestations. Clinical presentation of chronic/latent magnesium deficiency may vary from vague and non-specific symptoms to causing and/or exacerbating the progression of wide range of diseases such as cardiovascular pathology (CVS), primary hypertension and diabetes type two.

Magnesium is a physiological calcium antagonist and natural calcium channel blocker and thereby essential for normal neurological and muscular function [28,29]. In skeletal and smooth muscle, magnesium promotes relaxation whilst calcium stimulates contraction. A high calcium/magnesium ratio caused by magnesium deficiency and/or high calcium intake may affect this finely regulated homeostatic balance and may be a factor in the increased risk of cardiovascular events in patients receiving calcium supplementation [30,31]. Magnesium deficiency is implicated/present in almost all patients with hypokalaemia and those with magnesium-dependent hypocalcaemia [32-38].

A growing body of literature has demonstrated a wide pathological role for magnesium deficiency. In 221 peer reviewed studies published from 1990 to April 2015, magnesium deficiency was associated with increased risk and prevalence in the eleven conditions listed in Table 2 (irrespective of the nature, design, parameters, size and statistical approach of these studies). Such an inverse relationship was also demonstrable irrespective of the wide range of methods used to assess magnesium body stores.

Similarly, in 79 studies over the same period, magnesium deficiency was found to predict adverse events and a reduced risk of pathology were noted when supplementation/treatment was instituted. In a recent study [39] a direct aetiological link between magnesium deficiency, impaired glucose tolerance and CVS was demonstrated. In this study thirteen postmenopausal American women (12 Caucasian and 1 African-American) volunteered to reduce their dietary magnesium intake to ~one third of the recommended daily requirement (average 101 mg/day). In less than three months, five subjects had cardiac rhythm abnormalities and three exhibited atrial fibrillation/flutter that responded quickly to magnesium supplementation. Impaired glucose homeostasis was found in 10 volunteers who underwent intravenous glucose tolerance test (IV GTT). The clinical manifestation was reflected in reduced levels in red-cell membranes; however, serum levels remained within reference range. This study, though small, is consistent with epidemiological surveys, supplementation trials and animal studies [40,41] (Table 2 and [1,11]).

Electrolytes	Hypocalcaemia
	Hypokalaemia
CVS	Ventricular arrhythmias esp. Torsades de Pointes,
	Cardiac conduction abnormalities-SVTs,
	Abnormal vascular tone, Congestive cardiac failure
	Ischaemic heart disease/myocardial infarction
Hypertension	Pre-eclampsia/eclampsia, primary hypertension
Endocrine	Type II Diabetes Mellitus
Metabolic	The Metabolic syndrome
Bone	BMD and osteoporosis
Muscular	Muscle weakness, fatigue, numbness, tingling, spasms/cramps/tetany, fibromyalgia
Neurological	Irritability, depression, migraines, vertical and horizontal nystagmus
Cancer	Colorectal
Alcoholics	Exhibiting any of the above manifestations
Respiratory	Asthma

Table 2: Conditions associated with magnesium deficiency.

"Modus Vivendi" and Its Role in Identifying Potential Magnesium Deficiency

Potential causes of magnesium deficiency are outlined in Table 3. It may not be difficult to surmise potential magnesium deficiency from an individual's life-style as body stores are dependent on the balance between daily intake and renal loss [21,42-44]. Approximately 30-70% of dietary magnesium intake is absorbed by a healthy gut with negative magnesium store and high gastric acidity enhancing absorption [21,28,42-46]. The commonly recommended daily intake for adults is 320-400 mg/day (or 6 mg/kg/body weight for both genders) [47] and increases during pregnancy, lactation and regular strenuous exercise [48-50] which increases magnesium losses in urine and sweat. An average healthy daily diet supplies ~250 mg of magnesium (120 mg per 1000 calories) with green vegetables, cereals, fish and nuts are being a rich source (Table 4). Refined grains and white flour are generally low in magnesium. Unrefined sea salt is very rich in magnesium occurring at ~12% of sodium mass, however because this makes raw sea-salt bitter, magnesium (and calcium) are removed making purified table salt essentially ~99% sodium chloride.

Another important source is water [51,52], with some (but not all) hard tap water containing more magnesium than soft water. Local water supplier can provide information regarding magnesium concentration in tap water to each location (e.g. postcode area in the UK). The bioavailability of magnesium in water is generally good at ~60%; however its absorption from water significantly decline with age [53,54].

The magnesium content in tap and/or bottle water varies greatly. Hardness of water is caused by dissolved calcium and magnesium and is usually expressed as the equivalent quantity of calcium carbonate in mg/l (e.g. a hardness of 100 mg/l would contain 40 mg/l of elemental Ca and/or Mg and 60 mg as carbonate). Water containing >200 mg/l equivalent calcium carbonate is considered hard; medium hardness is between 100-200 mg/l; moderately soft <100 mg/l and soft <50 mg/l calcium carbonate equivalent. Hardness above 200 mg/l results in scale deposition on heating if large amount of calcium carbonate is present because it is less soluble in hot water.

Age; elderly absorb less and lose more magnesium
Daily diet low in magnesium
Soft drinking water, bottle or hard water low in magnesium
Refined salt for cooking and in food
Pregnancy, lactation and regular strenuous exercise
Regular alcohol intake esp. spirits
Malabsorption (also short bowel syndrome/intestinal surgery)
Drugs such as diuretics

Table 3: Factors contributing to chronic magnesium deficiency.

Magnesium-rich food contains >100 mg per measure. A measure is a cup of vegetables, grains, legumes or 2 oz (or 56 g) of nuts and seeds.
Vegetables; Green and leafy e.g. Spinach, seaweed and artichoke
Fish; Halibut (4 oz)
Grains; Barley, Wheat, Oat, Bran, (Whole grain bread)
Legumes; Soybean, Adzuki and black bean
Nuts; Almond, Brazil, Cashews, Pine, Peanuts (Peanut butter)
Seeds; (Dried) Pumpkin, Sunflower, watermelon

Table 4: Magnesium content in food.

It may be important to point out that the ratio of calcium to magnesium in hard water varies. Hard water may in some cases have predominantly high concentration of calcium but low in magnesium or vice versa. Furthermore, the type of anion in the calcium salt is important. For example, hard water which is rich in calcium carbonate is usually regarded as "temporary hardness" because on heating, calcium carbonate precipitates. In other forms of hard waters, magnesium and/or calcium may combine with anions other than carbonate, such as sulphate and in this case water is referred to as "permanently hard" because these elements are not affected by heating. All naturally occurring magnesium salts unlike those of calcium, are relatively more soluble in both cold and heated water, including magnesium carbonate. Although hard water is a general term which encompasses wide ratios of calcium to magnesium, the magnesium contents in most hard water (but not all) are 5-20 times more than in soft water and can potentially provide up to 30% of daily requirement.

The term soft water is straight forward because it is used to describe types of water that contain few calcium or magnesium ions. Soft Water usually comes from peat or igneous rock (volcanic rocks which make 95% of earth's crust after the cooling of magma); other sources are granite and sandstone. All such sedimentary rocks are usually low in calcium and magnesium. The magnesium content of soft drinking water is between 2-20 mg/l, average ~6 mg/l. The content of magnesium in bottled water varies from 0-126 mg/litre [55] while carbonated tonic and soda water contains little or no magnesium. One gram of instant coffee granules releases ~5 mg of magnesium in hot water; the corresponding figure for tea is ~0.6 mg [56].

Significant magnesium deficiency has been reported in both elderly self-caring in the community as well as in hospitalized Norwegians [57]. In a consensus survey involving 37,000 Americans, 39% were found to ingest less than 70% of the recommended daily magnesium intake and 10% of women over the age of 70 yrs consume less than 42% of the recommended dietary requirement [58-60]. When dietary magnesium intake is poor, the kidney can compensate by increasing fractional reabsorption to >99% of the filtered load, mainly in the loop of Henle with further reabsorption in the distal tubule. Normally, plasma magnesium is filtered at the glomeruli apart from the fraction bound to albumin. Reabsorption of the filtered load can vary depending on the body store, being lowest when body stores are adequate to maximum in deficiencies. Prolonged periods of poor dietary intake however would eventually lead to a decline in intracellular magnesium concentration.

Excessive renal loss is however a common cause of negative magnesium stores. Alcohol is a known cause, being magnesium diuretic as even moderate amounts produces magnesiuresis. Alcohol increases urinary magnesium loss above baseline by an average of 167% (range 90-357%) and its effect is rapid [61-66] and occurs even in individuals with an already negative magnesium balance. Alcohol consumption has increased with availability and cheaper cost [65,67] and in moderate amounts, is considered socially and culturally acceptable (taken as 2 to 4 units' i.e., 16-32 g of alcohol a day, though there is no standard definition). It may be of interest to point out that spirits such as gin, rum, brandy, cognac, vodka and whisky contain little or no magnesium; fermented apple ciders have 10-50 mg/l of magnesium while beer and wine have levels ranging from ~30-250 mg/l. Although drinks such as some ciders, beer and wine may be considered "magnesium-rich", they cannot be recommended as a reliable source. Furthermore, large consumption of magnesium rich beer and wine can have a laxative or even diarrheatic effect, potentially impeding bioavailability and absorption.

It appears reasonable therefore to suggest that a life-style associated with low dietary magnesium intake in food and drinking water, purified table salt for cooking and in-food, regular and strenuous exercise coupled with moderate and regular consumption of alcoholic drinks which cause a net renal magnesium loss can additively lead to negative balance over time. Magnesium deficiency can be further compounded with malabsorption and those receiving medications [68-72] such as diuretics (loop and thiazide), proton pump inhibitors, tacrolimus, chemotherapeutic agents such as cisplatin, ciclosporin, omeprazole, cetuximab and some phosphate-based drugs.

In summary, modus vivendi when carefully examined can determine the potential of latent magnesium deficiency which may be associated with a wide range of major pathologies. It is however a common practice for clinicians to rely more on laboratory tests in the diagnosis of magnesium deficiency.

Laboratory Tests and Assessment of Magnesium Deficiency

Assessment of magnesium status is biochemical. Serum magnesium is the most commonly requested test and is informative when magnesium is reduced indicating hypomagnesaemia. However, normal serum magnesium (commonly reported ~0.75 mmol/l to ~1.2 mmol/l) remained problematical because in patients suspected with magnesium deficiency serum concentration can be normal despite whole body deficiency [73-76]. This is not surprising because only 1% or less of body magnesium is in blood; the bulk of magnesium is intracellular bound to numerous subcellular components and these are the moieties which account for its biological role. In other words, it is the intracellular bound magnesium which expresses its primary biological role and normal serum magnesium (total or ionized) must be interpreted with caution [76]. Low serum magnesium (with normal albumin) in a fasting or random sample confirms significant deficiency warranting supplementation. For this reason, the practicable, inexpensive and commonly used serum magnesium must be regarded as potentially flawed test, capable of identifying magnesium deficiency in some (range from 2.5 to 15%) but not all patients with deficiency and negative body stores. A fraction of bone magnesium appears to be on a surface limited pool, present either within the hydration shell or else on the crystal lattice. Based largely on animal studies, it has been speculated that this form of bone surface magnesium may represent a limited buffering capacity.

To exclude with confidence latent/chronic magnesium deficiency in cases with high index of suspicion albeit normal serum magnesium, a dynamic study namely magnesium loading test would be appropriate if renal function is normal. This procedure is probably the best physiological "gold standard test" within the capability of all routine hospital laboratories. It involves the administration of elemental magnesium load (as sulphate or chloride) intravenously followed by assessment of the amount of elemental magnesium excreted in the urine in the following 24 hrs [77-81]. A large fraction of the given magnesium load is retained and a smaller amount of the given dose appears in the urine in patients with latent magnesium deficiency. Such a procedure in the experience of one of us was valuable, accurate and informative, however, it is time consuming and (understandably) not commonly used in clinical practice. It is also contra-indicated in individuals with renal impairment.

Magnesium Loading Test

The loading test measures the body's retention of magnesium and therefore reflects the degree of deficiency [77-81]. Attention to details is however paramount for valid interpretation of data. Patient should empty their bladder immediately before the test. The test involves intravenous administration of 30 mmol of elemental magnesium (1 mmol=24 mg) in 500 ml 5% dextrose over a period of 8-12 hours. A slow rate infusion is important because plasma magnesium concentration affects the renal reabsorption threshold and abrupt elevation of plasma concentration above the normal range would reduce magnesium retention and increases urinary excretion with its potential misinterpretation. Urine collection begins with the onset of magnesium infusion and continues over the next 24 hrs period, including a last void at end of this period.

Patients with adequate body magnesium stores retain less than 10% of the infused elemental magnesium load. Latent magnesium deficiency is considered present if less than 25 mmol of elemental magnesium are excreted in the 24 hrs collection. Repeat of magnesium loading test to check repletion can also be informative because average difference between two repeats is ~2%. Magnesium body stores are considered repleted when >90% of the elemental magnesium load is excreted in the following 24 hrs urine.

Magnesium loading test is contraindicated in patients with renal impediment, salt losing nephropathy, respiratory failure and medications which affect renal tubular function such as diuretics, cisplatin, ciclosporin, etc.

A number of studies attempted to simplify the magnesium loading test [82] by reducing the infused magnesium load to 0.1 mmol of elemental magnesium per kilogram body weight, reducing the infusion time to 1-2 hrs and collecting urine over shorter period of 12 hrs. Oral magnesium loading test was also described. However, although these modifications are simpler, their usage was limited and the 8-12 hour infusion of 30 mmol remained the standard test.

24-h Urinary Magnesium Excretion

Patients with magnesium deficiency, not on medications/alcoholic beverages and normal renal function, excrete small amounts of magnesium per day (usually <0.5 mmol or 12 mg). Considerable care and attention to completeness of 24-h urine collection is necessary [83].

Treatment Modalities in Patients with Magnesium Deficiency

Magnesium has low-toxicity in people with normal renal function. Deficiency however may not be corrected through nutritional supplementation only. The most common therapeutic modalities are intravenous infusion in patients with depletion manifesting as significant hypomagnesaemia; and orally (occasionally subcutaneously [84]) for individuals requiring long-term supplementation. Aerosolized magnesium sulphate was also used in patients with acute asthma [85,86].

Intravenous magnesium (up to ~30 mmol of elemental magnesium; 1 mmol=24 mg) is given over a period of hours. A slow rate infusion is important because plasma magnesium concentration affects the renal reabsorption threshold and abrupt elevation of plasma concentration above the normal range can reduce magnesium retention. Magnesium body stores are considered repleted when >90% of the elemental magnesium load is excreted in the following 24 hrs urine (see magnesium loading test). On the other hand, persistent elevation in serum magnesium in samples taken longer than 24 hrs after treatment would be indicative of over-treatment. Other analytes which may be associated with magnesium deficiency are calcium, potassium, phosphate and vitamin D [87].

Common oral magnesium supplement exists in two forms-chelated and non-chelated. In the chelated forms, magnesium is attached to organic radicals; in the non-chelated forms magnesium is in the form of sulphate, chloride or oxide. Magnesium attached to organic/aminoacid radicals appears to be better tolerated with superior bioavailability [88,89] than the commonly available magnesium oxide. Generally over-treatment leading to significant hypermagnesaemia is unlikely to occur in patients on the recommended oral magnesium supplement. This is because when the intake exceeds daily requirement, absorption of magnesium from the gut is reduced and its excretion can exceed 100% of the filtered load caused by active renal secretion in the urine.

It may be of interest to point out that net magnesium absorption rises with increasing intake, however fractional absorption falls as magnesium intake increases (e.g. from 65% at 40 mg intake to 11% at 960 mg). Magnesium absorption from the gut is slow with ~80% of oral magnesium being absorbed within 6-7 hrs [90]. Note also that calcium and magnesium competes for absorption, thus too much calcium in diet/medication can impede magnesium absorption. A ratio for calcium to magnesium of ~2:1 would allow adequate absorption of magnesium. However, high oral calcium intake or consumption of large amounts of calcium-rich products such as dairy foods which have a ratio of calcium to magnesium of ~10:1 can sufficiently alter the balance, potentially reducing magnesium absorption. Dosage regimen of oral magnesium should therefore take into account the degree of patients' magnesium deficiency in the first place, the basic chemical composition of oral magnesium supplement and its bioavailability plus other concurrent medications which can increase magnesium loss (e.g. diuretics, regular intake of spirits) and/or impede its absorption e.g. GI disorders. Sustained oral magnesium supplementation may be considered in individuals with life style below RDA intake.

Claims that Epsom salt can be absorbed through the skin are wide spread throughout the internet with numerous products which can be added to bath water, in oil, gel or lotions to be directly messaged to skin for "extra-relaxation, detoxification and exfoliation". However, no peer reviewed systematic or controlled studies could be found on this subject. In a widely quoted but rather limited, not peer-reviewed study involving 19 subjects (Waring R; School of Bioscience, Birmingham University, UK) who for one week bathed in water containing 1% Epsom salt at temperature of ~50°C for ~15 mins, 16 have increased their baseline serum magnesium concentration before the test by up to 40% and doubled their magnesium content in urine. However, in view of the dearth of scientifically peer-reviewed studies, transdermal absorption of magnesium should remain speculative.

Conclusion and Take-home Message

Magnesium deficiency is an underestimated multifactorial disorder, common particularly in the elderly. Magnesium deficiency can be associated with consequential morbidity and mortality especially in patients with other co-morbidities. Serum magnesium is a useful test because low serum concentration indicates significant deficiency warranting replacement. However, normal magnesium concentration must not be used to exclude negative body stores. Modus vivendi has an important role in identifying at risk patients, such as adults living in areas with soft drinking water or hard water with low magnesium contents plus other factors listed in Table 2, notably diet and diuretics. The most informative laboratory investigation is magnesium loading test.

Magnesium deficiency should always be considered in cases such as electrolyte disturbances (hypocalcaemia and/or hypokalaemia), arrhythmia, regular/excessive alcohol intake and muscular spasms/cramps in both normocalcaemic and hypocalcaemic patients. In other conditions however, it is important that patients at risk in each category are also identified. The limitations of serum magnesium, though well known among laboratorians is not widely disseminated nor emphasized to clinical practitioners. The perception that "normal" serum magnesium excludes deficiency has therefore contributed to the under-diagnosis of latent/chronic magnesium deficiency. Based on literature in the last two decades, magnesium deficiency remained common and undervalued, warranting a proactive approach because restoration of magnesium stores is simple, tolerable, and inexpensive and can be clinically beneficial.

References

1. Ismail Y, Ismail AA, Ismail AAA (2010) The underestimated problem of using serum magnesium measurements to exclude magnesium deficiency in adults; a health warning is needed for "normal" results. Clin Chem Lab Med 48: 323-327.
2. Moomaw AS, Maguire ME (2008) The unique nature of mg^{2+} channels. Physiology (Bethesda) 23: 275-285.
3. Maguire ME, Cowan JA (2002) Magnesium chemistry and biochemistry. Biometals 15: 203-210.
4. Bianconi E, Piovesan A, Facchin F, Beraudi A, Casadei R, et al. (2013) An estimation of the number of cells in the human body. Ann Hum Biol 40: 463-471.
5. Buchachenko A, Kouznetsov DA, Orlova MA, Markarian AA (2005) Magnetic isotope effect of magnesium in phosphoglycerate kinase phosphorylation. Prc Nat Acad Sci 102: 10793-10796.
6. Grubbs RD, Maguire ME (1987) Magnesium as a regulatory cation: criteria and evaluation. Magnesium 6: 113-127.
7. Laires MJ, Monteiro CP, Bicho M (2004) Role of cellular magnesium in health and human disease. Front Biosci 9: 262-276.
8. Alexander RT, Hoenderop JG, Bindels RJ (2008) Molecular determinants of magnesium homeostasis: insights from human disease. J Am Soc Nephrol 19: 1451-1458.
9. Rude RK (1998) Magnesium deficiency: a cause of heterogeneous disease in humans. J Bone Miner Res 13: 749-758.
10. Altura BM, Altura BT (1992) Cardiovascular risk factors and magnesium: relationships to atherosclerosis, ischemic heart disease and hypertension. Magnes Trace Elem 10: 182-192.
11. Al-Delaimy WK, Rimm EB, Willett WC, Stampfer MJ, Hu FB (2004) Magnesium intake and risk of coronary heart disease among men. J Am Coll Nutr 23: 63-70.
12. Touyz RM (2008) Transient receptor potential melastatin 6 and 7 channels magnesium transport and vascular biology: implications in hypertension. Am J Physiol Heart Circ Physiol 294: 1103-1118.
13. Larsson SC, Bergkvist L, Wolk A (2005) Magnesium intake in relation to risk of colorectal cancer in women. JAMA 293: 86-89.
14. Ismail AAA, Ismail AA, Ismail Y (2013) Clinical assessment of magnesium status in the adult; an overview. In magnesium in health and disease. In: Watson RR, Preedy V, Zibadi S (Eds.), Publisher Humana Press; Springer Science, USA.
15. Ismail AA, Thurston A (2010) How magnesium deficiency affects bone health. Osteoporosis Rev 8: 9-12.
16. Swaminathan R (2003) Magnesium metabolism and its disorders. Clin Biochem Rev 24: 47-66.
17. Murphy E (2000) Mysteries of magnesium homeostasis. Circ Res 86: 245-248.
18. Abed E, Moreau R (2007) Importance of melastatin-like transient receptor potential 7 and cations (magnesium, calcium) in human osteoblast-like cell proliferation. Cell Prolif 40: 849-865.
19. Kim BJ, Lim HH, Yang DK, Jun JY, Chang IY, et al. (2005) Melastatin-type transient receptor potential channel 7 is required for intestinal pacemaking activity. Gastroenterology 129: 1504-1517.
20. Wolf FI (2004) TRPM7: channeling the future of cellular magnesium homeostasis? Sci STKE 2004: pe23.
21. Bindels RJ (2010) 2009 Homer W. Smith Award: Minerals in motion: from new ion transporters to new concepts. J Am Soc Nephrol 21: 1263-1269.
22. Glaudemans B, Knoers NV, Hoenderop JG, Bindels RJ (2010) New molecular players facilitating Mg(2+) reabsorption in the distal convoluted tubule. Kidney Int 77: 17-22.
23. Killilea DW, Maier JA (2008) A connection between magnesium deficiency and aging: new insights from cellular studies. Magnesium Research 21: 77-82.
24. Barbagallo M, Belvedere M, Dominguez LJ (2009) Magnesium homeostasis and aging. Magnes Res 22: 235-246.
25. Musso CG (2009) Magnesium metabolism in health and disease. Int Urol Nephrol 41: 357-362.
26. Arinzon Z, Peisakh A, Schrire S, Berner YN (2010) Prevalence of hypomagnesemia (HM) in a geriatric long-term care (LTC) setting. Arch Gerontol Geriatr 51: 36-40.
27. Barbagallo M, Dominguez LJ (2010) Magnesium and aging. Curr Pharm Des 16: 832-839.
28. Saris NE, Mervaala E, Karppanen H, Khawaja JA, Lewenstam A (2000) Magnesium. An update on physiological, clinical and analytical aspects. Clin Chim Acta 294: 1-26.
29. Topf JM, Murray PT (2003) Hypomagnesemia and hypermagnesemia. Rev Endocr Metab Disord 4: 195-206.
30. Bolland MJ, Barber PA, Doughty RN, Mason B, Horne A, et al. (2008) Vascular events in healthy older women receiving calcium supplementation: randomsied controlled trial. BMJ 336: 262-266
31. Rowe WJ (2006) Calcium-magnesium-ratio intake and cardiovascular risk. Am J Cardiol 98: 140.
32. Hermans C, Lefebvre CH, Devogelaer JP, Lambert M (1996) Hypocalcaemia and chronic alcohol intoxication: Transient hypoparathyroidism secondary to magnesium deficiency. Clin Rheumatol 15: 193-196.
33. Loughrey CM (2002) Serum magnesium must also be known in profound hypokalaemia. BMJ 324: 1039-1040.
34. Whang R, Flink EB, Dyckner T, Wester PO, Aikawa JK, et al. (1985) Magnesium depletion as a cause of refractory potassium repletion. Arch Intern Med 145: 1686-1689.
35. Whang R, Whang DD, Ryan MP (1992) Refractory potassium repletion. A consequence of magnesium deficiency. Arch Intern Med 152: 40-45.
36. Jones BJ, Twomey PJ (2009) Comparison of reflective and reflex testing for hypomagnesaemia in severe hypokalaemia. J Clin Pathol 62: 816-819.
37. Srivastava R, Bartlett WA, Kennedy IM, Hiney A, Fletcher C, et al. (2010) Reflex and reflective testing: efficiency and effectiveness of adding on laboratory tests. Ann Clin Biochem 47: 223-227.
38. Ismail AA (2010) On the efficiency and effectiveness of added-on serum magnesium in patients with hypokalaemia and hypocalcaemia. Ann Clin Biochem 47: 492-493.
39. Nielsen FH, Milne DB, Klevay LM, Gallagher S, Johnson L (2007) Dietary magnesium deficiency induces heart rhythm changes, impairs glucose tolerance and decrease serum cholesterol in post-menopausal women. J Am Coll Nutr 26: 121-132.
40. Fung TT, Manson JE, Solomon CG, Liu S, Willett WC, et al. (2003) The association between magnesium intake and fasting insulin concentration in healthy middle-aged women. J Am Coll Nutr 22: 533-538.
41. Rumawas ME, McKeown NM, Rogers G, Meigs JB, Wilson PW, et al. (2006) Magnesium intake is related to improved insulin homeostasis in the framingham offspring cohort. J Am Coll Nutr 25: 486-492.
42. Ladefoged K, Hessov I, Jarnum S (1996) Nutrition in short-bowel syndrome. Scand J Gastroenterol 216: 122-131.
43. Rude RK (1993) Magnesium metabolism and deficiency. Endocrinol Metab Clin North Am 22: 377-395.
44. Quamme GA (2008) Recent developments in intestinal magnesium absorption. Curr Opin Gastroenterol 24: 230-235.

45. Ford ES, Mokdad AH (2003) Dietary magnesium intake in a national sample of US adults. J Nutr 133: 2879-2882.
46. Bialostosky K, Wright JD, Kennedy-Stephenson J, McDowell M, Johnson CL (2002) Dietary intake of macronutrients, micronutrients and other dietary constituents: United States 1988-94. Vital Heath Stat 11 ed: National Center for Health Statistics.
47. Rayssiguier Y, Durlach J, Boirie Y (2000) Apports Nutritionnels Conseille ́s pour la population francaise. A Martin coordonnateur, Paris: TEC DOC Lavoisier.
48. Bohl CH, Volpe SL (2002) Magnesium and exercise. Crit Rev Food Sci Nutr 42: 533-563.
49. Nielsen FH, Lukaski HC (2006) Update on the relationship between magnesium and exercise. Magnes Res 19: 180-189.
50. Laires MJ, Monteiro C (2008) Exercise, magnesium and immune function. Magnes Res 21: 92-96.
51. Rubenowitz E, Axelsson G, Rylander R (1998) Magnesium in drinking water and body magnesium status measured using an oral loading test. Scand J Clin Lab Invest 58: 423-428.
52. Monarca S, Donato F, Zerbini I, Calderon RL, Craun GF (2006) Review of epidemiological studies on drinking water hardness and cardiovascular diseases. Eur J Cardiovasc Prev Rehabil 13: 495-506.
53. Verhas M, de la Guéronnière V, Grognet JM, Paternot J, Hermanne A, et al. (2002) Magnesium bioavailability from mineral water. A study in adult men. Eur J Clin Nutr 56: 442-447.
54. Durlach J, Durlach V, Bac P, Rayssiguier Y, Bara M, et al. (1993) Magnesium and ageing. II. Clinical data: aetiological mechanism and pathophysiological consequences of magnesium deficit in the elderly. Magnesium Res 6: 379-394.
55. Garzon P, Eisenberg MJ (1998) Variation in the mineral content of commercially available bottled waters: implications for health and disease. Am J Med 105: 125-130.
56. Gillies ME, Birkbeck JA (1983) Tea and coffee as sources of some minerals in the New Zealand diet. Am J Clin Nutr 38: 936-942.
57. Gullestad L, Nes M, Rønneberg R, Midtvedt K, Falch D, et al. (1994) Magnesium status in healthy free-living elderly Norwegians. J Am Coll Nutr 13: 45-50.
58. Marier JR (1986) Magnesium content of the food supply in the modern-day world. Magnesium 5: 1-8.
59. Costello RB, Moser-Veillon PB (1992) A review of magnesium intake in the elderly. A cause for concern? Magnesium Research 5: 61-67.
60. Byrd RP Jr, Roy TM (2003) Magnesium: its proven and potential clinical significance. South Med J 96: 104.
61. Martin He, Mccuskey C Jr, Tupikova N (1959) Electrolyte disturbance in acute alcoholism: with particular reference to magnesium. Am J Clin Nutr 7: 191-196.
62. Rylander R, Mégevand Y, Lasserre B, Amstutz W, Granbom S (2001) Moderate alcohol consumption and urinary excretion of magnesium and calcium. Scand J Clin Lab Invest 61: 401-405.
63. Rivlin RS (1994) Magnesium deficiency and alcohol intake: mechanisms, clinical significance and possible relation to cancer development (a review). J Am Coll Nutr 13: 416-423.
64. kalbfleisch Jm, Lindeman Rd, Ginn He, Smith Wo (1963) Effects of ethanol administration on urinary excretion of magnesium and other electrolytes in alcoholic and normal subjects. J Clin Invest 42: 1471-1475.
65. Peele S (1997) Utilizing culture and behaviour in epidemiological models of alcohol consumption and consequences for Western nations. Alcohol Alcohol 32: 51-64.
66. Poikolainen K, Alho H (2008) Magnesium treatment in alcoholics: a randomized clinical trial. Subst Abuse Treat Prev Policy 3: 1.
67. Sheron N (2007) Alcohol in Europe: the EU alcohol forum. Clin Med (Lond) 7: 323-324.
68. Cundy T, Mackay J (2011) Proton pump inhibitors and severe hypomagnesaemia. Curr Opin Gastroenterol 27: 180-185.
69. Cao Y, Liao C, Tan A, Liu L, Gao F (2010) Meta-analysis of incidence and risk of Hypomagnesemia with Cetuximab for advanced cancer. Chemotherapy 56: 459-465.
70. Joo Suk O (2008) Paradoxical hypomagnesemia caused by excessive ingestion of magnesium hydroxide. Am J Emerg Med 26: 837.
71. Cundy T, Dissanayake A (2008) Severe hypomagnesaemia in long-term users of proton-pump inhibitors. Clin Endocrinol (Oxf) 69: 338-341.
72. Shabajee N, Lamb EJ, Sturgess I, Sumathipala RW (2008) Omeprazole and refractory hypomagnesaemia. BMJ 337: a425.
73. Liebscher DH, Liebscher DE (2004) About the misdiagnosis of magnesium deficiency. J Am Coll Nutr 23: 730S-1S.
74. Franz KB (2004) A functional biological marker is needed for diagnosing magnesium deficiency. J Am Coll Nutr 23: 738S-41S.
75. Arnaud MJ1 (2008) Update on the assessment of magnesium status. Br J Nutr 99: S24-S36.
76. Ismail AAA, Ismail Y, Ismail AA (2015) Deceptive potassium and magnesium measurements. Diagnosis 1: 272-282.
77. Ismail AAA (1983) In Biochemical Investigation in Endocrinology. Publ: Acad Press.
78. Rasmussen HS, Nair P, Goransson L, Balslov S, Larsen OG, et al. (1988) Magnesium deficiency in patients with ischaemic heart disease with and without acute myocardial infarction uncovered by an intravenous loading test. Arch Int Med 148: 329-332.
79. Goto K, Yasue H, Okumura K, Matsuyama K, Kugiyama K, et al. (1990) Magnesium deficiency detected by intravenous loading test in variant angina pectoris. Am J Cardiol 65: 709-712.
80. Gullestad L, Midtvedt K, Dolva LO, Norseth J, Kjekshus J (1994) The magnesium loading test: reference values in healthy subjects. Scand J Clin Lab Invest 54: 23-31.
81. Gullestad L, Dolva LO, Waage A, Falch D, Fagerthun H, et al. (1992) Magnesium deficiency diagnosed by an intravenous loading test. Scand J Clin Lab Invest 52: 245-253.
82. Seyfert T, Dick K, Renner F, Rob PM (1998) Simplification of the magnesium loading test for use in outpatients. Trace metals and Electrolytes 15: 120-126.
83. Ayuk J, Gittoes NJ (2014) Contemporary view of the clinical relevance of magnesium homeostasis. Ann Clin Biochem 51: 179-188.
84. Martinez-Riquelme A, Rawlings J, Morley S, Kindall J, Hosking D, et al. (2005) Self-administered subcutaneous fluid infusion at home in the management of fluid depletion and hypomagnesaemia in gastro-intestinal disease. Clin Nutr 24: 158-163.
85. Blitz M, Blitz S, Hughes R, Diner B, Beasley R, et al. (2005) Aerosolized magnesium sulfate for acute asthma: a systematic review. Chest 128: 337-344.
86. Villeneuve EJ, Zed PJ (2006) Nebulized magnesium sulfate in the management of acute exacerbations of asthma. Ann Pharmacother 40: 1118-1124.
87. Bringhurst FR, Demay MB, Krane SM, Kronenberg HM (2008) Bone and mineral metabolism in health and disease. In Harrison's principles of internal medicine. (17th edn.). In: Fauci AS, Braunwald E, Kasper DL, Hauser SL, Longo DL, Jameson JL, Loscalzo J (eds.), Publ McGraw Hill Medical.
88. Firoz M, Graber M (2001) Bioavailability of US commercial magnesium preparations. Magnes Res 14: 257-262.
89. Walker AF, Marakis G, Christie-byng M (2003) Magnesium citrate found more bioavailability than other magnesium preparations in a randomized double blind study. Mag Res 16: 183-191.
90. Graham LA, Caesar JJ, Burgen AS (1960) Gastrointestinal absorption and excretion of Mg 28 in man. Metabolism 9: 646-659.

3

Advances in Nutrition of Patients with Inflammatory Bowel Diseases

Dworzanski T[1], Celinski K[1,*], Dworzanska E[2] and Lach T[3]

[1]*Chair and Department of Gastroenterology, Medical University of Lublin, Poland*

[2]*Department of Pediatric Neurology, Medical University of Lublin, Poland*

[3]*Medical University of Lublin, Poland*

[*]**Correspondence address:** Celinski K, Chair and Department of Gastroenterology, Medical University of Lublin, Poland, E-mail: celinski.krzysztof@gmail.com

Abstract

Inflammatory bowel diseases (IBDs) are multifactorial disorders whose aetiology and pathogenesis have not been fully elucidated. Their occurrence is affected by genetic and environmental factors. Amongst the environmental factors, proper diet seems to be crucial, both in the healthy population and in patients during disease exacerbations and remissions. Depending on their severity, duration and extent of inflammatory lesions, IBD exacerbations result in some dietary deficits. Appropriate supplementation can effectively correct the deficits; in some cases, mainly in CD, nutritional therapy can be equally effective for inducing remissions as pharmacotherapy. Enteral feeding is recommended in each case without important contraindications for its use. Counteracting the caloric, protein and microelement deficiencies is pivotal for inhibition of disease pathogenesis and for enhancement of the anti-inflammatory response of the organism. The present paper is to present simply review and analyse of recent reports regarding nutrition in patients with CD and UC as well as to discuss recommended nutritional management in certain IBD course-associated conditions. Nutritional therapy is a key element of management of IBD patients.

Keywords: Enteral nutrition; Crohn`s disease; Ulcerative colitis; Diet in IBD; Nutrition de iciences in IBD

Introduction

Inflammatory bowel diseases (IBDs) are multifactorial disorders whose aetiology and pathogenesis have not been fully elucidated. Their occurrence is affected by genetic and environmental factors. The environmental factors that can influence the occurrence of the first symptoms and subsequent exacerbations include diet, changes in the intestinal microbiome associated with it, some drugs, particularly contraceptives, tobacco smoking, stress and lack of physical activity. In recent years, a relation between increased IBD incidence rates, perinatal and early childhood infections and infections caused by atypical pathogens has been highlighted. The latest genetic studies have revealed the occurrence of over hundreds loci of genes associated with the risk of Crohn`s disease (CD and ulcerative colitis (UC); nevertheless, the predisposition alone is not sufficient for the disease to develop [1]. Amongst the environmental factors mentioned above, diet seems crucial, both in the healthy population and in patients during disease exacerbations and remissions. Depending on their severity, duration and extent of inflammatory lesions, IBD exacerbations result in various dietary deficits. Appropriate supplementation can effectively correct the deficits. In some cases, mainly in CD, nutritional therapy can be equally effective for inducing remissions as pharmacology. The present paper is to review and analyse recent reports regarding nutrition in patients with CD and UC as well as to discuss recommended nutritional management in certain IBD course-associated conditions. We used several data base: Cochrane library, Scopus, Web of science and Pub-med. As a key words for search we used: ulcerative colitis, Crohn's disease, nutrition, enteral feeding.

Effects of diet on the IBD incidence and course

Study findings regarding the effects of diet on the IBD incidence are contradictory. It seems undeniable that increased incidence rates of IBDs in North America and Western Europe are related to consumption of highly processed food products containing large amounts of trans fats as well as simple sugars and limited intake of fibre, vegetables and fruits [2-6]. Moreover, some studies have demonstrated an inverse correlation between consumption of citrus fruits, fruit and vegetable juices vs. incidence of CD and UC [7,8]. According to the study carried out in Denmark in 118 patients with IBD and in several-hundred controls, high sugar intake significantly increased the risk of IBDs while consumption of large amounts of vegetables had protective effects [9]. To maintain the integrity of the intestinal mucosa, hence the intestinal barrier, it is essential to consume the products rich in fibre. The fibre after fermentation is metabolised by intestinal bacteria to short-chain fatty acids inhibiting the transcription factor involved in the production of pro-inflammatory cytokines [10]. In another study in 168 children, including 53 diagnosed with CD and 27 diagnosed with UC, diets of CD children have been found to contain higher amounts of meat, sugar, fats and lower amounts of vitamins [11]. The EpiCom study conducted on the population of 1560 patients with non-specific inflammatory bowel diseases has revealed that increased intake of sugars and fast food was associated with the earlier first episode of IBD and higher risk of severe course and surgery amongst patients with UC [12].

Patients often associate disease exacerbations with the diet and e.g. avoid vegetables they believe have adverse effects on their health. The New Zealand genes and diet in IBD study has indeed shown polymorphisms of single nucleotides correlated with intolerance of cruciferous vegetables in some patients with CD [13]. Determination of these changes in the population of CD patients could help to identify the group of individuals in which the vegetable diet would be indicated without increased risks of exacerbations [13]. Furthermore, a correlation between the consumption of hardened fatty acids, e.g. margarines, and granulomatous ileitis [14] and UC [15] has been observed. The observations in the Greenland Eskimo population consuming large amounts of polyunsaturated omega-3 fatty acids from sea fish oil and characterised by low incidence rates of IBDs enabled to formulate the thesis about anti-inflammatory properties of these substances, as opposed to pro-inflammatory properties of omega-6 fatty acids [16,17]. The further studies have confirmed that omega-6 acids are involved in the pathogenesis of IBDs through the metabolic pathway of arachidonic acid, a source of leukotriene B4 showing pro-inflammatory activity. According to Costea et al. [18] carriers of specific variants of genes responsible for metabolism of polyunsaturated fatty acids are at a higher risk of CD when their diets are rich in omega-6 acids and poor in omega-3 acids [18]. The above findings have drawn new attention to the importance of intake of suitable fats in inflammatory diseases, as fats are the main components of cell membranes, of both the gastrointestinal (GI) tract and immune system cells [19].

The IBD incidence shows high geographic differentiation with clearly rising rates in the north regions, both in America and Europe. Many researchers believe that this differentiation is associated with short exposure to sunlight in northern countries, hence vitamin D deficiency. Vitamin D acting through the nuclear receptor is a relevant factor of the signalling pathway responsible for regulation of innate immunity [20]. The Nurses' Health Study has confirmed this theory showing that the risk of UC in women growing up in southern latitudes was lower, as compared to the populations living in northern and mid- latitudes. No such a relation has been found for CD [21]. An animal model of colitis has demonstrated that lack of vitamin D or 1,25(OH)2D3 receptor results in higher susceptibility to GI tract damage [22].

Numerous studies have demonstrated that breast-feeding reduces the risk of CD and UC [23-26]. The study by Bergstrand et al. reveals a relation between reduced risk of CD and longer breast-feeding [25]. Unfortunately, the reports on this relation are conflicting. According to the study carried out in 222 patients with CD diagnosed before the age of 17 years, breast-feeding was a statistically significant risk factor of this disease [27]. Another meta-analysis based on 14 population case control studies has shown that breast-feeding had protective effects on UC incidence; no such a relation was found in the case of CD [28]. Moreover, there are studies demonstrating no effects of breast-feeding on the risk of IBDs [29]. Likely positive effects of breast-feeding result from the changes in bacterial flora of the newborn GI tract. The intestinal contents of children who were breast-fed was found to contain significantly higher numbers of bifidobacteria and statistically significantly lower amounts of anaerobic bacteria. Intestinal microbiota can undergo changes to the age of 2 years and therefore breast-feeding above the standard 6 months can be essential.

Some other studies report negative effects of cow milk consumption on the incidence of non-specific inflammatory bowel diseases. Specific antibodies are detected in the population consuming cow milk, as compared to the control group, whose level correlates with a CD activity index [30].

Despite the publications discussed above, an absolute correlation between diets and IBD etiopathogenesis has not been elucidated. Undeniale changes in the composition and method for processing food in developed countries are factors contributing to morbidity, yet other environmental factors that can affect these processes are not fully known.

Nutritional deficiencies in IBDs

In IBDs, especially in the course of CD involving the small intestine, patients develop various nutritional deficiencies. The degree of nutritional disorders depends on the location of inflammatory lesions, their extent and duration of exacerbation. Compared to UC, CD more frequently leads to protein deficiencies and certain nutritional disorders (avitaminosis, deficits of microelements) [31]. The study in IBD patients indicates that the problem regards 23% of ambulatory patients and even 85% of those requiring hospitalisation [32]. The problem is predominant in CD patients [31,33,34]. One of the nutritional status index of IBD patients is the level of albumins, which correlates with caloric-protein deficiencies and body weight loss. Significant weight losses are observed in 75% of patients hospitalised due to CD exacerbations whereas negative nitrogen balance is found in about 50% of cases [35,36].

The main factors predisposing to nutritional deficiencies are intolerance to multiple food products, abstaining from eating due to therapeutic reasons, increased calorie demands in the course of disease, malabsorption in the substantial fragment of the inflammation-affected intestine or interactions between food and drugs [37-39]. The less common factors include chronic diarrhoea and vomiting, chronic GI bleeding, enteropathy with loss of proteins, mucus and electrolytes, complicated infections, fistulae or impaired absorption of biliary salts in the case of bowel resection [40-44] (Table 1).

Causes of nutritional disorders in IBD patients	
Limited oral intake	Dietary restriction Lack of nutrition due to therapeutic reasons Related to diarrhoea, nausea, vomiting, abdominal pain [45] Changes in taste caused by drugs and vitamins taken and mineral deficiencies [43] Anorexia-like effects of pro-inflammatory cytokines [43]
Loss via the stomach or intestine	Diarrhoea Bloody stools Loss of mucus and microelements Enteropathy with loss of proteins

Increased energy demands	Inflammation Increased basal metabolism Infection complications Conditions after surgery
Metabolic disorders	Increased energy expenditure due to inflammation, fever, sepsis Increased oxidation of fatty acids
Drug interactions	Steroids and calcium re-absorption Steroids and protein catabolism Sulfasalazine and folic acid Methotrexate and folic acid Cholestyramine and fat-soluble vitamins Micro-organisms and vitamin K [46,47] IPP and iron [48]
Low absorption of food	Reduced absorption area due to ileal resection Blind loop syndrome and bacterial overgrowth Poor absorption of bile acids in ileitis or following resection Inflammation of the mucous membrane

Table 1: Causes of nutritional disorders in IBD patients.

Moreover, the pro-inflammatory cytokines (such as TNF- alpha, IL1, IL6), involved in the pathogenesis of IBDs, are responsible for worsened nutritional status due to catabolism-increasing effects. The most common deficiencies of microelements are those regarding iron reserves, vitamin B12 and folic acid manifesting in anaemia detected in laboratory tests. Folic acid deficiencies are observed in over half of IBD patients and most likely result from low-fibre diets, malabsorption or drug interactions, e.g. sulfasalazine or methotrexate. Some drugs exert adverse effects on the nutritional status of IBD patients; for instance, metronidazole can cause reduced intake due to dyspeptic symptoms or metallic taste in the mouth, steroids reduce calcium absorption from the GI tract and increase its loss through kidneys whereas cholestyramine impairs absorption of calcium, fats and vitamins dissolved in fats [32].

The study by Goh et al. has demonstrated that the folic acid deficiency is associated with increased risk of neoplasia in IBDs [31]. According to some other studies, the substance in question exhibits protective properties against the development of dysplasia and carcinogenesis in patients with long-term UC [49,50]. The deficiency of folic acid is also associated with increased risk of thromboembolic incidents in UC and CD via the effects on homocysteine metabolism [51]. Another factor affecting homocysteine metabolism, and indirectly increased risk, is vitamin B12, whose deficiency is detected in about 20-60% of patients with inflammation of the terminal ileum during CD.

Important immunological processes are impaired by zinc and selenium deficiencies. Zinc is essential for wound healing; therefore, its deficiency should be considered in the case of Crohn`s disease complicated by unhealing fistulae [52,53]. Moreover, zinc plays a crucial role in anti-oxidative processes since (being a co-factor of superoxide dismutase) it is involved in cell protection against harmful effects of active oxygen forms. Oxidative stress is positively correlated with the level of pro-inflammatory cytokines. Selenium, vitamins A, C and E also have anti-oxidative properties, positively affecting the limitation of inflammation [54,55].

The information concerning deficiencies of other microelements is sparse; nevertheless, they are likely to be involved in the immune response regulation, depending on their extent, frequency and duration.

The consequences of dietary deficiencies depend on the patient's age the disease develops in and the disease activity. Considering earlier occurrence of CD, as compared to UC, and its frequent development in the small intestine, the risk of clinical manifestations of dietary deficiencies is higher in CD patients. Nutritional deficiencies in children with IBDs often lead to growth inhibition and delayed maturation, which regards about 10% of UC children and about 75% of CD children [40]. Protein deficiencies induce disorders of hormonal and immunological metabolism, resulting in higher risk of infections due to the translocation of intestinal bacteria.

Disorders of bone metabolism are likely to be multifactorial and result from vitamin D deficiency, reduced calcium intake, steroid drugs, insufficient physical activity and impaired absorptive function of the intestinal villi affected [56].

Nutrition as therapeutic management in IBD

Nutritional therapy is a key element of management of IBD patients. Enteral feeding is recommended in each case without absolute contraindications for its use. Counteracting the caloric, protein and microelement deficiencies is pivotal for inhibition of disease pathogenesis resulting from those disorders and for enhancement of the anti-inflammatory response of the organism.

Liquid and semi-liquid preparations are used for enteral feeding, which can be divided into elementary, half-elementary and polymeric. The elementary mixtures contain only amino acids, glucose, fatty acids and microelements, i.e., components that do not require digestion.

Semielementary diets involve administration of mixtures of small peptides, oligosaccharides and medium-chain fatty acids whereas polymeric diets consist of the mixture of proteins, carbohydrates, medium- and long-chain fatty acids, vitamins and trace elements [57]. Nutritional therapy can be oral or through the nasogastric or nasointestinal tube, depending on the patient's condition. Benefits of enteral feeding are dependent on the location of inflammatory lesions, their extent and intensity. According to the guidelines available, total enteral nutrition was most commonly introduced for the period of 6-8 weeks; then the normal diet was gradually included [58]. The preparations applied most frequently, both elementary and polymeric, contained about 1 kcal/ml and only slightly varied in their composition–most commonly, proteins were a source of 14-22% of energy, carbohydrates of 50-82% and fats if up to 35% of calories [59-64].

Gassull et al. [62] compared the efficacy of two nutritional formulae and steroid therapy for induction of remission in the course of CD. Both mixtures differed only in the fatty acids contained predominantly– in the first one, it was oleic acid (monounsaturated fatty acid MUFA) and in the other one linolenic acid (polyunsaturated fatty acid PUFA). The study was discontinued prematurely because only 20% of oleic acid formula patients had remission after 4 weeks. The group treated with linoleic acid formula showed the 52% efficacy; the efficacy in the group administered steroids was found to be 79%. The authors suggest that the effectiveness in inducing remission is significantly affected by the composition of fatty acids in the nutritional formula and hypothesize that n-6 MUFAs are less effective as they are the precursors of pro-inflammatory factors.

Leiper et al. described their randomized trial comparing the efficacy of induction of CD active response to the polymeric diet with high (group 1) or low (group 2) content of long-chain triglycerides. In both groups, the response rate was above 50% and no significant intergroup differences were observed [65]. The study by Gorard et al. compared the efficacy of CD remission in the group of 22 patients receiving the enteral diet for 4 weeks and 20 patients treated with steroids in a dose of 0.75 mg/kg daily for 2 weeks with a subsequent dose reduction. Unfortunately, nine patients of group 1 discontinued treatment due t enteral feeding intolerance. Amongst the remaining patients in both groups, the effectiveness of remission was comparable; however, a statistically significant difference in favour of steroid therapy regarded possible 6-month remission, 0.67 vs. 0.28 [66].

Another study demonstrated comparable efficacy of nutritional therapy and steroid therapy in induction of CD remission in adults (80% vs. 88%) [67].

The available literature indicates that patients with small intestine CD benefit most from enteral nutrition. According to meta-analysis of randomized studies published by Fernandes-Baranes et al, enteral nutrition is equally effective for inducing remission in the case of active CD as steroid therapy [68]. Moreover, nutritional therapy enables to maintain CD remission [69-71] and statistically significantly delays the need for surgical intervention or possible re-intervention [72]. Furthermore, numerous publications revealed that total enteral nutrition was associated with higher mucosal healing [73], changed intestinal microflora [74] and quicker weight gain [75], higher concentration of vitamin D [76], improved bone metabolism [77], increased insulin-like growth factor [78] and better quality of life after treatment [79], as compared to steroid therapy.

The paediatric studies suggest that higher effectiveness of nutritional therapy are observed in children with newly diagnosed CD (80%) in comparison with therapy of exacerbations of long-lasting disease (58%) [75].

Despite the benefits of total nutritional therapy, the management is not univocally recommended in algorithms of IBD treatment instead of pharmacological therapy; it is only advocated as supplementary therapy [80,81]. In many studies, negative effects on the percentage of nutritional therapy efficacy resulted from more frequent abandonment of nutritional mixtures due to unacceptable taste or troublesomeness of long-term nutrition through the intestinal tube. Additionally, some patients on enteral feeding reported abdominal pain, flatulence and symptoms of reflux disease. The review of studies on total enteral nutrition presented by Wall et al. suggests that despite numerous promising reports, there is no evidence demonstrating higher efficacy of his therapy in patients with newly diagnosed CD and casus of ileum location. The authors suggest that the use of oral nutrition with polymeric diets of acceptable taste can markedly improve the percentage of patients following orders and result in higher percentage of induction of CD remission, improved nutritional status and effective control of deficiencies [82].

Most importantly, nutritional therapy has no significant adverse side effects, as opposed to pharmacological methods widely used in IBDs. There are no explicit data regarding the effects of nutritional therapy on CD confined to the large intestine. Moreover, benefits of this kind of therapy in UC have not been explicitly demonstrated. Rare studies on the role of nutrition in UC exacerbations indicate no distinct differences in the impact on the remission index or need of colostomy between enteral and parenteral nutrition in patients treated with steroids [83]. Enteral feeding in UC exacerbations shows anabolic action, is safe and justified when the nutritional status has to be improved and deficiencies corrected.

Enteral feeding mechanism of action

The mechanism of effects of enteral feeding on inhibition of the inflammatory reaction is multifactorial [46]. It is known that one of the elements of IBD pathogenesis is increased permeability of the mucosa, which improves as a result of nutritional therapy used. The available data suggest that the administration of nutritional preparations regulated impaired balance in the composition of intestinal bacterial flora, responsible for activation of improper immune response. The exposure to intestinal antigens from improper intestinal microbiota decreases; most likely, the expression of genes of the intestinal epithelial cells, which affect immune reactions changes [84,85]. The use of elementary mixtures considerably reduces the digestive effort, peristalsis and secretion related to the process of digestion, which beneficially affect the process of recovery [47]. Moreover, the elementary diet can reduce the number of commensal bacteria in the GI tract, which are likely to be involved in the induction of inflammation. The reports on this issue are not explicit; no positive effects of elementary diets were confirmed in scientific studies, which did not demonstrate the differences in therapeutic efficacy of elementary vs. non-elementary diets [86].

The knowledge about negative effects of improper dysbiosis on intestinal epithelial dysfunction, increased stimulation of the immune system and reduced resistance to damaging factors suggests high impact of properly chosen probiotics in the treatment of IBDs [87].

Nutritional therapy with probiotic preparations shows significant effects on maintenance of remission in UC patients and therapeutic benefits in the therapy of pouchitis.

In recent years, numerous studies were devoted to the effects of probiotics in maintenance of remission in IBD patients. They demonstrated the impact of short-chain fatty acids (SCFAs), such as butyrate, propionate and lactate, on the composition of intestinal microbiota. SCFAs are produced due to fermentation of fibres by some intestinal bacteria, e.g. lactobacillus or bifidobacterium and are a relevant substrate nourishing enterocytes and positively affecting on the properties of the intestinal epithelium. The best known prebiotic of proved anti-inflammatory action is butyrate [88,89].

Some reports suggest that the key therapeutic element of enteral nutrition is proper appropriate composition of fats [62,67]. However, there is no consensus as to the recommended composition and proportion of fatty components. It was explicitly demonstrated that dietary supplementation of omega-3 fatty AIDS beneficially affects the maintenance of remission in CD patients; no such a relation was confirmed in the case of UC [90-92]. Despite conflicting data regarding the efficacy of administration of fatty components in enteral nutrition, this kind of management is recommended due to therapeutic potential and lack of adverse side effects.

Analysis of reports on the effects of enteral nutrition on maintenance of remission in patients receiving biological therapy provides interesting information. In one of the studies, 56 patients with remission during infliximab treatment, the therapy was continued in a standard dose. Patients were divided in to the group additionally receiving night and day elementary diet and the group without dietary restrictions. The level of CDAI after the 56-week observations did not show differences, which indicated lack of effects of nutritional therapy on maintenance of remission in patients receiving supportive infliximab therapy [93]. In another study, the 85-week observation of patients receiving infliximab supportive therapy revealed that the additional use of nutritional therapy >600 kcal/24h with elementary and polymeric formula is an independent factor maintaining a stable response to the biological drug [94]. Positive effects of nutritional therapy on maintenance of CD remission in patients subjected to chronic infliximab therapy was described by Hirai et al. The cumulative remission index was significantly higher in the group additionally receiving, compared to the group without nutritional therapy; moreover, multi-variant analysis demonstrated that such management is the only relevant factor preventing the recurrence of disease [95].

Parenteral nutrition of patients with IBDs shows numerous adverse side effects with increased risk of systemic infections; and most importantly is not beneficial for IBD control [96,97]. No positive effects of parenteral nutrition on maintenance of remissions and in its induction were demonstrated in both CD and UC. This way of nutrition is the management of choice in cases with contraindication for enteral feeding, such as short bowel syndrome after extensive resection, megacolon toxicum, increased GI bleeding or CD complicated with difficult healing of fistulas [98,99].

Dietary guidelines in patients with IBD

Diverse diets rich in vegetables, fruits, meat, sea fish, olive oil and cold-pressed linseed and rapeseed oil is essential for nutrition of patients with IBDs.

Moreover, intake of high amounts of fibre is recommended except of patients with significant intestinal constriction, functional diarrhoea disorders, e.g., in concomitant irritable bowel syndrome or patients with highly active IBD exacerbations

In patients diagnosed with lactose intolerance and those with IBD exacerbations, it is recommended to withdraw milk and dairy products. To supplement calcium deficiencies, high-calcium soya products or feta cheese should be consumed.

In order to present frequent deficiencies in IBD patients, calcium (1000 mg/24h) and vitamin D (400-800 IU) should be controlled and supplemented, especially in patients undergoing long-term corticotherapy, whose risk of osteoporosis is higher. Moreover, the levels of iron and folic acid should be monitored as their deficiencies are the most common cause of anaemia; likewise, the level of vitamin B12 should be monitored, particularly in patients after resection of the terminal ileum segment.

It should be remembered that resection of the terminal ileum segment impairs the intestinal hepatic loop of circulation of biliary acids, which are crucial for digestion and absorption of fats and vitamins dissolved in fats (A,D,E,K). Patients with extensive active diseases of the small intestine or after resection of the terminal ileum segment are recommended to reduce the intake of fat and oxalates due to increased risk of renal calculosis [100,101].

Noteworthy, while choosing the nutritional preparations available on the market supporting IBD treatment, the patient's preferences should be considered (frequency of use, time, taste or the administration router in some cases). In patients with highly protein or corresponding to the high caloric demands elementary diets or partially elementary diets, nocturnal nutrition through the nasogastric tube should be considered.

Conclusions

Among the environmental factors affecting the incidence of IBD-proper diet is important both in the healthy population to reduce the risk of incidence of IBD, and also has a significant impact on the disease course and length of remission periods.

In the course of IBD a significant percentage of patients develop nutrition's disorders and relevant dietary deficiency. CD compared to UC leads to a higher protein deficiency and other nutrition's disorders such as deficiency of vitamins A, D, E, iron, vitamin B12, folic acid and trace elements like Zink and potassium.

It is necessary to carefully monitor the patient for early diagnosis of malnutrition and appropriate supplementation.

Enteral nutritional therapies restore impaired nutritional status in the population of IBD patients and positively modulate intestinal immune response.

This management is particularly recommended for children with CD and can prove sufficient to induce remission without corticotherapy.

In patients with CD and severe cases of UC, enteral nutrition is recommended as additional management supporting induction of remission and counteracting adverse effects of drugs [86]. In this group, nutritional therapy can be used to induce remission when corticotherapy is contraindicated [102].

Conflict of Interest

"The author(s) declare(s) that there is no conflict of interest regarding the publication of this paper."

References

1. Kabi A, Nickerson KP, Homer CR, McDonald C (2012) Digesting the genetics of inflammatory bowel disease: insights from studies of autophagy risk genes. Inflamm Bowel Dis 18: 782-792.
2. Reif S, Klein I, Lubin F, Farbstein M, Hallak A, et al. (1997) Pre-illness dietary factors in inflammatory bowel disease. Gut 40: 754-760.
3. Geerling BJ, Stockbrügger RW, Brummer RJ (1999) Nutrition and inflammatory bowel disease: an update. Scand J Gastroenterol Suppl 230: 95-105.
4. Thornton JR, Emmett PM, Heaton KW (1985) Smoking, sugar, and inflammatory bowel disease. Br Med J (Clin Res Ed) 290: 1786-1787.
5. Husain A, Korzenik JR (1998) Nutritional issues and therapy in inflammatory bowel disease. Semin Gastrointest Dis 9: 21-30.
6. Panza E, Franceschi S, La Vecchia C (1987) Dietary factors in the aetiology of inflammatory bowel disease. Ital J Gastroenterol 19: 205-209.
7. Thornton JR, Emmett PM, Heaton KW (1979) Diet and Crohn's disease: characteristics of the pre-illness diet. Br Med J 2: 762-764.
8. Bianchi Porro G, Panza E (1985) Smoking, sugar, and inflammatory bowel disease. Br Med J (Clin Res Ed) 291: 971-972.
9. Jakobsen C, Paerregaard A, Munkholm P, Wewer V (2013) Environmental factors and risk of developing paediatric inflammatory bowel disease -- a population based study 2007-2009. J Crohns Colitis 7: 79-88.
10. Maslowski KM, Mackay CR (2011) Diet, gut microbiota and immune responses. Nat Immunol 12: 5-9.
11. Tsiountsioura M, Wong JE, Upton J, McIntyre K, Dimakou D, et al. (2014) Detailed assessment of nutritional status and eating patterns in children with gastrointestinal diseases attending an outpatients clinic and contemporary healthy controls. Eur J Clin Nutr 68: 700-706.
12. Burisch J, Pedersen N, Cukovic-Cavka S, Turk N, Kaimakliotis I, et al. (2014) Environmental factors in a population-based inception cohort of inflammatory bowel disease patients in Europe--an ECCO-EpiCom study. J Crohns Colitis 8: 607-616.
13. Laing B, Han DY, Ferguson LR (2013) Candidate genes involved in beneficial or adverse responses to commonly eaten brassica vegetables in a New Zealand Crohn's disease cohort. Nutrients 5: 5046-5064.
14. Guthy E (1982) [Crohn's disease and nutritional lipids. Hypothesis on etiology of regional enteritis]. Dtsch Med Wochenschr 107: 71-73.
15. (1994) Dietary and other risk factors of ulcerative colitis. A case-control study in Japan. Epidemiology Group of the Research Committee of Inflammatory Bowel Disease in Japan. J Clin Gastroenterol 19: 166-171.
16. Bang HO, Dyerberg J, Sinclair HM (1980) The composition of the Eskimo food in north western Greenland. Am J Clin Nutr 33: 2657-2661.
17. Grimble RF, Tappia PS (1998) Modulation of pro-inflammatory cytokine biology by unsaturated fatty acids. Z Ernahrungswiss 37 Suppl 1: 57-65.
18. Costea (2014) Interaction between the dietary polyunsaturated fatty acid ratio and genetic factors determine susceptibility to pediatric Crohn's disease. Gastroenterology 146: 929-931.
19. Jeffery NM, Newsholme EA, Calder PC (1997) Level of polyunsaturated fatty acids and the n-6 to n-3 polyunsaturated fatty acid ratio in the rat diet alter serum lipid levels and lymphocyte functions. Prostaglandins Leukot Essent Fatty Acids 57: 149-160.
20. Jeffery NM, Newsholme EA, Calder PC (1997) Level of polyunsaturated fatty acids and the n-6 to n-3 polyunsaturated fatty acid ratio in the rat diet alter serum lipid levels and lymphocyte functions. Prostaglandins Leukot Essent Fatty Acids 57: 149-160.
21. Wang TT, Dabbas B, Laperriere D, Bitton AJ, Soualhine H, et al. (2010) Direct and indirect induction by 1,25-dihydroxyvitamin D3 of the NOD2/CARD15-defensin beta2 innate immune pathway defective in Crohn disease. J Biol Chem 285: 2227-2231.
22. Khalili H, Huang ES, Ananthakrishnan AN, Higuchi L, Richter JM, et al. (2012) Geographical variation and incidence of inflammatory bowel disease among US women. Gut 61: 1686-1692.
23. Ooi JH, Li Y, Rogers CJ, Cantorna MT (2013) Vitamin D regulates the gut microbiome and protects mice from dextran sodium sulfate-induced colitis. J Nutr 143: 1679-1686.
24. Whorwell PJ, Holdstock G, Whorwell GM, Wright R (1979) Bottle feeding, early gastroenteritis, and inflammatory bowel disease. Br Med J 1: 382.
25. Corrao G, Tragnone A (1998) Risk of inflammatory bowel disease attributable to smoking, oral contraception and breastfeeding in Italy: a nationwide case-control study. Cooperative Investigators of the Italian Group for the Study of the Colon and the Rectum (GISC). Int J Epidemiol 27: 397-404.
26. Bergstrand O, Hellers G (1983) Breast-feeding during infancy in patients who later develop Crohn's disease. Scand J Gastroenterol 18: 903-906.
27. Koletzko S, Sherman P, Corey M, Griffiths A, Smith C (1989) Role of infant feeding practices in development of Crohn's disease in childhood. BMJ 298: 1617-1618.
28. Baron S, Turck D, Leplat C, Merle V, Gower-Rousseau C, et al. (2005) Environmental risk factors in paediatric inflammatory bowel diseases: a population based case control study. Gut 54: 357-363.
29. Klement E, Cohen RV, Boxman J, Joseph A, Reif S (2004) Breastfeeding and risk of inflammatory bowel disease: a systematic review with meta-analysis. Am J Clin Nutr 80: 1342-1352.
30. Khalili H, Ananthakrishnan AN, Higuchi LM, Richter JM, Fuchs CS, et al. (2013) Early life factors and risk of inflammatory bowel disease in adulthood. Inflamm Bowel Dis 19: 542-547.
31. Knoflach P, Park BH, Cunningham R, Weiser MM, Albini B (1987) Serum antibodies to cow's milk proteins in ulcerative colitis and Crohn's disease. Gastroenterology 92: 479-485.
32. Goh J, O'Morain CA (2003) Review article: nutrition and adult inflammatory bowel disease. Aliment Pharmacol Ther 17: 307-320.
33. Triantafillidis JK, Vagianos C2, Papalois AE3 (2015) The role of enteral nutrition in patients with inflammatory bowel disease: current aspects. Biomed Res Int 2015: 197167.
34. Han PD, Burke A, Baldassano RN, Rombeau JL, Lichtenstein GR (1999) Nutrition and inflammatory bowel disease. Gastroenterol Clin North Am 28: 423-443, ix.
35. Gassull MA, Cabré E (2001) Nutrition in inflammatory bowel disease. Curr Opin Clin Nutr Metab Care 4: 561-569.
36. Gee MI, Grace MGA, Wensel RH (1985) "Nutritional status of gastroenterology outpatients: comparison of inflammatory bowel disease with functional disorders," JADA 85: 1591-1599.
37. Sousa Guerreiro C, Cravo M, Costa AR (2007) "A comprehensive approach to evaluate nutritional status in Crohn's patients in the era of biologic therapy: a case-control study," TAJG 102: 2551-2556.
38. Al-Jaouni R, Hébuterne X, Pouget I, Rampal P (2000) Energy metabolism and substrate oxidation in patients with Crohn's disease. Nutrition 16: 173-178.
39. Mingrone G, Capristo E, Greco AV, Benedetti G, De Gaetano A, et al. (1999) Elevated diet-induced thermogenesis and lipid oxidation rate in Crohn disease. Am J Clin Nutr 69: 325-330.
40. Klein S, Meyers S, O'Sullivan P, Barton D, Leleiko N, et al. (1988) The metabolic impact of active ulcerative colitis. Energy expenditure and nitrogen balance. J Clin Gastroenterol 10: 34-40.
41. García MVDAA, Álvarez HJ, Maqueda VE (2006) Soporte nutricional en la enfermedad inflamatoria intestinal. In: Bellido D, De Luis D, editors. Manual de Nutrición y Metabolismo. Madrid: Díaz de Santos, 333-348.
42. Onal IK (2014) Folate deficiency in Crohn's disease. Scand J Gastroenterol 49: 253-254.
43. Bartels U, Strandberg PN, Jarnum S (1978) "Iron absorption and serum ferritin in chronic inflammatory bowel disease," SJG 13: 649-656.

44. Massironi S, Rossi RE, Cavalcoli FA, Valle SD (2013) "Nutritional deficiencies in inflammatory bowel disease: therapeutic approaches," Clinical Nutrition 32: 904-910.
45. Wako-Czopnik D, Paradowski L (2012) The influence of deficiencies of essential trace elements and vitamins on the course of Crohn's disease. Adv Clin Exp Med 21: 5-11.
46. Wu T, Song HY, Ji G (2012) Abnormal bone metabolism in Crohn's disease. Front Biosci (Landmark Ed) 17: 2675-2683.
47. Ioannidis O, Varnalidis I, Paraskevas G, Botsios D (2011) Nutritional modulation of the inflammatory bowel response. Digestion 84: 89-101.
48. Teahon K, Smethurst P, Pearson M, Levi AJ, Bjarnason I (1991) The effect of elemental diet on intestinal permeability and inflammation in Crohn's disease. Gastroenterology 101: 84-89.
49. Triantafillidis JK, Douvi G, Agrogiannis G, Patsouris E, Gikas A, et al. (2014) "Effect of mesalamine and prednisolone on TNBS experimental colitis, following various doses of orally administered iron," BioMed Research International.
50. Lashner BA, Heidenreich PA, Su GL, Kane SV, Hanauer SB (1989) Effect of folate supplementation on the incidence of dysplasia and cancer in chronic ulcerative colitis. A case-control study. Gastroenterology 97: 255-259.
51. Lashner BA, Provencher KS, Seidner DL, Knesebeck A, Brzezinski A (1997) The effect of folic acid supplementation on the risk for cancer or dysplasia in ulcerative colitis. Gastroenterology 112: 29-32.
52. Talbot RW, Heppell J, Dozois RR, Beart RW Jr (1986) Vascular complications of inflammatory bowel disease. Mayo Clin Proc 61: 140-145.
53. McClain C, Soutor C, Zieve L (1980) Zinc deficiency: a complication of Crohn's disease. Gastroenterology 78: 272-279.
54. Kruis W, Rindfleisch GE, Weinzierl M (1985) Zinc deficiency as a problem in patients with Crohn's disease and fistula formation. Hepatogastroenterology 32: 133-134.
55. Reimund JM, Arondel Y, Escalin G, Finck G, Baumann R, et al. (2005) Immune activation and nutritional status in adult Crohn's disease patients. Dig Liver Dis 37: 424-431.
56. Reimund JM, Hirth C, Koehl C, Baumann R, Duclos B (2000) Antioxidant and immune status in active Crohn's disease. A possible relationship. Clin Nutr 19: 43-48.
57. Menchén L, Ripoll C, Bretón I, Moreno C, de la Cuerda C, et al. (2005) [Osteoporosis and inflammatory bowel disease]. Nutr Hosp 20: 26-37.
58. Silk DB (1999) Formulation of enteral diets. Nutrition 15: 626-632.
59. Whitten KE, Rogers P, Ooi CY, Day AS (2012) International survey of enteral nutrition protocols used in children with Crohn's disease. J Dig Dis 13: 107-112.
60. Zoli G, Carè M, Parazza M, Spanò C, Biagi PL, et al. (1997) A randomized controlled study comparing elemental diet and steroid treatment in Crohn's disease. Aliment Pharmacol Ther 11: 735-740.
61. Lindor KD, Fleming CR, Burnes JU, Nelson JK, Ilstrup DM (1992) A randomized prospective trial comparing a defined formula diet, corticosteroids, and a defined formula diet plus corticosteroids in active Crohn's disease. Mayo Clin Proc 67: 328-333.
62. Okada M, Yao T, Yamamoto T, Takenaka K, Imamura K, et al. (1990) Controlled trial comparing an elemental diet with prednisolone in the treatment of active Crohn's disease. Hepatogastroenterology 37: 72-80.
63. Gassull MA, Fernández BF, Cabré E, Papo M, Giaffer MH, et al. (2002) Fat composition may be a clue to explain the primary therapeutic effect of enteral nutrition in Crohn's disease: results of a double blind randomized multicentre European trial. Gut 51: 164-168.
64. Lochs H, Steinhardt HJ, Klaus-Wentz B, Zeitz M, Vogelsang H, et al. (1991) Comparison of enteral nutrition and drug treatment in active Crohn's disease. Results of the European Cooperative Crohn's Disease Study. IV. Gastroenterology 101: 881-888.
65. Malchow H, Steinhardt HJ, Lorenz-Meyer H, Strohm WD, Rasmussen S, et al. (1990) Feasibility and effectiveness of a defined-formula diet regimen in treating active Crohn's disease. European Cooperative Crohn's Disease Study III. Scand J Gastroenterol 25: 235-244.
66. Leiper K, Woolner J, Mullan MM, Parker T, van der Vliet M, et al. (2001) A randomised controlled trial of high versus low long chain triglyceride whole protein feed in active Crohn's disease. Gut 49: 790-794.
67. Gorard DA, Hunt JB, Payne-James JJ, Palmer KR, Rees RG, et al. (1993) Initial response and subsequent course of Crohn's disease treated with elemental diet or prednisolone. Gut 34: 1198-1202.
68. González-Huix F, de León R, Fernández-Bañares F, Esteve M, Cabré E, et al. (1993) Polymeric enteral diets as primary treatment of active Crohn's disease: a prospective steroid controlled trial. Gut 34: 778-782.
69. Fernández-Banares F, Cabré E, Esteve-Comas M, Gassull MA (1995) How effective is enteral nutrition in inducing clinical remission in active Crohn's disease? A meta-analysis of the randomized clinical trials. JPEN J Parenter Enteral Nutr 19: 356-364.
70. Wilschanski M, Sherman P, Pencharz P, Davis L, Corey M, et al. (1996) Supplementary enteral nutrition maintains remission in paediatric Crohn's disease. Gut 38: 543-548.
71. Hiwatashi N (1997) Enteral nutrition for Crohn's disease in Japan. Dis Colon Rectum 40: S48-53.
72. Akobeng AK, Thomas AG (2007) Enteral nutrition for maintenance of remission in Crohn's disease. Cochrane Database Syst Rev : CD005984.
73. Ikeuchi H, Yamamura T, Nakano H, Kosaka T, Shimoyama T, et al. (2004) Efficacy of nutritional therapy for perforating and non-perforating Crohn's disease. Hepatogastroenterology 51: 1050-1052.
74. Borrelli O, Cordischi L, Cirulli M, Paganelli M, Labalestra V, et al. (2006) Polymeric diet alone versus corticosteroids in the treatment of active pediatric Crohn's disease: a randomized controlled open-label trial. Clin Gastroenterol Hepatol 4: 744-753.
75. Andoh A, Tsujikawa T, Sasaki M, Mitsuyama K, Suzuki Y, et al. (2209) Faecal microbiota profile of Crohn's disease determined by terminal restriction fragment length polymorphism analysis. Aliment Pharmacol Ther 29: 75-82.
76. Day AS, Whitten KE, Lemberg DA, Clarkson C, Vitug-Sales M, et al. (2006) Exclusive enteral feeding as primary therapy for Crohn's disease in Australian children and adolescents: a feasible and effective approach. J Gastroenterol Hepatol 21: 1609-1614.
77. Levin AD, Wadhera V, Leach ST, Woodhead HJ, Lemberg DA, et al. (2011) Vitamin D deficiency in children with inflammatory bowel disease. Dig Dis Sci 56: 830-836.
78. Whitten KE, Leach ST, Bohane TD, Woodhead HJ, Day AS (2010) Effect of exclusive enteral nutrition on bone turnover in children with Crohn's disease. J Gastroenterol 45: 399-405.
79. Beattie RM, Schiffrin EJ, Donnet-Hughes A, Huggett AC, Domizio P, et al. (1994) Polymeric nutrition as the primary therapy in children with small bowel Crohn's disease. Aliment Pharmacol Ther 8: 609-615.
80. Afzal NA, Van Der Zaag-Loonen HJ, Arnaud-Battandier F, Davies S, Murch S, et al. (2004) Improvement in quality of life of children with acute Crohn's disease does not parallel mucosal healing after treatment with exclusive enteral nutrition. Aliment Pharmacol Ther 20: 167-172.
81. Dignass A, Van Assche G (2010) The second European evidence-based Consensus on the diagnosis and management of Crohn's disease: Current management. J Crohns Colitis 4: 28-62.
82. Lichtenstein GR, Hanauer SB, Sandborn WJ; Practice Parameters Committee of American College of Gastroenterology (2009) Management of Crohn's disease in adults. Am J Gastroenterol 104: 465-483.
83. Wall CL, Day AS, Gearry RB (2013) Use of exclusive enteral nutrition in adults with Crohn's disease: a review. World J Gastroenterol 19: 7652-7660.
84. Gonzalez-Huix F, Fernandez-Banares F, Esteve-Comas M (1993) "Enteral versus parenteral nutrition as adjunct therapy in acute ulcerative colitis," AJG 88: 227-232.
85. Gupta P, Andrew H, Kirschner BS, Guandalini S (2000) Is lactobacillus

GG helpful in children with Crohn's disease? Results of a preliminary, open-label study. J Pediatr Gastroenterol Nutr 31: 453-457.

86. Gionchetti P, Lammers KM, Rizzello F, Campieri M (2005) Probiotics and barrier function in colitis. Gut 54: 898-900.

87. Akobeng AK, Thomas AG (2007) Enteral nutrition for maintenance of remission in Crohn's disease. Cochrane Database Syst Rev : CD005984.

88. Bibiloni R, Fedorak RN, Tannock GW, Madsen KL, Gionchetti P, et al. (2005) VSL#3 probiotic-mixture induces remission in patients with active ulcerative colitis. Am J Gastroenterol 100: 1539-1546.

89. Steinhart AH, Hiruki T, Brzezinski A, Baker JP (1996) Treatment of left-sided ulcerative colitis with butyrate enemas: a controlled trial. Aliment Pharmacol Ther 10: 729-736.

90. Assumpção IR, Rodrigues M, Barbieri D (1999) [Treatment of unspecific ulcerative rectocolitis in a child with enemas containing butyrate. Case report]. Arq Gastroenterol 36: 238-243.

91. Belluzzi A, Brignola C, Campieri M, Pera A, Boschi S, et al. (1996) Effect of an enteric-coated fish-oil preparation on relapses in Crohn's disease. N Engl J Med 334: 1557-1560.

92. Turner D, Zlotkin SH, Shah PS, Griffiths AM (2007) Omega 3 fatty acids (fish oil) for maintenance of remission in Crohn's disease. Cochrane Database Syst Rev: CD006320.

93. Turner D, Steinhart AH, Griffiths AM (2007) Omega 3 fatty acids (fish oil) for maintenance of remission in ulcerative colitis. Cochrane Database Syst Rev CD006443.

94. Yamamoto T, Nakahigashi M, Umegae S, Matsumoto K (2010) "Prospective clinical trial: enteral nutrition during maintenance infliximab in Crohn's disease," J Gastroenterol 45: 24-29.

95. Sazuka S, Katsuno T, Nakagawa T (2012) "Concomitant use of enteral nutrition therapy is associated with sustained response to infliximab in patients with Crohns disease," EJCN 66: 1219-1223.

96. Hirai F, Ishihara H, Yada S, Esaki M, Ohwan T, et al. (2013) Effectiveness of concomitant enteral nutrition therapy and infliximab for maintenance treatment of Crohn's disease in adults. Dig Dis Sci 58: 1329-1334.

97. Greenberg GR, Fleming CR, Jeejeebhoy KN, Rosenberg IH, Sales D, et al. (1988) Controlled trial of bowel rest and nutritional support in the management of Crohn's disease. Gut 29: 1309-1315.

98. Lochs H, Meryn S, Marosi L, Ferenci P, Hörtnagl H (1983) Has total bowel rest a beneficial effect in the treatment of Crohn's disease? Clin Nutr 2: 61-64.

99. Duerksen DR, Nehra V, Bistrian BR, Blackburn GL (1998) Appropriate nutritional support in acute and complicated Crohn's disease. Nutrition 14: 462-465.

100. Khanna MP, Gordon PH (2000) Gastrocolic fistulization in Crohn's disease: a case report and a review of the literature. Can J Surg 43: 53-56.

101. Lucendo AJ, De Rezende LC (2009) "Importance of nutrition in inflammatory bowel disease," WJG 15: 2081-2088.

102. Rajendran N, Kumar D (2010) Role of diet in the management of inflammatory bowel disease. World J Gastroenterol 16: 1442-1448.

103. Triantafillidis JK, Vagianos C, Papalois AE (2015) The role of enteral nutrition in patients with inflammatory bowel disease: current aspects. Biomed Res Int 2015: 197167.

4

Quinoa (*Chenopodium quinoa* Willd), from Nutritional Value to Potential Health Benefits

Gordillo-Bastidas E[1], Díaz-Rizzolo DA[3], Roura E[2], Massanés T[2] and Gomis R[1,3-5,*]

[1]*Department of Endocrinology and Nutrition, Hospital Clínic, Barcelona, Spain*

[2]*Fundació Alícia, Barcelona, Spain*

[3]*Diabetes and Obesity Research Laboratory, IDIBAPS, Barcelona, Spain*

[4]*CIBER in Diabetes and Associated Metabolic Disorders (CIBERDEM), Barcelona, Spain*

[5]*University of Barcelona, Barcelona, Spain*

[*]**Corresponding author:** Gomis R, IDIBAPS, C/Rosselló, 149-153, 08036 - Barcelona, Spain, E-mail: ramon.gomis@idibaps.org

Abstract

Chenopodium quinoa Willd, known as quinoa, has been cultivated and consumed by humans for the last 5,000-7,000 years. Quinoa was important to pre-Columbian Andean civilizations, as the Incas considered it a gift from their gods. Quinoa has potential health benefits and exceptional nutritional value: a high concentration of protein (all essential amino acids highly bioavailable), unsaturated fatty acids, a low glycemic index; vitamins, minerals and other beneficial compounds; it is also gluten-free; furthermore, quinoa is a sustainable food, as plants exhibit a carbon and water food print that is between 30 and 60 times lower than that of beef. Quinoa is easy to cook, has versatility in preparation, and could be cultivated in different environments. For these reasons, quinoa, previously considered a food of low social prestige, is now the focus of attention of many countries worldwide. However, few studies exist on quinoa or quinoa compounds, *in vitro*, *in vivo* and clinical trials, for assessing its potential clinical applications supported by strong scientific evidence; thus, there is a need for well-designed clinical trials and increased scientific research in this field.

Keywords: Quinoa; Glycemic index; Gluten free; Essential amino acids; Healthy food

Abbreviations

20E: 20-Hydroxyecdysone; ACE: Angiotensin I Converting Enzyme; Ca: Calcium; Cx43: Connexin 43; DPPH: Ferric Thiocyanate and 1,1-Diphenyl-2-Picrylhydrazyl; Fe: Iron; GI: Glycemic Index; HbA1c: Hemoglobin A1c; HF: High Fat Diet; HF20E: High Fat Diet+20-Hydroxyecdysone; HFQ: High Fat Diet+Quinoa; IgE: Immunoglobulin E; K: Potassium; kcals: Kilocalories; Mg: Magnesium; MTT: 3-(4,5-Dimethylthiazol-2-yl)-2,5-Diphenyltetrazolium Bromide; NASA: National Aeronautics and Space Administration; P: Phosphorus; PAI-1: Plasminogen Activator Inhibitor-1; PEPCK: Phosphoenolpyruvate Carboxykinase

Introduction

Quinoa is a grain with exceptional nutritional value; it has been cultivated for the last 5,000-7,000 years in the Andean region of Bolivia and Peru. 2013 was declared by the United Nations as the International Year of Quinoa as recognition of its significant potential [1-4].

Quinoa has high concentrations of protein, all essential amino acids, unsaturated fatty acids, and a low glycemic index (GI); it also contains vitamins, minerals and other beneficial compounds, and is gluten-free by nature. Quinoa is easy to cook and has versatility in preparation [1-4].

In this article, we present an extensive review of quinoa, starting with its history, analyzing its botanical characteristics, and covering its nutritional profile. In addition, we offer a critical comparison with other grains and describe quinoa culinary applications and uses. We also provide an updated review of the scientific information available on quinoa or quinoa compound properties through *in vivo*, *in vitro* and clinical studies, in order to evaluate its potential translational applications.

History

Quinoa has been cultivated for thousands of years in the Andean region of Bolivia and Peru [5,6]. It is known by different local names, or simply quinoa or quinua (quinua is in Quechua) [4]. This plant was called "the mother grain" by the Incas and was considered a gift from their gods, used even for treating medical issues. Traditionally, quinoa seeds were roasted and cooked, added to soups, used as a cereal, and even fermented into beer or chichi (traditional drink of the Andes) [4,7,8].

After the Spanish conquest of South America, the colonists looked down on quinoa as a peasant food or food of the Indians; consequently, quinoa has been considered a food of low social prestige. In addition, the Catholic Church actively suppressed its cultivation after discovering that quinoa was used as a sacred drink (Mudai) during indigenous religious ceremonies. Thus, quinoa remained only where Europeans could not reach and replace it with other grains [4].

Botanical description and cultivation

The botanical name of quinoa is *Chenopodium quinoa* Willd and belongs to the Goosefoot family "Chenopodiaceae", which includes: Swiss chard (*Beta sp.*), spinach (*Spinacia oleracea*) and Lamb's quarters

(*Chenopodium album*). Quinoa is a dicot plant that can grow from 1 to 3m high; it is considered a pseudo-cereal, not a true grain but rather a fruit. The seeds are round and flat, about 1.5-4.0 mm in diameter and their color varies from white to grey and black, with tones of yellow, rose, red, purple and violet (Figure 1). Quinoa has demonstrated a strong tolerance to salty, acid or alkaline soils, in both cold (-5°C) or hot climates (up to 35°C) [4,5].

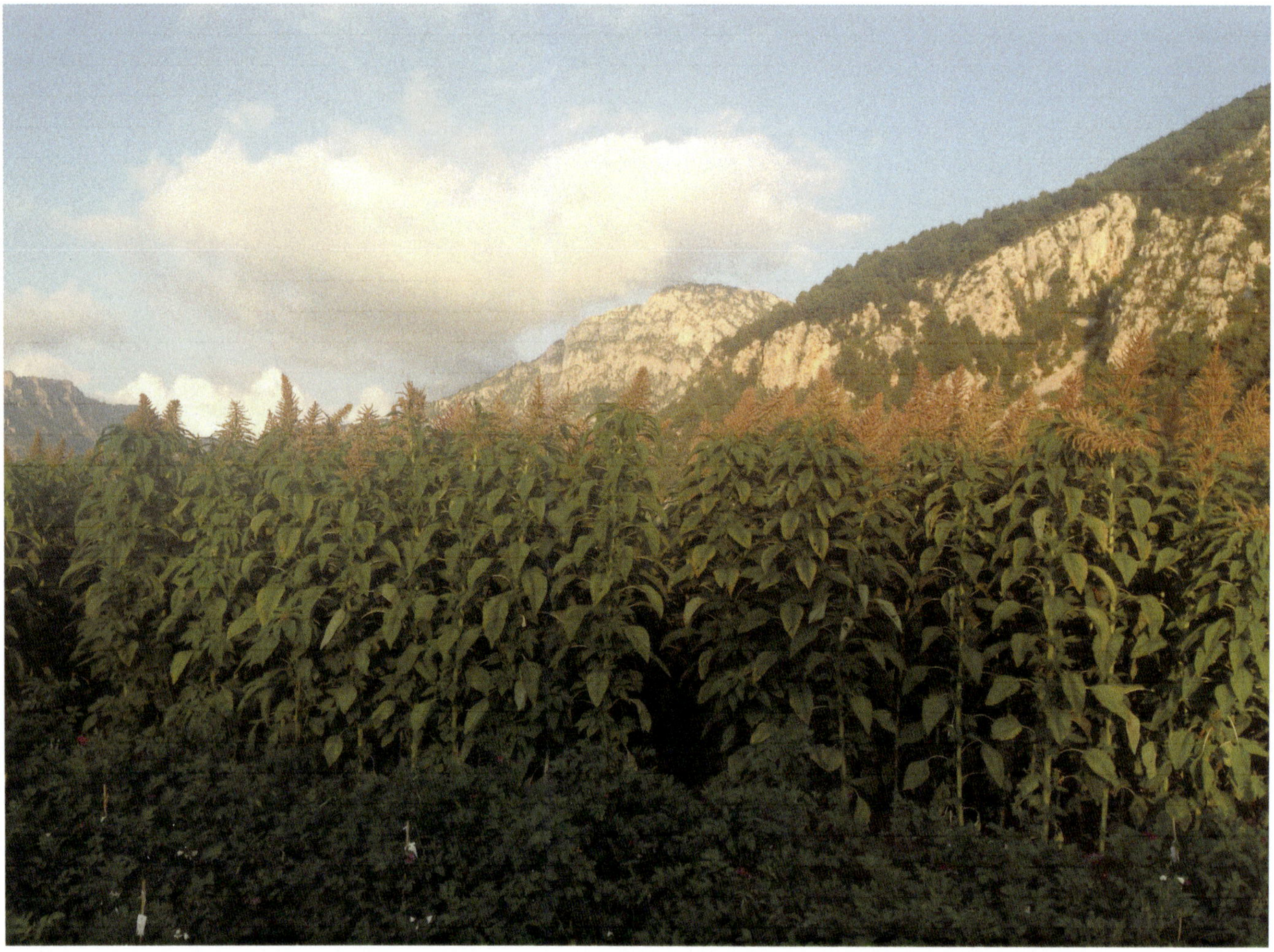

Figure 1: Quinoa plant, Quinoa is a pseudo-cereal. Its seeds can be different colors; its leaves are shaped like a goose's foot.

Quinoa is distributed worldwide and includes 250 varieties. Its classification is based on the color of the plant and fruits, or on plant morphology [4,5]. This grain has been authorized to be sown in Europe, North America, Asia and Africa. In Europe the project "Quinoa: a multipurpose crop for the European Community" was approved in 1993 [4].

Nutritional profile

The effects of globalization and urbanization have influenced dietary patterns and lifestyle behaviors among population groups throughout the world. Traditional food patterns rich in complex carbohydrates, micronutrients, fiber and phytochemicals are being replaced with diets high in animal fats and refined carbohydrates and oils, a situation that has made a direct impact on the prevalence of certain chronic diseases [9]. For this reason, many researchers devote their efforts to analyzing food or food components that may prove to be healthy for human consumption [5]; one example is the work of the HEALTHGRAIN Consortium, which, of note, has included quinoa in its list of healthy grains [10].

Quinoa is considered one of the best vegetal protein sources, as its protein levels are similar to those found in milk and higher than those present in cereals such as wheat, rice and maize. Quinoa also has been used by the National Aeronautics and Space Administration (NASA) due to its versatility in meeting the needs of humans during space missions [3,4,7,11,12].

Protein

Proteins and amino acids are major biological macromolecules that serve as structural constituents and as catalysts for enzymatic reactions, energy sources and protein synthesis in the body [13,14].

The protein biological value measures the proportion of protein absorbed from a food which then becomes incorporated into the proteins of the body. Quinoa has a high biological value (73%), similar to that of beef (74%), and higher than those of white rice (56%), wheat (49%) and corn (36%). Quinoa also contains all ten essential amino acids, and its protein content ranges from 12.9 to 16.5% [4,15-17]. Of primary interest is the high lys value, an essential amino acid that is deficient in many grains [16,18]. Quinoa is also high in the essential amino acid met, which is deficient in many legumes [19,20]. According to the daily recommended amounts of amino acids indicated by the Food and Agriculture Organization (FAO) of the United Nations and by the World Health Organization (WHO), quinoa fulfills the amino acid requirements for adults: 180% of histidine (his), 274% of isoleucine (ile), 338% of lysine (lys), 212% of methionine+cysteine (met+cys), 320% of phenylalanine+tyrosine (phe+tyr), 331% of threonine (thr), 228% of tryptophan (trp) and 323% of valine (val) (20). For these reasons, quinoa could represent a valuable source of nutrition, especially for infants and children, and may be used in nutritive foods and beverages [21].

Another feature of note is the high sustainability of plant food consumption due to their low carbon, water and ecological food prints. In this sense, quinoa is an excellent protein source such as beef, but it has a carbon and water food print that is between 30 and 60 times lower in value [22].

Carbohydrates

Carbohydrates are organic compounds comprised of carbon, hydrogen, and oxygen. Carbohydrates act as signaling molecules, energy sources and structural components [14].

Starch, as a carbohydrate, provides the major source of physiological energy in the human diet. The content of starch in quinoa ranges from 58.1% to 64.2% of dry matter, of which 11% is amylose. Moreover, quinoa has a high content of D-xylose and maltose and a low content of glucose and fructose.

100 g of quinoa contains: Glucose 1.70 mg, fructose 0.20 mg, saccharose 2.90 mg and maltose 1.40 mg [4,5,17]. In addition, there are studies that suggest that quinoa polysaccharides have antioxidant properties [23].

Lipids

Lipids are concentrated sources of energy as well as structural components of cell membranes that the body uses for performing a variety of normal functions [2,4]. A higher intake of vegetables is associated with a reduced risk of type 2 diabetes, due to their high unsaturated fat content, which is associated with lower inflammation [24,25].

The quality of lipids is very important. For example, it is known that omega-6 stimulates inflammatory activity in the body, while omega-3 performs anti-inflammatory functions. A lower ratio of omega-6: omega-3 fatty acids are more desirable for reducing the risk of cardiovascular disease, cancer, and inflammatory and autoimmune diseases [2,4,26].

The total lipid content of quinoa is 14.5%, with approximately 70%-89.4% being unsaturated (38.9%-57% of linoleic acid, 24.0%-27.7% of oleic acid and 4% of α-linolenic acid). The unsaturated fatty acid content is protected by vitamin E in this plant. The ratio between omega-6 and omega-3 in quinoa is about 6:1 [2,4].

Fiber

Dietary fiber is the indigestible portion of food derived from plants and has two main components: soluble and insoluble. Soluble fiber dissolves in water, is readily fermented in the colon into gases and physiologically active products, and has prebiotic properties. Insoluble fiber, which does not dissolve in water, is either metabolically inert and provides bulking mass, or it can be prebiotic and metabolically ferment in the large intestine. Bulking fibers absorb water, easing defecation [3,27].

Greater consumption of fiber-rich whole grains is associated with a lower risk of type 2 diabetes [24] and cardiovascular disease [28]. Quinoa is an excellent source of dietary fiber, comprising about 2.6%-10% of the total weight of the grain; about 78% of its fiber content is insoluble and 22% soluble [3,5,17,27,29].

Glycemic index (GI)

The GI is a ranking of carbohydrates on a scale from 0 to 100 according to their impact on blood sugar levels during the 2 h following consumption. Low GI (<55) foods produce gradual rises in blood sugar and insulin levels. Low GI diets have been shown to improve glucose and lipid levels and weight control because they help control appetite [30,31]. Low GI diets also reduce insulin resistance and the risk of cardiovascular diseases, diabetes and some cancers [9,24,32]. It is reported that fasting insulin is lower in individuals with higher dietary fiber intakes [33] and that the ingestion of complex carbohydrates promotes longevity [14]; and also that a high GI diet increases the levels of inflammation biomarkers. In patients with celiac disease, a reduced inflammatory state could provide certain protective mechanisms, thus, following a low GI diet could meliorate this disease [34].

The GI for quinoa ranges 35-53 depending on the cooking time; 150 g of quinoa, cooked, refrigerated and reheated in the microwave for 1.5 min has a GI of 53. Therefore, even when more or less "overcooked", quinoa maintains a low GI [32].

In Table 1 we present a summary of the nutritional profile of cooked quinoa, in comparison with common cereals (also cooked).

Food	Energy (kcals)	Proteins (g)	Essential amino acids (number)	Carbo-hydrates (g)	Lipids (g)	Unsaturated fatty acids (g)	Fiber (g)	GI
Quinoa	120	4.4	10/10	21.3	1.92	1.61	2.8	35-53
Rice (white, medium grain)	130	2.38	9/10	28.59	0.21	0.12	0.3	75-89
Wheat (soft, white)	113	3.6	10/10	25.12	0.66	0.35	4.23	48

Corn (sweet, yellow)	96	3.41	9/10	20.98	1.5	0.98	2.4	60

Table 1: General nutritional profile of quinoa, we observe the overall content of quinoa in comparison with that of other foods [35,36]. *Portion size is 100 g of each cooked food; as a norm, cooked food increases its size 3 times. kcal: Kilocalories, GI: Glycemic index.

Vitamins

Vitamins are compounds essential for the health of humans. Quinoa has many vitamins, with 100 g of this grain containing: 0.4 mg of thiamine, 78.1 mg of folic acid, 1.4 mg of vitamin C, 0.20 mg of vitamin B6, and 0.61 mg of pantothenic acid [4]. Its vitamin E content ranges 37.49-59.82 μg/g. Tocopherol isoforms have also been detected in this seed: γ-tocopherol (47-53 μg/g), α-tocopherol (17-26 μg/g), and β- and δ-tocopherol (<5 μm/g) [2,5].

Minerals

Dietary minerals are essential chemical elements that play a role in regulating electrolyte balance, glucose homeostasis, the transmission of nerve impulses and enzyme cofactors in the body [37].

Calcium, magnesium and potassium in quinoa are found in sufficient quantities and bioavailable forms necessary for maintaining a balanced human diet. Quinoa contains: 874 mg/kg of calcium (Ca) [4,5,38], iron (Fe) 948.5 mg/kg, phosphorus (P) 2735.0 mg/kg-4543.3 mg/kg, potassium (K) 9562.2 mg/kg and magnesium (Mg) 1901.5 mg/kg [3,5,39].

Betaine

Betaine is an essential osmolyte source of methyl groups and finds its source either in diet or in the oxidation of choline. Its metabolism methylates homocysteine into methionine, also producing N,N-dimethylglycine. Mammals use betaine to assist in cell volume regulation, and as a methyl donor for the remethylation of homocysteine into methionine [27,40-42].

Hyperhomocysteinemia makes a person more prone to endothelial cell injury by activating inflammation pathways and is thus a possible risk factor for coronary artery disease. For this reason, betaine consumption could prove beneficial, as it converts homocysteine into methione. Nevertheless, urinary excretion of betaine is minimal, even following a large betaine dose [43,44]. It is generally agreed that most people consume between 100 mg/day and 300 mg/day [5,41,45].

Betaine content of foods: cooked white rice 0 μg/g; cooked oatmeal 139 μg/g; cooked wheat spaghetti 287 μg/g; cooked quinoa approximately 1310 μg/g–2000 μg/g [45].

Polyphenols

Polyphenols are natural organic chemicals with large multiples of phenol structural units. They are commonly found in plant foods and represent the most abundant antioxidants found in the human diet [46].

Quinoa presents at least 23 phenolic compounds. The total phenolic content (mg/kg quinoa) is 466.99, 634.66 and 682.05 for white, red and black quinoa, respectively. The most abundant phenols are ferulic acid and quercetin [1,6,47]. Quinoa contains more phenols than whole cereals, including wheat, barley, millet, rice and buckwheat [11].

Isoflavones

Isoflavones are organic compounds that have a role in influencing sex hormone metabolism and biological activity through intracellular enzymes, protein synthesis, growth factor actions, malignant cell proliferations, differentiation and angiogenesis [48].
In particular, quinoa contains the isoflavones daidzein and genistein; these hormones could be recognized by human estrogen receptors and act as antagonists of vessel contraction and reduce arterial resistance [4].

Carotenoids

Carotenoids are organic pigments found in the chloroplasts and chromoplasts of plants. The function of carotenoids in plants is to protect chlorophyll from photodamage. In humans, they exhibit antioxidant activity [27,49].

The total carotenoid content of white, red and black quinoa seeds are 11.87, 14.97 and 17.61 μg/g, respectively [50,51]. The β-carotene content of quinoa leaves ranges from 4.3 μg/1 g-19.5 μg/1 g [38].

Gluten

Gluten is one of the most abundant components of food (including grains) [52]. Gluten is a composite of the proteins gliadin and glutenin [51].

Celiac disease is an immune-mediated reaction to gluten, characterized by an insufficient T- cell-mediated immune response that causes inflammatory injury to the small intestine [17,52]. Celiac disease patients must consume food with gluten substitutes or gluten-free grains [17,34,51,52].

Several gluten-free foodstuffs contain more salt and fat (saturated fat) but fewer minerals and vitamins than their gluten-containing counterparts. For this reason, quinoa is an excellent gluten-free grain, with a high content of vitamins and minerals that make it a potentially essential part of any healthy, gluten-free diet [7,17,34,53]; also quinoa complies with the Codex Alimentarius nomenclature of gluten-free products (gluten content <20 mg/kg) [51].

In Table 2, we present a summary of the principal quinoa compounds.

Vitamins		Minerals		Polyphenols	
Thiamine mg/100 g	0.4	Fe mg/kg	948.5	Total Phenolic Content mg/kg	467-682
Folic acid mg/100 g	78.1	Ca mg/kg	874	Ferulic acid mg/kg	37.5-58.4

Vitamin C mg/100 g	1.4	P mg/kg	2735	Quercetin mg/kg	5.3-13
B6 mg/100 g	0.2	K mg/kg	9562	Isoflavones	
Pantothenic acid mg/100 g	0.61	Mg mg/kg	1903	Daidzein mg/100 g	0.78-2.05
Vitamin E µg/1 g	37.49-59.82			Carotenoids	
Total carotenoids µg/g					11.87-17.61

Table 2: Summary of quinoa compounds. Quinoa contains several vitamins, minerals and antioxidant molecules. Fe: Iron, Ca: Calcium, P: Phosphorus, K: Potassium, Mg: Magnesium.

Anti-nutritional factors

Saponins are natural detergents made of glycosylated secondary metabolites that are utilized by the plant as a predator repellent [54].

Quinoa contains saponins with a bitter taste, which could cause gastric irritation; its content varies between 0.1% and 5%; quinoa could even be classified according to its free saponin content, into either sweet (<0.11%) or bitter quinoa (>0.11%). In addition, there are studies of methods for saponin removal without any significant modification of nutritional value, such as thoroughly washing it in cold water [55].

On the other hand, isolated saponins could also have certain health benefits, such as anti-inflammatory activity [4,5,56-58].

Phytic acid is a saturated cyclic acid and is the principal storage form of phosphorus in many plant tissues. If the content of phytic acid is high in the food, this acid binds minerals, thereby rendering them unavailable for metabolism [27,59]. But, if the phytic acid content is low, it could act as an antioxidant: chelates various metals (for example, suppresses damaging Fe-catalysed redox reactions), inhibits xanthine oxidase, suppresses oxidant damage to the intestinal epithelium, and interferes with the formation of ADP-Fe-oxygen complexes that initiate lipid peroxidation; prevents the formation of carcinogens and blocks the interaction of carcinogens with cells; controls cell division and reduces cell proliferation rate; increases the immune response by enhancing the activity of natural killer cells; may be involved in cellular and nuclear signalling pathways; important source of P; inhibitor for renal stone development; hypoglycaemic (for example, by chelating Ca, an a-amylase cofactor) and cholesterol-lowering (by binding Zn and decreasing Zn:Cu ratio) effects; affects the metabolic and detoxification capacity of the liver; reduces blood glucose and lipid, and hepatic lipid levels; inhibits calcification of cardiovascular system (lower level of Ca in aorta); prevention of platelet aggregation; high affinity for hydroxyapatite; adsorption onto Ca-based crystals; *in vitro* effect on gene expression through chromatin remodelling [27].

The general content of phytic acid in quinoa is low and ranges from 10.5 mg to 13.5 mg, in comparison with corn that contains 720 mg, wheat 390 mg and rice 60 mg [4].

Protease inhibitors are proteins that form very stable complexes with proteolytic enzymes in the body. The content of protease inhibitors in quinoa seeds is <50 ppm, which is very low and does not pose any serious concerns [4].

Allergenicity

Asao and others observed that quinoa consumption did not show a positive reaction against wheat protein antibodies and suggested that quinoa could be ingested by people who have allergies against wheat proteins [11]. However, Astier and others reported a case of anaphylaxis to quinoa in France: a 52 year old man developed a systemic reaction consisting of dysphagia, dysphonia, urticaria and angioedema after the ingestion of quinoa with fish and bread. They tested samples of the ingested food, and only quinoa showed Immunoglobulin E (IgE) reactivity in the patient's serum [60].

Current status in experimental and clinical research

As we have seen above, quinoa has outstanding potential for human nutrition. Therefore, in this section we will provide an updated review of scientific information available on quinoa or quinoa compounds in different models.

In vitro

Betaine: Lee and others tested a betaine pretreatment (2 mM) in H2.35 mouse hepatocyte cells. They observed an increase in cytochrome C oxidase activity and improved mitochondrial respiration (mitochondrial dysfunction is a commonly found in many pathological conditions and ageing) [40].

Polyphenols: Gawlik-Dziki and others cultured AT-2 and MAT-LyLu prostate cancer cells with quinoa leaf extract (rich in ferulic, sinapinic and gallic acid). They observed that cell proliferation was blocked, the expression of Connexin 43 (Cx43) was decreased, and lipid oxidation was prevented, inhibiting lipoxygenase activity. They also concluded that 80% of phenolics are available *in vitro* [61].

Quinoa flour: Extracts from quinoa flour and from that of whole cereals (wheat, barley, millet, rice, buckwheat) were used to evaluate antioxidant potential. The ferric thiocyanate and 1,1-diphenyl-2-picrylhydrazyl (DPPH) radical scavenging activity methods were used; also, the Angiotensin I Converting Enzyme (ACE) inhibitory activity was measured. Quinoa presented higher antioxidant potential and higher ACE inhibition activity (23.3%) in comparison with the same whole cereals. These results suggested that quinoa possesses potent free radical-scavenging compounds [11].

In vivo

Saponins: In mice, Verza and others reported that no lethality or local toxicity (local swelling, loss of hair, and piloerection) was observed after administering 300 µg of quinoa saponins [62].

20-hydroxyecdysone: Ecdysteroids are steroid hormones which have been implicated in plant repellence against insects, and in the control of the molting and reproduction processes of arthropods. The main phytoecdysteroid found in plants is 20-hydroxyecdysone (20E). Quinoa contains about 1.9% of 20E. These ecdysteroids have anabolic properties and help in controlling blood glucose levels. Graf and others tested an extract from quinoa seeds in obese mice and observed that fasting blood glucose levels were significantly lower [63].

Moreover, Foucault and others conducted a study on six-week-old male C57BL/6J mice. Mice were fed with a high-fat diet (HF) ad libitum, for 3 weeks. The high-fat diet group was supplemented or not with either quinoa powder (HFQ) or pure 20E (HF20E). The epididymal adipose tissue following treatment was significantly lower in the HFQ and in the HF20E vs. HF group. The HFQ showed a trend of reduced lipid storage capacity in the adipose tissue, increased LPL and PPAR-γ mRNA levels, and reduced expression of Phosphoenolpyruvate carboxykinase (PEPCK) and Plasminogen activator inhibitor-1 (PAI-1) in the adipose tissue, as well as decreased adipocyte hypertrophy [64,65].

Extract from seeds of quinoa: Meneguetti and others analyzed the effects of an extract from quinoa seeds in male Wistar rats assigned randomly to different groups: (1) a sedentary supplemented group, which received 2,000 mg/kg of the extract; (2) a sedentary control group, non-supplemented; (3) an exercise supplemented group with 2,000 mg/kg of the extract; and (4) an exercise control group non-supplemented. Follow-up was performed for 30 days. They observed beneficial effects in both supplemented groups (sedentary and exercise), as these groups showed a tendency of decreased food intake, body weight, fat deposition, and blood triglycerides (TG) levels [15].

Quinoa seeds in lipid profile and glucose levels: Pasko and others conducted a five week study with 24 male Wistar rats divided into different groups: a control group (corn starch); a control group with 31% of its dieting consisting of fructose; a group fed with a diet of quinoa seeds (310 g/kg); and a group fed with a diet of quinoa seeds (310 g/kg) and 31% of fructose. The group fed with quinoa showed significantly reduced serum total cholesterol (26%), LDL (57%), TG (11%) and glucose (10%). Fructose significantly decreased HDL (15%) levels in the control group, but when quinoa seeds were added to the diet, the decrease in HDL levels was inhibited [66]. The same research group analyzed fructose administration effects in the same animal groups, and they reported an increase in oxidative stress (high malondialdehyde) in the control group with 31% of its dieting consisting of fructose. In addition, the co-administration of quinoa seeds (310 g/kg fodder) decreased malondialdehyde in plasma [67].

Clinical studies

Quinoa and serum lipids: A prospective and double-blind study was conducted in overweight, postmenopausal women testing the effects of quinoa flakes vs corn flakes (25 g for 4 weeks). The group that consumed quinoa flakes showed a significant reduction in serum TG, a tendency of reduced total cholesterol and LDL and increased glutathione [68].

Quinoa and celiac disease: Zevallos and others conducted a study in nineteen celiac patients who consumed 50 g/day of quinoa for 6 weeks as part of their usual gluten-free diet. Duodenal biopsies and blood samples were obtained. Quinoa consumption was well-tolerated and did not exacerbate the clinical presentation of celiac disease. The study showed a positive trend toward improved histological parameters (the ratio of villus height to crypt depth improved from slightly below normal values 2.8:1 to normal levels 3:1, surface-enterocyte cell height improved from 28.76 µm to 29.77 µm and the number of intra-epithelial lymphocytes per 100 enterocytes decreased from 30.3 to 29.7 and serum total cholesterol [51].

Betaine and homocysteine in plasma: McRae conducted a meta-analysis of randomized placebo-controlled trials that used betaine supplementation. This analysis included five randomized controlled trials, published between 2002 and 2010. The studies used healthy adult participants who were supplemented with at least 4 g/d of betaine for a period between 6 and 24 weeks. The meta-analysis concluded that betaine supplementation decreased plasma homocysteine 1.23 µmol/L [69].

Betaine and metabolic syndrome: There is a significant negative association between markers of obesity (BMI, percent body fat and waist circumference) and plasma betaine concentrations in human cross-sectional data; in addition, more than 20% of patients with diabetes mellitus excrete abnormal amounts of betaine in their urine (41). Higher concentrations of plasma betaine were associated also with lower non-HDL cholesterol, TG, homocysteine and markers of inflammation [70].

Quinoa and diabetes: Jenkins and others tested a low GI diet (quinoa included). For 6 months, they performed follow-up on 210 patients divided into 2 groups (high cereal fiber diet or low GI diet). They observed a greater decrease of Hemoglobin A1c (HbA1c) in the low GI diet (-0.50%) and an increase in HDL (1.7 mg/dL) in a statistically significant manner [71].

To summarize the results presented in this section, quinoa emerges as a food of particular interest to celiac patients, as the potential cornerstone of a healthy, gluten-free diet. Furthermore, we hypothesize that including quinoa in the diet could decrease oxidative stress, improve serum lipid profile, help to control body weight and serum glucose, and decrease cardiovascular disease and type 2 diabetes risk factors; quinoa may even prove beneficial in reversing the effects of these diseases. However, until now, very few studies using quinoa or quinoa compounds *in vitro*, *in vivo* or clinical trials have taken place for determining translational applications based on strong scientific evidence.

In Table 3, we provide a complete summary of the potential health benefits of quinoa.

Compound	Dose	Model	Effect	Reference
Betaine	2 mM	H2.35 mouse hepatocyte cells	Improves mitochondrial respiration	[40]
Quinoa leaves extract	WI	AT-2 and MAT-LyLu prostate cancer cells	Cell proliferation was blocked, expression of Cx43 decreased, and lipid oxidation was prevented.	[61]
Quinoa flour	WI	Analysis of quinoa flour	ACE inhibition activity (23.3%), potent free radical-scavenging.	[11]
Saponins	300 µg	Mice	No lethality or local toxicity.	[62]

20-hydroxyecdysone	WI	C57BL/6J mice	Decreased epididymal adipose tissue. Trend of reduced lipid storage capacity in the adipose tissue, increased LPL and P-PARg, reduced expression of PEPCK and PAI-1 in adipose tissue, and also decreased adipocyte hypertrophy.	[64,65]
Extract from seeds of quinoa	2,000 mg/kg	Male Wistar rats	Tendency of decreased food intake, body weight, fat deposition, and blood TG levels.	[15]
Quinoa seeds	310 g/kg	Male Wistar rats	Reduction in total cholesterol (26%), LDL (57%), TG (11%), glucose (10%), and malondialdehyde in plasma.	[66,67]
Quinoa flakes	25 g	Postmenopausal women who were overweight	Reduction in serum TG, and tendency of decreased total cholesterol and LDL and increased glutathione.	[68]
Betaine	4 g	Healthy adults	Decreased plasma homocysteine 1.23 μmol/L.	[69]
Quinoa	50 g	Celiac patients	Good tolerance without any exacerbation of celiac disease. Trend toward improved histological parameters and serum total cholesterol.	[51]
Low GI diet that included quinoa	WI	Patients with type 2 diabetes	HbA1c decreased 50% and HDL increased 1.7 mg/dL.	[71]

Table 3: Potential health benefits of quinoa, we review the effects of quinoa or its components in *in vitro* and *in vivo* studies and in clinical trials. WI: Without information, ACE: Angiotensin I Converting Enzyme, LPL: Lipopolysaccharides, PAI-1: Plasminogen Activator Inhibitor-1, Hb1Ac: Hemoglobin A1c.

Culinary Issues

Quinoa is traditionally cooked as a whole grain similar to rice or milled into flour and made into pasta and breads [8]. This grain can also be processed by extrusion, drum-drying and autoclaving. Quinoa is very versatile in terms of culinary preparation: whole grains, uncooked or roasted flour, small leaves, meal, and instant powder can be prepared in a number of ways. There are numerous recipes available featuring approximately 100 preparations (Figure 2). Commercially available quinoa products exist such as pasta, bread, cookies, muffins, cereal, snacks, drinks, flakes, baby food, and diet supplements; in general, these have approximately 20% quinoa content [5,11,72-80]. The fresh leaves and tender shoots of the plant are eaten raw in salads, or cooked and eaten as a vegetable [1,5,20].

Quinoa cooking times varied from 11.9 to 19.2 min depending on the kind of seed (longer cooking time also correlated with higher protein content). Water uptake ratio varied from 2.5 to 4.0 fold [73].

Organoleptic properties

Organoleptic properties are the aspects of food as experienced by the senses, including taste, sight, smell, and touch. Food texture refers to those qualities of a food that can be felt with the fingers, tongue, palate, or teeth. In addition, the replacement of refined flour by whole grains such as quinoa could produce changes in the organoleptic properties of foods, like darker color due to the presence of bran, and may influence the consumer decisions.

Cooked quinoa normally has a texture described as creamy and smooth but, at the same time, slightly crunchy [79].

Conclusion

The use of pseudocereals such as quinoa represents a promising area of research, as its use could improve the intake of certain macromolecules and phytochemicals that are known to be beneficial to human health. Quinoa is an attractive, gluten-free alternative available to celiac patients, and including quinoa in the diet may prove to be a good strategy for consuming high biological value proteins as well as all bioavailable essential amino acids, something that other grains rarely offer. Quinoa also contains unsaturated lipids, fiber, complex carbohydrates and other beneficial compounds such as betaine, and may be used to improve the metabolic risk factor profile and help control type 2 diabetes. Quinoa may be useful for some other medical complications such as cancer, obesity and dyslipidemia. Furthermore, quinoa, as a plant food, is highly sustainable, with a carbon and water food print that is 30 to 60 times lower than that of beef.

Moreover, the anti-nutritional factors in the quinoa grain could easily be inactivated or reduced to safe health levels when appropriate techniques for industrial processing or household preparation of this food are used. As for culinary applications, the replacement of refined flour by whole grains such as quinoa raises several challenges that need to be addressed, including changes in organoleptic properties.

Finally, quinoa could represent a strategic crop used to complement the diet in rural/marginal regions where energy-protein malnutrition affects a greater part of the population in certain developing countries.

In summary, there are few *in vitro* or *in vivo* studies or clinical trials using quinoa or quinoa compounds; there is a justified need for well-designed clinical trials and increased scientific research in this field, in order to determine the most effective translational applications of quinoa based on solid scientific evidence. Quinoa, known as the "mother grain", represents an exotic and healthy rediscovered food in the developed world.

Acknowledgement

All authors have read and approved the final manuscript.

The authors thank Kimberly Katte for providing linguistic assistance and also Laura Brugnara and Serafin Murillo for manuscript proofreading.

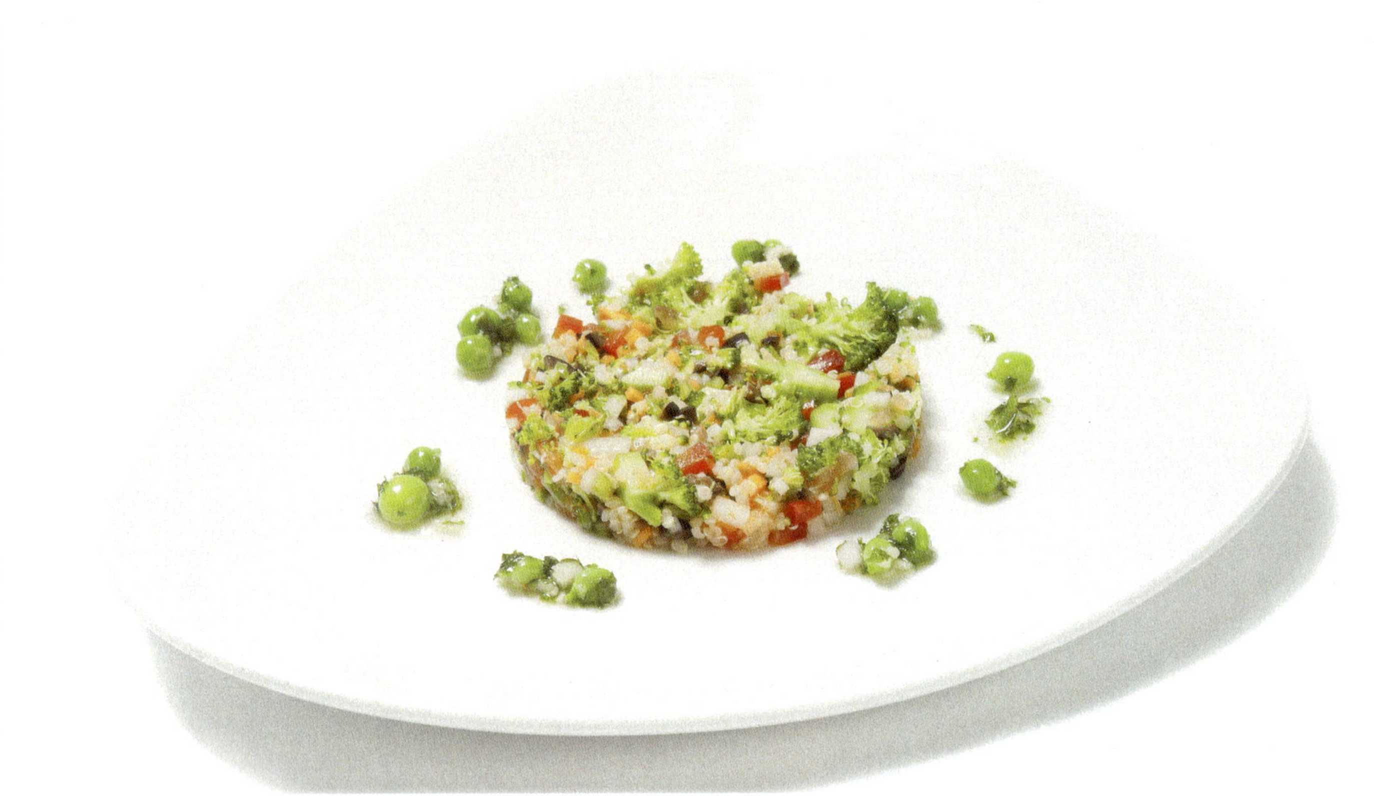

Figure 2: Quinoa salad, quinoa is very versatile in culinary preparation; in this picture quinoa is boiled in water and then mixed with vegetables.

Sources of Financial Support

This work was supported by Institut d'Investigacions Biomèdiques August Pi i Sunyer (IDIBAPS) and Fundaciò Catalunya-La Pedrera, both in Barcelona, Spain.

EGB is recipient of a postdoctoral fellowship from CONACYT (México). DADR has a doctoral fellowship form Resercaixa (Barcelona, Spain).

Potential Conflicts of Interest

The authors (EGB, ER, DADR, TM and RG) have no potential conflicts of interest relevant to this work.

References

1. Tang Y, Li X, Chen PX, Zhang B, Hernandez M, et al. (2015b) Characterisation of fatty acid, carotenoid, tocopherol/tocotrienol compositions and antioxidant activities in seeds of three *Chenopodium quinoa* Willd. genotypes. Food chemistry 174: 502-508.
2. Tang Y, Li X, Zhang B, Chen PX, Liu R, et al. (2015) Characterisation of phenolics, betanins and antioxidant activities in seeds of three *Chenopodium quinoa* Willd. genotypes. Food Chem 166: 380-388.
3. González Martín MI, Wells Moncada G, Fischer S, Escuredo O (2014) Chemical characteristics and mineral composition of quinoa by near-infrared spectroscopy. J Sci Food Agric 94: 876-881.
4. Vega-Gálvez A, Miranda M, Vergara J, Uribe E, Puente L, et al. (2010) Nutrition facts and functional potential of quinoa (*Chenopodium quinoa* Willd.), an ancient Andean grain: a review. J Sci Food Agric 90: 2541-2547.
5. Jancurová M, Minarovicova L, Dandar A (2009) Quinoa - A Review. Czech J Food Sci 27: 71-79.
6. Galvez Ranilla L, Apostolidis E, Genoveses MI, Lajolo FM, Shetty K (2009) Evaluation of Indigenous Grains from the Peruvian Andean Region for Antidiabetes and Antihypertension Potential Using *In Vitro* Methods. J Med Food 12: 704-13.
7. Cooper R (2015) Re-discovering ancient wheat varieties as functional foods. J Tradit Complement Med 5: 138-143.
8. Bazile D, Bertero D, Nieto C (2014) Estado del arte de la quinua en el mundo en 2013: FAO (Santiago de Chile) y CIRAD (Montpellier, Francia). Perspectivas Nutracéuticas de la Quinua: Propiedades Biológicas y aplicaciones funcionales. FAO pp: 341-57.
9. Schaffer-Lequart C, Lehmann U, Ross AB, Roger O, Eldridge AL, et al. (2015) Whole Grain in Manufactured Foods: Current use, Challenges and the way forward. Crit Rev Food Sci Nutr (ahead of print).
10. van der Kamp JW, Poutanen K, Seal CJ, Richardson DP (2014) The HEALTHGRAIN definition of 'whole grain'. Food Nutr Res 58.
11. Asao M, Watanabe K (2010) Functional and Bioactive Properties of Quinoa and Amaranth. Food Sci Technol Res 16: 163-8.
12. Koziol MJ (1992) Chemical Composition and Nutritional Evaluation of Quinoa (*Chenopodium quinoa* Willd.). J Food Comp Anal 5: 35-68.
13. Morrison CD, Laeger T (2015) Protein-dependent regulation of feeding and metabolism. Trends Endocrinol Metab 26: 256-262.
14. Lee D, Hwang W, Artan M, Jeong DE, Lee SJ (2015) Effects of nutritional components on aging. Aging Cell 14: 8-16.
15. Meneguetti QA, Brenzan MA, Batista MR, Bazotte RB, Silva DR, et al. (2011) Biological effects of hydrolyzed quinoa extract from seeds of *Chenopodium quinoa* Willd. J Med Food 14: 653-657.

16. Gesinski K, Nowak K (2011) Comparative analysis of the biological value of protein of *Chenopodium quinoa* Willd. and *Chenopodium album* L. Part I Amino acid composition of the seed protein. Acta Sci Pol Agricultura 10: 47-56.
17. Saturni L, Ferretti G, Bacchetti T (2010) The gluten-free diet: safety and nutritional quality. Nutrients 2: 16-34.
18. Yang H, Ludewig U (2014) Lysine catabolism, amino acid transport, and systemic acquired resistance: what is the link? Plant Signal Behav 9: e28933.
19. Sánchez-Chino X, Jiménez-Martínez C, Dávila-Ortiz G, Álvarez-González I, Madrigal-Bujaidar E (2015) Nutrient and Non-nutrient Components of legumes, and Its Chemopreventive Activity: A Review. Nutr Cancer 24: 1-10.
20. Schlick G, Bubenheim DL (1993) (Ames Research Center, Moffett Field, California). Quinoa: An Emerging "New" Crop with Potential for CELSS. NASA (US). Report No: 3422, pp: 1-6.
21. Abugoch LE, Romero N, Tapia CA, Silva J, Rivera M (2008) Study of some physicochemical and functional properties of quinoa (*Chenopodium quinoa* Willd) protein isolates. J Agric Food Chem 56: 4745-4750.
22. Ruini LF, Ciati R, Pratesi CA, Marino M, Principato L, et al. (2015) Working toward healthy and sustainable diets: the "Double Pyramid Model" developed by the Barilla center for Food and Nutrition to raise awareness about the environmental and nutritional impact of foods. Frontiers in Nutrition 2: 1-6.
23. Yao Y, Shi Z, Ren G (2014a) Antioxidant and Immunoregulatory Activity of Polysaccharides from Quinoa (*Chenopodium quinoa* Willd.). International Journal of Molecular Sciences 15: 19307-19318.
24. Maki KC, Phillips AK (2015) Dietary substitutions for refined carbohydrate that show promise for reducing risk of type 2 diabetes in men and women. J Nutr 145: 159S-163S.
25. Da Silva MS, Rudkowska I (2015) Dairy nutrients and their effect on inflammatory profile in molecular studies. Mol Nutr Food Res 59: 1249-1263.
26. Guadarrama-López AL, Valdés-Ramos R, Martínez-Carrillo BE (2014) Type 2 Diabetes, PUFAs, and Vitamin D: Their Relation to Inflammation. J Immuno Res 1-13.
27. Fardet A (2010) New hypotheses for the health-protective mechanisms of whole-grain cereals: what is beyond fibre? Nutr Res Rev 23: 65-134.
28. Wu Y, Qian Y, Pan Y, Li P, Yang J, et al. (2015) Association between dietary fiber intake and risk of coronary heart disease: A meta-analysis. Clin Nutr 34: 603-611.
29. Lamothe LM, Srichuwong S, Reuhs BL, Hamaker BR (2015) Quinoa (*Chenopodium quinoa* W.) and amaranth (*Amaranthus caudatus* L.) provide dietary fibres high in pectic substances and xyloglucans. Food Chem 167: 490-496.
30. Thomas D, Elliott EJ (2009) Low glycaemic index, or low glycaemic load, diets for diabetes mellitus. Cochrane Database Syst Rev: CD006296.
31. Thomas DE, Elliott EJ, Baur L (2007) Low glycaemic index or low glycaemic load diets for overweight and obesity. Cochrane Database Syst Rev: CD005105.
32. Atkinson FS, Foster-Powell K, Brand-Miller JC (2008) International tables of glycemic index and glycemic load values: 2008. Diabetes Care 31: 2281-2283.
33. Pereira MA, Jacobs DR Jr, Pins JJ, Raatz SK, Gross MD, et al. (2002) Effect of whole grains on insulin sensitivity in overweight hyperinsulinemic adults. Am J Clin Nutr 75: 848-855.
34. Pellegrini N, Agostoni C (2014) Nutritional aspects of gluten-free products. J Sci Food Agric 95: 1-6.
35. USDA (2015) National Nutrient database for Standard Reference Release 27. National Agricultural Library. Basic Report 20137 (consulted on March 2015).
36. The University of Sydney (2014) GI Foods advanced research. Sydney University's Glycemic Index Research Service (consulted on July 2015).
37. Granados-Silvestre Mde L, Ortiz-López MG, Montúfar-Robles I, Menjívar-Iraheta M (2014) Micronutrients and diabetes, the case of minerals. Cir Cir 82: 119-125.
38. Sharma KD, Bindal G, Rathour R, Rana JC (2012). β-carotene and mineral content of different Chenopodium species and the effect of cooking on micronutrient retention. Int J F Sci Nutr 63: 290-295.
39. Nascimento AC, Mota C, Coelho I, Gueifao S, Santos M, et al. (2014) Characterisation of nutrient profile of quinoa (*Chenopodium quinoa*), amaranth (*Amaranthus caudatus*), and purple corn (Zea mays L.) consumed in the North of Argentina: Proximates, minerals and trace elements. Food Chem 148: 420-426.
40. Lee I (2015) Betaine is a positive regulator of mitochondrial respiration. Biochem Biophys Res Commun 456: 621-625.
41. Lever M, Slow S (2010) The clinical significance of betaine, an osmolyte with a key role in methyl group metabolism. Clin Biochem 43: 732-744.
42. Shabala L, Mackay A, Tian Y, Jacobsen SE, Zhou D, et al. (2012) Oxidative stress protection and stomatal patterning as components of salinity tolerance mechanism in quinoa (*Chenopodium quinoa*). Physiologia Plantarum 146: 26-38.
43. Schartum-Hansen H, Ueland PM, Pedersen ER, Meyer K, Ebbing M, et al. (2013) Assessment of urinary betaine as a marker of diabetes mellitus in cardiovascular patients. PLoS One 8: e69454.
44. Wijekoon EP, Brosnan ME, Brosnan JT (2007) Homocysteine metabolism in diabetes. Biochem Soc Trans 35: 1175-1179.
45. Ross AB, Zangger A, Guiraud SP (2014) Cereal foods are the major source of betaine in the Western diet--analysis of betaine and free choline in cereal foods and updated assessments of betaine intake. Food Chem 145: 859-865.
46. Jakobek L (2015) Interactions of polyphenols with carbohydrates, lipids and proteins. Food Chem 175: 556-567.
47. Repo-Carrasco-Valencia R, Hellstrom JK, Pihlava JM, Mattila PH (2010) Flavonoids and other phenolic compounds in Andean indigenous grains: Quinoa (*Chenopodium quinoa*), kañiwa (*chenopodium pallidicaule*) and kiwicha (*Amaranthus caudatus*). Food Chemistry 120:128-133.
48. Messina M (2014) Soy foods, isoflavones, and health of postmenopausal women. Am J Clin Nutr 1: S423-S430.
49. Müller L, Caris-Veyrat C, Lowe G, Böhm V (2015) Lycopene and Its Antioxidant Role in the Prevention of Cardiovascular Diseases - A Critical Review. Crit Rev Food Sci Nutr .
50. Tang Y, Li X, Chen PX, Zhang B, Hernandez M, et al. (2014) Lipids, Tocopherols, and Carotenoids in Leaves of Amaranth and Quinoa Cultivars and a New Approach to Overall Evaluation of Nutritional Quality Traits. J Agric Food Chem 62: 12610-12619.
51. Zevallos VF, Herencia LI, Chang F, Donnelly S, Ellis HJ, et al. (2014) Gastrointestinal effects of eating quinoa (Chenopodium quinoa Willd.) in celiac patients. Am J Gastroenterol 109: 270-278.
52. Tovoli F, Masi C, Guidetti E, Negrini G, Paterini P, et al. (2015) Clinical and diagnostic aspects of gluten related disorders. World J Clin Cases 3: 275-284.
53. Peñas E, Uberti F, di Lorenzo C, Ballabio C, Brandolini A, et al. (2014) Biochemical and immunochemical evidences supporting the inclusion of quinoa (*Chenopodium quinoa* Willd.) as a gluten-free ingredient. Plant Foods Hum Nutr 69: 297-303.
54. Elekofehinti OO (2015) Saponins: Anti-diabetic principles from medicinal plants - A review. Pathophysiology 22: 95-103.
55. Maradini Filho AM, Ribeiro Pirozi M, Da Silva Borges JT, Pinheiro Sant´Ana HM, Paes Chaves JB, et al. (2015) Quinoa: Nutritional, functional and anti-nutritional aspects. Critical Reviews in Food Science and Nutrition (ahead of print).
56. Gómez-Caravaca AM, Iafelice G, Verardo V, Marconi E, Caboni MF (2014) Influence of pearling process on phenolic and saponin content in quinoa (Chenopodium quinoa Willd). Food Chem 157: 174-178.
57. Gómez-Caravaca AM, Iafelice G, Lavini A, Pulvento C, Caboni MF, et al. (2012) Phenolic compounds and saponins in quinoa samples

(*Chenopodium quinoa* Willd.) grown under different saline and nonsaline irrigation regimens. J Agric Food Chem 60: 4620-4627.

58. Yao Y, Yang X, Shi Z, Ren G (2014b) Anti-Inflammatory Activity of Saponins from Quinoa (Chenopodium quinoa Willd.) Seeds in Lipopolysaccharide-Stimulated RAW 264.7 Macrophages Cells. J Food Sci 79: H1018-H1023.
59. Gupta RK, Gangoliya SS, Singh NK (2015) Reduction of phytic acid and enhancement of bioavailable micronutrients in food grains. J Food Sci Technol 52: 676-684.
60. Astier C, Moneret-Vautrin DA, Puillandre E, Bihain BE (2009) First case report of anaphylaxis to quinoa, a novel food in France. Allergy 64: 819-820.
61. Gawlik-Dziki U, Åšwieca M, SuÅ‚kowski M, Dziki D, Baraniak B, et al. (2013) Antioxidant and anticancer activities of Chenopodium quinoa leaves extracts - in vitro study. Food Chem Toxicol 57: 154-160.
62. Verza SG, Silveira F, Cibulski S, Kaiser S, Ferreira F, et al. (2012) Immunoadjuvant activity, toxicity assays, and determination by UPLC/Q-TOF-MS of triterpenic saponins from Chenopodium quinoa seeds. J Agric Food Chem 60: 3113-3118.
63. Graf BL, Poulev A, Kuhn P, Grace MH, Lila MA, et al. (2014) Quinoa seeds leach phytoecdysteroids and other compounds with anti-diabetic properties. Food Chem 163: 178-185.
64. Foucault AS, Even P, Lafont R, Dioh W, Veillet S, et al. (2014) Quinoa extract Enriched in 20-Hydroxyecdysone affects energy homeostasis and intestinal fat absorption in mice fed a high-fat diet. Physiology and Behavior 128: 226-231.
65. Foucault AS, Mathé V, Lafont R, Even P, Dioh W, et al. (2011) Quinoa extract enriched in 20-hydroxyecdysone protects mice from diet-induced obesity and modulates adipokines expression. Obesity 20: 270-277.
66. Pasko P, Zagrodzki P, Barton H, Chlopicka J, Gorinstein S (2010a) Effect of quinoa seeds (Chenopodium quinoa) in diet on some biochemical parameters and essential elements in blood of high fructose-fed rats. Plant Foods Hum Nutr 65: 333-338.
67. Pasko P, Barton H, Zagrodzki P, Izewska A, Krosniak M, et al. (2010) Effect of diet supplemented with quinoa seeds on oxidative status in plasma and selected tissues of high fructose-fed rats. Plant Foods Hum Nutr 65: 146-151.
68. De Carvalho FG, Ovidio PP, Padovan GJ, Jordao Junior AA, Marchini JS, et al. (2014) Metabolic parameters of postmenopausal women after quinoa or corn flakes intake- a prospective and doublé-blind study. Int J Food Sci Nutr 65: 380-385.
69. McRae MP (2013) Betaine supplementation decreases plasma homocysteine in healthy adult participants: a meta-analysis. J Chiropr Med 12: 20-25.
70. Ross AB, Bruce SJ, Blondel-Lubrano A, Oguey-Araymon S, Beaumont M, et al. (2011) A whole-grain cereal-rich diet increases plasma betaine, and tends to decrease total and LDL-cholesterol compared with refined-grain diet in healthy subjects. British Journal of Nutrition 105: 1-12.
71. Jenkins DJ, Kendall CW, McKeown-Eyssen G, Josse RG, Silverberg J, et al. (2008) Effect of a low-glycemic index or a high-cereal fiber diet on type 2 diabetes: a randomized trial. JAMA 300: 2742-2753.
72. Carciochi RA, Manrique GD, Dimitrov K (2015) Optimization of antioxidant phenolic compounds extraction from quinoa (Chenopodium quinoa) seeds. J Food Sci Technol 52: 4396-4404.
73. Wu G, Morris CF, Murphy KM (2014) Evaluation of texture differences among varieties of cooked quinoa. J Food Sci 79: S2337-2345.
74. Bianchi F, Rossi EA, Gomes RG, Sivieri K (2015) Potentially synbiotic fermented beverage with aqueous extracts of quinoa (Chenopodium quinoa Willd) and soy. Food Sci Technol Int 21: 403-415.
75. Medina WT, de la Llera AA, Condori JL, Aguilera JM (2011) Physical properties and microstructural changes during soaking of individual corn and quinoa breakfast flakes. J Food Sci 76: E254-265.
76. Schumacher AB, Brandelli A, Macedo FC, Pieta L, Klug TV, et al. (2010) Chemical and sensory evaluation of dark chocolate with addition of quinoa (*Chenopodium quinoa* Willd.). J Food Sci Technol 47: 202-206.
77. Schoenlechner R, Drausinger J, Ottenschlaeger V, Jurackova K, Berghofer E (2010) Functional properties of gluten-free pasta produced from amaranth, quinoa and buckwheat. Plant Foods Hum Nutr 65: 339-349.
78. Del Castillo V, Lescano G, Armada M (2009) Foods formulation for people with celiac disease based on quinoa (*Chenopoduim quinoa*), cereal flours and starches mixtures. Arch Latinoam Nutr 59: 332-336.
79. Abugoch L, Castro E, Tapia C, Añón MC, Gajardo P, et al. (2009) Stability of quinoa flour proteins (*Chenoppodium quinoa* Willd.) during storage. Int J Food Sci Techno 44: 2010-2013.
80. Ruales J, de Grijalva Y, Lopez-Jaramillo P, Nair BM (2002) The nutritional quality of an infant food from quinoa and its effect on the plasma level of insulin-like growth factor-1 (IGF-1) in undernourished children. Int J Food Sci Nutr 53: 143-154.

Thermal Stability of β-Amylase Activity and Sugar Profile of Sweet-Potato Varieties during Processing

Mensah EO[1,2*], **Ibok O**[1], **Ellis WO**[1] **and Carey EE**[2]

[1]*Food Science and Technology Department, College of Science, Kwame Nkrumah University of Science and Technology, Kumasi, Ghana*

[2]*International Potato Centre (CIP), c/o CSIR-CRI, P.O. Box 3785, Kumasi, Ghana*

[*]**Corresponding author:** Mensah EO, Food Science and Technology Department, College of Science, Kwame Nkrumah University of Science and Technology, Kumasi, Ghana, E-mail: e.owusu@cgiar.org, kyofresh@gmail.com

Abstract

Sweet-potato root is a good source of β-amylase for food applications. β-amylase catalyses the conversion of soluble starch to sugars thus increasing the free sugar composition and sweetness of processed sweet-potato products. This study was undertaken to determine effects of temperature, time and their interactions on thermal stability of β-amylase and sugar profile of sweet-potato roots. Moreover, percentage variability of temperature, time, genotype and interactions on β-amylase was assessed. Temperature, genotype, time, and genotype x temperature interaction accounted for 50%, 26%, 11% and 8% of the variation respectively. Increasing temperature and heating time generally reduced β-amylase activity and enhanced maltose formation. Heating sweet-potato roots up to 75°C reserve relatively higher percentage of the endogenous amylases required for starch conversion and free sugar formation in the tempered product. The relatively high β-amylolytic potential of Santom Pona makes it a good raw material for the brewery and sugar syrup industry.

Keywords: β-amylase; Temperature; Genotype; Sweet-potato roots; Thermal stability

Introduction

Amylases are of fundamental importance to processing and eating qualities of sweet-potato roots [1,2]. Literature is replete with information on the presence and role of amylases in sweet-potato roots [1,3,4]. There are three major types of amylases in sweet-potato root; α-amylase, β-amylase and starch phosphorylase. However β-amylase is the most abundant [5,6] and important during processing [7]. Sweet-potato flour with high β-amylolytic activity has been successfully used to increase wort extract of sorghum beer [8]. Utilisation of native amylases in intact roots involves heating the roots to gelatinise the starch fraction, and activate the amylases for starch degradation to maltose and limit dextrins [4,9,10]. Rapid heating of sweet-potato mashes to 70°C may be optimal for starch conversion and subsequent ethanol production [6]. Effect of temperature on β-amylase activity of six sweet-potato lines of varying maltose content has been investigated and reported [6]. However the percentage variability of the temperature, time and more especially interactions with β-amylase activity were not fully investigated. This current study therefore sought to examine the impact of time of heating, concentrations of key sugars including sucrose, the predominant sugar in raw roots, and interactions during processing of four different sweet-potato varieties. The presence and synergistic effect of α-amylase, at relatively higher temperature, in sugar formation was also investigated. Such information would be useful in controlling free sugar composition during processing of sweet-potato roots.

Methodology

Experimental design

A factorial design with three replications was used for all the experimental runs. The main factors were genotype, temperature, and heating time. Variables measured included β-amylase activity, α-amylase activity and sugars (sucrose, maltose, glucose and fructose). The experimental levels were 4, 3 and 4 for the genotype, temperature and time respectively.

Materials

Four sweet-potato varieties *viz.*, Ligri, Santom Pona, Hi-Starch and Apomuden with varying dry matter content, and yield (Table 1) were supplied by the Council for Scientific and Industry Research (CSIR)-Crops Research Institute (CRI), Fumesua, Ghana. They were planted at the experimental field of CRI in Ohawu, Volta region of Ghana. The site falls within the coastal savannah agro-ecological zone. The roots were harvested at four months and stored under room conditions (25-27°C) for a week prior to analysis.

Sweetpotato variety	Dry matter content (%)	Yield (t/ha)
Apomuden	21.9	30
Santom Pona	34.4	17
Ligri	34	18.4
Hi-Starch	40	18

Table 1: Dry matter content, and yield of the four sweet-potato varieties.

Methods

Four medium-sized intact roots of each variety were washed, rinsed and air-dried (25-27°C). The roots were then quartered, rinsed in deionised water and dried with paper towel. Each quarter was sliced along its longitudinal axis into 1.0 cm thickness and composite samples within each variety divided into 13 sub-samples of 50 g each. One sub-sample was denoted as raw. The rest were tightly wrapped with aluminum foil and separated into four groups. Each group from the varieties were placed in a force-air temperature controlled oven (Genlab MINI/50/DKG) and heated at 65°C, 75°C and 85°C for 0, 10, 20 and 40 min. Termination of heating process was aided by submerging the heated sweet-potato root samples into ice bath for 20 min. The samples were peeled and frozen at -25°C to -28°C and freeze dried (YK-118/50, Taiwan) for 72 h. The dried samples were milled using Thomas Scientific laboratory Miller (model 3383 L70) and sieve through 40 mesh receiver (Thomas scientific, cat no. 3383N20).

Amylase extraction and determination

Extraction of amylases: To 0.5 g of freeze-dried and milled sweet-potato root sample was added 5 mL of 1 M Tris/HCL buffer (pH 8.0) containing disodium EDTA (20 mM) and cysteine HCL (100 mM). Amylase was extracted for a maximum of 1 h with intermittent vortexing at room temperature. The extracts were obtained by centrifuging the mixture in a bench centrifuge (800 D, China) at 4,000 r/min for 10 min. The supernatant was decanted into another labelled centrifuge tube. Approximately 0.1 mL of the supernatant was added to 2.0 mL dilution buffer (MES buffer, pH 6.2) and was used for total β-amylase assay. For α-amylase, 1.5 mL of sodium malate (1 M, pH 5.4) together with sodium chloride (1M), calcium chloride (40 mM) and sodium azide (0.1%) was added [11,12].

Amylase assay: Amylase extracts (0.1 mL) of each sample was dispensed to 15mL polypropylene tubes and pre-incubated for 5 min at 50°C and 60°C for β and α-amylase respectively together with the substrates; p-Nitrophenyl β-Maltotrioside (PNP β-G3) - for β - amylase and Block p-nitrophenyl Maltoheptaoside (BPNPG7) - for α-amylase. To each tube containing the amylase extracts, 0.1 mL of the substrate solution was added, stirred and incubated at 50°C and 60°C for exactly 10 min from time of addition. 1.5 mL of stopping reagents (1% Trizma base.) of pH 11.0 was added and stirred. The absorbance of the reaction mixtures and the reagent blanks were read at 400 nm. One unit of activity was defined as the amount of enzyme required, in the presence of excess β-glucosidase (for β-amylase) and α-glucosidase (for α-amylase), to release one micromole of p-nitrophenol from PNPβ-G3 or BPNPG7 in one minute under the defined assay conditions and termed a Betamyl-3 and Ceralpha Unit correspondingly. Betamyl-3 unit was converted to International unit (U/g) using a factor of 193.9. Ceralpha unit was also expressed as International unit (U/g) on starch substrate with a factor of 4.1 [11,12].

Sugars determination

Freeze-dried and milled sweet-potato samples were sent to the Quality Plant Product Laboratory (Department of Crop Science, University of Gottingen, Germany) for sugars analysis using High Performance Liquid Chromatography (HPLC). Water extract of the freeze-dried samples (0.1 g in 100 mL) was incubated in a water bath at 60°C for 1 h and treated with 0.2 mL Carrez I and Carrez II solution to remove proteins. The mixture was purified by centrifugation (Sorvall RC-5B Refrigated Superspeed, GMI, Ramsay, USA) for 10 min at 10000 rpm. Sugars were determined from the membrane-filtered supernatant (pores size 0.45 μm). Glucose, fructose, sucrose, and maltose were separated using a LiChrospher 100 NH_2 (5 μm) 4 × 4 mm pre-column in combination with a LiChrospher 100 NH2 (5 μm) 4 × 250 mm separation column (Merck KGaA, Darmstadt, Germany) and an acetonitrile: pure water solution (80:20 v/v) as mobile phase at a flow rate of 1.0 mL min^{-1} at 20°C and an injection volume of 20 μL. Sugars were detected with a Knauer differential refractometer 198.00 (Knauer, Berlin, Germany).

Results and Discussion

Variability of temperature, time and interactions on β-amylase activity of sweet-potatoes

The percentage variability due to temperature, time, genotype and their interactions on β-amylase activity during processing of sweet-potatoes is presented in Table 2. Temperature and genotype accounted for the largest proportion of the experimental variance of 50.37% and 25.94% respectively. Heating time contributed 11.25% while genotype by temperature interaction accounted for 7.95%. Temperature by time interaction and genotype by time interaction account for 2.49% and 1.44% respectively. The combined interaction effect of all the factors was also significant and explained 0.56% of the variance observed.

Source of Variation	+Variance (%)	F Value
Temperature (Temp)	50.37**	40775.6
Genotype (GT)	25.94**	20996.9
Time	11.25**	9103.84
GT*Temp	7.95**	6433.85
Temp*Time	2.49**	2021.17
GT*Time	1.44**	1167.02
GT*Temp*Time	0.56**	452.29

Table 2: Source of variation and percentage variance of genotype, temperature and time on β-amylase activity of sweet-potato root [**Significant at $p<0.05$; +Calculated from sum of squares].

These current findings correspond well with earlier reports that temperature has profound effect of β-amylase activity during processing [6]. It decreased the activity of beta amylase when six sweet-potato lines of varying maltose content were heated [4,6]. However, the percentage contributions from each of the factors (temperature, genotype and time) and their interaction have not been evaluated prior to this current work. The results of this study imply that thermal stability of β-amylase in sweet-potato roots is also significantly determined by the interaction between variety and the processing conditions including temperature and time.

Thermal stability rate of β-amylase activity in four sweet-potato varieties

Rates of thermal stability of β-amylase activity in four sweet-potato varieties profiled in the current study are presented in Figure 1 (A, B and C). Temperature-time combined treatment generally had a negative effect on β-amylase activities in all the varieties. Activity generally decreased when temperature and heating time were increased. The effect was more profound at 75°C and 85°C for longer holding times (40 min), where all the varieties lost nearly all of their β-amylase activity. β-amylase activities were relatively stable at 65°C throughout the holding times. Wide variation was however observed among the varieties at the onset of the heating regime at 65°C.

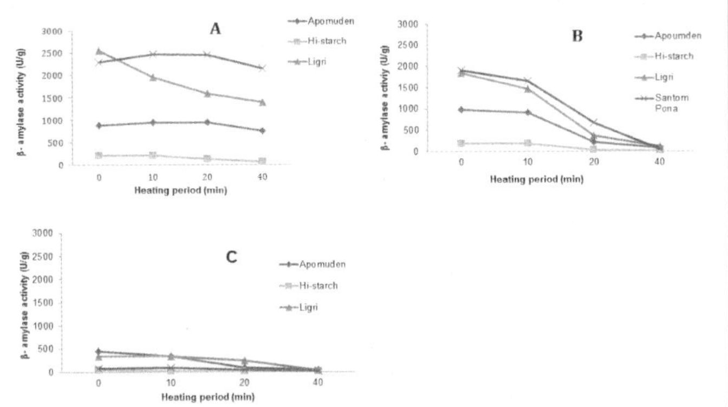

Figure 1: Changes in β-amylase activity during temperature-time heating regimes of four sweetpotato varieties: Santom Pona; Ligri; Apomuden; Hi-Starch. A - 65°C; B - 75°C; and C - 85°C. LSD=22.07.

Santom Pona and Ligri varieties had the highest amylase activity whilst Apomuden and Hi-Starch showed the moderate and the lowest activities respectively. The differences were maintained throughout the heating times except Ligri, which drop from first to second rank after 40 min of heating. The high amylase potential and retention rate of Santom Pona make it a good alternative source of amylase for food applications, which employ relatively mild processing temperature. At 75°C, beta amylase activity decreased steadily with time in all the varieties. Hi-Starch completely lost its activity whilst Apomuden, Ligri and Santom Pona retained 30% to 50% of its activity after 20 min of heating. All the varieties lost most of their activity after 40 min of heating. Beta-amylase activities were greatly reduced (less than 500 U/g) at the beginning of heating at 85°C. Only Apomuden and Ligri retained some activity and maintained the activity for 10 min and 20 min respectively. Activities in Santom Pona and Hi-Starch varieties were not detected even at the beginning of the 85°C treatment. From the study, Ligri and Apomuden retained some activity even at 85°C and can hence withstand high temperatures during mashing and liquefaction processes. It should be noted that gelatinization, a rate determining step in starch conversion, occurs at temperatures ≥ 60°C 18,21, hence raw materials selected for brewing and syrup production should have the ability to retain high amyase activity during heating.

Variability of temperature, genotype and interactions on sugar profile of sweet-potato roots

Influence of temperature, genotype and their interaction on sugar profile (sucrose, maltose, glucose and fructose) of sweet-potato roots during heating is showed in Table 3. Genotypic influence was the most intense and accounted for 99.71%, 99.01 and 97.84% of the variance observed in glucose, fructose and sucrose content respectively. The lowest effect was recorded in maltose (54.89%). Conversely, effect of temperature was highest in maltose (31.56%) formation. The rest of the sugars had less than 1.50% of the variance resulting from temperature. Moreover, the interaction effect was highest for maltose content (13.56%) and least for fructose (0.27%). Sucrose and fructose recorded 1.08% and 0.83% respectively.

	+Variance (%)			
Source of variation	**Sucrose**	**Maltose**	**Glucose**	**Fructose**
Genotype	97.84**	54.89**	99.71**	99.01**
Temperature	1.09**	31.56**	0.22**	0.91**
Genotype x Temperature	1.08**	13.56**	0.83**	0.27**

Table 3: Source of variation and percentage variance of sugars during heating of sweet-potato roots. [+Percentage variance was calculated from sum of squares; **Significant at p=0.0001]

The results indicate that except for maltose content, sugars in sweet-potatoes are greatly determined by the genomic makeup of the variety and do not substantially response to temperature during heating. Hence, the final concentration of these sugars (sucrose, glucose and fructose) is at least 97% proportional to the initial concentrations during processing of sweet-potato roots. Variation in endogenous sugars (sucrose, glucose and fructose) have been reported to be minimal after cooking [13-16] though their concentrations during heating have not been widely investigated prior to this studies. Fructose, glucose and sucrose levels in Jewel sweet-potato cultivar were not affected by baking temperature 20. Variation in maltose content, however, has been extensively investigated [9,13,14,16]. Reasons has been largely assigned to the increased in temperature, which activates the hydrolytic ability of native amylases found in the root resulting in increased of maltose content in the final product [4,15].

Effect of temperature on sugar profile of four sweet-potato varieties

Variation in sugar profile of the four sweet-potato varieties during heating is presented in Figures 2 and 3.

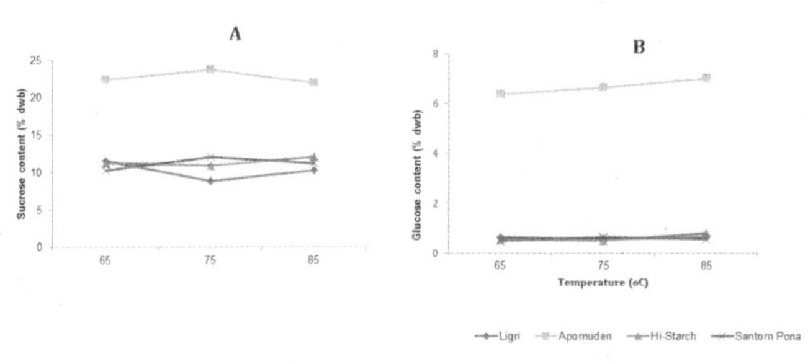

Figure 2: Changes in sucrose (A) and glucose (B) contents during heating of four sweet-potato varieties. LSD=0.07.

Sucrose, glucose and fructose concentrations in all the varieties were relatively stable throughout the heating period. Interaction effect was also minimal except at 75°C for sucrose contents. In all, Apomuden variety recorded the highest content of sucrose, fructose and glucose contents at 65°C and maintained the levels during the heating process. Effect of temperature was highly remarkable on maltose content, an observation confirming early conclusion that maltose content is greatly dependent of temperature (Table 3). Maltose, which was barely absent in all the varieties prior to heating, increased to 6.76% in Apomuden for instance at 75°C.

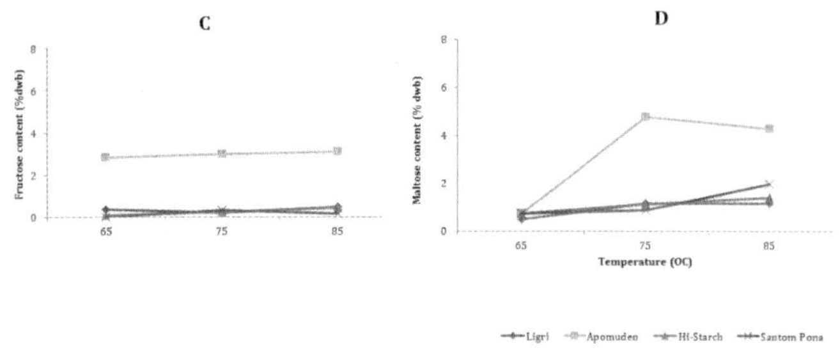

Figure 3: Changes in fructose (C) and maltose (D) contents during heating of four sweet-potato varieties. LSD=0.07.

Maltose content in Santom Pona began to increase substantially after 75°C. The presence and stability of beta amylase activity detected initially accounted for the variation in maltose content. Nevertheless, it should be noted that the optimum temperature of β-amylase falls below 75°C; hence the difference in maltose content at higher temperatures may be due to the activity of α-amylase [6,17]. Alpha amylase, which is relatively heat stable with optimum temperature of 71°C, rapidly degrades starch to lower molecular weight dextrins which are simultaneously hydrolysed into maltose by β-amylase [5,18].

Thermal stability of α-amylase activity was therefore assessed in order to ascertain its presence and synergistic contribution to β-amylase in sugar formation. The results revealed that the sweet-potato varieties also contained α-amylase (Figure 4).

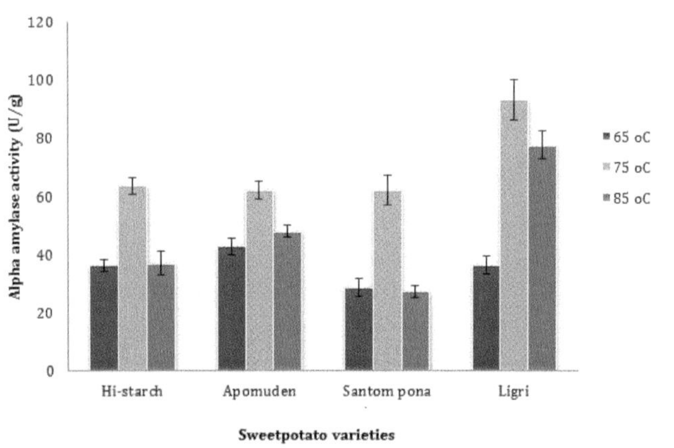

Figure 4: Alpha amylase activity of four sweet-potato varieties during heating at 65°C, 75°C and 85°C. Error bars represent standard deviations. LSD=2.31.

Alpha-amylase activity increased from 65°C to 75°C and declined at 85°C in all the varieties. Apomuden and Hi-Starch had the highest activity at 65°C while Santom Pona had the lowest. The activities were however not significantly different among the varieties at 75°C except Ligri. Ligri exhibited the highest activity of 90 U/g at 75°C, and also retained 75% of the activity at 85°C. Alpha-amylase had a higher optimum temperature (75°C) than β-amylase (65°C) demonstrating its ability to break down starch molecules at relatively higher temperature during processing. Variation in maltose content in this study hence resulted from the hydrolytic activity both α- and β-amylases.

Conclusion

The outcome of the study establishes that stability and hydrolytic power of β-amylase in sweet-potato roots is significantly influenced by the genetic composition of the variety, temperature, period of heating and the interaction between the amylase and processing conditions. Except maltose, final concentration of sugars was virtually directly proportional to the initial levels. Sucrose remained the major sugar after heating up to 85°C, though maltose content increased drastically. The sweet-potato varieties contained substantial amount of α-amylase and it presence may have enhanced the conversion of starch into maltose at higher temperatures.

Acknowledgement

The authors wish to acknowledge Mr Eric Owusu Danquah and Mr Kwadwo Adofo of Crops Research Institute (CRI), Fumesua, and Eric Kuna Dery of International Potato Centre for their diverse contributions toward the completion of the study.

References

1. Dziedoave NT, Graffham AJ, Westby A, Otoo J, Komlaga G (2010) Influence of variety and growth environment on β-amylase activity of flour from sweet potato (*Ipomoea batatas*). Food Control. 21: 162-165.
2. Kays SJ, Wang Y, McLaurin JW (2005) Chemical and Geographical assessment of the sweetness of the cultivated sweet-potato clones of the world. J Amer Soc Hort Sci 130: 591-591.
3. Nabubuya A, Namutebi A, Byaruhanga Y, Narvhu J, Stenstrom Y et al. (2012) Amylolytic activity in selected sweet-potato (*Ipomoea batatas* Lam) varieties during development and in storage. Food Nutr Sci 3: 660-668.
4. Hagenimana V, Vezina LP, Simard RE (1994) Sweet-potato α and β-amylases: Characterisation and kinetic studies with endogenous inhibitor. J Food Sci 59: 373-377.
5. Hagenimana V, Simard RE (1994) Amylolytic activity in germinating sweet-potato (*Ipomoea batatas* L.) roots. J Amer Soc Hort Sci 119: 313-320.
6. Takahata Y, Noda T, Naga ta T (1994) Effect of β-amylase stability and starch gelatinization during heating on varietal differences in maltose content in sweet-potatoes. J Agric Food Chem 42: 2564-2569.
7. Morrison TA, Pressey R, Kays SJ (1993) Changes in α and β-amylase during storage of sweet-potato lines with varying starch hydrolysis. J Amer Soc Hort Sci 118: 236-242.
8. Etim MU, EtokAkpan OU (1992) Sorghum brewing using sweet potato enzymatic flour to increase saccharification. World J Microbiol Biotechnol 8: 509-511.
9. Sawai J, Nakai T, Shimizu M (2009) Reducing sugar production in sweet potatoes heated by electromagnetic radiation. Food Sci Tech Int 15: 89-95.
10. Sawai J, Nakai T, Hashimoto A, Shimizu M (2004) A comparison of the hydrolysis of sweet-potato starch with β-amylase and infrared allows prediction of reducing sugar production. Inter J Food Sci Tech 39: 967-974.
11. Alpha-amylase assay procedure (Ceralpha method) for the measurement of plant and microbial alpha-amylase. Megazyme International Ireland.
12. Beta-amylase assay procedure (Betamyl-3 method) for the measurement of cereal grains, malt, food, beverages and fermentation products beta-amylase. Megazyme International Ireland.

13. Lewthwaite SL, Sutton KH, Triggs CM (1997) Free sugar composition of sweet-potato cultivars after storage. New Zealand J Crop and Hort Sci 25: 33-41.

14. Babu L (1994) Changes in carbohydrate fractions of sweet potato tubers on processing. Tropical agriculture 7: 71-73.

15. Picha DH (1985) HPLC determination of sugars in raw and baked sweet potatoes. J Food Sci 50: 1189-1190.

16. Sun JB, Severson RF, Kays SJ (1993) Effect of heating temperature and microwave pretreatment on the formation of sugars and volatile in jewel sweet-potato. J Food quality 17: 447-456.

17. Ikemiya M, Deobald HJ (1966) New characteristic alpha-amylase in sweet potatoes. J Agric Food Sci 14: 237-341.

18. Truong VD, Avula RY (2010) Sweet potato: Post harvest aspects in food. In: Ray RC, Tomlins KI (eds). Nova Science publishers. Inc., New York, pp: 117-161.

6

Anti-obesity effects of Lipid Extract from Sea-reared of Rainbow Trout (*Oncorhynchus mykiss*) Fed with Sea Squirt (*Halocynthia roretzi*) Tunic's Carotenoids and CLA

Rohmah Z[1], **Fitria L**[1], **Kang SJ**[2], **Kim JS**[2], **Lee JJ**[3], **Ha YL**[4] **and Choi BD**[2*]

[1]*Faculty of Biology, Universitas Gadjah Mada, Yogyakarta 55281, Indonesia*

[2]*Department of Seafood and Aquaculture Science, The Institute of Marine Industry, Gyeongsang National University, Tongyeong 53064, Korea*

[3]*Department of Food and Nutrition, Chosun University, Gwangju 61452, Korea*

[4]*Antiaging Institute, HK Biotech Co. Ltd., Jinju 52840, Korea*

[*]**Corresponding authors:** Choi BD, Department of Seafood and Aquaculture Science, Gyeongsang National University, Tongyeong 53064, Korea
E-mail: bdchoi@gnu.ac.kr ; Lee JJ, Department of Food and Nutrition, Chosun University, Gwangu 61452, Korea
E-mail: leejj80@chosun.ac.kr

Abstract

Purpose: In order to produce new functional seafood, rainbow trout were acclimation in seawater and fed with inclusion of CLA and carotenoid extract from sea squirt tunic. Lipid extract from the sea-reared rainbow trout muscle (RME) and viscera (RVE) were administered to rats simultaneously with normal or high fat diet for six weeks. We evaluated the effects of the dietary supplementation with CLA, carotenoids, and n-3 HUFA by the beneficial effects of anti-obesity activities.

Materials and method: Sea-reared rainbow trout (800 ± 20.5 g; 40.0 ± 1.7 cm) were fed with basal feed which supplemented with 10 mg/kg sea squirt tunic's carotenoids and 3% CLA (w/w) for three months. Lipid was extracted from rainbow trout muscle and viscera using chloroform/methanol (2/1). Forty eight male Sprague Dawley rats (400 ± 2.0 g) were randomly divided into six groups (n=8). Two types of diets, normal types (SN, RVN, RMN) and 45% of high fat research diets (SHF, RVHF, RMHF) were used. The excised liver and epididymal adipose tissues were fixed in 3% formaldehyde solution, embedded in paraffin. Organs sections were stained with hematoxylin-esosin. Histological examination on liver and adipose tissues sections were carried out with a light microscope.

Results: Sea farming and inclusion of CLA and carotenoids pigment extracted from the tunic of sea squirt, the content of C18:1n-9 was reduced to 32.5% in the muscle's lipid and 35.8% in the viscera's lipid. Serum lipid and liver enzymes activity in blood serum showed that RME and RVE have the liver protective ability.

Conclusion: RME and RVE have potency as weight reducer through fat burner routes as well as liver protective ability. Hence, it could be considered as anti-obesity supplement for the long period of administration.

Keywords: CLA; Carotenoids; Anti-obesity; Sea-reared rainbow trout; High fat diets

Introduction

Rainbow trout (*Oncorhynchus mykiss*, Walbaum 1792) is red muscle fish and known to accumulate carotenoids, especially astaxanthin, in its muscle. The degree of redness will determine the price of it. They are not synthesized in the animal's body, but are ingested from food. While wild rainbow trout naturally take in carotenoids from food, farmed rainbow trout should be supplemented with this substance from feed. The pigment inclusion into feed will increases the costs of the rainbow trout farming industry [1,2]. Sea squirts' tunic, a byproduct of seafood industry in Korea [3], contains many high value substances which one of those is carotenoids. It has 13 types of carotenoids isomers which 6 most abundance of those were alloxanthin, halocynthiaxanthin, diatoxanthin, diadinochrome, mytiloxanthinone, and astaxanthin, as well as minor concentration of lutein, mytiloxanthin, and β-carotene [4]. The sea squirt's tunic is a promising alternative of carotenoid for fish culture [5].

Conjugated linoleic acid (CLA) is one of the geometrical and position isomers of linoleic acid. It has been discovered that this compound naturally exists in diverse foods, such as dairy products or poultry. CLA has powerful anti-adiposity and decrease body fat deposition and changes the route of fat metabolism [6-8]. Body fat is a substance that causes an insulin resistance syndrome, similar to what is observed in type 2 diabetes [9]. Therefore, the effect of CLA intake was shown to reduce body fat while increasing the amount of muscle in mammals. According experiment on mouse models, feeding CLA with fish oil not only increased insulin sensitivity, but it also led to the accumulation of bone marrow fat, caused an inflammatory reaction, and reduced the oxidative stress associated with aging [6].

CLA was also reported to have chemo-protective effects in several tissues during multiple stages of carcinogenesis [10] as well as immune enhancing qualities [6] and possible anti-atherogenic properties [11]. Most of these experiments were used free CLA directly from plant. On the other hand, in this experiment we used CLA that have been incorporated into the muscle or viscera of sea-reared rainbow trout.

This study aimed to develop functional seafood, by combining the beneficial effects of anti-obesity activities of CLA, carotenoids, and n-3 HUFA from the sea-reared rainbow trout's lipid. The rainbow trout was fed with inclusion of sea squirt tunic's carotenoid and CLA, and then the fish oil extracted from sea-reared rainbow trout supplemented to male Sprague Dawley rats. The nutritional aspects were compared with normal and high fat diet group. The bioactivities of accumulated CLA and sea squirt tunic's carotenoid on rainbow trout's expectedly would be conveyed into secondary consumer. Therefore, our goal on tailoring value added fish would be achieved.

Materials and Method

Materials

The refined, bleached, deodorized CLA-rich soybean oil was provided by HK Biotech (Jinju, Korea). CLA FAME authentic standards (Sigma-Aldrich Inc., St. Louis, MO, USA) and FAME of menhaden oil standard (Sigma-Aldrich Inc., St. Louis, MO, USA) were used as comparison. All lipid extraction solvents and chemicals for analysis were analytical grade.

Animals, diets and experimental design

All procedures and experiments with animals in this study were done under animal ethics, supervised and approved by Chosun University Animal Care and Use Committee (CIACU2015-A0045). Forty eight male Sprague Dawley rats (400 ± 2.0 g) were obtained from Jungang Experimental Animal Co. Ltd. (Seoul, Korea). Animals' treatments were carried out at Animal Research Center Chosun University. Rats were randomly divided into 6 groups (n=8). Acclimation were done for 1 week prior of the feeding treatments. Two types of diets, normal type and 45% of high fat research diets were used in this experiment. These were supplemented with three different lipid extracts (soybean oil, rainbow trout viscera's lipid extract (RVE), and muscle lipid extract (RME)) which given orally. Experiment was carried out with randomized block design (Table 1) and done for 6 weeks. The doses of lipid extracts were calculated based on CLA daily dose for human diet (3.0 g/60 kg per day). Water and feed were given ad libitum. The rats' chambers were kept at constant temperature (18 ± 2°C) and 12 h photoperiods (08:00-20:00). The initial and final body weights of all rats were measured. Weight gain (g/day) was calculated by dividing final weight minus initial weight with days of treatment.

Rainbow trout lipid extraction and fatty acids analysis

Sea-reared rainbow trout (800 ± 20.5 g; 40.0 ± 1.7 cm) were fed with basal feed which supplemented with 10 mg/kg sea squirt tunic's carotenoids and 3% CLA (w/w) for 3 months. Lipid was extracted from rainbow trout muscle and viscera using chloroform/methanol (2/1) and total lipid was measured gravimetrically [12]. Fatty acids methyl ester (FAME) analysis was done with method as reported [13]. CLA FAME was analysis by method which briefly as follow: fifty milligrams of lipid extract was added with 1.5 mL 1.0 N NaOH. The mixture was heated at 100°C for 10 min and cooled to room temperature afterward [14]. Three milliliters of 1.0 N H_2SO_4 was added to solution and incubated at 55°C for 20 min. FAME was partitioned to isooctane by adding 1 mL of it to the mixture. The Isooctane fractions were analyzed with gas chromatography (Clarus 600, Perkin Elmer Co. Ltd., Waltham, MA, USA) and Omegawax-320 column (30 m × 0.32 mm ID) from Supelco Co. (Bellefonte, PA, USA). Injector and flame-ionization was set at 250°C. The carrier gas was helium with column-inlet pressure set at constant value, 1.0 kg/cm^2 and split ratio was 1:100. Oven temperature was set at 180°C for initial time 8 min to 230°C with increasing rate 3°C/min, the final temperature was kept for 15 min. FAME authentic standards of menhaden oil and CLA (Sigma-Aldrich Inc., St. Louis, MO, USA) were used as comparison.

Feed Supplement	Feed	
	Normal	High fat diet
Soybean oil	SN	SHF
Rainbow trout viscera lipid extract (RVE)	RVN	RVHF
Rainbow trout muscle lipid extract (RME)	RMN	RMHF

Fatty acids	RME (%)	RVE (%)
16:0	17.8 ± 0.5^a	17.4 ± 0.2^a
18:0	6.1 ± 0.3^a	5.6 ± 0.0^a
18:1n-9	32.5 ± 0.1^a	35.8 ± 0.3^b
18:2n-6	12.4 ± 0.5^a	13.3 ± 0.3^b
20:5n-3	1.5 ± 0.3^a	1.5 ± 0.3^a
22:6n-3	5.7 ± 0.3^a	6.5 ± 0.3^b
CLA[1]	9.1 ± 0.4^a	12.5 ± 0.2^b
- c9, t11	8.2 ± 0.1^a	9.1 ± 0.2^b
- t10, c12	0.5 ± 0.0^a	2.1 ± 0.0^b
- t8, t10	0.4 ± 0.0^a	1.3 ± 0.0^b
Σsaturates	27.1 ± 0.2^a	25.7 ± 0.3^b
Σmonoenes	42.0 ± 3.0^a	35.6 ± 0.3^b
Σpolyenes	30.9 ± 0.1^a	38.7 ± 0.2^b

Table 1: Experimental design of rat feeding regiment and fatty acids composition (%) of RME and RVE [Data are represented as mean ±SE (n=3). Means at same row that followed with different letters are significantly different at the 5% level of significance. [1]CLA: Conjugated linoleic acid and isomers].

Measurement of TG and TC concentrations in liver and adipose tissues

Lipid from liver, epididymal and mesenteric adipose tissues were extracted according to Folch's method [12]. After gravimetric analysis of the lipid extract, it was then divided into subsamples of 500 μL each. TG and TC contents of liver and adipose tissues were then measured [15, 16].

Determination of lipoprotein lipase (LPL) activity

Determination of LPL activity was done according to lipoprotein lipase method [17]. Briefly, 50 mg frozen epididymal and mesenteric adipose tissues were minced. These were then defrosted in 0.4 mL of Medium 199 (Gibco BRL, Carlsbad, CA, USA) containing 1% bovine serum albumin and 50 U/mL of heparin. The solutions were incubated in shaking incubator at 24°C for 45 min. LPL activity in the present of heparin was measured using the glycerol stabilized ^{3}H-triolein emulsion as substrate. One unit of LPL activity was defined as the release of 1 μmol of free fatty acid in 1 h.

Histologic procedure for hepatic tissue lipid accumulation assessment and measurement of adipocyte size

The excised liver and epididymal adipose tissues were fixed in 3% formaldehyde solution, embedded in paraffin. Organs sections were stained with hematoxylin-esosin. Histological examination on liver and adipose tissues sections were carried out with a light microscope (×100 magnifications). The diameters of adipocytes were measured in 10 randomly chosen adipocytes from 10 slides of organs of each independent animals using Olympus microscope system (www.olympus.co.kr) equipped with micrometer. Oil red O staining was used as special staining for hepatic lipid deposition. The fresh frozen liver was sections at 6 μm thick and mounted on slides. The fixation was done with 10% formalin. The slides were then wash with distilled water and let air dry. Absolute propylene glycol was use as dehydration agent. Slides were stained with pre-warmed Oil Red O solution (Sigma-Aldrich Inc.) for 8-10 minutes in 60°C oven. Differentiation was carried out in 85% propylene glycol solution for 2-5 minutes and rinsed with distilled water. Mayer's hematoxylin was used as counterstain. This were quantify by counting the number of lipid droplets (diameter>1 μm) in 5 randomly chosen microscopic area (100 μm^2) of liver of each independent animals.

Statistical analysis

The statistical analyses were carried out using Statistical Package for Social Science (SPSS Inc., Chicago, Il, USA, version 12.0) for in vivo assays and Minitab® 17.1.0 (Pennsylvania, USA). Each set of data was analyzed with one-way analysis of variance (ANOVA), Tukey's range test was performed as post-hoc test. The difference of the means was considered significant when p-value was less than 0.05.

Results and Discussion

Fatty acids composition of rainbow trout muscle extract (RME) and viscera extract (RVE)

The fatty acid composition of RME and RVE is described in Table 1. Although there were no significant differences in the fatty acid compositions of RME and RVE, the content of monoenoic and saturated fatty acid of the second was lower than the previous one. However, the content of polyenoic of RVE was higher than RME ($p<0.05$). The highest content of C18:1n-9 (oleic acid) and accumulated CLA was found in RVE. Oleic acid is often reported to be the most abundant MUFA in feed and shall be reflected on the fish fatty acid content. The abundance of oleic acid in feed was indirect result of replacement of fish oil with plant oil [18]. To date, researches indicate that up to 80-90% of fish oil can be replaced by vegetable oils and other fat resources in rainbow trout diets without affecting its growth. However, the n-3 PUFA of fish fillet can be affected by this feed alteration. Hence the fillet quality is importance for consumers can be altered and manipulated [19].

In this experiment, as a result of sea farming and inclusion of CLA and carotenoid pigment extracted from the tunic of sea squirt, the content of C18:1n-9 was reduced to 32.5% in the RME and 35.8% in the RVE. At the same time the content of C22: 6n-3 was increased to 5.7% and 6.5%, for RME and RVE respectively. This suggested that carotenoid extract of sea squirt tunic and dietary CLA would increase the quality of sea-reared rainbow trout lipid content.

Bioactivities of lipid extract from sea-reared rainbow trout treated with dietary sea squirt tunic's carotenoids and CLA on rats

Feeding RME and RVE to rats would increase it's the food efficiency ratio (FER) especially the one which was fed with high fat diets (Table 2). Table 2 also shows that RME and RVE would significantly ($p>0.05$) lower the weight gain on high fat groups, though it does not make significantly different for the normal diet groups ($p>0.05$). The decreasing of the rat body weight could be accounted to the effect of RME and RVE, given that the feed intake among the groups were not significantly different ($p>0.05$). This result was in agreement with Baraldi et al. [20] who investigated whether dietary supplementation of CLA and extra virgin olive oil (EVOO) would affect the mice metabolism. They reported that there were changes on body metabolism associated with mitochondrial energetics on male C57BI/6 mice. Even though there were no clear differences for weight gain among the groups.

The treatment groups (RVN, RMN, RVHF, and RMHF) had lower total lipid weight compare to high fat diet control group (SHF) (Table 2). The CLA content of RME and RVE was most prominent to affect the retroperitoneal adipose tissue mass. On the other hand, the treatment showed no effect on other adipose tissues in the body ($p>0.05$). Even though, some of the adipose tissues (perirenal and mesenteric) started to be decreased. This result was similar to those reported [20, 21]. Mice fed CLA- and CLA+EVOO-supplemented diet had less white adipose tissue weight compared to that of control mice [20].

The peritoneal adipose tissue was the most reactive toward CLA treatments [22]. In contrast of this finding that the epididymal adipose tissue is the less responsive, in this study epididymal adipose tissue is more responsive to the treatment than mesenteric and perirenal ones. Recent study suggested that supplementation CLA decreases fat deposition by inducing adipocyte apoptosis [23]. The anti-obesity effect of CLA has been ascribed to reduced adipocyte size, reduced adipocyte proliferation, increased adipocyte lipolysis and apoptosis, as well as to enhanced fatty acid oxidation and energy expenditure, which is particularly found to be higher in t10-CLA-fed mice [24].

Since the accumulation of neutral fat in fat cells due to the intake of a high fat diet is a result of increased fat cell diameter, measuring the size of fat cells is an effective way to prove anti-obesity effects [25]. Therefore, this study monitored the size of epididymal fat cells, and the results are shown in Figure 1 and Table 2. The size of the epididymal fat cells in the group that was orally administered the RME and RVE in the normal or high fat diet tended to decrease when compared to the SN and SHF groups, which were administered the soybean oil. According to the measurements (Table 2), the size of the fat cells was in the order of SHF≥RVHF≥RMHF≥SN>RVN>RMN ($p<0.05$). It appears that the size of the fat cells of the white mice that orally administered RME and RVE were decreased as a result of controlling fat accumulation (Figures 1C-1E).

	Groups					
	SN	RVN	RMN	SHF	RVHF	RMHF
Initial weight (g)	192.8 ± 4.8^{NS}	192.8 ± 4.2	192.8 ± 6.4	192.7 ± 4.9	193.0 ± 3.1	193.7 ± 4.5
Final weight (g)	460.0 ± 18.8^{NS}	456.3 ± 16.7	454.8 ± 14.8	495.9 ± 12.5	468.7 ± 11.3	433.0 ± 14.6
Weight gain (g/day)	6.4 ± 0.4^{ab}	6.3 ± 0.3^{ab}	6.2 ± 0.4^{ab}	7.2 ± 0.3^{a}	6.6 ± 0.2^{ab}	5.7 ± 0.4^{b}
Feed intake (g/day)	25.2 ± 1.1^{NS}	24.7 ± 1.0	24.8 ± 1.5	21.4 ± 1.6	21.3 ± 1.1	20.2 ± 0.9
FER[1]	0.25 ± 0.00^{c}	0.25 ± 0.01^{bc}	0.25 ± 0.01^{c}	0.34 ± 0.02^{a}	0.31 ± 0.01^{ab}	0.28 ± 0.01^{bc}
Liver (g)	14.0 ± 0.5^{NS}	13.9 ± 0.5	13.3 ± 0.4	15.2 ± 0.4	14.1 ± 0.6	13.7 ± 0.5
Weight of adipose tissue (g)						
- Epididymal	6.8 ± 0.8^{NS}	7.0 ± 0.6	6.8 ± 0.6	9.2 ± 0.5	8.8 ± 0.6	9.0 ± 0.5
- Mesenteric	4.6 ± 0.39^{NS}	4.4 ± 0.5	4.5 ± 0.6	5.6 ± 0.5	4.6 ± 0.5	4.6 ± 0.4
- Retroperitoneal	9.3 ± 0.6^{ab}	7.1 ± 0.47^{b}	8.3 ± 1.26^{ab}	11.6 ± 0.80^{a}	9.5 ± 0.84^{ab}	9.8 ± 0.53^{ab}
- Perirenal	2.4 ± 0.3^{NS}	2.4 ± 0.3	2.2 ± 0.4	3.5 ± 0.4	2.6 ± 0.4	2.3 ± 0.2
- Total	23.2 ± 1.7^{ab}	20.9 ± 1.6^{b}	21.8 ± 2.8^{ab}	29.9 ± 2.1^{a}	25.6 ± 2.1^{ab}	25.6 ± 1.1^{ab}
Adipocytes diameter (μm)	4.7 ± 0.6^{bc}	3.8 ± 1.0^{c}	4.0 ± 0.9^{c}	8.6 ± 1.4^{a}	5.5 ± 0.9^{b}	4.0 ± 0.6^{c}
Number of lipid droplet in liver	21.26.0^{b}	13.84.8^{cd}	12.83.0^{d}	28.82.6^{a}	21.42.4^{b}	20.61.7^{bc}

Table 2: Weight gain, feed intake, feed efficiency ratio (FER), liver, adipose tissue weights, and Adipocytes diameter of rats treated with RME and RVE. Data are represented as mean ±SE (n=6). Values with different superscripts in the same row are significantly different ($p<0.05$) from each other. NS: not significant. [1]FER (feed efficiency ratio): weight gain (g/day)/feed intake (g/day).

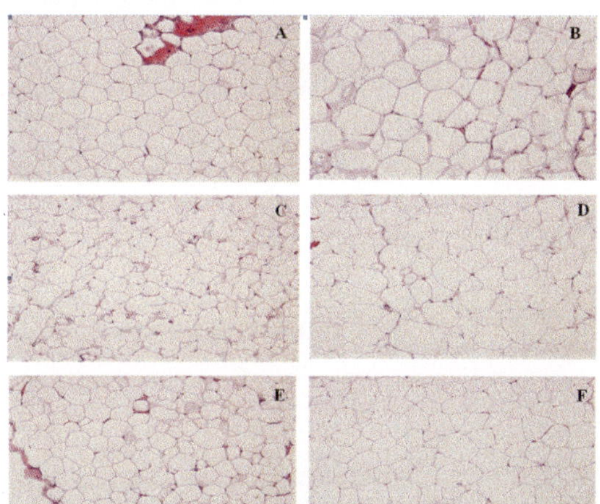

Figure 1: Representative histological slides of adipose tissue from rats. Treated with A. normal diet and soybean oil (SN), B. high fat diet and soy bean oil (SHF), C. normal diet and rainbow trout viscera lipid extract (SVN), D. high fat diet and rainbow trout viscera lipid extract (RVHF), E. normal diet and rainbow trout muscle lipid extract (RMN), and F. high fat diet and rainbow trout viscera muscle extract (RMHF). Tissue was processed with paraffin method and hematoxylin-eosin staining.

The result of the oil red O staining on liver is shown in Figure 2. Lipid was identified as red color droplet among hepatocytes. There was clear evidence of excessive of fat accumulation on the liver which can cause to fatty lipid [24]. The number and size of lipid droplet varied among treatment groups (Table 2 and Figure 2). Result revealed that SHF has the highest number of lipid droplets compare to other groups ($p<0.05$).

Biochemicals change of serum

Table 3 shows the analysis of the serum of the rat fed RME and RVE. Compared to the normal diet groups, the serum activity of alanine transaminase (ALT), aspartate transaminase (AST), alkaline phosphatase(ALP), and lactate dehydrogenase (LDH) all increased in the high fat diet groups (SHF, RVHF, and RMHF). It has been reported that the present and activities of ALT and AST in the serum corresponded to the liver function. The release of these enzymes from liver will be accelerated on as high-fat diets, high-cholesterol diets, and alcohol consumption. These diets and consumption caused fatty liver or the accumulation of liver toxic substances which damaged the liver tissues [26]. In this experiment, RVE significantly affected the concentration of ALT and AST compare to RME ($p<0.05$) in both normal diet and high fat diets. This result showed that RVE is good for health compare to RME.

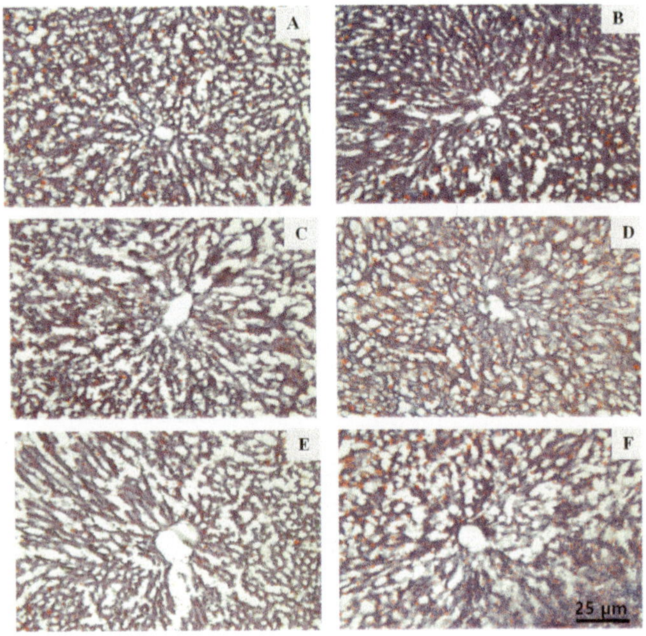

Figure 2: Representative histological slides of liver from rats. Treated with A) Normal diet and soybean oil (SN), B) High fat diet and soy bean oil (SHF), C) Normal diet and rainbow trout viscera lipid extract (SVN), D) High fat diet and rainbow trout viscera lipid extract (RVHF), E) Normal diet and rainbow trout muscle lipid extract (RMN), and F) High fat diet and rainbow trout viscera muscle extract (RMHF). Lipid could be observed as red droplets between plasma. Tissue was processed with oil red O staining.

The present of ALP in the blood serum was sign of biliary duct obstruction or hepatocytes membrane damage [27]. This could be repaired by increasing the concentration of cholesterol and elimination disorders of bile acid in the liver. In addition, LDH is an enzyme that is involved in both oxidation and reduction reactions at the final stage of the internal anaerobic process; the level of this enzyme is known to significantly increase in acute hepatitis, early hepatitis, myocardial infarction, pernicious anemia, and leukemia [28]. In this research however, there was no significant difference in the activity of AST and LDH among experimental groups (Table 3). The activity of ALT and ALP in the SHF were the highest compared to the other groups. This demonstrated that high fat diets could cause obstruction on liver function. Whilst, group fed the RME and RVE showed lower concentration of those enzymes. This revealed that CLA and carotenoid pigment extracted from sea squirt tunic exhibited liver-protective actions even though it has been accumulated in rainbow trout.

Table 4 shows the results of neutral lipid levels (TG), total cholesterol (TC), low-density lipoprotein (LDL) cholesterol and high-density lipoprotein (HDL) cholesterol in the serum, as well as the arteriosclerosis index and the cardiovascular index calculation. According to the analysis, the groups that fed the high fat diet had higher levels of TG, TC, and LDL-cholesterol, as well as high values for the arteriosclerosis index and cardiovascular index, but a low level of HDL-cholesterol when compared to those groups administered the regular diet. There was no significant ($p>0.05$) difference between the experimental groups in terms of TC, HDL-cholesterol levels, arteriosclerosis index values, and cardiovascular index values in the serum. On the other hand, the level of TG and the content of LDL-cholesterol in serum was significantly different ($p<0.05$).

In mammals, the effect of CLA on blood lipid levels was ever ambiguous. In mice, TG and TC levels and the (TC-HDL)/HDL ratio decreased, but HDL and lipoprotein lipase (LPL) levels increased with increasing CLA addition [29]. In the comparison among the groups that fed with high fat diet, SHF had the highest levels of TG and LDL-cholesterol compared to the others ($p<0.05$). In contrast, RMN had the significantly lowest levels of TG and LDL-cholesterol in serum compare to other groups. Addition of dietary CLA in the feed of obese juvenile *A. schrenckii* resulted in a lower growth rate [30]. Dietary CLA reduced body and liver lipid accumulation as well as lower lipid level in the blood. An inclusion of 2.0% CLA was found adequate to achieve the maximum effect.

Groups	Serum activity (IU/L)			
	Alanine amino transferase (ALT)	Aspartate amino transferase (AST)	Alkaline phosphatase (ALP)	Lactate dehydrogenase(LDH)
SN	18.3 ± 1.4^{b}	95.8 ± 5.7^{NS}	432.3 ± 32.0^{b}	493.8 ± 68.5^{NS}
RVN	18.8 ± 1.1^{b}	98.7 ± 4.5	514.7 ± 26.6^{ab}	453.8 ± 46.7
RMN	21.2 ± 0.9^{ab}	118.2 ± 9.0	421.0 ± 35.3^{b}	683.2 ± 79.5
SHF	27.8 ± 1.8^{a}	125.3 ± 5.14	678.2 ± 64.0^{a}	603.3 ± 87.4
RVHF	24.8 ± 1.7^{ab}	109.5 ± 12.8	654.5 ± 36.5^{a}	535.8 ± 87.1
RMHF	26.7 ± 2.7^{a}	124.7 ± 12.1	542.0 ± 42.2^{ab}	680.0 ± 113.0

Table 3: Serum activities of AST, ALT, ALP and LDH of rats treated with RME and RVE. Data are represented as mean ± SE (n=8). Values with different superscripts in the same column are significantly different ($p<0.05$). NS: Not significant.

Groups	Concentration (mg/dL)				AI[1]	CRF[2]
	Triglyceride	Total Cholesterol	LDL-cholesterol	HDL-cholesterol		
SN	78.7 ± 6.4^{b}	83.3 ± 3.0^{NS}	52.2 ± 3.4^{bc}	46.8 ± 1.7^{NS}	0.79 ± 0.08^{NS}	1.79 ± 0.08^{NS}
RVN	81.0 ± 7.3^{b}	84.0 ± 5.7	52.0 ± 7.8^{bc}	48.2 ± 5.3	0.88 ± 0.27	1.88 ± 0.27
RMN	75.3 ± 10.1^{b}	81.7 ± 3.0	46.7 ± 6.9^{c}	50.0 ± 5.8	0.78 ± 0.28	1.78 ± 0.28
SHF	135.2 ± 13.9^{a}	101.8 ± 5.8	89.0 ± 6.9^{a}	39.8 ± 2.0	1.59 ± 0.17	2.59 ± 0.17
RVHF	118.2 ± 3.8^{a}	88.2 ± 4.7	68.5 ± 3.8^{abc}	43.3 ± 3.5	1.07 ± 0.11	2.07 ± 0.11
RMHF	104.7 ± 6.6^{ab}	98.2 ± 6.9	75.1 ± 8.3^{ab}	44.0 ± 1.9	1.27 ± 0.22	2.27 ± 0.22

Table 4: Serum concentrations of triglyceride, total cholesterol LDL-cholesterol, HDL-cholesterol, AI and CRF of rats treated with RME and RVE. Data are represented as mean ±SE (n=8). Values with different superscripts in the same column are significantly different ($p<0.05$). NS: Not significant. [1]AI (atherosclerotic index)=(total cholesterol-HDL-cholesterol)/HDL-cholesterol. [2]CRF (cardiac risk factor)=total cholesterol/HDL-cholesterol.

Conclusions

New functional seafood based on sea-reared rainbow trout inclusion with CLA, carotenoids, and n-3 HUFA was developed. RME and RVE have potency as weight reducer through fat burner routes as well as liver protective ability. Hence, it could be considered as anti-obesity supplement of seafood for the long period of administration.

Acknowledgement

This research was a part of the project titled 'Production of functional sea-reared rainbow trout (*Oncorhynchus mykiss*) and development of products from this fish' funded by the Ministry of Oceans and Fisheriess of Korea (Grant Number: 2014-0647).

References

1. Bjerkeng B (2008) Carotenoids in aquaculture: fish and crustaceans. Carotenoids. Britton G, Liaaen-Jensen S, Pfander HH (eds.), Springer Co, NY, USA.
2. Jobling M, Tveiten H, Hatlen B (1998) Cultivation of Arctic char: An update. Aqua Interna 6: 181-196.
3. KMI (Korea Maritime Institute), Fisheries outlook.
4. Choi BD, Kang SJ, Choi YJ, Youm MG, Lee KH (1994) Utilization of ascidian (*Halocynthia roretzi*) tunic: Carotenoid composition of ascidian tunic. Korean J Fish Aqua Sci 27: 344-350.
5. Rohmah Z, Jeong UC, Ticar BF, Kim JS, Lee JJ, et al. (2016) Effect of ascidian (*Halocynthia roretzi*, Drasche 1884) tunics carotenoids on enhancing growth and muscle coloring of sea-reared rainbow trout (*Oncorhynchus mykiss*, Walbaum 1792). Aquaculture Reports 4: 22-29.
6. Cook ME, Miller CC, Park Y, Pariza MW (1993) Immune modulation by altered nutrient metabolism: Nutritional control of immune-induced growth depression. Poultry Sci 72: 1301-1305.
7. Poirier H, Shapiro JS, Kim RJ, Lazar MA (2006) Nutritional supplementation with trans-10, cis-12-conjugated linoleic acid induces inflammation of white adipose tissue. Diabetes 55: 1634-1641.
8. Terpstra AM, Javadi M, Beynen AC, Kocsis S, Lankhorst AE, et al. (2003) Dietary conjugated linoleic acids as free fatty acids and triacylglycerols similarly affect body composition and energy balance in mice. J Nutr 133: 3181-3186.
9. Boden G, Laakso M (2004) Lipids and glucose in type 2 diabetes: What is the cause and effect? Diabetes Care 27: 2253-2259.
10. Belury MA (1995) Conjugated dienoic linoleate: a polyunsaturated fatty acid with unique chemoprotective properties. Nutr Rev 53: 83-89.
11. Lee KN, Kritchevsky D, Pariza MW (1994) Conjugated linoleic acid and atheroscierosis in rabbits. Atheroscierosis 108: 19-25.
12. Folch J, Lees M, Sloane-Stanley G (1957) A simple method for the isolation and purification of total lipids from animal tissues. J Biol Chem 226: 497-509.
13. Sabetian M, Delshad ST, Moini S, Islami HR, Motalebi A (2012) Identification of fatty acid content, amino acid profile and proximate composition in rainbow trout (*Oncorhynchus mykiss*). J Am Sci 8: 670-677.
14. Park SJ, Park CW, Kim SJ, Kim JK, Kim YR, et al. (2002) Methylation methods for the quantitative analysis of conjugated linoleic acid (CLA) isomers in various lipid samples. J Agric Food Chem 50: 989-996.
15. Biggs HG, Erikson TM, Moorehead WR (1975) A manual colorimetric assay of triglyceride in serum. Clin Chem 21: 437-441.
16. Zlatkis A, Zak B (1969) Study of a new cholesterol reagent. Anal Biochem 29: 143-148.
17. Nilsson-Ehle P, Schotz MA (1976) A stable, radioactive substrate emulsion for assay of lipoprotein lipase. J Lipid Res 17: 536-541.
18. Baron CP, Svendsen GH, Lund I, Jokumsen A, Nielsen HH, et al. (2013) Organic plant ingredients in the diet of rainbow trout (*Oncorhynchusmykiss*): impact on fish muscle composition and oxidative stability. Eur J Lipid Sci Technol 115: 1367-1377.
19. Turchini GM, Hermon K, Cleveland BJ, Emery JA, Rankin T, et al. (2013) Seven fish oil substitutes over a rainbow trout grow-out cycle: I) Effects on performance and fatty acid metabolism. Aquac Nutr 19: 82-94.
20. Baraldi FG, Vicentini TM, Teodoro BG, Dalalio FM, Dechandt CRP, et al. (2016) The combination of conjugated linoleic acid (CLA) and extra virgin olive oil increases mitochondrial and body metabolism and prevents CLA-associated insulin resistance and liver hypertrophy in C57Bl/6 mice. J Nutr Biochem 28: 147-154.
21. Goonewardene LA, Mir PS, Wang Z, Okine EK, Mir Z, et al. (2004) Study of carcass, organ, muscle, fat tissue weight, and concentration in rats fed CLA or its precursors by principal component analysis. Can J Animal Sci 84: 537-543.
22. Azain MJ, Hausman DB, Sisk MB, Flatt WP, Jewell DE (2000) Dietary conjugated linoleic acid reduces rat adipose tissue cell size rather than cell number. J Nutr 130: 1548-1554.
23. Qi R, Yang F, Huang J, Peng H, Liu Y, Liu Z (2014) Supplementation with conjugated linoeic acid decreases pig back fat deposition by inducing adipocyte apoptosis. BMC Vet Res 10: 141-147.

24. Halade GV, Rahman MM, Fernandes G (2010) Differential effects of conjugated linoleic acid isomers in insulin-resistant female C57Bl/6J mice. J Nutr Biochem 21: 332-337.
25. Kim HS, Kim TW, Kim DJ, Hwang HJ, Lee HJ, et al. (2007) Effects of natural plants supplementation on adipocyte size of the epididymal fat pads in rats. J Korean Soc Food Sci Nutr 36: 419-423.
26. Sollof LA, Futenberg HL, Lacko AG (1973) Serum cholesterol esterification in patients with coronary artery disease. Am Heart J 85: 153-161.
27. Lim SS, Kim MH, Lee JH (1997) Effect of *Artemisia princeps* var *orientalis* and *Circium japonicas* var *ussuriense* on liver functions body lipid and bile acid hyperlipidemic rat. Korean J Nutr 30: 797-802.
28. Ki HY, Song SW, Ha CS, Han SS (1993) Effects of the population density on growth and various physiological values of Sprague-Dawley rats. J Animal Sci Technol 9: 71-82.
29. Xiuheng X, Zhigeng W, Juhua W, Lin M, Mi L (2006) Effect of fortified conjugated linoleic acid milk on body fat and plasma lipids in mice. Acta Nutrimenta Sini 28: 120-123.
30. Yang CG, Wen H, Jiang M, Liu W, Wu F, et al. (2014) Effect of dietary conjugated linoleic acid supplementation on the growth, lipid metabolism, and plasma lipid levels of juvenile Amur sturgeon (*Acipenser schrenckii* Brandt, 1869). J Appl Ichthyol 30: 1626-1631.

7

Nutraceutical-prophylactic and Therapeutic Role of Functional Food in Health

Rintu Das, Silpak Biswas and Ena Ray Banerjee*

Department of Zoology, University of Calcutta, India

***Corresponding author:** Ena Ray Banerjee, Associate Professor, Department of Zoology, Immunology and Regenerative Medicine Research Laboratory, University of Calcutta, 35, Ballygunge Circular Road, Kolkata-700019, West Bengal, India, E-mail: enaraybanerjee@gmail.com

Abstract:

This paper reviews the potential of functional foods in our daily life. A functional food with new ingredients gives an additional function to human health. Above their basic nutritional value functional foods deliver enhanced benefits. The functional food industry is growing rapidly in recent years. Epidemiological studies as well as *in vivo*, *in vitro*, and clinical data showed that plant-based functional foods are able to reduce the risk of different chronic disease, such as cancer. These biologically active plant chemicals are known as 'phytochemicals'. Not only phytochemicals, also there are other animal products considered as functional foods for their potential role in human health. Foods containing probiotics, prebiotics, or plant sterols are also considered as functional foods. The aim of this review was to focus on the role of functional foods on human health. The research work to understand the relationship between different beneficial foods and human health system and to explore the role of the functional foods against various diseases will be an important aspect scientifically, clinically as well as socio-economically. Finally, functional foods will be successful depending on several factors including their effectiveness, safety, and quality.

Keywords: Inflammation; Anti-oxidant; Phenolic compounds; Scavenger activities; Phytochemicals; Anti-carcinogenic agents

Introduction

The industrialized world of this century forced to deal with new challenges such as excess healthcare costs, longer life expectancy and changes in living manner. Nutritionists have enthusiastically accepted the idea of 'optimal nutrition', which focuses on optimising daily diet quality in terms of its nutraceutical value for the proper health. As a result, development of functional foods or nutraceuticals comes into play [1,2]. The demand of functional food is increasing due to more health awareness.

The term 'nutraceutical' coined by DeFelice in 1989 and the Foundation for Innovation in Medicine [3,4]. The term 'functional foods' was first introduced in Japan. The processed foods containing nutritious ingredients that support healthy body functions are known as functional foods [5,6]. According to International Food Information Council (IFIC) the functional foods are dietary components with a health benefit beyond basic nutrition [4,7]. On the other hand, International Life Sciences Institute of North America (ILSI) also defines functional foods as physiologically active food components which provide health benefits [5,8]. Another definition by Health Canada described the functional food which is capable to reduce the risk of chronic diseases. To improve its bioavailability some components of functional foods could be changed by applying new technology [9]. Scientific research is very useful aspect for the production of 'functional food'. According to some journal, functional food is a food with added or concentrated ingredients, which improves health [10]. European consensus publication regarded functional food as healthy food with beneficial and additional nutritional effects on human body. On 10th International Conference in Santa Barbara, CA, 2012, a new definition for 'functional food' announced as 'natural or processed foods that contains known or unknown biologically-active compounds with health benefit for the prevention, management, and/or treatment of chronic disease' [11].

Baby foods, sport drinks, enriched cereals, breads and other foods are considered as functional foods. There were some reports that, the Vitamin B-enriched flour was found to protect pellagra; vitamin D-enriched milk was effective in eliminating rickets and iodine-fortified salt decreased incidences of goitre [12]. Functional foods are different from medical foods and are distributed and regulated separately. Functional foods could be consumed freely as part of our everyday life, whereas medical foods and drugs are consumed when recommended by medical professionals (Table 1). The aim of this review was to focus on the role of functional foods on human health and to understand its use against different diseases and about its production in the industry.

Functional Foods from Plant Sources

Epidemiological evidence (*in vivo* and *in vitro*) and clinical trial data indicates that a plant-based diet can reduce the risk of various chronic diseases. In 1992, a review of 200 epidemiological studies demonstrated that risk of cancer was half to the people who consumed more fruits [13]. This work demonstrated that, bioactive compounds of plant based diets can reduce risk of cancer. Cereals and its ingredients are very good source of dietary fibre, proteins, energy, minerals, vitamins. Wheat, oat, barley, flaxseed, brown rice and soy products are important cereal based functional food and nutraceuticals [14]. The fermented cereals can be used for the growth of probiotic microorganisms also [15]. This review demonstrates health benefits of some plant based functional food.

Difference	Functional foods	Medical foods	Prescription drugs
Uses	Energy enhancement; weight management; bolster gut, bone or heart health; disease risk reduction; memory improvement	Dietary management of a disease or condition with distinctive nutritional requirements (e.g. difficulty swallowing, loss of appetite, nutrition repletion post-surgery)	Treatment of disease, symptom, or condition
Method of obtainment	No prescription or supervision needed; consumer selects	Used with medical supervision	Prescribed by health provider
Distribution channels	Supermarkets, drugstores, online, major retailers	Hospitals, pharmacies, drugstores, online	Pharmacies, hospitals
Regulatory body	No specific body, but is considered food and is therefore subject to FDA regulation (FDA regulates any specific health claims that might be made)	No additional FDA review/approval needed, but must abide by regulations concerning foods, e.g. labeling (FDA regulates any specific health claims that might be made)	FDA approval needed, a multiyear, multistage review process
Amount consumed	As desired	As needed	As prescribed

Table 1: Comparing functional foods with medical foods and drugs.

Oats

Oats, commonly known as *Avena sativa* are considered as a minor cereal crop which comes under Poaceae family. Higher level of protein, lipids, vitamins, minerals antioxidants and phenolic compounds accounts for the nutritional significance of oats (Table 2) [16]. Oat products are good source of β-glucan, a soluble fibre which has the cholesterol-lowering capacity [17], reduce low density lipoprotein [7], contain antioxidant compounds [17], and improves gastrointestinal function and glucose metabolism [18]. Human clinical trials conducted on hyper-cholesterolemic subjects demonstrated 5% reduction in serum cholesterol due to intake of 60 g oatmeal or 40 g oat bran containing 3 g of β-glucan [7].

Components	Oat groat	Oat gum	Oat bran	Oat hull fibre
Total dietary fibre	60-90	-	120-240	900-970
β-glucan	35-50	600-800	55-90	-

Table 2: Composition of oat fibre and β-glucan (g/kg dry weight) [16,18].

Soy

Asian countries are consuming soy foods for centuries [19]. Soy has been in the spotlight during the 1990s. Soybean (*Glycine max*) consists of mainly isoflavones which are a group of naturally occurring heterocyclic phenols which perform several health-promoting functions [20]. Soy contains high quality protein and it plays preventive and therapeutic roles against diseases like cardiovascular disease (CVD), cancer, osteoporosis, and the alleviation of menopausal symptoms [7,21]. The cholesterol-lowering effect of soy is the well-documented physiological effect. There is strong evidence that soy-based diets consumption leads to decrease total cholesterol, LDL cholesterol, serum lipid concentration, and triglyceride levels [22]. According to meta-analysis of 38 separate studies (involving 743 subjects), consumption of soy protein significantly reduced LDL cholesterol (12.9%), total cholesterol (9.3%), and triglycerides (10.5%) [23]. Isoflavones is the key component for the cholesterol-lowering effect of soy. Soy proteins help to decrease LDL synthesis in liver and it can reduce insulin/glucagon ratio [24]. Isoflavones are heterocyclic phenols structurally similar to the estrogenic steroids. Among the isoflavone, genistein and daidzein are the most notable and soybeans are the significant dietary source [7,25]. Various studies reported that isoflavones can prevent intestine, prostate, stomach and breast cancers [26-29]. Another study described that soybeans contain several classes of anti-carcinogens, including protease inhibitors, phytosterols, phenolic acids, saponins, isoflavones and phytic [26,30,31]. The molecular structure of Isoflavones is similar to human estrogens and bind to both estrogen receptors ERα and ERβ but prefer ERβ [32]. Reports demonstrated that, consumption of soy decreases the chance of estrogen-dependent cancer [33]. Soy increases bone density [34,35] and also helps to reduce menopausal symptoms.

Rice

Rice is the most significant cereal crops and a staple food for most of the world's population. Rice is a very good reservoir of hypoallergenic protein and lysine. Protein quality of rice superior to that of wheat and corn [36]. Amino acid composition of rice protein was better than soy protein and casein [37]. It can be a suitable ingredient for infant food formulations [38]. Rice based fermented foods are highly acceptable because of its calorie value [39]. Chung et al. [40] stated that white rice with combination of 8% pigmented giant embryonic rice (Keunnunjami) is functional food which has strong hypolipidemic and anti-obesity properties. Choi et al. [41] described the anti-diabetic property of germinated brown rice extract.

Wheat

The most widely cultivated cereal crop in the World is wheat which is mainly used for milling and baking [42]. Wheat was cultivated first about 10000 years ago [43]. Common wheat (*Triticum aestivum*), also known as bread wheat, is suitable for biscuits [44]. Free and esterified phenolic acids of wheat have the greatest potential health benefit [36,45,46]. Whole wheat and wheat bran based cereals are significant source of dietary antioxidants. Red wheat generally contains higher levels of antioxidants than white wheat [47]. Wheat is a source of zinc, iron and selenium [43]. Recently it was demonstrated that whole wheat flour and bread have more antioxidant capacity then refined flour [48]. Wheat bran are rich in phytochemical like phenolic acids and betaine which are beneficial for [49].

Maize

Among the versatile emerging crops, maize is the most important because of its adaptability with varied agro-climatic conditions. Globally, it is considered as queen of cereals for its highest genetic yield potential. After rice and wheat, maize is the third most important cereal for human food stuff by contributing 9% to Indian basket and 5% to World's dietary energy supply [50]. Decortications by abrasion are feasible to obtain smooth texture of cooked products from maize because of its hardness and size and fine grinding is essential [51]. In Pharmaceutical industry, to release tablet formulation immediately pre-gelatinized maize starch was used and it was also considered for sustained release formulations [52,53].

Barley

Barley (*Hordeum vulgare*) grain is used as feed, malt, and food [36]. Barley is used as flour, as semolina, and as whole-dehulled grain. Barley is rich in dietary fibre, both insoluble and soluble fibre. Fibre constituents of barley have protective and therapeutic effects against various metabolic disorder like cardiovascular diseases, certain cancers and type-2 diabetes [54-57] β-glucan, which is a key component of soluble fibre implicated in hypercholesterolemia, hypoglycemia, and decreases the incidence of chemically induced colon cancer in preclinical model, lowers postprandial plasma glucose and ameliorates insulin resistance [58,59]. Multiple varieties of dishes such as soups, couscous and bread are made by barley products [60].

Millets (*Eleusine coracana*)

Millets belongs to the family Poaceae. Millets are small seeded, annual cereal grasses which can survive in less fertile soil [61]. Millets include sorghum (Jowar), proso millet (Chena), pearl millet (Bajra), foxtail millet (Kakum), finger millet (Ragi), little millet (Kutki), kodo millet (Kodon), barnyard millet (Sanwa), and brown top millet [61,62].

Eleusine coracana is widely cultivated in the arid areas of Africa and Asia. Finger millet is one of the oldest crops in India [63]. In India, it is cultivated over an area of 2.65 million hectares [64]. Milet is considered as one of the important staple foods in some parts of Africa and India (FAO). In India, finger millet was processed by grinding, malting, and fermentation for products like beverages, idli, dosa, and roti [65]. Germinated finger millet can be a good substrate for statins (anti-hypocholestrolemic metabolites) production [66]. Various *in vitro* and *in vivo* studies demonstrated its blood glucose lowering, cholesterol lowering and wound healing properties [67]. It can be used for the preparation of dietetic foods for anaemia patients and geriatric food formulation [68]. Several work demonstrated the antioxidant properties of millet [69-74]. Finger millet also possesses antimicrobial activities [72,75,76]. Protein glycation, one of the complications of diabetes, was inhibited by methanolic extract of finger millet [67,77]. Chethan et al. [78] reported that finger millet phenolics can inhibit aldose reductase and snake venom phospholipases (PLA2) too. Among the cereals and millets, finger millet is the richest source of calcium (344 mg%) and potassium (408 mg%).

Sorghum (Sorghum bicolor)

Sorghum is a cereal which belongs to the family Poaceae. It is considered as major source of carbohydrates and proteins. Sorghum is used as human food worldwide [79]. Pigmented sorghum is a good source of dietary phenolics, mainly flavones, flavanones and deoxyanthocyanidins. Several research has demonstrated anti-cancer activities of phenolic compounds of sorghum, especially 3-deoxyanthocyanidins and it is effective on various cancer such as skin melanoma, liver, colon, breast, esophagus, and bone marrow [80-86]. Other than cancer, sorghum also effective against several diseases such as diabetes, dyslipidemia, hypertension, obesity and inflammation [87].

Table 3 showing composition of different varieties of cereals expressed as 100 g of edible portion.

Parameter	Rice	Wheat	Maize	Sorghum	Millets
Water (%)	12	12	13.8	11	11.8
Protein (g)	7.5	13.3	8.9	11	9.9
Fat (g)	1.9	2	3.9	3.3	2.9
Carbohydrates (g)	77.4	71	72.2	73	72.9
Fibre (g)	0.9	2.3	2	1.7	3.2
Ash (g)	1.2	1.7	1.2	1.7	2.5
Ca (mg)	32	41	22	28	20
P (mg)	221	372	268	287	311
Fe (mg)	1.6	3.3	2.1	4.4	68
K (mg)	214	370	284	350	430
Mg (mg)	88	113	147	n.d.	162
Riboflavin (mg)	0.05	0.12	0.12	0.15	0.38
Niacin (mg)	1.7	4.3	2.2	3.9	2.3
Thiamin (mg)	0.34	0.55	0.37	0.38	0.73

Table 3: Composition of different varieties of cereals expressed as 100 g of edible portion [88].

Fig (Ficus carica)

Figs belongs to the Moraceae family. Semi-arid climate is suitable for fig. Figs are usually dried and stored for later consumption. Medicinal value of figs already documented in various research papers and it has been demonstrated that figs has positive impact to treat respiratory, anti-inflammatory disorders, anti-cancer, antiviral, cardiovascular, aphrodisiac, hairnutritive [89,90], anti-diabetic, hypolipidemic [91,92], antipyretic [93], antibacterial [94,95], antifungal [96], scavenging activity and immune response [97]. It was demonstrated that ripe dried fig has potential effect on gastrointestinal, inflammatory disorders [98], and anti-infertility [99,100]. The Wildlife Conservation Society of New York reported that, wild figs are considered as 'keystone' fruit due to its high calcium content [101]. Hepatoprotective activity of figs has been demonstrated previously [102]. Other than fruits, latex of fig also has various medicinal importance. Leaves of fig tree are very useful to treat diabetes and contact dermatitis [92].

Fenugreek (Methi)

Fenugreek (*Trigonella foenum-graceum*) is a semi-arid crop belongs to Fabaceae family and is cultivated worldwide [103,104]. Fenugreek seeds and green leaves are used in food as well as in medicinal application. Fenugreek paste, locally termed as 'Cemen' is a popular food in Turkey [105], which is prepared from ground fenugreek seeds. Crushed fenugreek seed is used to make ball to make clarified butter. Fenugreek has strong spicy and seasoning type sweet flavour [106]. Aromatic and flavourful fenugreek is a popular spice and is widely used for well-known medicinal properties [107]. India is a major producer of fenugreek and also a major consumer of it for its medicinal application. It is used as a functional food, traditional food and nutraceuticals. Singhal et al. [108] demonstrated hypo-cholesterolemic activities of fenugreek seeds and Basch et al. [109] reported that fenugreek seeds lowered serum cholesterol, low-density lipoprotein (LDL) and triglyceride in hypercholesterolemic patients. According to Basch et al. [109] Fenugreek consumption in diet reduced triglyceride accumulation in the liver. Fenugreek also used as an antibacterial, anticancer, antiulcer, antioxidant, and antidiabetic agent. It helps to improve digestion. Fenugreek contains different alkaloids, flavonoids and saponins [110,111]. Grover et al. [112] reported that fenugreek seeds showed hypoglycaemic and anti-hyperglycaemic activity in diabetic mice. The aqueous extract of fenugreek showed significant positive effect on ulcer. It has soothing effect on gastric and gastritis ulcer [113]. Fenugreek possess various bioactive compounds, among them trigonelline, galactomannan, diosgenin, 4-hydroxyisoleucin, and soluble dietary fibre fraction are important [114,115]. Several study revealed anti-diabetic property of diosgenin in animal model [116-118]. Recently, Bahmani et al. [119] demonstrated that, trigonelline which is bioactive compound of fenugreek is responsible for anti-diabetic property of fenugreek and it decreases blood cholesterol too. Diaszhenin is one of the important bioactive compounds of fenugreek and it is used as contraceptive pills [119]. Dietary fibre of fenugreek seed is used for cooking [120,121] and it is very active to reduce postprandial hyperglycemia in preclinical model and decrease serum lipids [122,123]. Fenugreek provides natural food fibre and other nutrients required for human body [124]. Saponins are found to be in maximum concentration in the fenugreek [125] and Cholin content is very high in fenugreek [126]. Fenugreek seed is riched in multivitamin such as Vitamins-A (1040 IU per 100 g), B1 (0.41 mg per 100 g), B2 (0.36 mg per 100 g), C (12.0 mg per 100 g), nicotinic acid (1.1 mg per 100 g) and niacin (6.0 mg per 100 g) [127].

Cordyceps mushroom

Cordyceps militaris is widely distributed in China, Tibetan Plateau, Bhutan, Nepal and north east India at high altitude. In traditional Chinese medicine it is used as a tonic herb [128]. *C. militaris* has traditionally been used as a functional food and several bioactive compounds like adenosine, cordycepin, polysaccharides, mannitol, and ergosterol have been isolated from it [129,130]. It can be used to treat various inflammatory disorders and boosting the immune system [131]. Several researches demonstrated its promising activity in various inflammatory disease models like ovalbumin-induced asthma, dextran sodium sulphate (DSS)-induced colitis, and croton oil-induced ear oedema [132]. Humoral immune hyper-function was inhibited by cultivated Cordyceps and it improved liver function of post-hepatic cirrhosis patients by up regulate the level of the serum complement [133]. Recently, *C. militaris* cultivated on germinated soybean (GSC) extract and it was very effective against allergy and Type I hypersensitive animal model [132,134]. Cordycepin isolated from hot water extracts of C. Sinensis might be a good drug candidate against anticancer and antimetastatic [135]. 100 g of *Cordyceps militaris* contains 2.01 g manitol and 24.71 g trehalose free sugar. It is rich in polyunsaturated fatty acids (68.87%) than saturated fatty acids (23.40%). Various organic acids were found in this mushroom as oxalic, citric and fumaric acids (0.33, 7.97 and 0.13 g/100 g, respectively). Among the phenolic acids, only 0.02 mg p-Hydroxybenzoic acid was found in 100 g of this mushroom and d-tocopherol concentration was 55.86 lg/100 g [136]. This functional food has been used as drug and need further research by modern scientific approach for accurate phytochemical and bioactive compounds.

Flaxseed:

Flax (*Linum usitassimum*) is a blue flowering annual herb comes to Linaceae family. It produces golden yellow to reddish brown coloured flat seed. It has been used for medicinal purposes for over 5000 years [137,138]. More than 50 countries cultivate flaxseed [138,139]. According to Oomah [140], World's largest producer and exporter of flaxseeds is Canada. Scientific research has focused on fibre-associated compounds known as lignans. The richest source of mammalian lignan precursors is flaxseed [141,142]. Flexseeds are very effective in several diseases like diabetes, arthritis, neurological disorders, osteoporosis, cardiovascular disease, cancer and various chronic non-communicable [143-145]. Consumption of flaxseed has also been shown to lower LDL cholesterol [146,147] and platelet aggregation [148]. Several researches supported the chemo protective activities of the omega-3s and lignan phytoestrogens of flaxseed in human and animals [149-171]. Estrogen-dependent cancers can be prevented by mammalian lignans. In rodents, flaxseed has been shown to decrease tumours of the colon and mammary gland [155,164,172-176] as well as of the lung [177]. Different studies demonstrated that, consumption of flaxseed reduce breast [168,178,179] and prostate cancer [180-182]. It has also been reported that the ingestion of 10 g of flaxseed daily elicited several hormonal changes associated with reduced breast cancer risk [183]. Recent study revealed the anti-hepatotoxicity property of flaxseed oil [184]. *In vivo*, *in vitro* and *in silico* study reported that, dietary flaxseed might be a good approach to treat muscle dystrophies [185].

Tomatoes (*Solanum lycopersicum*)

Tomato is an important vegetable because of lycopene which is the primary carotenoid found in this fruit [186]. Different products are obtained from tomato, such as ketchup, sauces, and soups [187,188]. The tomatoes are rich in various bioactive compounds such as lycopene, β-carotene, phenolic compounds, flavonoids, glycoalkaloids, tomatine pro-vitamin A and vitamins C and E [189-197]. A clinical study by Giovannucci et al. [198] demonstrated that, tomato can reduce developing advanced prostate cancer [198]. Recent study revealed dietary lycopene consumption protect from prostate cancer by ERG protein expression [199]. Other than prostate cancer, it also has positive effect on breast, digestive tract, cervix, bladder, and skin cancer [200,201]. Along with peroxyl radicals scavenging capacity lycopene can also scavenge nitrogen dioxide and hydrogen peroxide [202,203]. Lycopene is the most effective as singlet oxygen quencher in biological systems [204]. Several work demonstrated that lycopene bioavailability of processed tomato is more than unprocessed tomato [205-207]. Recent study showed the hypolipidemic activities of processed tomato juice in animal model [208]. Tomato drink can reduce about 42% DNA damage in lymphocyte caused by oxidative stress [209].

Pumpkin (*Cucurbita pepo*)

Cucurbita pepo (pumpkin) comes under the family Cucurbitaceae. Cultivation of pumpkin originated in central Africa on 5500 BC

[210-212]. Pumpkin is one of the well-known plants which have been used as functional food [213]. It is very rich source of fatty acids like palmitic (C 16:0), stearic (C 18:0), oleic (C 18:1) and linoleic (C 18:2), linolenic (C18:3), sterols, gamma aminobutyric acids, proteins and peptides, polysaccharides, para-aminobenzoic acid and fixed oils, essential fatty acid such as omega 6 and omega 9, phytosterols, and antioxidants such as tocopherols, carotenoids, vitamin A and vitamin E [214-222]. Various ethnopharmacological studies demonstrated that *Cucurbita pepo* is used as antiviral, analgesic urinary disorders, anti-microbial, anti-ulcer, antidiabetic, anti-cancer, and antioxidant in various diseases [212,223-230]. Low dose pumpkin showed hypoglycaemic activity by decreasing triglycerides, LDL and CRP (C-reactive protein) and high dose pumpkin decreased cholesterol [231]. Pumpkin is used as anti-diabetic traditionally medicine worldwide [232,213]. Several studies reported that pumpkin exhibits anti-diabetic activities in mice model [233-238]. Another research demonstrated anti-diabetic effect of tocopherol fraction of pumpkin seed oil in Wistar rats [239,240]. Pumpkin helps to improve pancreas β cells functionality by increasing the number of insulin positive cells [241]. It is also very effective against alcohol induced hepatic damage [242-244]. Recent research stated that, the pumpkin seeds are very useful to manage the benign prostatic hyperplasia [245].

Garlic

Garlic (*Allium sativum*) was originated in Central Asia [246] and is used universally as a flavouring agent as well as traditional medicine and a functional food to enhance physical and mental health [247]. The health benefits of garlic are numerous, including anti-diabetic, cholesterol-lowering properties, chronic inflammation, cancer chemopreventive anti-aging, antibiotic, and anti-hypertensive, increase blood circulation, anti-gastric cancer, antioxidant [246,248-254]. Garlic mixed with calcium hydroxide to form paste and applied to treat carbuncle [255]. Garlic has various medicinal values due to its oil-and water-soluble, sulphur-containing elements [256-262]. The whole garlic bulb contains alliin, a derivative of the amino acid cysteine. Alliin is converted to allicin by allinase [13]. Allicin is responsible for the pungent odour of fresh garlic [263,264]. Alliin was the first natural compound which has both carbon and sulfur-centered stereochemistry [265]. Allicin have been investigated for their chemo-preventive activity [7]. Water content is 65% of fresh weight of garlic and the bulk of the dry weight is composed of mainly fructans, a fructose-containing carbohydrates, followed by other compounds like fibre, sulfur compounds, free amino acids and protein [266]. Several work demonstrated that, garlic extract capable to reduce diet-induced hyper-cholesterolemia [267]. Garlic has also been used for the prevention of CVD. The cardio protective effects are more likely due to its cholesterol-lowering effect. A meta-analysis [268] demonstrated that, an average of 900 mg garlic/day can reduce 9% serum cholesterol. Some authors suggested that garlic can reduce total cholesterol levels by 12% [269,270]. Although another study reported that, 12 weeks of garlic treatment was ineffective to reduce cholesterol in hypercholesterolemia subject [271,272]. Anti-tumorigenesis activity of garlic has been demonstrated in several preclinical models [250]. Several epidemiological studies demonstrated that, stomach cancer risk can be reduced by increasing allium intake [273]. In a clinical study with more than 40,000 postmenopausal women showed that, garlic consumption can reduce nearly 50% risk of colon cancer [274]. Antimicrobial activity of garlic has been documented from long time and Mr. Louis Pasteur also demonstrated the same [247,275-285]. Several recent studies also reported the promising effect of aqueous garlic extracts against various bacteria as antibacterial agent [286-289]. Recent study demonstrated that, allicin and other organosulfur compounds from garlic showed promising antibacterial effect on methicillin-resistant *Staphylococcus aureus* (MRSA) which are now considered as a major hospital acquired pathogen all over the world [290]. It has been shown hepatoprotective activities of garlic in several studies also [291-293]. Due to hepatoprotective effect of garlic, it can be a very good supplementation with first line anti-TB drugs [294]. Antimicrobial activity of garlic against *Mycobacterium tuberculosis* was firstly documented in 1946 [295]. Another study reported that, being promising antimicrobial agent, aqueous extract of garlic can be useful for dental caries and periodontitis [296].

Cranberry (*Vaccinium macrocarpon*)

Cranberry belongs to the Ericaceae family and 90% of total production of it contributed by North America and Canada [297]. Intake of cranberry juice significantly increases plasma antioxidant level [298-300]. Cranberry juice has been recognized as efficacious in the treatment of urinary tract infections since 1914 [301]. Several investigations have exhibited the ability of proanthocyanidins of cranberry juice to inhibit the attachment of *Escherichia coli* to uroepithelial cells [302-305]. Cranberry is beneficial to various diseases like cardiovascular disease, lipoprotein oxidation, and atherosclerosis [299,306,307]. Several *in vitro* studies supported the anti-cancer property of cranberries [308-313].

Cocoa (*Theobroma cacao*)

Theobroma cacao is commonly known as cacao tree or cocoa tree. The cocoa tree originated from ancient Central America [314]. Cocoa and cocoa-rich chocolates are very popular and widely consumed food component [315-317]. Cocoa is beneficial on blood pressure, vascular, platelet function and insulin resistance [315]. Cocoa beans and their parts are important ingredients for making chocolate. Cocoa is among the richest sources of polyphenols [318] and the total polyphenol content of the cocoa bean is about 6-8% by dry weight. Flavonoids, polyphenols, and procyanidins are the most important bioactive compounds with disease preventive characteristics [314]. Cocoa and cocoa products are recognized for health benefits related to hypertension, diabetes, anaemia, cardiovascular diseases, atherosclerosis, obesity, tuberculosis, fever, gout, kidney stones, mental fatigue, poor sexual appetite, neurodegenerative diseases and cancer [314,319-324]. Recent metaanalysis study stated the blood pressure lowering property of cocoa rich food [325] and it has been found that, in addition to the hypotensive effects, cocoa flavonols reduce adipose tissue by stimulating thermo genesis and lipolysis [326]. Recent research demonstrated that, cacao osmotin and its derived peptides might be a good drug candidate against pathogenic fungi [327].

Peanut

Peanut is an important crop worldwide and by-products of peanut contain vitamins, proteins, antioxidants, fibers, polyphenols, and minerals. These ingredients are used in many processed foods. Some reports described that, peanuts are also source of flavonoids, phytosterols and phenolic acids which are able to block the absorption of cholesterol from diet. Peanut also contains 20 amino acids and known for its disease preventive properties [328].

Strawberry

Strawberries, a rich source of phytochemicals and vitamins are considered as functional food for their preventive and therapeutic health benefits. Strawberry is also known for its antioxidant capacity [329,330]. Many studies found its anti-inflammatory, antihyperlipidemic, antihypertensive, or antiproliferative effects principally via downregulation of NF-kB activity [331-336]. Strawberries are a significant source of flavonoids. Flavonoids have been shown to have direct antibacterial activity [337-339]. Different epidemiological studies support the protective effects of strawberries against cancer, inflammation, cardiovascular mortality and hypertension [335,340]. Some studies demonstrated that, strawberries can reduce oxidant stress [341,342]. Different epidemiological and clinical studies observed cardio-protective effects of strawberries. Pinto et al. [343] using *in vitro* models reported the role of strawberry phytochemicals in managing hyperglycemia and hypertension. Another report demonstrated berry polyphenols as a potential phytotherapy in obesity and hyperglycemia [344]. Strawberry has been shown to exert anticarcinogenic effects [331,345]. Stoner et al. [346,347] showed the effects of freeze-dried strawberries on the inhibition of tumors in rodents.

Tannins (a specific strawberry polyphenols) showed significant anticancer effects in human breast, cervix, and colon carcinoma cells [348,349]. Ellagic acid found in strawberries demonstrated anticarcinogenic effects in several human cancer cell models in some studies [350,351]. Several studies described the role of strawberries in curing age-related neurodegenerative disorders [352-354].

Table 4 showing examples of foods with higher content of specific nutraceutical substances.

Diosgenin	Fenugreek
Allyl sulfur compounds	Garlic
Isoflavones (e.g. genestein, daidzein)	Soybeans and other legumes
Quercetin	Citrus fruit
Capsaicinoids	Pepper fruit
EPA and DHA	Fish oils
Lycopene	Tomatoes and tomato products
Isothiocyanates	Cruciferous vegetables
β-Glucan	Oat bran
CLA Beef and dairy	Beef and dairy
Catechins	berries
Adenosine	Garlic
Curcumin	Tumeric
Ellagic acid	Strawberries
Cellulose	Most plants (component of cell walls)
Monounsaturated fatty acids	Tree nuts, olive oil
Inulin, Fructooligosaccharides (FOS)	Whole grains, garlic
Lactobacilli, Bifidobacteria	Yogurt and other dairy
Catechins	Cocoa
Lignans	Flax
Cyclic peptides, cordycepin, 10-membered macrolides, cepharosporolides C, E and F, pyridine-2,6-dicarboxylic acid and 2-carboxymethyl-4-(30-hydroxybutyl) furan, dipicolinic acid	*Cordyceps militaris*

Table 4: Examples of foods with higher content of specific nutraceutical substances.

Functional Foods from Animal Sources

Some animal products with potential beneficial effects on human health are considered as functional foods. Some examples are as follows:

Fish

Fish contain animal protein. Fish oils contain the omega-3 (n-3) polyunsaturated fatty acids, vitamins and minerals [355]. The omega-3 fatty acid is an essential class of polyunsaturated fatty acids (PUFAs). Omega-3 fatty acids can reduce the rate of cardiovascular diseases or CVD [356] and it can also lower triglyceride level [357]. Studies by Kris-Etherton et al. [358] reported the effects of omega-3 fatty acids to reduce the incidence of CVD. Some observational studies report a decrease in cardiovascular disease with higher fish oil intake [359]. Omega-3 fatty acids also decrease the risk of thrombosis [360].

Consumption of 35 g of fish per day has been shown to reduce the risk of total mortality by cardiovascular disease [361]. Fish oil also plays role in decreasing weight and waist circumference [362]. The evidence of fish oil supplements lowering triglycerides has been found in dialysis patients [363]. Saccone and Berghella reported that, fish oil supplements appeared to be associated with greater weight at birth of the child [364]. Another report demonstrated that, supplementation of fish oil improves the quality of life in patients with chronic heart failure [365]. Some studies reported that, patients with a higher consumption of fish are less likely to have type 2 diabetes as compared to patients with lower fish consumption [366]. Recent randomized, controlled clinical trial by Pase et al. [367] showed the effects of long-chain omega-3 fish oils on cognitive and cardiovascular function.

Dairy products

Dairy products are considered as functional foods as they are rich of calcium. Fermented dairy food products could prevent diseases such as hypertension. Calcium helps preventing osteoporosis and possibly colon cancer. Other than calcium, many other components in fermented dairy products are known as probiotics. Probiotics are microorganisms with health benefits to the host animal by improving its intestinal microorganisms. Probiotics are termed as functional foods which can alter and modify pre-existing intestinal flora [368,369].

Both beneficial (e.g. *Bifidobacterium* and *Lactobacillus*) and detrimental (e.g. Enterobacteriaceae and *Clostridium* spp.) bacteria inhabit the human gastrointestinal tract. Among these bacteria, lactic acid bacteria are used in food fermentation [370-372]. Probiotics are known for their anti-carcinogenic, hypo-cholesterolemic and antagonistic actions against gut pathogens. Probiotics are used in colon cancer risk reduction [373,374]. This is because lactic acid cultures are able to alter the activity of faecal enzymes such as β-glucuronidase, azoreductase, nitroreductase which plays a role in the development of colon cancer [375,376].

The prebiotics are defined as 'non-digestible food ingredients that beneficially affect the host by selectively stimulating the growth and/or activity of one or a few number of bacteria in the colon and thus improves host health' [377]. These include starches, dietary fibres, sugar alcohols, and oligosaccharides [378]. Among these prebiotics oligosaccharides found naturally in many fruits and vegetables and have received great attention for their health benefits [379]. Prebiotics as food additives are valuable for functional foods and also helps in preventing diet-related diseases [380]. The prebiotic concept has been further extended to understand the effect of the synbiotics which is a mixture of pro-and prebiotics [377]. Many such synbiotic products are currently on the market in different countries. Recently our group demonstrated the use of combination of probiotic microbial strains supplemented in food as possible therapeutic and prophylactic agent to fight against inflammation and degeneration in Inflammatory Bowel Diseases (IBD) [381].

Beef

Meat and meat products contain important source of protein, fat, and several functional compounds [382]. Thomas and others [383] described the importance of animal meat for the high quality proteins as well as for its contribution to food security in the rural livelihoods. In 1987, conjugated linoleic acid (CLA) was first isolated from beef. CLA is an anti-carcinogenic fatty acid and it is a mixture of isomers of linoleic acid. CLA consists mixture of two isomers, cis-9, trans-11 and trans-10, cis-12. Conjugated linoleic acid has been approved as GRAS (generally recognized as safe) in USA since 2008 [384]. CLA increases in cooked foods and it acts as a weight-reduction agent. Reports showed that, CLA acts as a protective agent in mammary carcinogenesis and aberrant colonic crypt foci in rats [385]. On the other hand, dairy cow milk contains conjugated linoleic acid by dietary modification [386]. Conjugated linoleic acid isomers also reported to block lipogenic genes expression in rats [387]. Meat processing and preservation technologies are essential for food security and also to supply good-quality and affordable meat products. Many authors have reported different methods and technologies to extend the shelf life of fresh meat [388].

Animal foods

Some animal foods such as vitamin-like substances, coenzyme Q10, α-lipoic acid and others are considered as physiologically active compounds. According to some reports carnitine is an essential nutrient in infancy [389]. Coenzyme Q10 is a vitamin-like substance and plays an important role in the generation of cellular energy in the human body. It also helps in healthy cardiovascular effects [390]. α-Lipoic acid has been known for its antioxidant activity [391].

Table 5 showing some examples of nutraceutical substances grouped by food source and Table 6 showing some of the food ingredients approved by Food Safety and Standards Authority of India (FSSAI) in India.

Plants	Animal	Microbial
α-Glucan,	Conjugated Linoleic Acid (CLA)	*Saccharomyces boulardii* (yeast)
Ascorbic acid	Coenzyme Q10	*Bifidobacterium bifidum*
γ-Tocotrienol	Eicosapentaenoic acid (EPA)	*B. longum*
Quercetin	Docosahexenoic acid (DHA)	*Lactobacillus acidophilus*(LC1)
Luteolin	Spingolipids	*L. acidophilus* (NCFB 1748)
Gallic acid	Choline	*Streptococcus salvarius* (subs.
Indole-3-carbonol	Calcium	Thermophilus)
Indole-3-carbonol	Selenium	
Pectin	Creatine	
Daidzein	Zinc	
Glutathione	Minerals	
Potassium		
Allicin		
δ-Limonene		
Genestein		
Lycopene		
Hemicellulose		
Lignin		
Capsaicin		
Geraniol		
β-Ionone		
α-Tocopherol		
β-Carotene		
Nordihydrocapsaicin		
Selenium		
Zeaxanthin		
Minerals		
MUFA		

Table 5: Examples of nutraceutical substances grouped by food source [10].

Impact of Urbanization on Health and Functional Food Market

The direct and indirect beneficial effects of functional food depend on environmental factors such as place and time of cultivation. The benefits and risks of functional foods to individuals and populations as a whole must be determined carefully.

Industrialization, globalization and urbanization, these three factors influences Indian life-styles and food habit. In India, incidence of lifestyle related health problems such as diabetes, cardiovascular diseases, hypertension and obesity increasing rapidly [392]. Day by day people are becoming disease prone due to the stressful work and less physical activity [393]. Work related stress leads to many diseases such as hypertension and cardiovascular diseases [392]. Choice of foods and diet structure such as fast food and added sugar in the diet gradually changing the human health quality [394]. In this current scenario functional food plays an important promising role in the healthy human life. Indian consumers' markets are increasing for a healthy food as well as demand of functional foods are increasing in Indian food industry.

Ingredient	Industry Usage	Health Claims
Omega 3 and 6	Functional foods (fortified foods): e.g. omega fortified malted beverages	Prevention from inflammatory and autoimmune diseases, also reducing cholesterol, and hence, various heart risks.
Probiotics	Functional foods: e.g. probiotic Yogurt/dahi improve intestinal microflora and aid better digestive health.	Improve intestinal microflora and aid better digestive health.
Beta glucan	Functional beverages: e.g. soya milk drinks	Soluble fibre that soaks up the cholesterol.
Phytoestrogens	Functional foods: e.g. rice bran fortifies oil	Reduce the risk of many kinds of cancers, cholesterol and risk of coronary heart disease.
Tocopherols	Functional foods: e.g. rice bran fortifies oil	Cholesterol lowering potential. Prevent or delay heart disease and related Complications, cataracts, macular degeneration, prostrate and other cancers.
Ginseng	Dietary supplements: e.g. Tonicsand stimulants	Cures lethargy, arthritis, impotence, senility, ani-aging properties.
Beta-carotene	Dietary supplements: e.g. Beta-carotene in antioxidants	Prevent night blindness, skin problem, enhance immunity, protect toxins and cancers

Table 6: Some of the food ingredients approved by food safety and standards authority of India (FSSAI) in India.

Indian Functional Food and Nutraceutical Market Size and Growth

Among the developing countries, India is the most potential market for nutraceuticals and dietary supplement products. Nutraceuticals market is growing rapidly in comparison to other sectors of Indian food market.

According to Ernst and Young study, Indian functional food market in 2008 was about INR 30 billion, apart from the dietary supplements and it has grown at a CAGR (compound annual growth rate) of 18% as compared to a world average of 7% [392]. Indian functional food market deals with products like fruits, vegetables, fortified juices, energy drinks, fresh dairy products, confectionary, breakfast cereals, and fibre rich foods which imparting the desired health benefits and physiological changes. Main ingredients of these products are probiotics, prebiotics, omega fatty acids fortified foods, tocopherols, phytoestrogens, xylitol, soy, gluten and whey proteins. In 2010, about 116 new functional food products were launched in India [395]. Out of these, 80 products were targeted at enhancing the cardio vascular functioning and the rest 36 at promoting the immunity.

Conclusion

Functional foods are an important part of healthy lifestyle that also includes a balanced diet and physical activity. Functional foods will be successful depending on several factors including their effectiveness, safety, and quality. Our understanding of functional foods by scientific research will enhance the knowledge on long-term health benefits. Some functional dairy products support healthy heart by lowering blood pressure. Epidemiological studies needed to cope with enormous amount of inquiries and demands for functional food all around the world. Probiotics supply necessary bacteria which act as commensals in the gut and form a biofilm by colonizing specific tissue locations. Through quorum sensing these heterogeneous food products provide additional physiological fortification as well as developmental signals. Phytochemicals, micronutrients in food and animal resources, microbes and their metabolic by-products directly or indirectly help mobilize the body's physiological network encompassing the neuro-immuno-endocrine cycles and help maintain optimum health. More future research on food items will expand the existing knowledge of functional food as well as developing specific strategy in the biodiversity management.

References

1. Ashwell M (2002) Concepts of functional foods. International Life Sciences Institute (ILSI) Europe Concise Monograph Series, Brussels.
2. Pushpangadan P, George V, Sreedevi P, Biney AJ, Anzar S, et al. (2014) Functional foods and nutraceuticals with special focus on mother and child care. Annals of Phytomedicine 3: 4-24.
3. DeFelice SL (2002) FIM Rationale and proposed guidelines for the nutraceutical research and education act-NREA.
4. Kalra EK (2003) Nutraceutical--definition and introduction. AAPS PharmSci 5: E25.
5. Henry CJ (2010) Functional foods. Eur J Clin Nutr 64: 657-659.
6. Kumar J, Pal A (2015a) An Overview of Prospective study on Functional Foods. International Journal of Recent Scientific Research Research 6: 5497-5500.
7. Hasler CM (1998) Functional foods: their role in disease prevention and health promotion. Food Technology 52: 57-62.
8. Bagchi D (2008) Neutraceutical and Functional Food Regulations. Elsevier: New York.
9. Roberfroid MB (1999) What is beneficial for health? The concept of functional food. Food Chem Toxicol 37: 1039-1041.
10. Keservani RK, Kesharwani RK, Vyas N (2010) Nutraceutical and Functional Food as Future Food: A Review. Der Pharmacia Lettre 2: 106-116.
11. Texas (2015) Functional Food Center, Dallas, Texas.
12. (2013) USA Food and Beverage Market Study.
13. Block G, Patterson B, Subar A (1992) Fruit, vegetables, and cancer prevention: a review of the epidemiological evidence. Nutr Cancer 18: 1-29.
14. Truswell AS (2002) Cereal grains and coronary heart disease. Eur J Clin Nutr 56: 1-14.
15. Charalampopoulos D, Wang R, Pandiella SS, Webb C (2002) Application of cereals and cereal components in functional foods: a review. Int J Food Microbiol 79: 131-141.
16. Wani SA, Tajamul SR, Bazaria B, Ahmad NG, Amir G, et al. (2014) Oats as a functional food: a review. Universal Journal of Pharmacy 3: 14-20.

17. Malkki Y, Myllymaki O, Teinila K, Koponen S (2004) Method for preparing an oat product and a foodstuff enriched in the content of beta-glucan. US Patent 6: 797-307.
18. Malkki Y, Virtanen E (2001) Gastrointestinal effects of oat bran and oat gum: A review. Lebensm WisS Technol 34: 337-347.
19. Xiao CW (2008) Health effects of soy protein and isoflavones in humans. J Nutr 138: 1244S-9S.
20. Jackson CJC, Dini JP, Lavandier C, Rupasinghe HPV, Faulkner H, et al. (2002) Effects of processing on the content and composition of isoflavones during manufacturing of soy beverage and tofu. Process Biochemistry 37: 1117-1123.
21. Zheng X, Lee SK, Chun OK (2016) Soy Isoflavones and Osteoporotic Bone Loss: A Review with an Emphasis on Modulation of Bone Remodeling. J Med Food 19: 1-14.
22. Song WO, Chun OK, Hwang I, Shin HS, Kim BG, et al. (2007) Soy isoflavones as safe functional ingredients. J Med Food 10: 571-580.
23. Anderson JW, Johnstone BM, Cook-Newell ME (1995) Meta-analysis of the effects of soy protein intake on serum lipids. N Engl J Med 333: 276-282.
24. Davidson M (2008) A review of the current status of the management of mixed dyslipidemia associated with diabetes mellitus and metabolic syndrome. Am J Cardiol 102: 19L-27L.
25. Chen TR, Wei QK (2008) Analysis of bioactive aglycone isoflavones in soybean and soybean products. Nutrition Food Science 38: 540-547.
26. Messina M, Barnes S (1991) The role of soy products in reducing risk of cancer. J Natl Cancer Inst 83: 541-546.
27. Rowland I, Faughnan M, Hoey L, Wähälä K, Williamson G, et al. (2003) Bioavailability of phyto-oestrogens. Br J Nutr 89: S45-S58.
28. Fang CY, Tseng M, Daly MB (2005) Correlates of soy food consumption in women at increased risk for breast cancer. J Am Diet Assoc 105: 1552-1558.
29. Uifălean A, Schneider S, Ionescu C, Lalk M (2015) Soy Isoflavones and Breast Cancer Cell Lines: Molecular Mechanisms and Future Perspectives. Molecules 21: E13.
30. Romani A, Vignolini P, Galardi C, Aroldi C, Vazzana C, et al. (2003) Polyphenolic content in different plant parts of soy cultivars grown under natural conditions. J Agric Food Chem 51: 5301-5306.
31. Rostagno MA, Villares A, Guillamón E, García-Lafuente A, Martínez JA (2009) Sample preparation for the analysis of isoflavones from soybeans and soy foods. J Chromatogr A 1216: 2-29.
32. Messina M, McCaskill-Stevens W, Lampe JW (2006) Addressing the soy and breast cancer relationship: review, commentary, and workshop proceedings. J Natl Cancer Inst 98: 1275-1284.
33. Messina M, Barnes S, Setchell KD (1997) Phyto-oestrogens and breast cancer. Lancet 350: 971-972.
34. Tew BY, Xu X, Wang HJ, Murphy PA, Hendrich S (1996) A diet high in wheat fiber decreases the bioavailability of soybean isoflavones in a single meal fed to women. J Nutr 126: 871-877.
35. Anderson JJB, Garner SC (1997) The effects of phytoestrogens on bone. Nutr Res 17: 1617-1632.
36. Das A, Raychaudhuri U, Chakraborty R (2012) Cereal based functional food of Indian subcontinent: a review. J Food Sci Technol 49: 665-672.
37. Wang M, Hettiarachchy NS, Qi M, Burks W, Siebenmorgen T (1999) Preparation and functional properties of rice bran protein isolate. J Agric Food Chem 47: 411-416.
38. Gurpreet KC, Sogi DS (2007) Functional properties of rice bran protein concentrates. J Food Eng 79: 592-597.
39. Steinkraus KH (1994) Nutritional significance of fermented foods. Food Res Int 27: 259.
40. Chung SI, Rico CW, Lee SC, Kang MY (2016) Instant rice made from white and pigmented giant embryonic rice reduces lipid levels and body weight in high fat diet-fed mice. Obes Res Clin Pract.
41. Choi HD, Kim YS, Choi IU, Park YK, Park YD (2009) Hypotensive effect of germinated brown rice on spontaneously hypertensive rats. Korean Journal of Food Science and Technology 38: 448-451.
42. Kumar J, Kumar J, Singh SP, Tuli R (2014) Association of satellites with a mastrevirus in natural infection: complexity of Wheat dwarf India virus disease. J Virol 88: 7093-7104.
43. Shewry PR (2009) Wheat. J Exp Bot 60: 1537-1553.
44. Sapirstein HD, David P, Preston KR, Dexter JE (2007) Durum wheat bread making quality: Effects of gluten strength, protein composition, semolina particle size and fermentation time. Journal of Cereal Science 45: 150-161.
45. Baublis AJ, Lu C, Clydesdale FM, Decker EA (2000) Potential of wheat-based breakfast cereals as a source of dietary antioxidants. J Am Coll Nutr 19: 308S-311S.
46. Ötles A, Cagindi Ö (2006) Cereal based functional foods and nutraceuticals. Acta Sci Pol Technol Aliment 5: 107-112.
47. Kim KH, Tsao R, Yang R, Cui SW (2006) Phenolic acid profiles and antioxidant activities of sheat bran extracts and the effect of hydrolysis conditions. Food Chem 95: 466-473.
48. Yu L, Nanguet AL, Beta T (2013) Comparison of Antioxidant Properties of Refined and Whole Wheat Flour and Bread. Antioxidants (Basel) 2: 370-383.
49. Shewry PR, Hey SJ (2015) The contribution of wheat to human diet and health. Food and Energy Security 4: 178-202.
50. Saikumar R, Kumar B, Kaul J, Kumar A (2012) Maize research in India-historical prospective and future challenges. Maize Journal 1: 1-6.
51. Nout MJ (2009) Rich nutrition from the poorest-cereal fermentations in Africa and Asia. Food Microbiol 26: 685-692.
52. Lenaerts V, Moussa I, Dumoulin Y, Mebsout F, Chouinard F, et al. (1998) Cross-linked high amylose starch for controlled release of drugs: recent advances. J Control Release 53: 225-234.
53. Autamashih M, Isah AB, Allagh TS, Ibrahim MA (2011) Effects of selected diluents and maize starch mucilage binder on the tablets formulation of the crude aqueous extract of Vernonia galamensis. Int J Pharm Technol 3: 2746-2756.
54. Brennan CS, Cleary LJ (2005) The potential use of cereal (103) (104)-b-D-glucans as functional food ingredients. J Cereal Sci 42: 113.
55. Pins JJ, Kaur H (2006) A review of the effects of barley b-glucan on cardiovascular and diabetic risk. Cereal Foods World 51: 811.
56. Wood P (2010) Oat and rye b-glucan: properties and function. Cereal Chem 87: 315330.
57. Izydorczyk MS, McMillan T, Bazin S, Kletke J, Dushnicky L (2014) Milling of Canadian oats and barley for functional food ingredients: Oat bran and barley fibre-rich fractions. Can J Plant Sci 94: 573-586.
58. Bhatty RS (1999) The potential of hull-less barley. Cereal Chem 76: 589-599.
59. Behall KM, Scholfield DJ, Hallfrisch JG (2002) Fasting glucose and insulin and measures of insulin resistance of men after consumption of whole wheat/brown rice or barley. J Am Col Nutr 21: 486.
60. Amri A, Ouammou L, Nassif F (2005) Barley-Based Food in Southern Morocco. In: Grando S and Gomezmacpherson H (eds.), Food Barley: Importance, Uses, and Local Knowledge. ICARDA, Aleppo.
61. Hulse JH, Laing EM, Pearson OE (1980) Sorghum and the millets: Their composition and nutritive value. London: Academic Press.
62. Gopalan C, Sastri RBV, Balasubramanian SC (2009) Nutritive value of Indian foods. Hyderabad, India: National Institute of Nutrition, Indian Council of Medical Research.
63. Achaya KT (2009) The illustrated food of India A-Z. New Delhi, India: Oxford University Press.
64. Rane AG, Vora JD, Priyanka J (2014) A review on the biochemical, antimicrobial and organoleptic studies on the germination profile of finger millet (Eleusine coracana). Int J Food Sci Nutr Diet 3: 129-133.
65. Malathi D, Nirmalakumari A (2007) Cooking of small millets in Tamil Nadu. In: Krishne Gowda KT, Seetharam A, Food uses of small millets and avenues for further processing and value addition: Indian Council of Agricultural Research. Project Coordination cell, All India Co-ordinated small millets improvement project. Indian Council of Agricultural Research, UAS, GKVK, Bangalore, India.

66. Venkateswaran V, Vijayalakshmi G (2010) Finger millet (Eleusine coracana)-An economically viable source for antihypercholesterolemic metabolites production by Monascus purpureus. Journal of Food Science and Technology 47: 426-431.
67. Shobana S, Sreerama YN, Malleshi NG (2009) Composition and enzyme inhibitory properties of finger millet (Eleusine coracana L.) seed coat phenolics: Mode of inhibition of a-glucosidase and a-amylase. Food Chemistry 115: 1268-1273.
68. Hemalatha S, Platel K, Srinivasan K (2007) Influence of germination and fermentation on bioaccessibility of zinc and iron from food grains. Eur J Clin Nutr 61: 342-348.
69. Sripriya G, Chandrasekharan K, Murthy VS, Chandra TS (1996) ESR spectroscopic studies on free radical quenching action of finger millet (Eleusine coracana). Food Chemistry 57: 537-540.
70. Rao SMV, Muralikrishna G (2002) Evaluation of the antioxidant properties of free and bound phenolic acids from native and malted finger millet (Ragi, Eleusine coracana Indaf-15). Journal of Agricultural and Food Chemistry 50: 889-892.
71. Hegde PS, Rajasekaran NS, Chandra TS (2005) Effects of the antioxidant properties of millet species on oxidative stress and glycemic status in alloxan-induced rats. Nutrition. Research 25: 1109-1120.
72. Varsha V, Urooj A, Malleshi NG (2009) Evaluation of antioxidant and antimicrobial properties of finger millet (Eleusine coracana) polyphenols. Food Chemistry 114: 340-346.
73. Chandrasekara A, Shahidi F (2011) Determination of antioxidant activity in free and hydrolyzed fractions of millet grains and characterization of their phenolic profiles by HPLC-DAD-ESI-MSn. J Functional Foods 3: 144-158.
74. Veenashri BR, Muralikrishna G (2011) In vitro anti-oxidant activity of xylooligosaccharides derived from cereal and millet brans-A comparative study. Food Chemistry 126: 1475-1481.
75. Antony U, Moses LG, Chandra TS (1998) Inhibition of Salmonella typhimurium and Escherichia coli by fermented flour of finger millet. World. J Microbiology Biotechnology 14: 883-886.
76. Chethan S, Malleshi NG (2007) Finger millet polyphenols: Characterization and their nutraceutical potential. American. Journal Food Technology 2: 582-592.
77. Hegde PS, Chandrakasan G, Chandra TS (2002) Inhibition of collagen glycation and crosslinking in vitro by methanolic extracts of finger millet (Eleusine coracana) and kodo millet (Paspalum scrobiculatum). The Journal of Nutritional Biochemistry 13: 517-521.
78. Chethan S, Dharmesh MS, Malleshi NG (2008) Inhibition of aldose reductase from cataracted eye lenses by finger millet (Eleusine coracana) polyphenols. Bioorganic. Medicinal. Chemistry 16: 10085-10090.
79. Lazaro EL, Favier JF (2000) Alkaline debranning of sorghum and millet. American Association of Cereal Chemists 77: 717-719.
80. Shih CH, Siu SO, Ng R, Wong E, Chiu LC, et al. (2007) Quantitative analysis of anticancer 3-deoxyanthocyanidins in infected sorghum seedlings. J Agric Food Chem 55: 254-259.
81. Awika JM, Yang L, Browning JD, Faraj A (2009) Comparative antioxidant, antiproliferative and phase II enzyme inducing potential of sorghum (Sorghum bicolor) varieties. LWT-Food Science and Technology 42: 1041-1046.
82. Yang L, Browning JD, Awika JM (2009) Sorghum 3-deoxyanthocyanins possess strong phase II enzyme inducer activity and cancer cell growth inhibition properties. Journal of Agricultural and Food Chemistry 57: 1797-1804.
83. Devi PS, Kumar MS, Das SM (2011) Evaluation of antiproliferative activity of red sorghum bran anthocyanin on a human breast cancer cell line (mcf-7). Int J Breast Cancer 2011: 891481.
84. Woo HJ, Oh IT, Lee JY, Jun DY, Seu MC (2012) Apigeninidin induces apoptosis through activation of Bak and Bax and subsequent mediation of mitochondrial damage in human promyelocytic leukemia HL-60 cells. Process Biochemistry 47: 1861-1871.
85. Park JH, Darvin P, Lim EJ, Joung YH, Hong DY, et al. (2012) Hwanggeumchal sorghum induces cell cycle arrest, and suppresses tumor growth and metastasis through Jak2/STAT pathways in breast cancer xenografts. PLoS One 7: e40531.
86. Hwang JM, Choi KC, Bang SJ, Son YO, Kim BT, et al. (2013) Anti-oxidant and anti-inflammatory properties of methanol extracts from various crops. Food Science and Biotechnology 22: 265-272.
87. Cardoso LM, Pinheiro SS, Martino SHD, Pinheiro-Sant'Ana HM (2015) Sorghum (sorghum bicolor l): nutrients, bioactive compounds, and potential impact on human health. Critical Reviews in Food Science and Nutrition.
88. Severson DK (1998) Lactic acid fermentations. In: Nagodawithana TW and Reed G (eds.), Nutritional Requirements of Commercially Important Microorganisms. Milwaukee: Esteekay Associates, pp: 258-297.
89. Rubnov S, Kashman Y, Rabinowitz R, Schlesinger M, Mechoulam R (2001) Suppressors of cancer cell proliferation from fig (Ficus carica) resin: isolation and structure elucidation. J Nat Prod 64: 993-996.
90. Jeong MR, Cha JD, Lee YE (2005) Antibacterial activity of Korean Fig (Ficus carica L.) against food poisoning bacteria. Korean J Food Cookery Sci 21: 84-93.
91. Perez C, Dominguez E, Ramiro JM, Campillo JE, Torres MD (1998)A study on the glycemic balance in streptozotocin-diabetic rats treated with an aqueous extract of Ficus carica (fig tree) leaves. Phytotherapy Research 10: 82-83.
92. Canal JR, Torres MD, Romero A, Pérez C (2000) A chloroform extract obtained from a decoction of Ficus carica leaves improves the cholesterolaemic status of rats with streptozotocin-induced diabetes. Acta Physiol Hung 87: 71-76.
93. Patil VV, Bhangale SC, Patil VR (2010) Evaluation of antipyretic potential of Ficuscarica Leaves. Int J of Pharmaceutical Sciences Review and Research 2: 48.
94. Mi-Ran J, Kim HY, Dan JC (2009) Antimicrobial activity of methanol extract from Ficuscarica leaves against oral bacteria. Journal of Bacteriology and Virology 39: 97-102.
95. Al-Yousuf HHH (2012) Antibacterial activity of Ficus carica L. extract against six bacterial strains. Int J Drug Dev and Res 4: 307-310.
96. Aref HL, Salah KB, Chaumont JP, Fekih A, Aouni M, et al. (2010) In vitro antimicrobial activity of four Ficus carica latex fractions against resistant human pathogens (antimicrobial activity of Ficus carica latex). Pak J Pharm Sci 23: 53-58.
97. Yang XM, Yu W, Ou ZP, Ma HL, Liu WM, et al. (2009) Antioxidant and immunity activity of water extract and crude polysaccharide from Ficus carica L. fruit. Plant Foods Hum Nutr 64: 167-173.
98. Gilani AH, Mehmood MH, Janbaz KH, Khan AU, Saeed SA (2008) Ethnopharmacological studies on antispasmodic and antiplatelet activities of Ficus carica. J Ethnopharmacol 119: 1-5.
99. Trifunschi SI (2012) Determination of the antioxidant activity of Ficuscarica aqueous extract. Proceedings of the National Academy of Sciences 122: 25-31.
100. Naghdi M, Maghbool M, Seifalah-Zade M, Mahaldashtian M, Makoolati Z, et al. (2016) Effects of common fig (Ficus carica) leaf extracts on sperm parameters and testis of mice intoxicated with formaldehyde. Evidence-Based Complementary and Alternative Medicine 2016: 1-9.
101. O'Brien TG, Kinniar MF, Silver SC (1998) What's so special about figs? Nature 392: 668.
102. Gond NY, Khadabadi SS (2008) Hepatoprotective Activity of Ficus carica Leaf Extract on Rifampicin-Induced Hepatic Damage in Rats. Indian J Pharm Sci 70: 364-366.
103. Saxena A, Vikram NK (2004) Role of selected Indian plants in management of type 2 diabetes: a review. J Altern Complement Med 10: 369-378.
104. Wang E, Wylie-Rosett J (2008) Review of selected Chinese herbal medicines in the treatment of type 2 diabetes. Diabetes Educ 34: 645-654.
105. Ramesh HP, Yamaki K, Ono H, Tsushida T (2001) Two-dimensional NMR spectroscopic studies of fenugreek (Trigonella foenum-graecum L.) galactomannan without chemical fragmentation. Carbohydrate Polymers

45: 69-77.
106. Blank I (1996) The flavor principle of fenugreek. Nestlé research center. 211th ACS Symposium, New Orleans.
107. Senthil A, Mamatha BS, Vishwanath P, Bhat KK, Ravishankar GA (2011) Studies on development and storage stability of instant spice adjunct mix from seaweed (Eucheuma). J Food Sci Technol 48: 712-717.
108. Singhal PC, Gupta RK, Joshi LD (1982) Hypocholesterolmic effect of seeds. Current Science 51: 136-137.
109. Basch E, Ulbricht C, Kuo G, Szapary P, Smith M (2003) Therapeutic applications of fenugreek. Altern Med Rev 8: 20-27.
110. Uemura T, Goto T, Kang MS, Mizoguchi N, Hirai S, et al. (2011) Diosgenin, the main aglycon of fenugreek, inhibits LXRα activity in HepG2 cells and decreases plasma and hepatic triglycerides in obese diabetic mice. J Nutr 141: 17-23.
111. Kumar P, Kale RK, McLean P, Baquer NZ (2012) Antidiabetic and neuroprotective effects of Trigonella foenum-graecum seed powder in diabetic rat brain. Prague Med Rep 113: 33-43.
112. Grover JK, Yadav S, Vats V (2002) Medicinal plants of India with anti-diabetic potential. J Ethnopharmacol 81: 81-100.
113. Srinivasan K (2006) Fenugreek (Trigonella foenum-graecum): A Review of Health Beneficial Physiological Effects. Food Reviews International 22: 203-224.
114. Koupý D, Kotolová H, Rudá Kučerová J (2015) [Effectiveness of phytotherapy in supportive treatment of type 2 diabetes mellitus II. Fenugreek (Trigonella foenum-graecum)]. Ceska Slov Farm 64: 67-71.
115. Fuller S, Stephens JM (2015) Diosgenin, 4-hydroxyisoleucine, and fiber from fenugreek: mechanisms of actions and potential effects on metabolic syndrome. Adv Nutr 6: 189-197.
116. Sangeetha MK, ShriShri Mal N, Atmaja K, Sali VK, Vasanthi HR (2013) PPAR's and Diosgenin a chemico biological insight in NIDDM. Chem Biol Interact 206: 403-410.
117. Tharaheswari M, Reddy JN, Kumar R, Varshney KC, Kannan M, et al. (2014) Trigonelline and diosgenin attenuate ER stress, oxidative stress-mediated damage in pancreas and enhance adipose tissue PPARgamma activity in type 2 diabetic rats. Mol Cell Biochem 396: 161-174.
118. Saravanan G, Ponmurugan P, Deepa MA, Senthilkumar B (2014) Modulatory effects of diosgenin on attenuating the key enzymes activities of carbohydrate metabolism and glycogen content in streptozotocin-induced diabetic rats. Can J Diabetes 38: 409-414.
119. Bahmani M, Shirzad H, Mirhosseini M, Mesripour A, Rafieian-Kopaei M (2016) A Review on Ethnobotanical and Therapeutic Uses of Fenugreek (Trigonella foenum-graceum L). J Evid Based Complementary Altern Med 21: 53-62.
120. Roberts KT (2011) The potential of fenugreek (Trigonella foenum-graecum) as a functional food and nutraceutical and its effects on glycemia and lipidemia. J Med Food 14: 1485-1489.
121. Kumar P, Bhandari U, Jamadagni S (2014) Fenugreek seed extract inhibit fat accumulation and ameliorates dyslipidemia in high fat diet-induced obese rats. Biomed Res Int 2014: 606021.
122. Hannan JM, Rokeya B, Faruque O, Nahar N, Mosihuzzaman M, et al. (2003) Effect of soluble dietary fibre fraction of Trigonella foenum graecum on glycemic, insulinemic, lipidemic and platelet aggregation status of Type 2 diabetic model rats. J Ethnopharmacol 88: 73-77.
123. Hannan JMA, Ali L, Rokeya B, Khaleque J, Akhter M, et al. (2007) Soluble dietary fibre fraction of Trigonella foenumgraecum (fenugreek) seed improves glucose homeostasis in animal models of type 1 and type 2 diabetes by delaying carbohydrate digestion and absorption, and enhancing insulin action. Br J Nutr 97: 514-521.
124. Thomas JE, Bandara M, Lee EL, Driedger D, Acharya S (2011) Biochemical monitoring in fenugreek to develop functional food and medicinal plant variants. N Biotechnol 28: 110-117.
125. Singh V, Garg AN (2006) Availability of essential trace elements in Indian cereals, vegetables and spices using INAA and the contribution of spices to daily dietary intake. Food Chem 94: 81-89.
126. Meghwal M, Goswami TK (2012) A Review on the Functional Properties, Nutritional Content, Medicinal Utilization and Potential Application of Fenugreek. J Food Process Technol 3: 9.
127. Leela NK, Shafeekh KM (2008) Fenugreek, Chemistry of Spices. CAB International, Pondicherry, India.
128. Li SP, Zhang GH, Zeng Q, Huang ZG, Wang YT, et al. (2006) Hypoglycemic activity of polysaccharide, with antioxidation, isolated from cultured Cordyceps mycelia. Phytomedicine 13: 428-433.
129. Yue K, Ye M, Zhou Z, Sun W, Lin X (2013) The genus Cordyceps: a chemical and pharmacological review. J Pharm Pharmacol 65: 474-493.
130. Tuli HS, Sharma AK, Sandhu SS, Kashyap D (2013) Cordycepin: a bioactive metabolite with therapeutic potential. Life Sci 93: 863-869.
131. Paterson RR (2008) Cordyceps: a traditional Chinese medicine and another fungal therapeutic biofactory? Phytochemistry 69: 1469-1495.
132. Han ES, Oh JY, Park HJ (2011) Cordyceps militaris extract suppresses dextran sodium sulfate-induced acute colitis in mice and production of inflammatory mediators from macrophages and mast cells. J Ethnopharmacology 134: 703-710.
133. Zhu JL, Liu C (1992) Modulating effects of extractum semen Persicae and cultivated Cordyceps hyphae on immuno-dysfunction of inpatients with posthepatitic cirrhosis. Zhongguo Zhong Xi Yi Jie He Za Zhi 12: 207-209.
134. Park DK, Choi WS, Park HJ (2012a) Antiallergic activity of novel isoflavone methylglycosides from Cordyceps militaris grown on germinated soybeans in antigen-stimulated mast cells. Journal of Agricultural and Food Chemistry 60: 2309-2315.
135. Nakamura K, Shinozuka K, Yoshikawa N (2015) Anticancer and antimetastatic effects of cordycepin, an active component of Cordyceps sinensis. J Pharmacol Sci 127: 53-56.
136. Reis FS, Barros L, Calhelha RC, Ciric´A, Van Griensven LJLD, et al. (2013) The methanolic extract of Cordyceps militaris (L.) Link fruiting body shows antioxidant, antibacterial, antifungal and antihuman tumor cell lines properties. Food Chemical and Toxicology 62: 91-98.
137. Tolkachev ON, Zhuchenko AA Jr (2000) Biologically active substances of flax: medicinal and nutritional properties (a review). Pharmaceutical Chemistry Journal 34: 360-367.
138. Singh KK, Mridula D, Rehal J, Barnwal P (2011) Flaxseed: a potential source of food, feed and fiber. Crit Rev Food Sci Nutr 51: 210-222.
139. Oomah BD, Mazza G (1998) Compositional changes during commercial processing of flaxseed. Ind Crop Prod 9: 29-37.
140. Oomah BD (2001) Flaxseed as a functional food source. J Sci Food Agric 81: 889-894.
141. Thompson LU, Robb P, Serraino M, Cheung F (1991) Mammalian lignan production from various foods. Nutr Cancer 16: 43-52.
142. Kamal-Eldin A, Peerlkamp N, Johnsson P, Andersson R, Andersson RE, et al. (2001) An oligomer from flaxseed composed of secoisolariciresinoldiglucoside and 3-hydroxy-3-methyl glutaric acid residues. Phytochemistry 58: 587-590.
143. Maggio M, Artoni A, Lauretani F, Borghi L, Nouvenne A, et al. (2009) The impact of omega-3 fatty acids on osteoporosis. Curr Pharm Des 15: 4157-4164.
144. Rodriguez-Leyva D, Dupasquier CM, McCullough R, Pierce GN (2010) The cardiovascular effects of flaxseed and its omega-3 fatty acid, alpha-linolenic acid. Can J Cardiol 26: 489-496.
145. Goyal A, Sharma V, Upadhyay N, Gill S, Sihag M (2014) Flax and flaxseed oil: an ancient medicine and modern functional food. J Food Sci Technol 51: 1633-1653.
146. Bierenbaum ML, Reichstein R, Watkins TR (1993) Reducing atherogenic risk in hyperlipemic humans with flax seed supplementation: a preliminary report. J Am Coll Nutr 12: 501-504.
147. Cunnane SC, Ganguli S, Menard C, Liede AC, Hamadeh MJ, et al. (1993) High alpha-linolenic acid flaxseed (Linum usitatissimum): some nutritional properties in humans. Br J Nutr 69: 443-453.
148. Allman MA, Pena MM, Pang D (1995) Supplementation with flaxseed oil versus sunflowerseed oil in healthy young men consuming a low fat diet: effects on platelet composition and function. Eur J Clin Nutr 49: 169-178.
149. Setchell KD, Lawson AM, Mitchell FL, Adlercreutz H, Kirk DN, et al.

(1980) Lignans in man and in animal species. Nature 287: 740-742.

150. Setchell KD, Lawson AM, Borriello SP, Harkness R, Gordon H, et al. (1981) Lignan formation in man--microbial involvement and possible roles in relation to cancer. Lancet 2: 4-7.
151. Adlercreutz H, Fotsis T, Bannwart C, Hämäläinen E, Bloigu S, et al. (1986) Urinary estrogen profile determination in young Finnish vegetarian and omnivorous women. J Steroid Biochem 24: 289-296.
152. Adlercreutz H (1988) Lignans and phytoestrogens. Possible preventative role in cancer. In: Frontiers of Gastrointestinal Research, Rozen P, Karger, Basel.
153. Adlercreutz H (1990) Western diet and Western diseases: some hormonal and biochemical mechanisms and associations. Scand J Clin Lab Invest Suppl 201: 3-23.
154. Adlercreutz H, Honjo H, Higashi A, Fotsis T, Hämäläinen E, et al. (1991) Urinary excretion of lignans and isoflavanoid phytoestrogens in Japanese men and women consuming a traditional Japansese diet. American Journal of Clinical Nutrition 54: 1093-1100.
155. Serraino M, Thompson LU (1992) The effect of flaxseed supplementation on the initiation and promotional stages of mammary tumorigenesis. Nutr Cancer 17: 153-159.
156. Kashtan H, Stern HS, Jenkins DJ, Jenkins AL, Thompson LU, et al. (1992) Colonic fermentation and markers of colorectal-cancer risk. Am J Clin Nutr 55: 723-728.
157. Mousavi Y, Adlercreutz H (1992) Enterolactone and estradiol inhibit each other's proliferative effect on MCF-7 breast cancer cells in culture. Journal of Steroid Biochemistry and Molecular Biology 41: 615-619.
158. Sathyamoorthy N, Wang TT, Phang JM (1994) Stimulation of pS2 expression by diet-derived compounds. Cancer Res 54: 957-961.
159. Adlercreutz H (1995) Phytoestrogens: epidemiology and a possible role in cancer protection. Environ Health Perspect 103: 103-112.
160. Westcott ND, Muir AD (1996) Variation in the concentration of the flax seed lignan concentration with variety, location and year. In: Proceedings of the 56th Flax Institute of the United States Conference, Flax Institute of the United States, Fargo, ND.
161. Thompson LU, Seidl MM, Rickard SE, Orcheson LJ, Fong HH (1996) Antitumorigenic effect of a mammalian lignan precursor from flaxseed. Nutr Cancer 26: 159-165.
162. Adlercreutz H (1996a) Lignans and isoflavonoids: Epidemiology and a possible role in prevention of cancer. In: Natural Antioxidants and Food Quality in Atherosclerosis and Cancer Prevention. Kumpulainen, Salonen JT, The Royal Society of Chemistry, London.
163. Adlercreutz H (1996b) Phytoestrogens from biochemistry to prevention of cancer and other diseases. In: The 8th International Congress on Menopause, Sydney, Australia.
164. Jenab M, Thompson LU (1996) The influence of flaxseed and lignans on colon carcinogenesis and beta-glucuronidase activity. Carcinogenesis 17: 1343-1348.
165. Ingram D, Sanders K, Kolybaba M, Lopez D (1997) Case-control study of phyto-oestrogens and breast cancer. Lancet 350: 990-994.
166. Muir AD, Westcott ND, Prasad K (1999) Extraction, purification and animal model testing of an anti-artherosclerotic lignan secoisolariciresinol digluoside from flaxseed (Linum usitatissmum). Acta Hort 501: 245-248.
167. Thompson LU (1999) Role of lignans in carcinogenesis, in phytochemicals in human health protection, nutrition, and plant defense. In: Romeo JT (ed.), Recent Advance in Phytochemistry, Kluwer, New York.
168. Rickard SE, Yuan YV, Thompson LU (2000) Plasma insulin-like growth factor I levels in rats are reduced by dietary supplementation of flaxseed or its lignan secoisolariciresinol diglycoside. Cancer Lett 161: 47-55.
169. Morris DH (2001) Essential nutrients and other functional compounds in flaxseed. Nutrition Today 36: 159-162.
170. Ohr ML (2002) A growing arnesal against cancer. Food Technology 56: 67-71.
171. Westcott ND, Muir AD (2003) Chemical studies on the constituents of Linuum spp. In: Flax, The Genus Linum Muir, AD and Westcott, Taylor and Francis, London.
172. Thompson LU (1995) In: Flaxseed in Human Nutrition. Cunnane SC and Thompson LU (eds.), Champaign, IL: AOCS Press.
173. Thompson LU, Rickard SE, Cheung F, Kenaschuk EO, Obermeyer WR (1997) Variability in anticancer lignan levels in flaxseed. Nutr Cancer 27: 26-30.
174. Oikarinen SI, Pajari AM, Salminen I, Heinonen SM, Adlercreutz H, et al. (2005) Effects of a flaxseed mixture and plant oils rich in alpha-linolenic acid on the adenoma formation in multiple intestinal neoplasia (Min) mice. Br J Nutr 94: 510-518.
175. Bommareddy A, Arasada BL, Mathees DP, Dwivedi C (2006) Chemopreventive effects of dietary flaxseed on colon tumor development. Nutr Cancer 54: 216-222.
176. Bommareddy A, Zhang X, Schrader D, Kaushik RS, Zeman D, et al. (2009) Effects of dietary flaxseed on intestinal tumorigenesis in Apc(Min) mouse. Nutr Cancer 61: 276-283.
177. Yan L, Yee JA, Li D, McGuire MH, Thompson LU (1998) Dietary flaxseed supplementation and experimental metastasis of melanoma cells in mice. Cancer Lett 124: 181-186.
178. Bergman JM, Thompson LU, Dabrosin C (2007) Flaxseed and its lignans inhibit estradiol-induced growth, angiogenesis, and secretion of vascular endothelial growth factor in human breast cancer xenografts in vivo. Clin Cancer Res 13: 1061-1067.
179. Mason JK, Thompson LU (2014) Flaxseed and its lignan and oil components: can they play a role in reducing the risk of and improving the treatment of breast cancer? Appl Physiol Nutr Metab 39: 663-678.
180. Lin X, Gingrich JR, Bao W, Li J, Haroon ZA, et al. (2002) Effect of flaxseed supplementation on prostatic carcinoma in transgenic mice. Urology 60: 919-924.
181. Boccardo F, Lunardi G, Guglielmini P, Parodi M, Murialdo R, et al. (2004) Serum enterolactone levels and the risk of breast cancer in women with palpable cysts. Eur J Cancer 40: 84-89.
182. Demark-Wahnefried W, Polascik TJ, George SL, Switzer BR, Madden JF, et al. (2008) Flaxseed supplementation (not dietary fat restriction) reduces prostate cancer proliferation rates in men presurgery. Cancer Epidemiol Biomarkers Prev 17: 3577-3587.
183. Phipps WR, Martini MC, Lampe JW, Slavin JL, Kurzer MS (1993) Effect of flax seed ingestion on the menstrual cycle. J Clin Endocrinol Metab 77: 1215-1219.
184. Hendawi MY, Alam RT, Abdellatief SA (2016) Ameliorative effect of flaxseed oil against thiacloprid-induced toxicity in rats: hematological, biochemical, and histopathological study. Environ Sci Pollut Res Int 23: 11855-11863.
185. Carotenuto F, Costa A, Albertini MC, Luigi Rocchi MB, Rudov A, et al. (2016) Dietary flaxseed mitigates impaired skeletal muscle regeneration: in vivo, in vitro and in silico Studies. International Journal of Medical Sciences 13: 206-219.
186. Gerster H (1997) The potential role of lycopene for human health. J Am Coll Nutr 16: 109-126.
187. Santos-Sánchez NF, Valadez-Blanco R, Salas-Coronado R (2013) Factors affecting the antioxidant content of fresh tomatoes and their processed products. In: Tomatoes: Cultivation, Varieties and Nutrition. Higashide T, Nova Science Publishers, Hauppauge, NY, USA.
188. Luna-Guevara ML, Hernández-Carranza P, Luna-Guevara JJ, Flores-Sánchez R, Ochoa-Velasco CE, et al. (2015) Effect of sonication and blanching postharvest treatments on physicochemical characteristics and antioxidant compounds of tomatoes: Fresh and refrigerated. Academia Journal of Agricultural Research 3: 127-131.
189. Takagi K, Toyoda M, Shimizu M, Satoh T, Saito Y (1994) Determination of tomatine in foods by liquid chromatography after derivatization. J Chromatogr A 659: 127-131.
190. Leonardi C, Ambrosino P, Esposito F, Fogliano V (2000) Antioxidative activity and carotenoid and tomatine contents in different typologies of fresh consumption tomatoes. J Agric Food Chem 48: 4723-4727.

191. Friedman M (2002) Tomato glycoalkaloids: role in the plant and in the diet. J Agric Food Chem 50: 5751-5780.
192. Giovanelli G, Paradiso A (2002) Stability of dried and intermediate moisture tomato pulp during storage. J Agric Food Chem 50: 7277-7281.
193. George B, Kaur C, Khurdiya DS, Kapoor HC (2004) Antioxidants in tomato (Lycopersium esculentum) as a function of genotype. Food Chem 84: 45-51.
194. Toor RK, Savage GP (2005) Antioxidant activity in different fractions of tomatoes. Food Res Int 38: 487-494.
195. Canene-Adams K, Campbell JK, Zaripheh S, Jeffery EH, Erdman JW Jr (2005) The tomato as a functional food. J Nutr 135: 1226-1230.
196. Juroszek P, Lumpkin HM, Yang RY, Ledesma DR, Ma CH (2009) Fruit quality and bioactive compounds with antioxidant activity of tomatoes grown on-farm: comparison of organic and conventional management systems. J Agric Food Chem 57: 1188-1194.
197. Slimestad R, Verheul M (2009) Review of flavonoids and other phenolics from fruits of different tomato (Lycopersicon esculentum Mill.) cultivars. J Sci Food Agric 89: 1255-1270.
198. Giovannucci E, Ascherio A, Rimm EB, Stampfer MJ, Colditz GA, et al. (1995) Intake of carotenoids and retinol in relation to risk of prostate cancer. J Natl Cancer Inst 87: 1767-1776.
199. Graff RE, Pettersson A, Lis RT, Ahearn TU, Markt SC, et al. (2016) Dietary lycopene intake and risk of prostate cancer defined by ERG protein expression. Am J Clin Nutr 103: 851-860.
200. Clinton SK (1998) Lycopene: chemistry, biology, and implications for human health and disease. Nutr Rev 56: 35-51.
201. Weisburger JH (1998) International Symposium on Lycopene and Tomato Products in Disease Prevention: an introduction. Proc Soc Exp Biol Med 218: 93-94.
202. Böhm F, Tinkler JH, Truscott TG (1995) Carotenoids protect against cell membrane damage by the nitrogen dioxide radical. Nat Med 1: 98-99.
203. Woodall AA, Lee SW, Weesie RJ, Jackson MJ, Britton G (1997) Oxidation of carotenoids by free radicals: relationship between structure and reactivity. Biochim Biophys Acta 1336: 33-42.
204. Di Mascio P, Kaiser S, Sies H (1989) Lycopene as the most efficient biological carotenoid singlet oxygen quencher. Arch Biochem Biophys 274: 532-538.
205. Chang KJ, Cheong SH (2007) The effect of fermented milk supplement with tomato (Lycopersion esculentum) on blood lipid profiles in ovariectomy-induced hyperlipidemic female rats. FASEB J 21: 1086.
206. Hsu YM, Lai CH, Chang CY, Fan CT, Chen CT, et al. (2008) Characterizing the lipid-lowering effects and antioxidant mechanisms of tomato paste. Biosci Biotechnol Biochem 72: 677-685.
207. Friedman M (2013) Anticarcinogenic, cardioprotective, and other health benefits of tomato compounds lycopene, a-tomatine, and tomatidine in pure form and in fresh and processed tomatoes. J Agric Food Chem 61: 9534-9550.
208. Lee LC, Wei L, Huang WC, Hsu YJ, Chen YM, et al. (2015) Hypolipidemic Effect of Tomato Juice in Hamsters in High Cholesterol Diet-Induced Hyperlipidemia. Nutrients 7: 10525-10537.
209. Das D, Vimala R, Das N (2010) Functional foods in Natural Origin-An Overview. Indian Journal Natural Products Resources 1: 136-142.
210. Satyavati GV, Raina MK, Sharma M (1976) Medicinal Plants of India. Indian Council of Medical Research, New Delhi 1: 201-206.
211. Bradley PR (1992) British Herbal Compendium. British Herbal Medicine Association, Bournemouth, Dorset, UK.
212. Chonoko UG, Rufai AB (2011) Phytochemical screening and antibacterial activity of Cucurbita pepo(Pumpkin) against Staphylococcus aureus and Salmonella typhi. Bayero Journal of Pure and Applied Sciences 4: 145-147.
213. Caili F, Huan S, Quanhong L (2006) A review on pharmacological activities and utilization technologies of pumpkin. Plant Foods Hum Nutr 61: 73-80.
214. Eynard AR, Cejas V, Silva R, Quiroga P, Muñoz S (1992) Histopathology of essential fatty acid-deficient mice. Nutrition 8: 37-40.
215. Murkovic M, Hillebrand A, Winkler J, Pfannhauser W (1996) Variability of vitamin E content in pumpkin seeds (Cucurbita pepo L.). Eur Food Res Technol 202: 275-278.
216. Liu HW (2001) Determination of 4-aminobutyric acid in pumpkin powder by high performance liquid chromatography. Se Pu 19: 532-533.
217. Lovejoy JC (2002) The influence of dietary fats in insulin resistance. Curr Diab Rep 2: 430-440.
218. Stevenson DG, Eller FJ, Wang L, Jane JL, Wang T, et al. (2007) Oil and tocopherol content and composition of pumpkin seed oil in 12 cultivars. J Agric Food Chem 55: 4005-4013.
219. Kulaitiene J, Jariene E, Danilcenko H (2007) Oil pumpkins seeds and their quality. Pol J Food Nutr Sci 57: 349-352.
220. Gossell-Williams M, Lyttle K, Clarke T, Gardner M, Simon O (2008) Supplementation with pumpkin seed oil improves plasma lipid profile and cardiovascular outcomes of female nonovariectomized and ovariectomized Sprague-Dawley rats. Phytotherapy Res 22: 873-877.
221. Ardabili G, Farhoosh R, Khodaparast MHH (2011) Chemical composition and physicochemical properties of pumpkin seeds (Cucurbita pepo Subsp. pepo Var. Styriaka) grown in Iran. J Agr Sci Tech 13: 1053-1063.
222. Srbinoska M, Hrabovski N, Rafajlovska V, Fišer SS (2012) Characterizaation of the seed and seed extracts of the Pompkins Cucurbita maxima and Cucurbita pepo L. from Macedonia. Macedonian Journal of Chemistry and Chemical Engineering 31: 65-78.
223. Smith BD (1997) The initial domestication of Cucurbita pepo in the Americas 10,000 years ago. Sci 276: 932-934.
224. Wang XL, Liu J, Chen ZHB, Gao F, Liu JX, et al. (2001) Preliminary study on pharmacologically effect of Curcurbita pepo cv Dayanggua. J Trad Chin Vet Med 20: 6-9.
225. Park SC, Lee JR, Kim JY, Hwang I, Nah JW, et al. (2010) Pr-1, a novel antifungal protein from pumpkin rinds. Biotechnol Lett 32: 125-130.
226. Gill NS, Bali M (2011) Isolation of anti ulcer cucurbitane type triterpenoid from the seeds of Cucurbita pepo. Research Journal of Phytochemistry 5: 70-79.
227. Shrivastava A, Gupta VB (2012) Various treatment options for benign prostatic hyperplasia: A current update. J Midlife Health 3: 10-19.
228. Rathinavelu A, Levy A, Sivanesan D, Gossell-Williams M (2013) Cytotoxic effect of pumpkin (Cucurbita pepo) seed extracts in LNCAP prostate cancer cells is mediated through apoptosis. Current Topics in Nutraceutical Research 11: 137.
229. Tomar PP, Kumar N, Singh A, Selvakumar P, Roy P (2014) Characterization of anticancer, DNase and antifungal activity of pumpkin 2S albumin. Biochemical and Biophysical Research Communications 448: 349-354.
230. Vorobyova OA, Bolshakova AE, Pegova RA, Kol'chik OV, Klabukova IN, et al. (2014) Analysis of the components of pumpkin seed oil in suppositories and the possibility of its use in pharmaceuticals. Journal of Chemical and Pharmaceutical Research 6: 1106-1116.
231. Sedigheh A, Jamal MS, Mahbubeh S, Somayeh K, Mahmoud RK, et al. (2011) Hypoglycaemic and hypolipidemic effects of pumpkin (Cucurbita pepo L.) on alloxan-induced diabetic rats. African Journal of Pharmacy and Pharmacology 5: 2620-2626.
232. Jia W, Gao W, Tang L (2003) Antidiabetic herbal drugs officially approved in China. Phytother Res 17: 1127-1134.
233. Alarcon-Aguilar FJ, Hernandez-Galicia E, Campos-Sepulveda AE (2002) Evaluation of the hypoglycemic effect of Cucurbita ficifolia Bouche (Cucurbitaceae) in different experimental models. J Ethnopharmacol 82: 185-189.
234. Xia T, Wang Q (2007) Hypoglycaemic role of Cucurbita ficifolia (Cucurbitaceae) fruit extract in streptozotocin induced diabetic rats. J Sci Food Agric 87: 1753-1757.
235. Jian Z, Du Q (2011) Glucose-lowering activity of novel tetrasaccharide glyceroglycolipids from the fruits of Cucurbita moschata. Bioorg Med Chem Lett 21: 1001-1003.
236. Díaz-Flores M, Angeles-Mejia S, Baiza-Gutman LA, Medina-Navarro R,

Hernández-Saavedra D, et al. (2012) Effect of an aqueous extract of Cucurbita ficifolia Bouché on the glutathione redox cycle in mice with STZ-induced diabetes. J Ethnopharmacol 144: 101-108.

237. Jin H, Zhang YJ, Jiang JX, Zhu LY, Chen P, et al. (2013) Studies on the extraction of pumpkin components and their biological effects on blood glucose of diabetic mice. Journal of food and drug analysis 21: 184-189.

238. Teugwa CM, Boudjeko T, Tchinda BT, Mejiato PC, Zofou D (2013) Anti-hyperglycaemic globulins from selected Cucurbitaceae seeds used as antidiabetic medicinal plants in Africa. BMC Complement Altern Med 13: 63.

239. Bharti SK, Kumar A, Sharma NK, Prakash BO, Kumar S, et al. (2013) Tocopherol from seeds of Cucurbita pepo against diabetes: Validation by in vivo experiments supported by computational docking. J Formosan Med Assoc 112: 676-690.

240. Gutierrez RMP (2016) Review of Cucurbita pepo (Pumpkin) its phytochemistry and pharmacology. Med Chem 6: 12-21.

241. Acosta-Patiño JL, Jiménez-Balderas E, Juárez-Oropeza MA, Díaz-Zagoya JC (2001) Hypoglycemic action of Cucurbita ficifolia on Type 2 diabetic patients with moderately high blood glucose levels. J Ethnopharmacol 77: 99-101.

242. Fruhwirth GO, Hermetter A (2007) Seeds and oil of the Styrian oil pumpkin: Components and biological activities. Eur J Lipid Sci Technol 109: 1128-1140.

243. Makni M, Fetoui H, Gargouri NK, Garoui el M, Jaber H, et al. (2008) Hypolipidemic and hepatoprotective effects of flax and pumpkin seed mixture rich in omega-3 and omega-6 fatty acids in hypercholesterolemic rats. Food Chem Toxicol 46: 3714-3720.

244. Seif HAS (2014) Ameliorative effect of pumpkin oil (Cucurbita pepo L.) against alcohol-induced hepatotoxicity and oxidative stress in albino rats. Beni-suef University Journal of Basic and Applied Sciences 3: 178-185.

245. Medjakovic S, Hobiger S, Ardjomand-Woelkart K, Bucar F, Jungbauer A (2016) Pumpkin seed extract: Cell growth inhibition of hyperplastic and cancer cells, independent of steroid hormone receptors. Fitoterapia 110: 150-156.

246. Rahman K (2003) Garlic and aging: new insights into an old remedy. Ageing Res Rev 2: 39-56.

247. Wu X, Santos RR, Fink-Gremmels J (2015a) Analyzing the antibacterial effects of food ingredients: model experiments with allicin and garlic extracts on biofilm formation and viability of Staphylococcus epidermidis. Food Sci Nutr 3: 158-168.

248. Dorant E, van den Brandt PA, Goldbohm RA, Hermus RJ, Sturmans F (1993) Garlic and its significance for the prevention of cancer in humans: a critical view. Br J Cancer 67: 424-429.

249. Srivastava KC, Bordia A, Verma SK (1995) Garlic (Allium sativum) for disease prevention. S Afr J Sci 91: 68-77.

250. Reuter HD, Koch HP, Lawson LD (1996) Therapeutic effects and applications of garlic and its preparations. Garlic: The Science and Therapeutic Application of Allium sativum L. In: Koch HP and Lawson LD (eds.), Baltimore, MD, USA.

251. Amagase H (2006) Clarifying the real bioactive constituents of garlic. J Nutr 136: 716S-725S.

252. Vazquez-Prieto MA, Lanzi CR, Lembo C, Galmarini CR, Miatello RM (2011) Garlic and onion attenuates vascular inflammation and oxidative stress in fructose-fed rats. J Nutr Metab 2011: 475216.

253. Borlinghaus J, Albrecht F, Gruhlke MC, Nwachukwu ID, Slusarenko AJ (2014) Allicin: chemistry and biological properties. Molecules 19: 12591-12618.

254. Kodali RT, Eslick GD (2015) Meta-analysis: Does garlic intake reduce risk of gastric cancer? Nutr Cancer 67: 1-11.

255. Das DC, Mahato G, Das M, Lal Pati M (2015a) Investigation of ethno medicinal plants for the treatment of Carbuncles from Purulia District of West Bengal. Int J Bioassays 4: 3896-3899.

256. Hussain SP, Jannu LN, Rao AR (1990) Chemopreventive action of garlic on methylcholanthrene-induced carcinogenesis in the uterine cervix of mice. Cancer Lett 49: 175-180.

257. Perchellet JP, Perchellet EM, Belman S (1990) Inhibition of DMBA-induced mouse skin tumorigenesis by garlic oil and inhibition of two tumor-promotion stages by garlic and onion oils. Nutr Cancer 14: 183-193.

258. Rao AR, Sadhana AS, Goel HC (1990) Inhibition of skin tumors in DMBA-induced complete carcinogenesis system in mice by garlic (Allium sativum). Indian J Exp Biol 28: 405-408.

259. Sumiyoshi H, Wargovich MJ (1990) Chemoprevention of 1,2-dimethylhydrazine-induced colon cancer in mice by naturally occurring organosulfur compounds. Cancer Res 50: 5084-5087.

260. Ip C, Lisk DJ, Stoewsand GS (1992) Mammary cancer prevention by regular garlic and selenium-enriched garlic. Nutr Cancer 17: 279-286.

261. Reddy BS, Rao CV, Rivenson A, Kelloff G (1993) Chemoprevention of colon carcinogenesis by organosulfur compounds. Cancer Res 53: 3493-3498.

262. Schaffer EM, Liu JZ, Milner JA (1997) Garlic powder and allyl sulfur compounds enhance the ability of dietary selenite to inhibit 7,12-dimethylbenz(a)anthracene-induced mammary DNA adducts. Nutr Cancer 27: 162-168.

263. Bautista DM, Movahed P, Hinman A, Axelsson HE, Sterner O, et al. (2005) Pungent products from garlic activate the sensory ion channel TRPA1. Proc Natl Acad Sci U S A 102: 12248-12252.

264. Salazar H, Llorente I, Jara-Oseguera A, García-Villegas R, Munari M, et al. (2008) A single N-terminal cysteine in TRPV1 determines activation by pungent compounds from onion and garlic. Nat Neurosci 11: 255-261.

265. Block E (2009) Garlic and other alliums: the lore and the science. Royal Society Chemistry.

266. [No authors listed] (1996) Book review. Platelets 7: 367-370.

267. Slowing K, Ganado P, Sanz M, Ruiz E, Tejerina T (2001) Study of garlic extracts and fractions on cholesterol plasma levels and vascular reactivity in cholesterol-fed rats. J Nutr 131: 994S-999S.

268. Warshafsky S, Kamer RS, Sivak SI (1993) Effect of garlic on total serum cholesterol: a-meta-analysis. Annals of International medicine 119: 599-615.

269. Silagy C, Neil A (1994) Garlic as a lipid lowering agent--a meta-analysis. J R Coll Physicians Lond 28: 39-45.

270. Vincent C, Furnham A (2001) Complementary medicine-A research prospective. John Willey and Sons.

271. Isaacsohn JL, Moser M, Stein EA, Dudley K, Davey JA, et al. (1998) Garlic powder and plasma lipids and lipoproteins: a multicenter, randomized, placebo-controlled trial. Arch Intern Med 158: 1189-1194.

272. Canogullari S, Baylan M, Erdogan Z (2010) The effects of dietary garlic powder on performance, egg yolk and serum cholesterol concentrations in laying quails. Czech J Anim Sci 55: 286-293.

273. You WC, Blot WJ, Chang YS, Ershow AG, Yang ZT, et al. (1988) Diet and high risk of stomach cancer in Shandong, China. Cancer Res 48: 3518-3523.

274. Steinmetz KA, Kushi LH, Bostick RM, Folsom AR, Potter JD (1994) Vegetables, fruit, and colon cancer in the Iowa Women's Health Study. Am J Epidemiol 139: 1-15.

275. Uchida Y, Takahashi T, Sato N (1975) [The characteristics of the antibacterial activity of garlic (author's transl)]. Jpn J Antibiot 28: 638-642.

276. Cellini L, Di Campli E, Masulli M, Di Bartolomeo S, Allocati N (1996) Inhibition of Helicobacter pylori by garlic extract (Allium sativum). FEMS Immunol Med Microbiol 13: 273-277.

277. Sivam GP, Lampe JW, Ulness B, Swanzy SR, Potter JD (1997) Helicobacter pylori-in vitro susceptibility to garlic (Allium sativum) extract. Nutr Cancer 27: 118-121.

278. Jain RC (1998) Anti tubercular activity of garlic oil. Indian J Pathol Microbiol 41: 131.

279. Ankri S, Mirelman D (1999) Antimicrobial properties of allicin from garlic. Microbes Infect 1: 125-129.

280. Ross ZM, O'Gara EA, Hill DJ, Sleightholme HV, Maslin DJ (2001) Antimicrobial properties of garlic oil against human enteric bacteria:

evaluation of methodologies and comparisons with garlic oil sulfides and garlic powder. Appl Environ Microbiol 67: 475-480.

281. Tsao SM, Yin MC (2001) In vitro antimicrobial activity of four diallyl sulphides occurring naturally in garlic and Chinese leek oil. J Med Microbiol 50: 646-649.

282. Martin KW, Ernst E (2003) Herbal medicines for treatment of bacterial infections: a review of controlled clinical trials. J Antimicrob Chemother 51: 241-246.

283. Shuford JA, Steckelberg JM, Patel R (2005) Effects of fresh garlic extract on Candida albicans biofilms. Antimicrob Agents Chemother 49: 473.

284. Shokradeh M, Ebadi AG (2006) Antibacterial effect of garlic (Allium sativum) on Staphylococcus. Pak J boil Sci 9: 158-1579.

285. Low CF, Chong PP, Yong PV, Lim CS, Ahmad Z, et al. (2008) Inhibition of hyphae formation and SIR2 expression in Candida albicans treated with fresh Allium sativum (garlic) extract. J Appl Microbiol 105: 2169-2177.

286. Mozaffari Nejad AS, Shabani S, Bayat M, Hosseini SE (2014) Antibacterial Effect of Garlic Aqueous Extract on Staphylococcus aureus in Hamburger. Jundishapur J Microbiol 7: e13134.

287. Li G, Ma X, Deng L, Zhao X, Wei Y, et al. (2015) Fresh Garlic Extract Enhances the Antimicrobial Activities of Antibiotics on Resistant Strains in Vitro. Jundishapur J Microbiol 8: e14814.

288. Gheni AI, Noori MY, Shekhany AL, Smail HO (2016) Inhibitory Effects of Aqueous Garlic Extract (AGE) against multidrug resistant from Staphylococcus aureus and Escherichia coli. International Journal of Advanced Research 4: 928-933.

289. Saha S, Saha SK, Hossain MA, Paul SK, Gomes RR, et al. (2016) Anti-Bacterial effect of Aqueous Garlic Extract (AGE) determined by Disc Diffusion Method against Escherichia coli. Mymensingh Med J 25: 23-26.

290. Viswanathan V, Phadatare AG, Mukne A (2014) Antimycobacterial and Antibacterial Activity of Allium sativum Bulbs. Indian J Pharm Sci 76: 256-261.

291. Patrick-Iwuanyanwu KC, Wegwu MO, Ayalogu EO (2007) Prevention of CCl4-induced liver damage by ginger, garlic and vitamin E. Pak J Biol Sci 10: 617-621.

292. Ademiluyi AO, Oboh G, Owoloye TR, Agbebi OJ (2013) Modulatory effects of dietary inclusion of garlic (Allium sativum) on gentamycin-induced hepatotoxicity and oxidative stress in rats. Asian Pacific Journal of Tropical Biomedicine 3: 470-475.

293. Shin JH, Lee CW, Oh SJ, Yun J, Kang MR, et al. (2014) Hepatoprotective effect of aged black garlic extract in rodents. Toxicol Res 30: 49-54.

294. Nasiru A, Hafsat IG, Sabo AA (2012) Effect of anti-tuberculosis drugs co-administered with garlic homogenate on rat liver enzymes. International Conference on Biological and Life Sciences 40: 96-99.

295. Rao RR, Rao SS (1946) Inhibition of Mycobacterium tuberculosis by garlic extract. Nature 157: 441.

296. Houshmand B, Mahjour F, Dianat O (2013) Antibacterial effect of different concentrations of garlic (Allium sativum) extract on dental plaque bacteria. Indian J Dent Res 24: 71-75.

297. Vattem DA, Ghaedian R, Shetty K (2005) Enhancing health benefits of berries through phenolic antioxidant enrichment: focus on cranberry. Asia Pac J Clin Nutr 14: 120-130.

298. Pedersen CB, Kyle J, Jenkinson AM, Gardner PT, McPhail DB, et al. (2000) Effects of blueberry and cranberry juice consumption on the plasma antioxidant capacity of healthy female volunteers. Eur J Clin Nutr 54: 405-408.

299. Chu YF, Liu RH (2005) Cranberries inhibit LDL oxidation and induce LDL receptor expression in hepatocytes. Life Sci 77: 1892-1901.

300. Skrovankova S, Sumczynski D, Mlcek J, Jurikova T, Sochor J (2015) Bioactive Compounds and Antioxidant Activity in Different Types of Berries. Int J Mol Sci 16: 24673-24706.

301. Blatherwick NR (1914) The specific role of foods in relation to the composition of the urine. Arch Int Med 14: 409-450.

302. Schmidt DR, Sobota AE (1988) An examination of the anti-adherence activity of cranberry juice on urinary and nonurinary bacterial isolates. Microbios 55: 173-181.

303. Griffiths P (2003) The role of cranberry juice in the treatment of urinary tract infections. Br J Community Nurs 8: 557-561.

304. Ermel G, Georgeault S, Inisan C, Besnard M (2012) Inhibition of adhesion of uropathogenic Escherichia coli bacteria to uroepithelial cells by extracts from cranberry. J Med Food 15: 126-134.

305. Sun J, Marais JPJ, Khoo C, LaPlante K, Vejborg RM, et al. (2015) Cranberry (Vaccinium macrocarpon) oligosaccharides decrease biofilm formation by uropathogenic Escherichia coli. J Funct Foods 17: 235-242.

306. McKay DL, Blumberg JB (2007) Cranberries (Vaccinium macrocarpon) and cardiovascular disease risk factors. Nutr Rev 65: 490-502.

307. Novotny JA, Baer DJ, Khoo C, Gebauer SK, Charron CS (2015) Cranberry juice consumption lowers markers of cardiometabolic risk, including blood pressure and circulating C-reactive protein, triglyceride, and glucose concentrations in adults. J Nutr 145: 1185-1193.

308. Bomser J, Madhavi DL, Singletary K, Smith MA (1996) In vitro anticancer activity of fruit extracts from Vaccinium species. Planta Med 62: 212-216.

309. Krueger CG, Porter ML, Weibe DA, Cunningham DG, Reed JD (2000) Potential of cranberry flavonoids in the prevention of copper-induced LDL oxidation. Polyphenols Communications 2: 447-448.

310. Seeram NP, Adams LS, Hardy ML, Heber D (2004) Total cranberry extract versus its phytochemical constituents: Antiproliferative and synergistic effects against human tumor cell lines. J Agric Food Chem 52: 2512-2517.

311. Sun J, Hai Liu R (2006) Cranberry phytochemical extracts induce cell cycle arrest and apoptosis in human MCF-7 breast cancer cells. Cancer Lett 241: 124-134.

312. Vattem DA, Jang HD, Levin R, Shetty K (2006) Synergism of cranberry phenolics with ellagic acid and rosmarinic acid for antimutagenic and DNA protection functions. J Food Biochem 30: 98-116.

313. Vu KD, Carlettini H, Bouvet J, Côté J, Doyon G, et al. (2012) Effect of different cranberry extracts and juices during cranberry juice processing on the antiproliferative activity against two colon cancer cell lines. Food Chem 132: 959-967.

314. Baharum Z, Akim AM, Hin TY, Hamid RA, Kasran R (2016) Theobroma cacao: Review of the Extraction, Isolation, and Bioassay of Its Potential Anti-cancer Compounds. Trop Life Sci Res 27: 21-42.

315. Corti R, Flammer AJ, Hollenberg NK, Lüscher TF (2009) Cocoa and cardiovascular health. Circulation 119: 1433-1441.

316. Khan N, Khymenets O, Urpí-Sardà M, Tulipani S, Garcia-Aloy M, et al. (2014) Cocoa polyphenols and inflammatory markers of cardiovascular disease. Nutrients 6: 844-880.

317. Kumar R, Bhayana S, Kapoor S (2015b) The Role of Functional Foods for Healthy Life: Current Prospectives. Int J Pharm Bio Sci 6: 429-443.

318. Cooper KA, Donovan JL, Waterhouse AL, Williamson G (2008) Cocoa and health: a decade of research. Br J Nutr 99: 1-11.

319. Dillinger TL, Barriga P, Escárcega S, Jimenez M, Salazar Lowe D, et al. (2000) Food of the gods: cure for humanity? A cultural history of the medicinal and ritual use of chocolate. J Nutr 130: 2057S-72S.

320. Pearson DA, Paglieroni TG, Rein D, Wun T, Schramm DD, et al. (2002) The effects of flavanol-rich cocoa and aspirin on ex vivo platelet function. Thromb Res 106: 191-197.

321. Othman A, Ismail A, Abdul Ghani N, Adenan I (2007) Antioxidant capacity and phenolic content of cocoa beans. Food Chemistry 100: 1523-1530.

322. Erdman JW Jr, Carson L, Kwik-Uribe C, Evans EM, Allen RR (2008) Effects of cocoa flavanols on risk factors for cardiovascular disease. Asia Pac J Clin Nutr 17: 284-287.

323. Maskarinec G (2009) Cancer protective properties of cocoa: a review of the epidemiologic evidence. Nutr Cancer 61: 573-579.

324. Buijsse B, Weikert C, Drogan D, Bergmann M, Boeing H (2010) Chocolate consumption in relation to blood pressure and risk of cardiovascular disease in German adults. Eur Heart J 31: 1616-1623.

325. Ried K, Sullivan TR, Fakler P, Frank OR, Stocks NP (2012) Effect of cocoa on blood pressure. Cochrane Database Syst Rev.

326. Osakabe N, Hoshi J, Kudo N, Shibata M (2014) The flavan-3-ol fraction of cocoa powder suppressed changes associated with early-stage metabolic syndrome in high-fat diet-fed rats. Life Sci 114: 51-56.
327. Falcao LL, Silva-Werneck JO, Ramos Ade R, Martins NF, Bresso E, et al. (2016) Antimicrobial properties of two novel peptides derived from Theobroma cacao osmotin. Peptides 79: 75-82.
328. Arya SS, Salve AR, Chauhan S (2016) Peanuts as functional food: a review. J Food Sci Technol 53: 31-41.
329. Meyer AS, Heinonen M, Frankel EN (1998) Antioxidant interactions of catechin, cyanidin, caffeic acid, quercetin, and ellagic acid on human LDL oxidation. Food Chem 61: 71-75.
330. Aaby K, Ekeberg D, Skrede G (2007) Characterization of phenolic compounds in strawberry (Fragaria x ananassa) fruits by different hplc detectors and contribution of individual compounds to total antioxidant capacity. J Agric Food Chem 55: 4395-4406.
331. Meyers KJ, Watkins CB, Pritts MP, Liu RH (2003) Antioxidant and antiproliferative activities of strawberries. J Agric Food Chem 51: 6887-6892.
332. McDougall GJ, Ross HA, Ikeji M, Stewart D (2008) Berry extracts exert different antiproliferative effects against cervical and colon cancer cells grown in vitro. J Agric Food Chem 56: 3016-3023.
333. Lee IT, Chan YC, Lin CW, Lee WJ, Sheu WH (2008) Effect of cranberry extracts on lipid profiles in subjects with Type 2 diabetes. Diabet Med 25: 1473-1477.
334. Erlund I, Koli R, Alfthan G, Marniemi J, Puukka P, et al. (2008) Favorable effects of berry consumption on platelet function, blood pressure, and HDL cholesterol. Am J Clin Nutr 87: 323-331.
335. Cheplick S, Kwon YI, Bhowmik P, Shetty K (2010) Phenolic-linked variation in strawberry cultivars for potential dietary management of hyperglycemia and related complications of hypertension. Bioresour Technol 101: 404-413.
336. Giampieri F, Forbes-Hernandez TY, Gasparrini M, Alvarez-Suarez JM, Afrin S, et al. (2015) Strawberry as a health promoter: an evidence based review. Food Funct 6: 1386-1398.
337. Ozçelik B, Orhan I, Toker G (2006) Antiviral and antimicrobial assessment of some selected flavonoids. Z Naturforsch C 61: 632-638.
338. Orhan DD, Ozçelik B, Ozgen S, Ergun F (2010) Antibacterial, antifungal, and antiviral activities of some flavonoids. Microbiol Res 165: 496-504.
339. Daglia M (2012) Polyphenols as antimicrobial agents. Curr Opin Biotechnol 23: 174-181.
340. Basu A, Rhone M, Lyons TJ (2010) Berries: emerging impact on cardiovascular health. Nutr Rev 68: 168-177.
341. Burton-Freeman B (2010) Postprandial metabolic events and fruit-derived phenolics: a review of the science. Br J Nutr 104: S1-S14.
342. Henning SM, Seeram NP, Zhang Y, Li L, Gao K, et al. (2010) Strawberry consumption is associated with increased antioxidant capacity in serum. J Med Food 13: 116-122.
343. Pinto Mda S, de Carvalho JE, Lajolo FM, Genovese MI, Shetty K (2010) Evaluation of antiproliferative, anti-type 2 diabetes, and antihypertension potentials of ellagitannins from strawberries (Fragaria × ananassa Duch.) using in vitro models. J Med Food 13: 1027-1035.
344. McDougall GJ, Shpiro F, Dobson P, Smith P, Blake A, et al. (2005) Different polyphenolic components of soft fruits inhibit alpha-amylase and alpha-glucosidase. J Agric Food Chem 53: 2760-2766.
345. Wang SY, Feng R, Lu Y, Bowman L, Ding M (2005) Inhibitory effect on activator protein-1, nuclear factor-kappab, and cell transformation by extracts of strawberries (Fragaria x ananassa Duch.). J Agric Food Chem 53: 4187-4193.
346. Stoner GD, Chen T, Kresty LA, Aziz RM, Reinemann T, et al. (2006) Protection against esophageal cancer in rodents with lyophilized berries: potential mechanisms. Nutr Cancer 54: 33-46.
347. Stoner GD, Wang LS, Seguin C, Rocha C, Stoner K, et al. (2010) Multiple berry types prevent N-nitrosomethylbenzylamine-induced esophageal cancer in rats. Pharm Res 27: 1138-1145.
348. Kasimsetty SG, Bialonska D, Reddy MK, Ma G, Khan SI, et al. (2010) Colon cancer chemopreventive activities of pomegranate ellagitannins and urolithins. J Agric Food Chem 58: 2180-2187.
349. Stanojkovic TP, Konic-Ristic A, Juranic ZD, Savikin K, Zdunić G, et al. (2010) Cytotoxic and cell cycle effects induced by two herbal extracts on human cervix carcinoma and human breast cancer cell lines. J Med Food 13: 291-297.
350. Zhang Y, Seeram NP, Lee R, Feng L, Heber D (2008) Isolation and identification of strawberry phenolics with antioxidant and human cancer cell antiproliferative properties. J Agric Food Chem 56: 670-675.
351. Sharma M, Li L, Celver J, Killian C, Kovoor A, et al. (2010) Effects of fruit ellagitannin extracts, ellagic acid, and their colonic metabolite, urolithin A, on Wnt signaling. J Agric Food Chem 58: 3965-3969.
352. Joseph JA, Shukitt-Hale B, Denisova NA, Prior RL, Cao G, et al. (1998) Long-term dietary strawberry, spinach, or vitamin E supplementation retards the onset of age-related neuronal signal-transduction and cognitive behavioral deficits. J Neurosci 18: 8047-8055.
353. Shukitt-Hale B, Lau FC, Joseph JA (2008) Berry fruit supplementation and the aging brain. J Agric Food Chem 56: 636-641.
354. Joseph JA, Shukitt-Hale B, Willis LM (2009) Grape juice, berries, and walnuts affect brain aging and behavior. J Nutr 139: 1813S-1817S.
355. Tacon AGJ, Metian M (2013) Fish matters: importance of aquatic foods in human nutrition and global food supply. Reviews in Fisheries Science 21: 22-38.
356. Bang HO, Dyerberg J (1972) Plasma lipids and lipoproteins in Greenlandic west coast Eskimos. Acta Med Scand 192: 85-94.
357. Harris WS (1996) n-3 fatty acids and lipoproteins: comparison of results from human and animal studies. Lipids 31: 243-252.
358. Kris-Etherton PM, Hecker KD, Bonanome A, Coval SM, Binkoski AE, et al. (2002) Bioactive compounds in foods: their role in the prevention of cardiovascular disease and cancer. Am J Med 113: 71S-88S.
359. Wang C, Harris WS, Chung M, Lichtenstein AH, Balk EM, et al. (2006) n-3 fatty acids from fish or fish oil supplements, but not alpha-linolenic acid, benefit cardiovascular disease outcomes in primary-and secondary-prevention studies: a systematic review. American Journal of Clinical Nutrition 84: 5-17.
360. Bessell E, Jose MD, McKercher C (2015) Associations of fish oil and vitamin B and E supplementation with cardiovascular outcomes and mortality in people receiving haemodialysis: a review. BMC Nephrol 16: 143.
361. Albert CM, Hennekens CH, O'Donnell CJ, Ajani UA, Carey VJ, et al. (1998) Fish consumption and risk of sudden cardiac death. JAMA 279: 23-28.
362. Bender N, Portmann M, Heg Z, Hofmann K, Zwahlen M, et al. (2014) Fish or n3-PUFA intake and body composition: a systematic review and meta-analysis. Obes Rev 15: 657-665.
363. Zhu W, Dong C, Du H (2014) Effect of fish oil on serum lipid profile in dialysis patients: a systematic review and meta-analysis of randomized controlled trials. Lipids in Health and Disease 13: 127.
364. Saccone G, Berghella V (2015) Omega-3 supplementation to prevent recurrent preterm birth: a systematic review and meta-analysis of randomized controlled trials. American Journal of Obstetrics and Gynecology 213:135-140.
365. Wu C, Kato TS, Ji R, Zizola C, Brunjes DL, et al. (2015) Supplementation of l-Alanyl-l-Glutamine and Fish Oil Improves Body Composition and Quality of Life in Patients With Chronic Heart Failure. Circ Heart Fail 8: 1077-1087.
366. Kutner NG, Clow PW, Zhang R, Aviles X (2002) Association of fish intake and survival in a cohort of incident dialysis patients. Am J Kidney Dis 39: 1018-1024.
367. Pase MP, Grima N, Cockerell R, Stough C, Scholey A, et al. (2015) The effects of long-chain omega-3 fish oils and multivitamins on cognitive and cardiovascular function: a randomized, controlled clinical trial. J Am Coll Nutr 34: 21-31.
368. Fuller R (1994) History and development of probiotics. In: R. Fuller (ed.), Probiotics, Chapman and Hall, NY, USA.

369. Pandey KR, Naik SR, Vakil BV (2015) Probiotics, prebiotics and synbiotics-a review. J Food Sci Technol 52: 7577-7587.
370. Gerritsen J, Smidt H, Rijkers GT, de Vos WM (2011) Intestinal microbiota in human health and disease: the impact of probiotics. Genes Nutr 6: 209-240.
371. Fontana L, Bermudez-Brito M, Plaza-Diaz J, Muñoz-Quezada S, Gil A (2013) Sources, isolation, characterisation and evaluation of probiotics. Br J Nutr 109: S35-S50.
372. Zhang YJ, Li S, Gan RY, Zhou T, Xu DP, et al. (2015) Impacts of gut bacteria on human health and diseases. Int J Mol Sci 16: 7493-7519.
373. Liong MT (2008) Roles of probiotics and prebiotics in colon cancer prevention: Postulated mechanisms and in-vivo evidence. Int J Mol Sci 9: 854-863.
374. Pearson JR, Gill CI, Rowland IR (2009) Diet, fecal water, and colon cancer--development of a biomarker. Nutr Rev 67: 509-526.
375. Wollowski I, Rechkemmer G, Pool-Zobel BL (2001) Protective role of probiotics and prebiotics in colon cancer. Am J Clin Nutr 73: 451S-455S.
376. Uccello M, Malaguarnera G, Basile F, D'agata V, Malaguarnera M, et al. (2012) Potential role of probiotics on colorectal cancer prevention. BMC Surg 12: S35.
377. Gibson GR, Roberfroid MB (1995) Dietary modulation of the human colonic microbiota: introducing the concept of prebiotics. J Nutr 125: 1401-1412.
378. Gibso GR, Saavedra JM, Macfarlane S (1996) Probiotics and intestinal infection. In (Fuller R ed.), Probiotics: Therapeutic and Other Beneficial Effects, Chapman and Hall, London.
379. Tomomatsu H (1994) Health effects of oligosaccharides. Food Technol 48: 61-65
380. Florowska A, Krygier K, Florowski T, Dłużewska E (2016) Prebiotics as functional food ingredients preventing diet-related diseases. Food Funct 7: 2147-2155.
381. Das R, Trafadar B, Das P, Kar S, Mitra S, et al. (2015b) Anti-Inflammatory and Regenerative Potential of Probiotics to Combat Inflammatory Bowel Disease (IBD). J Biotechnol Biomater 5: 181.
382. Pighin D, Pazos A, Chamorro V, Paschetta F, Cunzolo S, et al. (2016) A Contribution of Beef to Human Health: A Review of the Role of the Animal Production Systems. ScientificWorldJournal 2016: 8681491.
383. Thomas C, Scollan N, Moran D (2014) A road map for the beef industry to meet the challenge of climate change-a discussion document. Animal Frontiers 1: 6-9.
384. Kim JH, Kim Y, Kim YJ, Park Y (2016) Conjugated Linoleic Acid: Potential Health Benefits as a Functional Food Ingredient. Annu Rev Food Sci Technol 7: 221-244.
385. Ip C, Scimeca JA (1997) Conjugated linoleic acid and linoleic acid are distinctive modulators of mammary carcinogenesis. Nutr Cancer 27: 131-135.
386. Kelly ML, Berry JR, Dwyer DA, Griinari JM, Chouinard PY, et al. (1998) Dietary fatty acid sources affect conjugated linoleic acid concentrations in milk from lactating dairy cows. J Nutr 128: 881-885.
387. Maslak E, Buczek E, Szumn A, Szczepnski W, Franczyk-Zarow M, et al. (2015) Individual CLA isomers, c9t11 and t10c12, prevent excess liver glycogen storage and inhibit lipogenic genes expression induced by high-fructose diet in rats. Biomed Res Int.
388. Zhou GH, Xu XL, Liu Y (2010) Preservation technologies for fresh meat-a review. Meat Sci 86: 119-128.
389. Giovannini M, Agostoni C, Salari PC (1991) Is carnitine essential in children? J Int Med Res 19: 88-102.
390. Overvad K, Diamant B, Holm L, Holmer G, Mortensen SA, et al. (1999) Coenzyme Q10 in health and disease. Eur J Clin Nutr 53: 764-770.
391. Packer L, Witt EH, Tritschler HJ (1995) alpha-Lipoic acid as a biological antioxidant. Free Radic Biol Med 19: 227-250.
392. Sharma M (2013) Functional Foods: Marketing 'Health' To Modern India. International Journal of Innovative Research and Development 2: 720-739.
393. Ayyagari R, Grover V, Purvis R (2011) Technostress: Technological Antecendents and Implications. MIS Quarterly 35: 831-858.
394. Popkin BM (2004) The nutrition transition: an overview of world patterns of change. Nutr Rev 62: S140-S143.
395. Banerjee A, Banerjee B (2000) Effective retail promotion management: use of point of sales information resources. Vikalpa 25: 52-59.

8

Nutritional Potential of Four Seaweed Species Collected in the Barbate Estuary (Gulf of Cadiz, Spain)

Garcia JS*, Palacios V and Roldán A

Department of Chemical Engineering and Food Technology, University of Cádiz, PB 40, Poligono Rio San Pedro, Puerto Real 11510, Cádiz, Spain

***Corresponding author:** Garcia JS, Department of Chemical Engineering and Food Technology, Faculty of Sciences, University of Cádiz, PB 40, Poligono Rio San Pedro, Puerto Real 11510, Cádiz, Spain, E-mail: fini.sanchez@uca.es

Abstract

The Gulf of Cádiz has great socio-economic importance given its high fishing activity and high diversity and abundance of marine resources including a wide variety of seaweeds not used as food. Four macro-algae (*Ulva* spp., *Codium* spp., *Halymenia floresia* and *Saccorhiza polyschides*) collected in the Gulf of Cádiz near the Barbate estuary were analyzed for moisture, proteins, lipids, carbohydrates, ash, dietary fiber, caloric content, minerals, amino acids and fatty acids. The algae showed variations in all of the parameters analyzed. However, high concentrations of lipids and macro and micro-minerals and low concentrations of fiber and carbohydrates were related to the salinity, water temperature and nitrate contents of the collection areas. All four species had a high nutritional value, and these macro-algae have great potential for human consumption.

Keywords: Seaweed; *Ulva* spp.; *Codium* spp.; *Halymenia f oresia*; *Saccorhiza polyschides*; Chemical composition

Introduction

Seaweeds have a long tradition in Asia as a food source, are commonly used as sushi wrapping, seasonings, condiments and vegetables and can constitute between 10 and 25% of food intake by most Japanese [1,2]. The production of macroalgae is limited to the brown species, Kombu, Wakame, Hijiki and Nori, marketed in China, Japan and Korea. However, in recent years, interest in these products and their consumption has increased in countries such as Chile, Brazil, Mexico, France, Germany and Spain, thereby increasing their collection and cultivation. World production is estimated at just over 25,000,000 tons of dry weight and total consumption of raw materials amounting to some 150,000 tons [3].

The abundance, diversity and commercial value of algae give it a large number of industrial applications, such as sources of human and animal food [4], biologically active phytochemicals (e.g., carotenoids, phycobilins, fatty acids, polysaccharides, vitamins and sterols) [5] and phycocolloids (e.g., alginates, carrageenan and agar) [6]. In the food industry, algae are currently used as raw materials for food in raw salads, soups, cookies, meals and condiments [7]. Algae can be used as a nutritional or functional ingredient to supplement food with natural antioxidants, antimicrobials or texturing agents, including chitin, chitosan, omega-3 oils, carotenoids, vitamins and minerals [4-6]. Thus, algae are used to develop new fortified foods such as bakery, dairy confectionary and pasta products [5].

The nutritional composition of macroalgae has been extensively studied [7-10]. These authors have highlighted its high water content, which varies between 70% and 90% of the fresh weight, protein content between 7% and 47%, carbohydrate content between 4% and 70%, lipids between 0.2% and 20% and ash content between 11% and 43%. Moreover, algae are appealing because of their high dietary fiber content (30-70%) which is higher than that found in common fruits and vegetables (1-5%) [8,10,11].

Macroalgae species are generally rich in essential amino acids, such as glycine, arginine, alanine, aspartic acid and glutamic acid [11], and in 3 and 6 PUFAs, of which the most abundant are C16:0, C18:19, C20:46, and C20:53 [12-14]. Macroalgae contain higher amounts of both macrominerals (Na, K, Ca and Mg) and trace elements (Fe, Zn, Cu and Mn) [15], but their concentrations vary by species and geographical origin [7,10,16,17].

Macroalgae are considered to be a highly nutritious food source, but their nutritional composition varies with species, habitat, growth stage, geographical origin, season and environmental conditions in the collection area (i.e., temperature, salinity and nutrients) [7,8,11,15,18-20].

The Gulf of Cádiz (southwestern coast of Spain) is an important fishing ground with a high diversity and productivity of exploited species [21]. This area connects the Atlantic Ocean with the Mediterranean Sea, and there are important estuaries and salt marshes associated with the mouths of rivers, such as the Guadiana, Piedras, Tinto-Odiel, Guadalquivir, Guadalete and Barbate, that feed in freshwater and other dissolved or suspended substances from the continent and increase the physiographic biodiversity of this area [22]. Moreover, the combination of warm nutrient-rich waters and wind regimes favors the diversity and abundance of marine resources [23], including a wide variety of seaweeds.

Although the Gulf of Cádiz marine ecosystem has great socio-economic importance given its high fishing activity [23], macroalgae is not yet collected and exploited. In fact, there is a lack of knowledge about the species that develop in this area, their characteristics and their food use.

The main goal of the present work was to determine the potential and value of Gulf of Cadiz macroalgae for human consumption. *Ulva* spp., *Codium* spp. (Chlorophyceae), *Halymenia floresia* (Rhodophyceae) and *Saccorhiza polyschides* (Phaeophyceae) collected in the Gulf of Cádiz near the Barbate estuary were evaluated in terms of their nutritional composition (i.e., moisture, proteins, carbohydrates, lipids, ash, dietary fiber, minerals, free amino acids and fatty acids) and caloric value and were compared to other species reported in the literature.

Materials and Methods

Raw materials

Macroalgae samples, *Ulva* spp., *Codium* spp., *Halymenia floresia* and *Saccorhiza polyschides*, were obtained from staff at Innova Vegetalia del Mar, S.L., who had experience in diving and seaweed harvesting. The samples were manually collected in autumn (2011) at 12-15 m depth near the Barbate estuary, Gulf of Cádiz, Spain (36°16 ′N, 5°89′W). This area is characterized by salinity values between 36.2 and 36.45 and temperatures between 19°C and 22°C at 20 m depth [24].

After collection, macroalgae samples were rinsed with seawater, tap water and distilled water. For all analyses except the moisture analysis, samples were freeze-dried and milled into a fine powder to homogenize them prior to use. The homogenized macroalgae samples were stored in a desiccator until analysis. The moisture content was determined by drying below 100°C in an oven to a constant weight [25].

Analytical methods

Chemical analysis of seaweeds

Protein content: Protein content was determined using the Kjeldahl method in Marsham. Samples were digested in an automated digester, model DK6 (Velp Scientific, Italy), and distilled by steam distillation, model UDK127 (Velp Scientific, Italy). The protein content was calculated using a nitrogen conversion factor of 6.25 (following previous studies of seaweeds, as Norziah and Ching [11], and Ortiz et al. [8], and the results were expressed as a percentage of dry weight.

Carbohydrate content: Carbohydrates were determined using the Clegg manual anthrone method [25]. Following extraction, the sample was reacted with anthrone reagent (0.1%) and a high concentration of sulfuric acid (96%). The absorbance was read at 630 nm on a spectrophotometer, model Genesys10v (Thermo Fisher Scientific Inc., USA). The amount of carbohydrate was estimated using a standard curve of d-glucose.

Dietary fiber: Fiber content was determined by acid digestion using the Scharrer–Kürschner method [25].

Fat and fatty acid content: Fat content was determined by the Soxhlet method [25] using an automated SER 148 Soxhlet extraction unit (Velp Scientific, Italy) and n-hexane as the extraction solvent.

Fatty acids were determined by gas-liquid chromatography after derivatization to methyl esters (FAMEs) according to the IUPAC standard method [26]. Analysis of FAMEs was performed on a Hewlett-Packard 5890 Series II GC with an FID detector and a capillary column: Teknokroma TBR-WAX (30 m × 0.25 m × DF ID 0.25 m). The column temperature was programed from 190°C to 250°C at 2°C/min. Reference fatty acid methyl esters (FAMEs) of marine products (SIGMA, Spain) were used to identify and quantify FAMEs by comparing the retention times of the peaks with those of the standards.

Ash and mineral contents: Ash content was determined by incineration of 1 g of freeze-dried sample in a muffle oven at 550°C [25]. The ashes were dissolved in HNO_3 [27], and the mineral constituents (i.e., Ca, K, Na, Mg, Fe, Zn and Cu) were determined by inductively coupled plasma atomic emission spectroscopy (Iris Intrepid ICP-AES, Thermo Scientific, Maryland, USA).

Caloric value determination: The caloric value was calculated using energy conversion factors specified in EU Directive 90/496, as shown in Livesey et al. [28].

Free amino acid analysis: Amino acids were determined by high-performance liquid chromatography (HPLC) according to the method described in Pereira et al. [29] with slight modifications. The samples extracts were derivatized pre-column using OPA (Panreac, Spain) as the derivatization reagent. The chromatographic conditions were as follows: flow rate of 1 ml/min; LiChrospher 100 RP-18 (5 µm) column thermostated at room temperature; solvents, A, sodium acetate buffer (50 mM, pH 6.8): methanol (9:1) with 2% tetrahydrofuran and B, methanol with 0.5% tetrahydrofuran. The gradient consisted of 85-72% of A to B for 3 min, 56% A (25 min), 44% A (35 min) and 20% A (45 min). Fluorometric detection was performed at excitation and emission wavelengths of 324 and 420 nm, respectively, using an Intelligent Fluorescence detector, model FP-2020 (Jasco Europe s.r.l., Italy). Identification and quantification of amino acids were performed by comparing the retention times of the peaks with those of standards (Sigma Chemicals).

Expression of data and statistical analysis

All analytical determinations were performed at least in triplicate. The data were expressed as means ± standard deviations, and reported on a dry matter basis.

Results and Discussion

Chemical composition

The proximal composition of the macroalgae considered in this study is shown in Table 1. The macroalgae had different compositions that were primarily species-specific.

Components	*Ulva spp.*	*Codium spp.*	*H. floresia*	*S. polyschides*
Moisture[b]	84.3 ± 0.3	98.6 ± 1.2	91.9 ± 0.7	94.3 ± 0.9
Protein	7.2 ± 0.0	15.6 ± 1.4	9.4 ± 0.0	7.3 ± 0.1
Lipid	3.4 ± 0.4	7.1 ± 0.1	12.3 ± 1.1	8.2 ± 0.1
Fibre	9.5 ± 0.7	1.4 ± 0.1	1.7 ± 0.0	16.6 ± 0.4
Carbohydrate	11.7 ± 0.4	8.8 ± 0.4	15.5 ± 1.5	6.3 ± 0.1
Ash	34.2 ± 0.7	30.7 ± 1.1	50.2 ± 1.1	30.7 ± 0.8
Caloric value[c]	106.5 ± 1.3	161.4 ± 2.3	210.6 ± 2.1	128.2 ± 0.9

Table 1: Chemical characteristics and caloric value of seaweeds studied (g/100 g on dry weight)[a]. [a]All values given are means of three determinations (X ± SD); SD: standard deviation. [b] Moisture content is expressed as percentage of fresh weigh. [c]Caloric value is expressed as kcal/100 g of dry weight.

The moisture content of fresh macroalgae ranged from 84.3% (*Ulva* spp.) to 98.6% (*Codium* spp.). *Ulva* spp., whose structure is laminar, had the lowest value, while *Codium* spp., with a tubular structure and water-holding capacity, had the highest water content. *Saccorhiza polyschides* and *Halymenia floresia*, which have laminar structures, had similar moisture contents (94.2 and 91.9%, respectively). The moisture content, of other species studied by Dawczynski et al. [9], including *Porphyra* sp., *Undaria pinnatifida* and *Laminaria* sp., ranged from 89.3-93.5%. These species have the same structure as *Saccorhiza polyschides* and *Halymenia floresia* and had similar moisture contents. Therefore, this content appears to be related to the morphology and structure of the species.

The protein contents ranged from 7.2-15.6% and were much higher in *Codium* spp. (15.6%). The rest of the macroalgae contained similar values ranging from 7-9%. These results were similar to other studies in other species. Gressler et al. [29] reported protein contents in *G. domingensis, G. birdiae, L. filiformis* and *L. intricate* macroalgae that ranged from 4.6-18.3%. Gómez-Ordoñez et al. [10] reported contents from 10.9-25.7% in brown macroalgae and 15.5-21.3% in red species. Protein content may vary according to the species, geographic area, season and environmental conditions [10,30]. The macroalgae studied were collected in the same geographic area, season and environmental conditions; thus, the protein content appears to be related to the species in this study. Of all the species evaluated, *Codium* spp. had the highest protein content, which could be related to its enhanced ability to assimilate nitrogen [31,32].

Lipid contents in all of the species studied in this work were higher than 7%, except in *Ulva* spp. (3.4%). These values are higher than that determined by Wong & Cheung [33] (1.42-1.64%), Ortiz et al. [8] (0.3-0.8%) and Gómez-Ordoñez et al. [10] (0.3-0.9%), but similar to those reported by other authors [7,9,20]. A review by Miyashita et al. showed that lipids vary in brown macroalgae based on species, geography, season, temperature, salinity and light intensity, as well as interactions between these factors. These authors reported that tropical species have significantly lower lipid contents than cold-water species. Additionally, Floreto et al. [34,35] showed that high levels and a lack of nitrate and high salinity and light intensity led to high lipid levels. Therefore, the high fat content in the macroalgae of the present study could be related to the salinity (36.4%), water temperature (19.5-20.4°C) or nitrate content (45M NO_3^-; [36]) of the collection area However, the observed differences between the macroalgae in the present study were species-specific.

Carbohydrate contents ranged from 6.3-15.5% and were higher in *Ulva* spp. (11.7%) and *Halymenia floresia* (15.5%). These values were similar to that reported by Wong & Cheung [33] for *H. japonica, H. charoides* and *U. lactuca* (4.3, 7.02 and 14.6%, respectively). However, Ortiz et al. [8] found higher values in *Durvillaea antarctica* (70.9%), *Ulva lactuca* (61.5%) and *Ulva fasciata* (34.8%). According to Macler [37], there is an inverse relationship between the N content of water and the carbohydrate content of macroalgae. Therefore, the high nitrogen content in the collection area [36] could explain the low levels of carbohydrates found in the four species studied.

Most previous studies have found that fiber is the most abundant component of seaweeds [9,10,30,33]. However, in the present work, fiber contents were less than 20% in all macroalgae. In fact, the highest value was observed in *Saccorhiza polyschides* (16.6%) followed by *Ulva* spp. (9.5%), and the lowest values were in *Codium* spp. and *Halymenia floresia* (1.4% and 1.7%, respectively). Norziah and Ching [11] observed that the fiber content may be related to geography, water temperature, and collection time and collection depth. More specific studies [10] have shown that the fiber content decreases in nitrogen-rich areas. Seaweeds collected in the studied area had significantly lower fiber contents than samples reported in other studies, a finding that could again be related to the high nitrogen content in the collection area [36].

Ash contents of *Ulva* spp., *Codium* spp. and *Saccorhiza polyschides* were high and ranged from 30.7-50.2% (*Codium* spp. and *S. polyschides*) (*H. floresia*). These results were similar to those obtained by Gressler et al. [20] in *G. domingensis, G. birdiae, L. filiformis* and *L. Intricate* (ranged 22.5-38.4%) and by Aguilera-Morales et al. [7] in *Enteromorpha* sp. (36.8%). The ash content varies between species, geography and seasons, but a general feature of macroalgae are their high ash contents [10]. The Barbate Estuary is an area that promotes accumulation fluvial sediments rich in minerals [37] and, therefore, their accumulation in algae. However, accumulation in our samples depended on the species because *Halymenia floresia* (50.2%) contained the highest amount of ash.

Caloric values of the studied macroalgae were calculated from protein, fat and carbohydrate contents following a previously reported method [28]. As shown in Table 1, caloric values ranged between 106.5 and 210.6 kcal/100 g of dry sample and were determined by the protein content. *Halymenia floresia* had the highest value (210.6 kcal/100 g dry sample) because of its high lipid and carbohydrate contents, followed by *Codium* spp. (161.4 Kcal/100 g), in which the caloric value was primarily determined by the protein content. *Ulva* spp. and *Saccorhiza polyschides* had the lowest caloric values because of their low protein contents, but they were rich in fiber.

Free amino acid composition

Free amino acids (mg/g protein) in the four species are shown in Table 2.

Amino acids	*Ulva spp.*	*Codium spp.*	*H. floresia*	*S. polyschides*
Aspartic acid	340.3 ± 1.5	28.5 ± 1.4	n.d.	n.d.
Threonine[b]	19.1 ± 0.8	7.5 ± 1.2	8.3 ± 0.2	n.d.
Serine	n.d.	105.1 ± 2.1	n.d.	2.8 ± 1.1
Glutamic acid	8.8 ± 0.3	15.2 ± 1.4	8.1 ± 0.1	n.d.
Lysine[b]	5.5 ± 0.5	0.2 ± 0.0	10.1 ± 0.3	0.7 ± 0.3
Arginine	210.2 ± 0.9	56.8 ± 2.7	42.4 ± 0.9	10.8 ± 0.7
Glycine	1.50 ± 1.0	0.5 ± 0.9	1.4 ± 0.0	0.2 ± 0.0
Phenylalanine[b]	18.4 ± 0.1	29.8 ± 1.6	4.9 ± 0.0	15.5 ± 0.8
Tryptophan[b]	89.8 ± 1.1	41.9 ± 2.6	17.6 ± 0.3	4.3 ± 1.2
Methionine[b]	0.1 ± 0.0	n.d.	6.1 ± 0.1	n.d.
Cysteine	29.1 ± 0.9	8.3 ± 2.1	6.6 ± 0.1	0.4 ± 0.0
Isoleucine[b]	23.6 ± 0.5	11.1 ± 1.9	3.4 ± 0.0	6.6 ± 0.8
Leucine[b]	26.3 ± 0.5	3.1 ± 1.6	5.3 ± 0.0	10.9 ± 1.4
Histidine	14.7 ± 0.1	8.4 ± 0.9	4.9 ± 0.2	17.6 ± 0.6
Valine[b]	1.1 ± 0.0	3.4 ± 1.1	0.1 ± 0.0	5.4 ± 0.7

TAA	788.5 ± 7.2	319.8 ± 5.4	119.2 ± 4.8	75.2 ± 6.1
TEAA	198.6 ± 2.3	105.4 ± 4.2	55.8 ± 6.1	61.0 ± 3.7
TEAA/TAA	0.25	0.33	0.47	0.81

Table 2: Amino acid contents of seaweeds studied (mg/g protein)[a]. TAA, total amino acids; TEAA, total essential amino acids; n.d., not detectable. [a] All values given are means of three determinations ($\bar{X}$ ± SD); SD: standard deviation. [b] Essential amino acid (EAA).

Seventeen amino acids were detected including essential amino acids such as threonine, lysine, phenylalanine, tryptophan, methionine, cysteine, isoleucine, leucine, histidine and valine. Alanine and tyrosine were not detected in any of the macroalga samples studied. Nevertheless in other studies if they were detected [8,33].

Levels of the different amino acids varied according to species and ranged from 0.1 ± 0.0 to 340.3 ± 1.5 (mg/g protein) in *Ulva* spp., from 0.2 ± 0.0 to 105.1 ± 2.1 (mg/g protein) in *Codium* spp., from 0.1 ± 0.0 to 42.4 ± 0.9 (mg/g protein) in *H. floresia*, and from 0.2 ± 0.0 to 17.6 ± 0.6 (mg/g protein) in *S. polyschides*.

Total free amino acids (TAA) were highest in *Ulva* spp. (788.5 mg/g protein), followed by *Codium* spp. (319.8 mg/g protein), *Halymenia floresia* (119.2 mg/g protein) and *Saccorhiza polyschides* (75.2 mg/g protein). The total free amino acids in *Ulva* spp. were significantly higher than those reported by Wong & Cheung [33] in other species. However, *Codium* spp., *Halymenia floresia* and *Saccorhiza polyschides* had lower values than those reported by Wong & Cheung [33] (range from 7.1-19.0% of protein), Ortiz et al. [8] (range from 10.4-12.6% of protein) and Dawczynski et al. [9] (range from 7.5-31.4% of protein).

The total protein and free amino acid contents of the different species are shown in Tables 1 and 2, respectively. The free amino acid contents in *Ulva* spp. and *Codium* spp. were 5.7 g/kg and 5 g/kg of dry weight sample, respectively, and nitrogen in both species principally consisted of free amino acids (78.9% and 32.0%, respectively). However, in *Saccorhiza polyschides* and *Halymenia floresia*, the contents of nitrogen present as free amino acids were 1.1 g/kg and 0.5 g/kg of dry weight sample, respectively (12.0% and 7.5%, respectively).

All macroalgae studied showed pronounced differences between the amino acid profiles and high levels of essential amino acids (TEAA), especially in *Ulva* spp. (382.5 mg/g protein), which stands out with its high level of tryptophan, followed of cysteine, isoleucine and leucine. *Codium* spp. contained high amounts of tryptophan (41.9 mg/g protein) and phenylalanine (29.8 mg/g protein), while *H. floresia* stood out for its lysine and methionine contents (17.6 mg/g and 6.1 mg/g protein, respectively). *S. polyschides* had the highest histidine and valine levels (17.6 mg/g and 5.4 mg/g protein, respectively).

Although the higher TEAA contents were observed in *Ulva* spp. and *Codium* spp., the relative TEAA/TAA value was higher in *Halymenia floresia* (0.8) because of its low amount of non-essential amino acids.

In terms of the non-essential free amino acids, *Ulva* spp. had the most complete amino acid profile and the highest levels of aspartic acid and arginine (340.3 mg/g and 210.2 mg/g, respectively). *Codium* spp. stood out for its serine, arginine and aspartic and glutamic acid contents (105.1, 56.8, 28.5 and 15.2 mg/g, respectively).

According to several authors [38,39], high levels of aspartic and glutamic acids may be responsible for organoleptic characteristics in macroalgae, including the intense flavor and taste. Therefore, the high level of aspartic acid in *Ulva* spp. (340.3 mg/g protein) could be related to its intense flavor and characteristic aroma.

Fatty acid composition

The fatty acid compositions of the macroalgae under study are given in Table 3.

Fatty acids	Methyl ester (%)			
	Ulva spp.	*Codium spp.*	*H. floresia*	*S. polyschides*
C 14:0	n.d.	n.d.	n.d.	n.d.
C 16:0	0.6 ± 1.0	0.3 ± 0.1	1.2 ± 0.5	0.5 ± 0.1
C 17:0	5.4 ± 1.8	0.9 ± 0.9	5.4 ± 0.7	1.9 ± 0.7
C 18:0	6.4 ± 0.2	3.9 ± 0.4	5.2 ± 0.3	8.7 ± 0.4
C 20:0	10.7 ± 2.3	11.5 ± 7.6	5.6 ± 3.7	7.3 ± 0.6
C 22:0	n.d.	n.d.	1.4 ± 0.4	n.d.
C 24:0	0.9 ± 1.7	0.4 ± 0.7	n.d.	2.1 ± 1.8
C $14:1_{\omega5}$	44.6 ± 2.6	48.4 ± 7.7	32.6 ± 2.9	35.8 ± 0.4
C $16:1_{\omega7}$	0.9 ± 1.4	n.d.	4.4 ± 2.9	1.8 ± 0.8
C $18:1_{\omega7}$	n.d.	n.d.	n.d.	n.d.
C $20:1_{\omega9}$	n.d.	n.d.	n.d.	n.d.
C $24:1_{\omega9}$	n.d.	0.3 ± 0.1	n.d.	n.d.
C $18:2_{\omega6}$	14.7 ± 1.8	19.3 ± 1.0	28.6 ± 2.3	21.8 ± 0.9
C $20:2_{\omega6}$	n.d.	n.d.	n.d.	n.d.
C $18:3_{\omega3}$	n.d.	n.d.	n.d.	0.6 ± 0.2
C $20:3_{\omega9}$	5.9 ± 3.7	1.1 ± 0.4	2.9 ± 0.1	3.9 ± 1.0
C $20:4_{\omega6}$	n.d.	n.d.	n.d.	n.d.
C $20:5_{\omega3}$	3.6 ± 1.7	6.6 ± 0.0	1.1 ± 0.7	1.4 ± 0.2
C $22:6_{\omega3}$	n.d.	0.2 ± 0.4	n.d.	n.d.
SFA	24.0 ± 1.1	17.0 ± 2.3	18.8 ± 0.8	20.5 ± 2.5
MUFA	45.5 ± 1.6	48.7 ± 2.6	37.0 ± 3.3	37.6 ± 0.6
PUFA	24.2 ± 3.6	27.2 ± 0.1	32.6 ± 1.7	27.7 ± 0.1
$\Sigma_{(MUFA+PUFA)}/\Sigma_{SFA}$	2.9 ± 0.3	4.5 ± 0.9	3.7 ± 0.1	3.2 ± 0.2
$PUFAs_{\omega6}$	14.7 ± 1.8	19.3 ± 1.0	28.6 ± 2.3	21.8 ± 0.9
$PUFAs_{\omega3}$	3.6 ± 1.8	6.8 ± 0.4	1.1 ± 0.7	2.0 ± 1.0
$Ratio_{\omega6/\omega3}$	4.1 ± 0.1	2.8 ± 0.3	26.0 ± 0.4	10.9 ± 0.9

Table 3: Fatty acid composition of seaweeds studied (g/100 g of total fatty acid)[a]. SFA, saturated fatty acids; MUFA, monounsaturated fatty acids; PUFA, polyunsaturated fatty acids; nd, not detectable. [a]All values given are means of three determinations ($\bar{X}$ ± SD); SD: standard deviation.

The saturated fatty acid content (SFA) was between 17.0% and 24.0%, and monounsaturated fatty acids (MUFA) and polyunsaturated fatty acids (PUFA) ranged from 37.0-48.7% and 24.2-32.6%, respectively. SFA levels in these macroalgae were lower than those found by Johns et al. [12] in green (23.9%), brown (27.9%) and red (33.8%) macroalgae or by Ortiz et al. [8] in *U. lactuca* and *D. Antarctica* (33.7% and 36.3%, respectively).

However, levels of MUFAs ranging 37.0-48.7% were higher than those observed in other species [8,12], while PUFA levels ranging 24.2-32.6% were similar to those found by other authors [8,9]. All macroalgae under study had higher total levels of polyunsaturated fatty acids (MUFA+PUFA) than saturated fatty acids (SFA) due to the high MUFA levels, and the unsaturated/saturated ratios ($\Sigma_{(MUFA+PUFA)}/\Sigma_{SFA}$) ranged from 2.9 in *Ulva* spp. to 4.5 in *Codium* spp. The fatty acid content and proportion of saturated and unsaturated fatty acids vary with seasons, geography [14], weather conditions and genetic variability [8,39]. According to Khairy and El-Shafay, MUFA levels in three macroalgae were highest in autumn. In the present study, seaweeds were collected in autumn, which could explain the high levels of fatty acids observed and the high 6/3 ratio, especially in *H. floresia* (26.0) and *S. polyschides* (10.9).

The four macroalgae studied contained C14:15 (myristoleic acid) and the essential fatty acid C18:26 (linoleic acid) as the major monounsaturated and polyunsaturated fatty acids, respectively. Arachidic acid (C20:0), followed by stearic acid (C18:0), were the main saturated fatty acids found in the studied species, ranging from 5.6-11.5% and 3.9-8.7%, respectively. These fatty acids levels were higher than those found in other macroalgae [8,9,30], in which the major fatty acids were C16:0 (palmitic acid), C18:1 (oleic acid) and C20:5 (eicosapentaenoic acid, EPA). However, C18:3 (linolenic acid) was only found in *Saccorhiza polyschides*, C22:0 (Behenic acid) only in *Halymenia floresia* and C22:6 (docosahexaenoic acid, DHA) and C24:1 (nervonic acid) only in *Codium* spp., indicating that some fatty acids seem to be species-specific in algae.

Overall, the algal species in the present study had low amounts of SFAs, high levels of MUFAs and a relationship with the $\omega 6/\omega 3$ fatty acids >1, which could be related to the species, conditions in collection area and season.

Mineral content

As shown in Table 4, the macroalga samples were rich in macrominerals (i.e., Na, K, Ca and Mg), with values ranging from 9690-14500 mg/100 g dry weight. These results are similar to those obtained by Rupérez (2002) in different species of brown (*Fucus vesiculosus, Laminaria digitata, Undaria pinnatifida*) and red (*Chondrus crispus, Porphyra tenera*) macroalgae, with values ranging from 8097-17885 mg/100 g dry weight.

Mineral	***Ulva spp.***	***Codium spp.***	***H. floresia***	***S. polyschides***
Na	3670 ± 216.4	3960 ± 106.8	5540 ± 763.5	2650 ± 176.9
K	3770 ± 114.6	4500 ± 182.4	5960 ± 861.3	10170 ± 112.4
Ca	1030 ± 321.5	820 ± 253.6	730 ± 283.4	1120 ± 94.2
Mg	2040 ± 34.7	410 ± 18.8	900 ± 162.7	560 ± 32.4
Σ macro elements	10510 ± 171.8	9690 ± 140.4	13130 ± 517.7	14500 ± 103.9
Fe	36.28 ± 0.49	45.14 ± 0.82	14.34 ± 0.39	25.12 ± 1.52
Zn	1.91 ± 0.65	0.78 ± 0.14	2.11 ± 0.01	8.57 ± 0.39
Cu	0.71 ± 0.37	0.45 ± 0.25	0.62 ± 0.23	0.94 ± 0.4
Σ microelements	38.9 ± 0.50	46.4 ± 0.40	17.1 ± 0.21	34.6 ± 0.19

Table 4: Mineral composition and trace elements of seaweeds studied (mg/100 g dry weight)[a]. [a]All values given are means of three determinations ($\bar{X}$ ± SD); SD: standard deviation.

However, the concentrations of Na, K, Ca and Mg varied slightly depending on the algal species. Na and K were the most abundant elements in all macroalgae, ranging from 2650 to 5540 and 3770-10170 mg/g dry weight, respectively, but Na/K ratios were below 1.0 in all samples (0.26-0.97). These ratios are similar to those found by Rupérez [10] in brown and red macroalgae. According to this author, a low ratio Na/K is interesting from a nutritional point of view. Since the instability of mineral salts of sodium and potassium is one of the most frequent causes of hypertension appears [40].

Sodium (5540 mg/100 g dry weight) was the most abundant element in *Halymenia floresia*, followed by potassium (10170 mg/100 g dry weight) in *Saccorhiza polyschides* and magnesium (2040 mg/100 g dry weight) in *Ulva* spp., whereas Ca contents were similar (0.7-1.1 mg/100 g dry weight) in the four species.

Microelement concentrations (i.e., Fe, Zn and Cu) also varied with the species. *Halymenia floresia* had the lowest levels (17.1 mg/100 g dry weight), and *Codium* spp. had the highest (46.4 mg/100 g dry weight). According to Ryan et al., these variations could be due to morphological and physiological differences in macroalge and their affinities for different metals [41].

Among the microelements analyzed, Fe was highest in all samples, ranging from 14.3 to 45.1 mg/100 g dry weight. This amount conforms to that reported by Yaich et al. [30] for *Ulva lactuca* and some of the species analyzed by Subba et al. [16].

Ulva spp. and *Codium* spp. contained significant amounts of Fe (36.3 and 45.1 mg/100 g dry weight, respectively), whereas *Saccorhiza polyschides* had the highest contents of Zn (8.57 mg/100 g dry weight) and Cu (0.9 mg/100 g dry weight). The ability of the four macroalga species to concentrate metals varied according to both species and type of metal accumulated. Similar results were obtained by Besada et al. [17] and Ryan et al., [41] that highlighted the complexity of the inter-relationships between metabolism, growth rate and metal uptake [17].

The high concentrations of macro and microminerals in *Ulva* spp., *Codium* spp., *Halymenia floresia* and *Saccorhiza polyschides* could be explained by the consumption and accumulation of nutritive elements in the collection medium. Studies by Martínez-Veláscо et al. [36] showed that the mouth of the Barbate River is rich in minerals, and the presence of Zn and Cu in both water and sediments was demonstrated by Gutiérrez-Mas et al. [37]. There are wealth of trace elements associated with fluvial mineral accumulation in the Barbate River and existing wetlands in the area, likely resulting in the richness of minerals found in macroalgae sampled.

Conclusion

The moisture content of fresh macroalgae (84.3-98.6%) could be related to the morphology and structure of the species. Macroalgae with tubular structures such as *Codium* spp. had the highest moisture content, while the other seaweeds, which had laminar structures, had lower contents. Protein contents exhibited high variability (7.2-15.6%), which could be related to the species and their ability to assimilate nitrogen. Lipid levels were greater than 7% in all species studied, except *Ulva* spp. These high contents could be related to the particular conditions of the collection area (i.e., salinity, water temperature and nitrate content). Carbohydrate and fiber concentrations were lower than in samples reported in other studies because of the high nitrogen content in our collection area. This area is characterized by fluvial accumulation of sediments, and therefore, the ash content and macro and microelements were especially high. Na, K, Fe, Zn and Cu concentrations varied between species, which could be due to morphological and physiological differences in the macroalgae and their affinities for different metals [41-44].

All macroalgae studied contained high levels of essential amino acids (75.2-788.5 mg/g protein) and different amino acid profiles.

Levels of MUFAs in these macroalgae (37.0-48.7%) were higher than those observed in other species. The main saturated fatty acids were arachidic acid (5.6-11.5%) and stearic acid (3.9-8.7%).

These results highlight the nutritional potential of these macroalgae as food, either as fresh produce or as a processed food ingredient, and development of seaweed farming in this area should be evaluated.

Acknowledgment

We thank Innova Vegetalia del Mar S.L. for supplying the fresh macroalgae samples.

References

1. Skibola C (2004) The effect of Fucus vesiculosus, an edible brown seaweed, upon menstrual cycle length and hormonal status in three pre-menopausal women: a case report. Complement Altern Med 4: 10-17.
2. Teas J (1981) The consumption of seaweed as a protective factor in the etiology of breast cancer. Medical Hypotheses 7: 601-613.
3. (2014) FAO.
4. Gupta S, Abu-Ghannam N (2011) Recent development in the application of seaweeds or seaweed extracts as a means for enhancing the safety and quality attributes of foods. Innov Food Sci. & Emerg Technol 12: 600-609.
5. Kadam SU, Prabhasankar P (2010) Marine foods as functional ingredients in bakery and pasta products. Food Res Int 1975-1980.
6. Devi KP, Suganthy N, Kesika P, Pandian SK (2008) Bioprotective properties of seaweeds: In vitro evaluation of antioxidant activity and antimicrobial activity against food borne bacteria in relation to polyphenolic content. Complement Altern Med KP 8: 38.
7. Aguilera-Morales M, Casas-Valdez M, Carrillo-Domínguez S, González-Acosta B, Pérez-Gil F (2005) Chemical composition and microbiological assays of marine algae Enteromorpha spp. as a potential food source. J Food Compos Anal 18: 79-88.
8. Ortiz J, Romero N, Robert P, Aray J, Lopez-Hernández J, et al. (2006) Dietary fiber, amino acid, fatty acid and tocopherol contents of the edible seaweeds Ulva lactuca and Durvillaea antarctica. Food Chem 99: 98-104.
9. Dawczynski C, Schubert R, Jahreis G (2007) Amino acids, fatty acids and dietary fibre in edible seaweed products. Food Chem 103: 891-899.
10. Gómez-Ordóñez E, Jiménez-Escrig A, Rupérez P (2010) Dietary fibre and physicochemical properties of several edible seaweeds from the northwestern Spanish coast. Food Res Int 43: 2289-2294.
11. Norziah MH, Ching CY (2000) Nutritional composition of edible seaweed Gracilaria changgi. Food Chem 68: 69-76.
12. Johns RB, Nichols PD, Perry GJ (1979) Fatty acid composition of ten marine algae from Australian waters. Phytochem 18: 799-802.
13. Sánchez-Machado DI, López-Cervantes J, López-Hernández J, Paseiro-Losada P (2004) Fatty acids, total lipid, protein and ash contents of processed edible seaweeds. Food Chem 85: 439-444.
14. Denis C, Morançais M, Li M, Deniaud E, Gaudin P, et al. (2010) Study of the chemical composition of edible red macroalgae Grateloupia turuturu from Brittany (France). Food Chem 119: 913-917.
15. Rúperez P (2002) Mineral content of edible marine seaweeds. Food Chem 79: 23-26.
16. Subba PV, Mantri VA, Ganesan K (2007) Mineral composition of edible seaweed Porphyra vietnemensis. Food Chem 102: 215-218.
17. Besada V, Andrade JM, Schultze F, González JJ (2009) Heavy metals in edible seaweeds commercialised for human consumption. J Marine Syst 75: 305-313.
18. Lartigue L, Sherman T (2002) Field assays for measuring nitrate reductase activity in Enteromorpha sp. (Chloropphyceae), Ulva spp. (Chlorophyceae), and Gelidium sp. (Rhodophyceae). J Phycol 38: 971-982.
19. Marinho-Soriano E, Fonseca PC, Carneiro MA, Moreira WS (2006) Seasonal variation in the chemical composition of two tropical seaweeds. Bioresour Technol 97: 2402-2406.
20. Gressler V, Yokoya NS, Toyota MT, Colepicolo P, Mancini J, et al. (2010) Lipid, fatty acid, protein, amino acid and ash contents in four Brazilian red algae species. Food Chem 120: 585-590.
21. Sobrino JA, Li Z, Stoll MP, Becker F (1994) Improvements in the split-window technique for land surface temperature determination. IEEE Trans Geosci Remote Sens 32: 243-253.
22. Sobrino I, Silva L, Bellido JM, Ramos F (2002) Rainfall, river discharges and sea temperature as factors affecting abundance of two coastal benthic cephalopod species in the gulf of Cadiz (SW Spain). Bull Mar Sci 71: 851-865.
23. Torres MA, Coll M, Heymans JJ, Christensen V, Sobrino I (2013) Food-web structure of and fishing impacts on the Gulf of Cadiz ecosystem (South-western Spain). Ecological Modelling 265: 26-44.
24. Anfuso E, Ponce R, González-Castro C, Forja JM (2010) Coupling between the thermohaline, chemical and biological fields during summer 2006 in the northeast continental shelf on the Gulf of Cadiz (SW Iberian Peninsula). Sci Mar 74: 47-56.
25. AOAC (2000) Official methods of analysis of AOAC international, (17th edn.) Gaithersburg, USA.
26. International Union of Pure and Applied Chemistry (IUPAC) (1992) In: Paquot C, Hautfenne A (eds) Standard method for the analysis of oils, fats and derivatives (7th edn.) London: Blackwell Scientific Publications.
27. AFNOR (1996) Dosage des minéraux-méthodes par spectrométrie d'émission de flamme. NF-T-90-019. Association Française de Normalisation (AFNOR), La Défense, France.
28. Livesey G, Buss D, Coussement P, Edwards DG, Howlett J, et al. (2000) Suitability of traditional energy values for novel foods and food ingredients. Food Control 11: 249-289.
29. Pereira L, Armado AM, Critchley AT, Van de Velde F, Ribeiro-Claro PJA (2009) Identification of selected seaweed polysaccharides (phycocolloids) by vibrational spectroscopy (FTIR-ATR and FT-Raman). Food Hydrocoll 23: 1903-1909.
30. Yaich H, Garna H, Besbes S, Paquot M, Blecker C, et al. (2011) Chemical composition and functional properties of Ulva lactuca seaweed collected in Tunisia. Food Chem 128: 895-901.
31. McHugh DJ (2003) A guide to the seaweed industry. FAO Fish Tech Pap 441: 105.
32. Navarro-Angulo L, Robledo D (1999) Effects of nitrogen source, N: P ratio and N-pulse concentration and frequency on the growth of Gracilaria cornea (Gracilariales, Rhodophyta) in culture. Hydrobiologia 399: 315-320.
33. Wong KH, Cheung PCK (2000) Nutritional evaluation of some

subtropical red and green seaweed. Part I- proximate composition, amino acid profiles and some physico-chemical properties. Food Chem 71: 475-482.

34. Floreto EAT, Teshima S, Ishikawa M (1996) Effects of nitrogen and phosphorus on the growth and fatty acid composition of Ulva pertusa Kjellman (Chlorophyta). Bot Mar 39: 69-74.
35. Floreto EAT, Teshima S (1998) The fatty acid composition of seaweeds exposed to different levels of light intensity and salinity. Bot Mar 41: 467-481.
36. Martínez-Velasco C, Forja JM, Gómez-Parra A (1999) Hydrochemistry characterisation of protected marine ecosystems in Cadiz. Bol Inst Esp Oceanogr 15: 451-456.
37. Gutiérrez-Mas JM, Moral JP, Sánchez A, Domínguez S, Muñoz-Pérez JJ (2003) Multicycle sediments on the continental shelf of Cadiz (SW Spain). Estuar. Coast. Shelf Sci 57: 667-677.
38. Mabeau S, Fleurence J (1993) Seaweed in food products: Biochemical and nutritional aspects. Trends Food Sci Technol 4: 103-107.
39. Macler BA (1986) Regulation of carbon flow by nitrogen and light in the red alga Gelidium coulteri. Plant Physiol 82: 136-141.
40. Geleijnse, Kok (2003) Grobbee, Blood pressure response to changes in sodium and potassium intake: a metaregression analysis of randomised trials. J Hum Hypertens 17: 471-480.
41. Ryan S, McLoughlin P, O'Donovan O (2012) A comprehensive study of metal distribution in three main classes of seaweed. Environ Pollut 167: 171-177.
42. Peinado I, Girón J, Koutsidis G, Ames JM (2014) Chemical composition, antioxidant activity and sensory evaluation of five different species of Brown edible seaweeds. Food Res Int 66: 36-44.
43. Fleurence J (1990) "Seaweeds proteins: Biochemical nutritional aspects and potential uses". Trends Food Sci & Tech 10: 25-28.
44. Pereira V, Pontes M, Câmara JS, Marques JC (2008) Simultaneous analysis of free amino acids and biogenic amines in honey and wine samples using in loop orthophthalaldeyde derivatization procedure. J Chromatogr A 1189: 435-443.

Tolerability Study of a Free Amino Acid-based Formula in Children with Cow's Milk Allergy

Jentzsch NS[1*], Silveira FJF[1], Cruz LL[2], Wainstein APDL[1] and Previato HDRA[3]

[1]*Faculty of Medical Sciences of Minas Gerais, Belo Horizonte/MG, Brazil*

[2]*School of Nutrition, Federal University of Ouro Preto, Ouro Preto/MG, Brazil*

[3]*Department of Food and Nutrition, School of Food Engineering, University of Campinas, Campinas/SP, Brazil*

[*]**Corresponding author:** Jentzsch NS, Department of Medical Sciences, Federal University of Minas Gerais, Brazil, E-mail: nulmasj@gmail.com

Abstract

Background: The prevalence of food allergy has increased worldwide. Cow's milk allergy is a very common type of allergy in childhood. In non-breast-fed infants, with extremely severe or life-threatening symptoms, an amino acid-based formula may be considered the first choice for the dietary treatment. This study aimed to assess the tolerance to a new Brazilian amino acid-based formula and the nutritional status in children affected by cow's milk allergy fed with this formula.

Objective: To assess the tolerance to an amino acid-based formula and its nutritional status impact on children affected by cow's milk allergy.

Method: This is a clinical study conducted with a sample of 15 children, less than 5 years old with a clinical cow's milk allergy diagnosis. The children were followed-up, in a Pediatric Outpatient Clinic. Anthropometric, clinical, epidemiological data were collected at the baseline and it was also prescribed the amino acid-based formula. Throughout the treatment, which lasted five months, the clinical response was assessed based on the remission of symptoms initially presented and the evolution of nutritional status, using the WHO child growth standards charts.

Results: The sample included predominantly boys with a mean age of 28.1 months and 66.7% IgE-mediated. The average age of onset of the allergic symptoms was 2.15 ± 2.33 months. Symptoms were reported in different systems (cutaneous, gastrointestinal and respiratory). In every child, there was complete remission of allergy symptoms initially presented and proper evolution of nutritional status.

Conclusion: This new free amino acid-based formula can safely be used for the dietary treatment for children with cow's milk allergy. The subjects studied showed adequate children's nutritional status evolution.

Keywords: Amino acids; Child nutritional status; Infant formula; Hypersensitivity; Milk protein; Cow's milk allergy

Introduction

The prevalence of allergic diseases has increased worldwide and it can be highlighted the prevalence of food allergies that consists of any adverse reaction, immune mediated, reproducible, that is triggered by a contact with a specific food [1,2].

Among food allergies, cow's milk protein allergy (CMPA) is the first allergic disease in childhood, which is why it is the most prevalent in that age range. However, its real rate it is not well known, predominantly due to methodological differences described in the scientific literature report, as well as the diagnostic criteria vary from each other. In Brazil, the prevalence in early childhood is 5.4% [2-4].

CMPA can present a wide spectrum of clinical reactions such as cutaneous, gastrointestinal, respiratory, or systemic symptoms that might be caused by immunoglobulin (Ig)E-mediated, non-IgE-mediated, or mixed.

Diagnosis is based on the child's clinical history associated with physical examination, clinical symptoms, quantification of specific IgE to food and the oral challenge, the last one is considered the gold standard [2].

The basic treatment of CMPA consists of the complete avoidance of milk and dairy products. Milk substitutes are needed and, in general, specific infant formula or hypoallergenic diets are recommended. The purpose is to avoid triggering of symptoms and the disease progression, besides providing child a suitable growth and development pattern. The recommended formulas are: extensively or partially hydrolyzed cow's milk protein formulas (casein or whey protein), soy formula (isolated or hydrolyzed) or other vegetable milk. However only free amino acid-based formula are considered to be non-allergenic [1,2].

In Brazil, the predominant suppliers of these formulas are multinational companies. The Brazilian government is the main purchaser and the deal is made through public biddings. The important demand for national formulas rather than the foreign ones due, among other issues, the reduction of public expenditures, led a

Brazilian food industry to develop and produce an amino acid-based formula, called Amix®, to treat children with CMPA.

The current study aimed to evaluate the tolerance to this new formula and its ability to provide the nutritional needs for children with CMPA, without risks to the patient's health.

Methods

According to research design, it was conducted, from August 2013 to June 2015, a self-controlled clinical study in a pediatric clinic, at Faculdade de Ciências Médicas de Minas Gerais (FCMMG). The research protocol and informed consent form were approved by the Ethics Committee of the FCMMG in accordance with Brazilian regulations [5]. After informing the children's parents or guardians about the research goals and all the procedures which would be conducted throughout the study, an informed consent was obtained from them.

Children from Belo Horizonte and metropolitan region, who were admitted to the pediatric clinic at FCMMG, presenting signs and symptoms of CMPA that had not improved with the consumption of extensively hydrolyzed cow's milk protein formulas were eligible for the study. The study enrolled 15 children, from birth to 5 years old.

The study consisted of two stages: a screening and a follow-up one. In the first stage, CMPA's diagnosis was confirmed based on a detailed clinical history and physical examination. Clinical evidence presented by the children while they were consuming cow's milk or cow's milk protein formulas, followed by remission of signs and symptoms after the introduction of exclusion diet, according to children guardians' reports and/or proven through medical reports were considered. In addition to the diagnosis, measurement of serum total and milk-protein IgE were assessed.

Through a questionnaire of sociodemographic, clinical and anthropometric data (such as date of birth, gender, type of delivery), information about breastfeeding, presented symptoms, type of allergic (IgE-mediated and not mediated), weight and length at birth, and also the current weight, length and head circumference, were also obtained at the first stage. From mothers were collected date of birth, educational background, and pregnancy complications. Before leaving the clinic, patients received the nutritionally complete and non-allergenic free amino acid-based formula, Amix®.

Each child attended 5 medical appointments. The follow-up stage, consisted of the assessment, at each visit, of clinical response of patients through presence or remission of gastrointestinal, respiratory and cutaneous symptoms initially presented, as well as formula acceptability, through the volume ingested. The evolution of nutritional status was also assessed by measurements of weight, length and head circumference. The variables weight and height were used to evaluate the body mass index for age (BMI/A). The WHO child growth standard charts were used to classify the nutritional status [6].

Data collection was carried out by two researchers and medicine students from FCMMG previously trained and qualified in accordance with the SISVAN's anthropometric rules [7]. Children under two years were weighed and measured completely naked. For those measurements, the digital pediatric scale Urano® and the infantometer Indaiá® were used. To measure the weight and height of children older than 2 years, Filizola® scale with stadiometer was used. Head circumference was measured using an inelastic and tape measure body.

Data obtained were deposited in a database and then processed and analyzed using WHO Anthro software, version 3.2.2 [8], WHO Anthro Plus, version 1.0.4 [9] and free software R version 3.1.3 [10]. The considered confidence interval was 95% with a 5% significance level ($p \leq 0.05$).

In the statistical analysis, the descriptive statistics were used to present variables collected at the first medical appointment (gender age in months, types of allergies, type of delivery, gestational complications, weight and length, gestational age and maternal age). For categorical variables were presented absolute and relative frequencies and for continuous variables, average, standard deviation and amplitude. The formula tolerability was evaluated by comparing the results of weight, height, length, head circumference and the symptoms observed at the first and last follow-up medical appointment. The McNemar Chi-square (χ^2) test was applied to compare paired categorical data. The Wilcoxon test compared paired continuous data.

Results

Table 1 presents the descriptive statistics of data collected in the first medical appointment. The sample was predominantly made up of boys (53.3%) with a mean age of 28.1 months (± 18.1) and non-IgE-mediated allergy (66.7%). The average birth weight was 2.89 kg (± 0.89 kg) and the most frequent type of delivery was the cesarean section (73.3%). With relation to pregnancy, the mean gestational age was 37 weeks (± 3.34 weeks), and prematurity, caused by a variety of factors such as premature placental abruption, constant bleeding, and maternal hypertension, occurred in 20% of cases (n=3). Some complications associated with pregnancy and childbirth were reported by 46.66% of mothers (n=7) and include pre-eclampsia and HELLP syndrome, constant bleeding, maternal hypertensive crisis and gestational diabetes.

Variables	**n**	**%**
Gender		
Male	8	53.3
Female	7	46.7
Age (months)		
Mean ± SD*	28.1 ± 18.1	
Minimum; Maximum	9.9; 78.2	
Birth weight (kg)		
Mean ± SD	2.89 ± 0.89	
Minimum; Maximum	1.10; 4.28	
Length weight (cm)		
Mean ± SD	47.50 ± 4.67	
Minimum; Maximum	36; 53	
Delivery mode		
Vaginal delivery	4	26.7
Cesarean section	11	73.3
Gestacional age (weeks)		

Mean ± SD	36.70 ± 3.34	
Minimum; Maximum	28; 41	
Pregnancy Complications		
No	8	53.3
Yes	7	46.7
Maternal age (age)		
Mean ± SD	31.21 ± 5.24	
Minimum; Maximum	21; 40	
Allergy		
Non-IgE-mediated	10	66.7
IgE mediated	5	33.3
*SD: Standard Deviation		

Table 1: Descriptive variables of the study population, Belo Horizonte, Brazil, 2015.

In the study population, 93.33% (n=14) of the children were breastfed, and 53.33% (n=7) remained on exclusive breastfeeding for the average period of 42 ± 66.64 days (1.4 ± 2.22 months). The average duration of full breastfeeding was 174.14 ± 172.0 days (5.80 ± 5.74 months).

The average age of introduction of whole cow's milk or infant formula was 69.27 ± 71.66 days (2.31 ± 2.39 months). In 60% (n=9) children milk-based formula was introduced, in 20% (n=3) whole cow's milk, in 13.33% (n=2) a free amino acid-based formula and in 6.66% (n=1) a formula with extensively hydrolyzed protein. In some cases, mothers were asked to do the elimination diet to continue breastfeeding.

Table 2 depicts the comparison of the occurrence of symptoms according to the duration of full and exclusive breastfeeding. There was no significant difference in the occurrence of symptoms in the first and fifth medical appointment to any of full breastfeeding groups. However, comparing the occurrence of symptoms according to exclusive breastfeeding, there was a significant reduction in the occurrence of gastrointestinal symptoms in children who had not been on exclusive breastfeeding (p=0.010).

Variable	Breast feeding duration	1st appointment		5th appointment		P-value
		n	%	n	%	
Full breast feeding duration						
Gastrointestinal symptoms	<6 months (n=7)	4	57.1	0	0	0.076*
	≥ 6 months (n=8)	4	50	0	50	0.056*
Respiratory symptoms	<6 months (n=7)	3	42.9	2	28.6	1.000*
	≥ 6 months (n=8)	2	25	0	0	0.450*
Cutaneous symptoms	<6 months (n=7)	2	28.6	0	0	0.445*
	≥ 6 months (n=8)	4	50	1	12.5	0.281*
Exclusive breast feeding duration						
Gastrointestinal symptoms	No (n=8)	6	75	0	0	0.010*
	Yes (n=8)	3	37.5	0	0	0.200*
Respiratory symptoms	No (n=8)	4	50	2	25	0.606*
	Yes (n=8)	1	12.5	1	12.5	1.000*
Cutaneous symptoms	No (n=8)	3	37.5	0	0	0.200*
	Yes (n=8)	4	50	1	12.5	0.281*
*P-value McNemar chi-square test to paired categorical data						

Table 2: Comparison of CMPA symptoms occurrence according to the duration of breastfeeding in the 1st and 5th medical appointment, Belo Horizonte, Brazil, 2015.

The average age at onset of CMPA symptoms was 2.15 ± 2.33 months (64.47 ± 69.75 days). Symptoms reported were grouped into three major groups: Cutaneous (atopic dermatitis, hives, rashes, itching and perianal rash), respiratory (wheezing and bronchospasm) and gastrointestinal (cramps, gas and bloating, vomiting, nausea, diarrhea containing mucus and blood, hematochezia, constipation, gastroesophageal reflux and severe constipation).

The average age of the children at the beginning and end of treatment with infant formula Amix® was 13 ± 13.58 months and 18 ± 14 months, respectively. All children presented good tolerance of the study formula. Average weight gain was 361.95 g/month and height gains 2.49 cm/month. In 60% of cases (n=9) both gains were higher than theoretically expected; in 26.67% (n=4) children only the length reached the expectation, and in 13.33% (n=2), only the weight gain was higher than expected for the age group.

Table 3 presents the comparison between the measurements of weight, height, head circumference and symptoms of children in the first and fifth medical appointment. There was a significant reduction in gastrointestinal symptoms, presented by nine of 15 children in the first medical appointment (60%), and in the fifth medical appointment, these symptoms were not observed in any children (p-value=0.000). Cutaneous symptoms were presented by 7 of 15 children in the first medical appointment (46.7%), only 1 child (6.7%) presented them in the fifth one (p-value=0.016). There was a significant increase in weight, height and head circumference of children.

Variables	1st appointment		5th appointment		P-value
	n	%	n	%	
Gastrointestinal symptoms	9	60	0	0.0	0.000**
Respiratory symptoms	5	33.3	3	20.0	0.433**
Cutaneous symptoms	7	46.7	1	6.7	0.016**
Weight (kg)					
Mean ± SD*	8.80 ± 3.37		10.40 ± 2.87		0.001***
Lenght (cm)					
Mean ± SD*	70.71 ± 12.72		78.81 ± 10.90		0.001***
Head Circumference (cm)					
Mean ± SD*	44.48 ± 3.99		46.19 ± 2.79		0.006***

*SD=standard deviation; ** P-value McNemar chi-square test to paired tegorical data; ***P-value Wilcoxon test to compare paired continuous data

Table 3: Comparison of weight, height, head circumference and symptoms presented by the children sampled in the 1st and 5th medical appointment, Belo Horizonte, Brazil, 2015.

BMI index for age (BMI/A) at the beginning and at the end of treatment with infant formula Amix® compared to the WHO standard distribution (2006) presented a good improvement in nutritional status (Figure 1). The mean BMI Z-score at the first visit (Figure 1A) and five months later (Figure 1B) were 0.015 ± 1.34 and 0.067 ± 1.33, respectively (p-value=0.89) corroborating the efficacy of Amix® formula.

Discussion

The available treatment for children diagnosed with CMPA currently described is the strict avoidance of milk and dairy products [11]. Therefore, there is great concern among health professionals and guardians in relation to the dietary intake and nutritional status of these children. If an adequate hypoallergenic diet is not implemented, the treatment may promote energy, protein and micronutrients deficits [12].

In situations which the maintenance of breastfeeding is not possible, the use of hydrolyzed cow's milk protein formulas or soy protein formulas is considered a recommended alternative to the treatment [2]. In the case of soybeans, unfortunately, about 30-50% of children who are intolerant to milk protein are also allergic to soy protein. Furthermore, the use of soy milk is not recommended for children under 6 months of age [2,13].

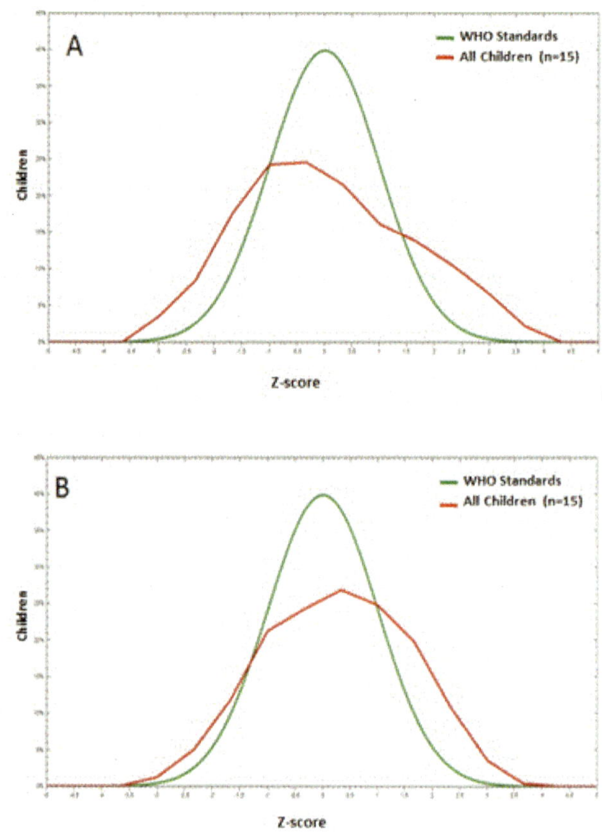

Figure 1: Index BMI/A distribution at the beginning (A) and the end (B) of treatment compared to the reference population, Belo Horizonte, Brazil, 2015.

The formulas containing milk proteins partially hydrolyzed or extensively are alternative options for the treatment of CMPA because they are less susceptible to induce an immune reaction. However, it should be considered that formulas containing partially hydrolyzed protein may cause allergy in one-third to half of allergic individuals and therefore cannot be considered hypoallergenic. Many researchers have already reported hypersensitivity reactions to these formulas, and also corroborated that this is a relatively common problem among children [14,15]. On the other hand, formulas containing extensively hydrolyzed proteins are well tolerated by approximately 95% of allergic individuals [16].

When patients do not respond to treatment with these products, free amino acid-based formulas, the only one considered non-allergenic, are indicated [2,17]. In general, the use of these formulas consists of an effective and safe method, able to promote adequate children's weight gain, growth and the remission of allergy symptoms initially presented [17,18].

Therefore, the development of a nutritionally complete free amino acid-based formula is an advance in the treatment of CMPA when hypersensitivity to intact or hydrolyzed proteins occurs. However, studies are needed to confirm the tolerability and nutritional adequacy of these formulas in children [19].

This work presents the first study to assess the tolerability to a new free amino acid-based formula for children with CMPA, called Amix®, available in the Brazilian market. The tolerability to amino acid-based formula, in some cases can be vital since, although most children respond to the avoidance of milk protein and to the introduction of extensively hydrolyzed formulas and diets, there are some situations or more severe cases in which only the free amino acid-based diets can solve the signs and symptoms of CMPA [2,14,20].

According to Bahna [19], to be considered hypoallergenic, the formula should be well tolerated by at least 90% (with 95% confidence) of individuals who are already allergic to milk protein. This study showed, with 95% confidence that all children with CMPA who participated in the study tolerated the free amino acid-based formula, Amix®.

At the end of treatment, it was observed that one child presented signs of atopic dermatitis. However, the manifestation of this symptom does not mean lack of tolerance to the infant formula Amix®, since this patient has not had other symptoms of CMPA, presented at the beginning of the treatment. These symptoms may be associated with increased synthesis of IgE, which is common in atopic children. The natural history of atopic manifestations is characterized by a typical sequence of IgE antibody responses and clinical symptoms which may appear early in life, persist over years and often remit spontaneously with age, called atopic march. So even with the exclusion of cow's milk and dairy products, the child may present other manifestations such as asthma, rhinitis, and dermatitis [21].

During the last physical examination, it was observed sibilant rhonchus, in three children with viral infection when undergoing chest auscultation. Despite this respiratory symptom also be suggestive of CMPA, its clinical manifestation in these cases is not associated with lack of tolerability to the infant formula Amix®. It is known that during the winter, due to climatic conditions, either the low temperature or the dry season, there is an increase in hospital admissions for complications related to the respiratory system [22].

As observed in other studies, digestive symptoms showed the highest prevalence among studied children [23,24]. Most children (66.7%) were diagnosed with non-IgE mediated reactions, which are characterized by symptoms of delayed onset, involving preferably the gastrointestinal tract, reinforcing the results observed at the first medical appointment when 60% of children had gastrointestinal symptoms.

The most common type of delivery was cesarean section and prematurity occurred in 20% of cases. These two variables are considered, among other maternal and perinatal characteristics, potential risk factors for the CMPA. Therefore, these findings contributed to reinforcing results already reported by other researchers, which the mode of delivery and prematurity contribute to the increased prevalence of CMPA [25,26]. The introduction of milk based infant formula (60%) reflects the early occurrence, not only the weaning but also the allergen presence on children feeding. The average time of exclusive breastfeeding (42 days) and full breastfeeding (approximately 180 days) observed in this study, is fall far shorter than the current WHO recommendations, which states that infant should be exclusively breastfed up to six months of age with continued breastfeeding along with appropriate complementary food up to two years of age or beyond [27]. This condition is also associated with an increased risk of developing CMPA [26].

The significant reduction in the occurrence of gastrointestinal symptoms in children, who were exclusively breastfed, does not mean that exclusive breastfeeding should not be encouraged in cases of CMPA. On the opposite, breastfeeding should be recommended due to many beneficial effects in the short and long terms for both mother and child, including as a protective agent for food allergies. Regarding this, mothers should be oriented to do the elimination diet [2].

What may explain this finding is that often the compliance to exclusion diet is not simple. Most of the time the mother consciously do not consume milk, dairy or traces, but an accidental ingestion can happen or also the lack of knowledge, especially when reading the labels of processed foods. It is for this reason that mothers and families need to receive nutritional counseling, which should address the possible cross-contamination and read not only food but also cosmetics and medicaments labels [28].

The WHO child growth standard charts were used for nutritional assessment, because they represent a prescriptive approach to how children around the world should grow and they are considered an adequate and robust instrument for assessing the nutritional status of children under five years, regardless of their ethnic and cultural characteristics, by the fact that, under optimal conditions, all children show similar growth pattern [29].

We conclude that there was an adequate improvement in children's nutritional status as well as weight gain ($p<0,001$), and improvement in other parameters, which prove the effectiveness of the formula Amix®. Therefore this formula can be used for the dietary management of children with CMPA, without prejudice to their nutritional status and without triggering immediate or late allergic symptoms.

Acknowledgement

The authors acknowledge Fundação de Amparo à Pesquisa do Estado de Minas (FAPEMIG) for the financial support, Dra. Isabel Gomes for statistical advice, and academic medical students of the Faculdade de Ciências Médicas de Minas Gerais for data collection.

Authors Note

This clinical trial was registered in "ClinicalTrials.gov Protocol Registration System", under the identification number: NCT02536482.

References

1. Vandenplas Y, De Greef E, Devreker T (2014) Treatment of Cow's Milk Protein Allergy. Pediatr Gastroenterol Hepatol 17: 1-5.
2. Solé D, Amâncio OMS, Jacob CMA, Cocco RR, Sarni ROS, et al. (2012) Practical guide to diagnosis and treatment of cow's milk protein allergy mediated by immunoglobulin E. Braz J Allergy Immunopathol 35: 203-233.
3. Lins MGM, Horowitz MR, Silva GAP, Motta MEFA (2010) Oral food challenge test to confirm the diagnosis of cow's milk protein allergy. Pediatr J 86: 285-289.
4. Oliveira VCD (2013) Cow's milk protein allergy and lactose intolerance: nutritional approach and perceptions of health professionals. Thesis to obtain the master's degree, University of Juiz de Fora, Brazil, pp: 1-104
5. National Health Council (2013) Resolution No. 466 of 12 December 2012. Approves regulatory standards for research involving human beings. Official Diary of the Union, Brazil.

6. World Health Organization (2006) Multicentre Growth Reference Study Group. WHO child growth standards based on length/height, weight, and age. Acta Ped 95: 76-85.
7. Fagundes AA, Barros DC, Duar HA, Sardinha, LMV, Pereira MM, et al. (2004) Food and Nutrition Surveillance: Basic guidelines for the collection, processing, data analysis and information in healthcare. Ministry of Health, Brazil.
8. World Health Organization (2007) WHO Anthro for personal computers, version 2, 2007: Software for assessing growth and development of the world's children. WHO, Geneva.
9. World Health Organization (2009) WHO AnthroPlus for personal computers Manual: Software for assessing the growth of the world's children and adolescents. WHO, Geneva.
10. R Development Core Team (2011) R: A language and environment for statistical computing. R Foundation for Statistical Computing, Vienna, Austria.
11. Host A, Halken S (2014) Cow's Milk Allergy: Where have we Come from and where are we Going? Endocrine, Metabolic and Immune Disorders-Drug Targets 14: 2-8.
12. Alves JQN, Mendes JFR (2013) Dietary intake and nutritional status in children with allergy to cow's milk protein. Health Science 24: 65-72.
13. Dias A, Santosa A, Pinheiro JA (2010) Persistence of cow's milk allergy beyond two years of age. Allergol Immunopathol 38: 8-12.
14. Frisner H, Rosendal A, Barkholt V (2000) Identification of immunogenic maize proteins in a casein hydrolysate formula. Pediatr Allergy Immunol 11: 106-110.
15. Isolauri E, Sutas Y, Makinen-Kiljunen S, Oja SSIR, Turjanmaa K (1995) Efficacy and safety of hydrolyzed cow milk and amino acid-derived formulas in infants with cow milk allergy. J Pediatr 127: 550-557.
16. Vanderhoof JA (2015) In time, improper and excessive use of amino acid formulas in allergy to cow's milk. Paul Pediatr J 34: 1-2.
17. Host A, Koletzko B, Dreborg S, Muraro A, Wahn U, et al. (1999) Dietary products used in infants for treatment and prevention of food allergy. Arch Dis Child 81: 80-84.
18. Hill DJ, Murchw SH, Raffertyz K, Wallisz P, Greenz CJ (2007) The efficacy of amino acid-based formulas in relieving the symptoms of cow's milk allergy: a systematic review. Clin Exp Allergy 37: 808-822.
19. Bahna SL (2008) Hypoallergenic formulas: optimal choices for treatment versus prevention. Ann Allergy Asthma Immunol 101: 453-459.
20. Koletzko S, Niggemann YB, Arato ZA, Dias JA, Heuschkel JJR, et al. (2012) Diagnostic Approach and Management of Cow's-Milk Protein Allergy in Infants and Children: ESPGHAN GI Committee Practical Guidelines. JPGN 55: 221-229.
21. Oliveira AKK, Ribeiro MR, Kalil J, Motta AA (2010) Dermatologic manifestations in respiratory atopic patients. Braz J Allergy Immunopathol 33: 203-208.
22. Amorim JRG, Oliveira AM, Neves D, Oliveira GP (2013) Association between environmental variables and respiratory diseases (asthma and bronchitis) in children in Macapa-AP city in the period 2008 to 2012. Planet Amazon: Int J Env Law Public Policy 5: 141-153.
23. Aguiar ALO, Maranhão CM, Spinelli LC, Figueiredo RM, Maia JMC, et al. (2013) Clinical and evolutionary evaluation of children in care program to use formulas for allergy to cow's milk protein. Paul Pediatr J 31: 152-158.
24. Canani RB, Nocerino R, Leone L, Di Costanzo M, Terrin G, et al. (2013) Tolerance to a new free amino acid-based formula in children with IgE or non-IgE-mediated cow's milk allergy: a randomized controlled clinical trial. BMC Pediatr 13: 1-6.
25. Metsala J, Lundqvist A, Kaila M, Gissler M, Klaukkay T, et al. (2010) Maternal and Perinatal Characteristics and the Risk of Cow's Milk Allergy in Infants up to 2 Years of Age: A Case-Control Study Nested in the Finnish Population. Am J Epidemiol 171: 1310-1316.
26. Monjaraz EMT, Mayans JAR, Bustamante RC, Morales EG, Rosales AM, et al. (2015) Perinatal factors associated with the development of cow's milk protein allergy. J Gastroenterol Mexico 80: 27-31.
27. World Health Organization (2000) Collaborative Study Team on the Role of Breastfeeding on the Prevention of Infant Mortality. Effect of breastfeeding on infant and child mortality due to infectious diseases in less developed countries: a pooled analysis. Lancet 355: 451-455.
28. Fiocchi A, Brozek J, Schunemann H, Bahna SL, Von Berg A, et al. (2010) World Allergy Organization (WAO) Diagnosis and Rationale for Action against Cow's Milk Allergy (DRACMA) Guidelines. WAO Journal 5: 57-161.
29. Bagni UV, Luiz RR, Veiga GV (2012) Distortions in the nutritional diagnosis of children related to the use of multiple growth curves in a developing country. Rev Paul Pediatr J 30: 544-552.

10

Tepary Bean: A Climate Smart Crop for Food and Nutritional Security

Jiri O[*] and Mafongoya P

School of Agricultural, Earth and Environmental Sciences, University of KwaZulu-Natal, Private Bag X01, Scottsville, Pietermaritzburg, 3209, South Africa

[*]**Corresponding author:** Jiri O, School of Agricultural, Earth and Environmental Sciences, University of KwaZulu-Natal, Private Bag X01, Scottsville, Pietermaritzburg, 3209, South Africa, E-mail: obertjiri@yahoo.co.uk

Abstract

The variability of climate demands the use of a variety of agronomic strategies and crop choices. Traditional drought tolerant crops such as sorghum are often chosen when drought seasons are anticipated. However, there are crops, tepary bean (*Phaseolus acutifolias*), such as that could help increase diversity of crops that can be grown in changed climates. Trials were conducted to determine the growth of tepary bean on station and in the field. In the field it was compared to other commonly used legumes such as cowpea, Bambara nut, groundnut and pigeon pea. Tepary bean matured in 54 days after planting, the earliest among all the legumes. A second experiment was done to determine the effects of inorganic fertilizer and rhizobium inoculation on the growth and grain yield of field grown tepary bean. This was conducted in a randomized complete block design with three replications at the University of Zimbabwe Crop Science fields. The treatments were: basal fertilizer with top dressing, basal fertilizer only, top dressing fertilizer only, rhizobium with top dressing fertilizer, rhizobium only and neither control with no rhizobium or any inorganic fertilizer (control). There were significant differences in biomass yield between the treatment with basal fertilizer+top dressing and the control ($P<0.05$). Podding showed significant differences between treatments ($P<0.05$). Results showed that a combination of ammonium nitrate with either compound D or rhizobium produced similar yield. Rhizobium with top dressing fertilizer had a mean yield of 0.57 t/ha whilst basal fertilizer with top dressing had 0.60 t/ha. We conclude that resource poor farmers, affected by drought effects of climate change, can use rhizobium for optimum production of tepary bean, in variable climate and drought seasons and still get a yield. This is crucial for food and nutritional security of vulnerable households affected by climate change and variability.

Keywords: Tepary bean; Climate smart crop; Drought; Smallholder farmers

Introduction

Leguminous crops are important in nutrition, particularly amongst resource poor people. Inclusion of legumes in the diet is important in control and prevention of various metabolic diseases such as colon cancer, diabetes mellitus and coronary heart disease. Legumes are sources of slow release dietary fibre (carbohydrates) and are rich in proteins (18%-25%). In Africa, legumes are the cheapest sources of supplementary proteins, besides being sources of minerals and vitamins. Legumes grain is an important food source used to cover dietary protein and energy requirements. They have high dietary fibre content and low lipid, with emerging evidence emphasizing the importance of legume grain as carriers of polyphenols, saponins, oxalates, lectins, phytosterols and enzyme inhibitors. Further evidence also suggests the importance of pulses in human health, particularly in prevention on coronary heart disease and diabetes.

Lately grain legumes have come out of the shadows in research and extension because of their highly valued and multiple benefits for the farmer and the farming systems across the developing world. For semi-arid regions in particular, inadequate and highly variable rainfall and short growing periods limit yield potential and create a risky primary production environment. Evidence from the Intergovernmental Panel on Climate Change (IPCC) is now overwhelmingly convincing that climate change poses one of the greatest challenges to agriculture and food security especially in sub-Saharan Africa (SSA). This is because the region is very widely recognized as one of the most vulnerable in the world due to adaptive capacity which is extremely low, which is linked to acute poverty levels and poor infrastructure, as reflected in a high dependence of rainfall agriculture [1,2]. Among the most significant impacts of climate change is the potential increase of food insecurity and malnutrition. Projections suggest that the number of people at risk of hunger will increase by 10%-20% by 2050 due to climate change, with 65% of this population in sub-Saharan Africa. The number of malnourished children could increase by up to 21% (24 million children), with the majority being in Africa [3]. These negative impacts of climate change and variability are presenting new challenges to the majority of smallholder farmers in the absence of appropriate response measures, hence the need to address the challenges. Food and nutrition strategies that bring co-benefits in terms of enhanced production of and access to food should be explored and tested. Focusing exclusively on increasing agricultural productions is too short sighted in the context of sustainable food and nutrition security under climate change because producing more food does not necessarily lead to a better access to food or to an improved nutritional status of those who need it most [3]. Adaptation is increasingly seen as an inevitable answer to the challenges posed by climate change. Diversification into new crop types and cultivars is one adaptation that has been identified as a potential farm level response to climate change and variability [4,5]. Integration of N_2-fixing legumes and other high value crops within smallholder farming systems has been identified as one of the climate change coping strategies. The potential for grain legumes as a food resource and for soil fertility replenishment has been widely researched [6-8]. Drought tolerant crops and high protein leguminous crops that include tepary bean (*Phaseolus acutifolius*) have over the years been largely ignored and neglected by research as minor crops could also be potential candidate to be included in the adaptation strategy by providing greater resilience in coping with climate change. Studies indicated that current global debates on climate change adaptation options for smallholders need also to consider benefits for human nutrition. Fageria et al. [9] reported that production of traditional crops such as small grains could be a strategy for reducing micronutrients deficiencies in humans. Finger millet and sorghum contain high content of minerals and vitamins [10]. Changes in climatic conditions have already affected the production of some staple crops. Maize (*Zea mays.* L), the staple food of Zimbabwe, is the most widespread grain crop grown under rainfed conditions in the smallholder cropping systems. As such, food security in Zimbabwe is generally defined in terms of maize but average maize yields remain low (<0.5 tha^{-1}) and continue to decline thus threatening household food security, yet in terms of nutritional importance, maize make up 49.5% of the daily calorie intake in the country [11]. Yet cereal grain alone does not provide enough nutritional value. Grain legumes complement household dietary requirements since they have high protein levels [12,13]. Physiologically, it is not only the quantity of food but also its quality and the combination into a varied, balanced diet which are crucial [14].

The human race is faced with many issues related to need for nutritious and adequate amounts of food. According to McCaffrey [15], there is no other food which has a more health-supportive nutrient profile than beans. This is because they contain nearly equal amounts of protein and fibre, which is a unique combination that is rarely found in other plant foods. This combination together with the antioxidant content of beans has proved to be a powerful weapon against today's common diseases. However, tepary bean has been noted to be better than all other bean crops. Because of the high fiber content, tepary beans have the lowest glycemic index (the rate at which a food raises blood sugar levels) of all beans [16].

Studies in the United States and Mexico suggest the importance of lectin toxins and other compounds from tepary beans in chemotherapy, halting the growth of cancer [17]. Furthermore, recent studies from the same region suggest that tepary beans are useful for treating cancer, and they could be ten times more effective than chemotherapy [15]. Tepary bean seeds were shown to contain at least two different groups of bioactive proteins with dissimilar effects on cancer cells. The lectins in tepary bean exhibited an anti-proliferative effect on non-transformed cells and on some cancer cells [18,19].

Due to the higher amounts of calcium, iron, zinc, magnesium, phosphorus and potassium, tepary bean has less digestive discomfort and gassiness as compared to other beans. Tepary beans are lower in polyunsaturated fat and in the anti-enzymatic compounds which make common beans hard to digest [16]. Phaseolus beans are amongst the major legumes for food consumption, especially in Latin America, Africa and Asia [20]. Organoleptic evaluation of tepary bean products by students native to the area of recipe origin indicated its dishes to be moderately to highly acceptable [21]. Tepary bean is mainly grown for its mature dry seeds, which are eaten after boiling, steaming, frying or baking. They are used in stews and soups, and mixed with whole-grain maize. In Uganda, the dry seeds are usually boiled and then coarsely ground before being added to soup. Occasionally, it is eaten as a green bean or as bean sprouts. The leaves are considered edible in Malawi, but are tougher than those of common bean (*Phaseolus vulgaris* L.) and take longer to cook. Tepary beans are high in protein (23%-25%) [22] and are also rich in carbohydrates according to [23].

In Zimbabwe little is known about tepary bean (*Phaseolus acutifolias*) except that is grown for subsistence by a few smallholder farmers in the eastern part of the country. With increasing climate change stress in southern Africa, tepary beans may prove to be a valuable and well adapting crop. Tepary bean has been identified as an important grain legume crop among resource poor farmers in semi-arid south eastern Kenya [24], and has been recommended as a suitable dry-season crop for the tropics [25]. Tepary bean is a short life cycle annual desert legume native to south-western United States of America and North-western Mexico [16,25]. It is a viny plant with a taproot system and nodulates well with *Rhizobium* sp. Strain R3254 fixing up to 260 kg N ha^{-1} [24]. Besides having the potential to contribute to soil fertility, the protein rich grains of legume can prevent malnutrition commonly associated with cereal based diets. Furthermore, legumes can provide market possibility, thereby providing farmers the opportunity to improve their income and livelihoods [6], which is needed to truly combat hunger and malnutrition besides an increase in total food production.

Consequently, there is the potential for the use of drought tolerant legumes such as tepary beans in agriculture to provide adequate food and nutrition security. However, there is no documented evidence on how tepary bean grows in Zimbabwe. There is need for testing the agronomic performance of tepary bean against commonly grown grain legumes. We also tested the effect of rhizobium inoculation and inorganic fertiliser application on the growth and grain yield of tepary bean.

Materials and Methods

The research was done at University of Zimbabwe Crop Science fields and at Makoholi Research Station in Masvingo Province, Zimbabwe. At Makoholi, tepary bean was grown together with other commonly grown legumes: cowpea, Bambara nut, groundnut and pigeon pea. The crops were fertilized at the known recommended rates. At Crop Science tepary bean was grown under the following treatments: Basal fertilizer only (compound D fertilizer - 7:14:7 - N: P: K); Top dressing (Ammonium Nitrate - 34.5% N) only; Rhizobium only; Rhizobium+top dressing; Basal fertilizer+top dressing; and a control with neither fertilizer nor inoculant.

Methodology

At both sites, the land was ploughed and diced. Planting was done by hand by means of a pre-marked wire cable in marking the planting stations at a spacing of 0.45 m between rows and 0.05 m within rows, with row length of 6 m. Each plot size was 27 m^2. Four seeds were hand planted per station then thinned to two plants per planting station after 2 weeks. For the rhizobium treatments, sugar was dissolved in 250 ml of water and mixed with the inoculant and mixed with 20 g of seed, and the seeds were sown immediately. Compound D was applied at a rate of 150 kg/ha before planting in the respective sub plots. Ammonium nitrate, at a rate of 100 kg/ha was applied as soon as flowering started. Mechanical weed control methods were used throughout the season to keep the crops weed free. For the tepary bean response experiment, agronomic and yield data was collected.

Experimental design and data analysis

For both trials the experimental design used was a randomized complete block design with 6 treatments and 3 replications. Data was analyzed using the statistical package R and Genstat 14.

Results

Tepary bean was the earliest maturing crop amongst all the legumes. Although the crops were established late, Tepary bean managed to produce a yield (Table 1), compared to other legumes.

Crop	Agronomic parameter				
	Day to 50% emergence	Days to 50% flowering	Pod yield (kg/ha)	Biomass (dry) (kg/ha)	Grain yield (kg/ha)
Tepary bean	5a	36a	151.1a	200.0a	245.9a
Cowpea	4a	51b	877.0b	502.2b	568.1b
Bambara nut	12b	46b	-	404.4b	0
Pigeon pea	11b	148c	-	493.3b	0
Common bean	12b	54b	14.8c	51.5c	227.0a
Groundnut	8b	38a	-	1,412.6d	0

Table 1: A field comparison of tepary bean agronomic performance compared with other legume crops in Masvingo Province, Zimbabwe. Means with the same letter are not significantly different from each other.

Tepary bean growth

In all the treatments germination took 5 days from the day of sowing. It took 32 days to flowering in all the treatments. The crop took 40 days to podding in all treatments. The crop took 57 days to maturity.

Tepary bean biomass yield

Figure 1 shows biomass accumulation in all the treatments. There is a clear trend of biomass increase from week 1 up to week 6 in all the treatments. However, there is a decrease in the increase in biomass at week 6 for treatments with rhizobium+top dressing and basal fertilizer only treatment. Top dressing only as well as the no fertilizer, no inoculant treatment (control) treatments showed continuous biomass accumulation even after week 6. Significant treatment differences were between the control and the basal+top dressing fertilizer treatment ($P<0.05$).

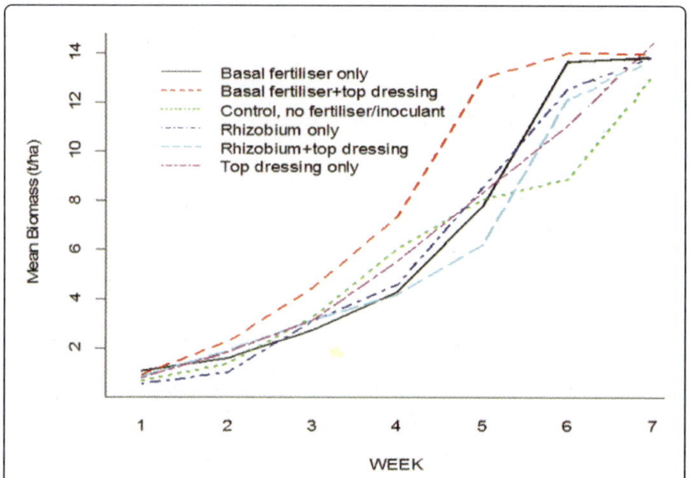

Figure 1: Effect of rhizobium inoculation and inorganic fertilizer application on tepary bean biomass yield.

Tepary bean pod number

There were significant differences in the treatments ($P<0.05$). The results as shown in Figure 2 indicate an increase in the pod number for all the treatments up to week 2 where the increase becomes steady except for treatment 4 which shows continuous increase up to week 3. Inoculating and applying top dressing fertilizer only produced the highest mean pod number whilst the lowest was recorded for the control. Analysis for each week did not show any significant differences.

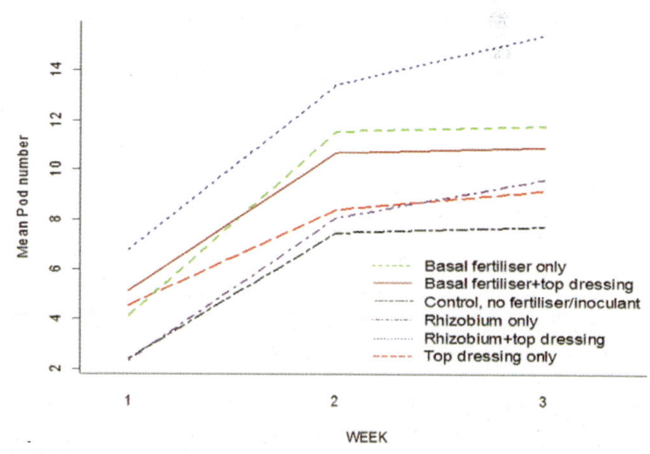

Figure 2: Effect of rhizobium inoculation and inorganic fertilizer application on the tepary bean pod number.

Tepary bean final grain yield

Figure 3 shows the final grain yield. There were no significant differences in the mean yields of basal fertilizer only and topdressing only treatments to that of the control (no fertilizer, no inoculant). Inoculant only, Inoculant+topdressing, and basal+top dressing treatments did not show any significant differences but they were significantly different from the control (P<0.05).

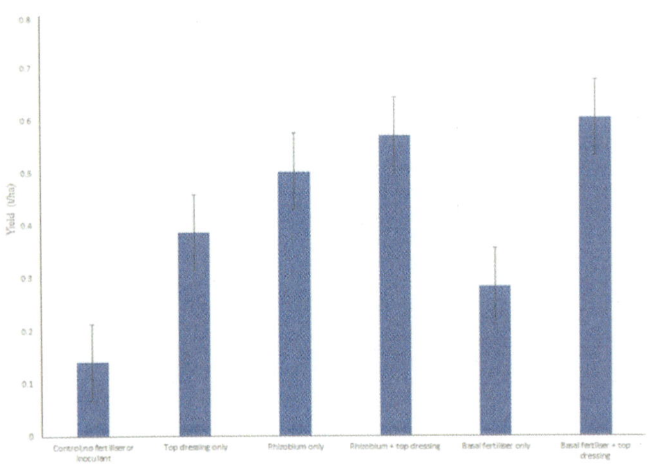

Figure 3: Effect of rhizobium inoculation and inorganic fertilizer application on final Tepary bean grain yield. Note: Error bars show LSD=0.15 (P<0.05).

Discussion

Comparison of tepary bean with other legumes

The results show that tepary bean compares well with other commonly grown legumes in the smallholder farming systems (Table 1). This is important as farmers diversify crops as a coping strategy to climate change and variability [26]. CGIAR [27] mentions important legumes for smallholder farmers as Bambara nut (*Vigna subterranea* (L.) Verdc.), Lentil (*Lens culinaris* Medic.), Chickpea (*Cicer arietinum* L.), Lima bean (*Phaseolus lunatus* L.) Common bean (*Phaseolus vulgaris* L.), Mung bean (Vigna radiata var. radiata (L.) R. Wilczek), Cowpea (*Vigna unguiculata* (L.) Walp.), Pea (*Pisum sativum* L.), Faba bean (*Vicia faba* L.) Pigeonpea (*Cajanus cajan* (L.) Millsp.), Grass pea (*Lathyrus sativus* L.), Soybean (*Glycine max* (L.) Merr.), Groundnut (*Arachis hypogaea* L.) and Tepary bean (*Phaseolus acutifolius* (A. Gray)). The majority of these pulses are already being grown worldwide, for instance common bean and groundnut, while others are concentrated in a few regions, for instance cowpea (sub-Saharan Africa), faba bean (East and North Africa, West Asia), pigeon pea (South Asia, East Africa), and mung bean (South and South East Asia). Tepary bean particularly provides hope to smallholder bean farmers affected by climate change in southern Africa as it has naturally evolved with resistances to drought and high temperature conditions [28]. Weil [16] emphasises the importnace of legumes as a cost-effective option for bettering diets of low-income consumers who cannot easily afford other sources of protein. This generates substantial benefits to the well-being of smallholder farm families. With many of the poorest countries deriving 10%-20% or more of their total dietary protein from grain legumes, the importance of low resource legumes such as tepary bean cannot be overemphasized [27]. Cereal diets, such as maize-based diets in eastern and southern Africa, are low in lysine content relative to human amino acid balance. Legumes, particularly tepary bean, are superior sources of lysine, and increase the biological value of the combined protein. The current WHO-endorsed index for protein quality is the protein digestibility-corrected amino acid score (PDCAAS) which estimates the true value of dietary protein. Experts recommend that foodstuffs of at least 70% PDCAAS should be consumed [27]. Cereals have a low PDCAAS value of about 35%, indicating their low protein quality when consumed in isolation; while a cereal legume combination in the proportions of 70/30 (weight/weight) can usually reach or exceed this PDCAAS threshold [27]. Thus, even in countries where a cereal is the dominant source of protein, every gram of legume protein potentiates another gram of cereal protein. Tepary bean seeds contain 24% protein as compared to average values of 22.3% in navy, 22.5% in red kidney, and 20.9% in pinto bean [16]. This makes tepary bean a key low cost and adaptable legume for the climate affected low potential regions of southern Africa.

Legume proteins are rich in globulins and albumins and generally have isoelectric points of 4.2 to 4.4 [28]. These protein fractions are rich in lysine and other essential amino acids but generally low in sulfur containing amino acids; therefore, they complement protein quality of cereal-based foods [29]. Several authors (e.g. in Weil [16]) have researched the production of protein isolates with approximately 90% protein from wild legumes such as lupins (*Lupinus albus* and *Lupinus mutabilis*) and Tepary beans (*Phaseoulus acutifolius*). The resulting isolates are utilized to upgrade protein concentration in foods and to impart different functionality to food systems such as water and oil absorption, foaming, emulsifying and gelation capacities [16]. This makes Tepary bean a key crop in this regard.

Other health benefits of legumes include enhanced iron concentration in beans [30]. The average iron concentration in tepary bean seed (10.7%) is higher than that in navy (6.4%), red kidney (6.7%), and pinto (5.9%) bean [16]. Grain legumes exhibit low glycemic index thus reducing the risk of obesity and diabetes [27]. A tepary bean diet, with exercise, was shown to decrease typical changes in weight gain, glycemia and lipid profile [30]. The adoption of such a program in individuals showing signs of T2D would also likely serve to protect against these physiological changes. Tepary bean seeds contain 1.8% oil as compared to values of 1.3, 1.1, and 1.1% for navy, kidney, and pinto beans, respectively. Tepary bean seed oil contains 33% saturated, 67% unsaturated, 24% mono-unsaturated, and 42% polyunsaturated fatty acids [31]. Thus consumption of tepary bean would have positive effects on colon and breast cancer and cardiovascular disease. Preliminary tests with HIV/AIDS victims fed grain legumes shows an increase in cell counts of CD4 cells, a primary element of the immune system [27]. This may imply further importance of tepary bean in diets.

Often legume crops are cultivated by women; harvests are consumed at home and sold to generate family income. In addition, tepary bean, like other grain legumes, provides on-farm agronomic benefits through biological nitrogen fixation. By complementing cereals in cropping systems of smallholder farmers, legumes can help intensify and diversify systems, particularly as an adaptation measure to climate variability and change, while improving diet and curbing malnutrition [32]. The fast growth of tepary bean not only improves soil protective cover and soil fertility, but also helps to break pest, disease and weed cycles in cereal cropping systems. Diversification of cropping choices with legumes such as tepary bean could reduce risks of harvest losses, thus increasing farmers' adaptive capacity and resilience to climate change and variability.

The climate change challenge and low soil fertility are major abiotic limitations for crop production, particularly for legume crops that are cultivated as escape crops and usually on marginal lands. Research has, however, placed legume crops to improve genetic adaptation to drought through an innovative combination of approaches such as trait based selection across different species; genomics combined with a thorough understanding of adaptation mechanisms; crop simulation modeling to help navigate the biological complexity; and interspecific crosses with desert species, *Phaseolus acutifolius*, in the case of common bean [15,33,34] This could prove to be a major breakthrough in combating devastating effects of climate induced hunger and malnutrition, particularly in hard-hit areas of southern Africa.

Tepary bean is perhaps the most drought resistant legume species in the whole world according to [16]. Gary [35] highlighted that tepary bean is recognized for its resistance to heat, drought and many diseases. It is capable of giving a notable yield with annual precipitation of less than 400 mm. These characteristics make it an ideal crop in parts of tropical production. Tepary beans' taproot is twice as long as common beans' (*Phaseolus vulgaris*), and this allows for efficient uptake of even small amounts of soil moisture [36]. The stress caused by shortage of water is believed to be the triggering factor to fruition [16]. It needs moisture to begin growing but is low on water use after it starts growth. Thus, it is an excellent xeriscape food plant [34]. Compared to common bean, it is shown to be superior in combining desirable traits that make it well adapted to drought stress [22].

Effect of rhizobium inoculation and inorganic fertilizer application on biomass yield

Basal fertilizer+top dressing had a significant effect on the biomass as shown in Figure 1. Significant differences were seen between this treatment and the control which had neither fertilizer nor inoculant. Interestingly, top dressing only treatment had the highest mean biomass yield. The basal fertilizer (compound D, 7:14:7) that was applied has more phosphorus than nitrogen and potassium. According to [37], phosphorus forms part of complex nucleic acid structure of plants, which controls protein synthesis as well as stimulating root growth. Potassium is also involved in protein synthesis [38]. The two nutrients are, therefore, important in cell division and development of new tissue. Phosphorus is also recommended for increasing early growth.

Tepary bean is known to have low root length density, which constraints nitrogen uptake [24]. However, the treatment that had compound D applied to it probably had a more extensive root network because of the phosphorus which enabled the crop to absorb nutrients from a greater area than the other treatments. It, therefore, led to the reason why this treatment had a more vigorous growth from week 1. Top dressing (Ammonium nitrate) has a higher percentage of nitrogen (33%-34%) [39] in the form of nitrates and ammonium which are readily available to the plant. It is known to increase growth [23,25,40]. The combination of basal fertilizer and top dressing consequently resulted in higher biomass yield for the most part of the plant's growth phase. Interestingly, the control and treatment 2 which had top dressing showed a continuous rise in biomass when all the other treatments were starting to show a decline in the biomass. Ammonium nitrate is known to promote vegetative growth because of its high percentage of nitrogen. Nitrogen is the most critical nutrient needed to support plant growth according to [41]. In this case it may have been the response of the crop to the ammonium nitrate.

In reference to a similar study done in Croatia, biomass yield in non-inoculated plants was significantly lower (8.01%-9.7%) compared to biomass yield in inoculated plants [42]. It is known that the synthesis of plant organic matter is promoted by inoculation.

Effect of rhizobium inoculation and inorganic fertilizer application on podding

Figure 2 shows a clear ascending trend in the number of pods for all the treatments as the weeks progressed from week one to week three. Rhizobium inoculation and inorganic fertilizer application had a significant effect on the number of pods. The crop responded to Rhizobium+top dressing more than the other treatments. Inoculation has an effect of fixing nitrogen, whilst ammonium nitrate is a source of nitrogen as well. This nitrogen may have caused the significant podding. Ammonium is a cation, so it competes with other cations like potassium, calcium and magnesium for uptake by the roots. An unbalanced fertilization might result in calcium and magnesium deficiencies. Potassium uptake is less affected by the competition [33]. Calcium is an important nutrient in the formation of pods and if in any case it was rendered unavailable by excess nitrogen then it might be the reason why the treatment with top dressing only had a low number of pods. An important point to note is the continuous increase in pod number which is shown in Figure 2 in all the treatments. The yield might have been a bit higher than the ones noted if the crops were left for some more weeks to reach their maximum capacity of podding. However, the weather conditions were not favorable as there was continuous rainfall which would have caused further losses in grain yield.

Effect of rhizobium inoculation and inorganic fertilizer application on final grain yield

The highest final grain yield was recorded for the treatment with basal fertilizer+top dressing and this was not significantly different to the treatment which had rhizobium+top dressing and the one with top dressing only as well as rhizobium only as denoted by Figure 3. This observation contradicts with a research done in Kenya in which nitrogenous fertilizer did not have significance on the yield of tepary bean [24]. This might mean that the effects of the rhizobium and basal fertilizer are the same if combined with ammonium nitrate. Basal fertilizer provides the plant with starter nutrients that are needed for early growth. However, according to [35] phosphorus does not increase grain yield. The nutrient may have played an indirect role of promoting a good root network which enabled the crop to absorb nutrients efficiently. Biological fixation of nitrogen by rhizobium contributes large amounts of plant usable nitrogen to the soil nitrogen pool [43]. This plant usable nitrogen might have an effect in the early growth of the crop which is equally as good as that provided by the basal fertilizer.

The treatment that had basal fertilizer only yield was not significantly different from that of the control. Compound D is known to be effective in the soil for the first four weeks after application. The low yield for this treatment may be attributed to this. By the time the crop was harvested basal fertilizer might have been exhausted and the crop was already thriving under nutrient deficiency conditions. Ahmad [44] states that balanced use of inputs like fertilizers and moisture is essential for improving harvest index of grain crops. Yields obtained in this study consummate with those obtained elsewhere, estimated to reach 200 kg to 900 kg per hectare; variations come as a result of differences in sowing density and rainfall [31].

These results show that tepary beans are a resilient food resource, able to survive in drought climates. This agrees with Albala [23] who reported that the plant is highly drought and disease resistant, and provides a quick harvest that is high in nutritional value. They are also small and develop quickly, soaking up a lot of water early on and protecting it within a hard, thick skin [36]. During the course of the experiment, at both sites, Tepary bean was not attacked by mildew or smut (*Xanthomonas phaseoli*), which commonly attach other grain legumes. This is supported by Gary [35] who concluded that the fact that tepary bean is not attacked by mildew or smut diseases makes it a useful species for improvement of other food legumes via genetic introgression. It is, therefore, expected to have significant potential for introduction into semi-arid areas [35]. IPCC reported that, with climate change, droughts would become more frequent and more severe in southern Africa and drought affected areas are projected to increase in extent. Drought ranks as the single most common cause of severe food shortages, particularly in developing countries, and represents one of the most important natural triggers of malnutrition and famine affects the four dimensions of food security, availability, stability, access and utilisation [45,46].

Conclusion and Recommendation

Tepary bean is among the most drought resistant legume species that can be grown in the smallholder drought prone farming areas. It is capable of giving a notable yield with annual precipitation of less than 400 mm. Furthermore, small-holder farmers can be recommended to grow tepary bean and inoculating it with rhizobium. Further research on rhizobium strain efficacy is recommended to determine the strain that has more effectiveness in terms of giving a higher Tepary bean yield. There will be need for further testing of other agronomic practices particularly planting dates and densities to determine the optimum yield. It is further recommended that a similar study be carried in other soil types to establish the effect of different soils on yield. Even though tepary bean is known to produce a nutritious seed that is suitable for human consumption composition of tepary bean seed produced in Zimbabwe is not known. There is need to characterize the protein and mineral composition of tepary bean seeds and to compare the composition of mature raw tepary bean seed to some of legumes commonly grown by smallholder farmer in Southern Africa.

References

1. Brooks N, Adger WN, Kelly PM (2005) The determinants of vulnerability and adaptive capacity at national and implications for adaptation. Global Environ Change 15: 151-163.
2. Ikeme J (2003) Climate change adaptation deficiencies in developing countries: The case of Sub-Saharan Africa. MASGC 8: 29-52.
3. Parry M, Evans A, Rosegrant MW, Wheeler T (2009) Climate Change and Hunger: Responding to the challenge. Rome, Italy: WFP.
4. Sheeran J (2010) How to end hunger. Washington Quarterly. April.
5. Pouilotte J, Mit B, Wexterhoff (2009) Adaptation and Development: Livelihood and climate change in Surbanabad, Bangladesh. CCD 1: 31-46.
6. Giller KE (2001) Nitrogen Fixation in Tropical Cropping Systems. (2ndedn) CAB International, Wallingford, UK.
7. Mapfumo P (2011) Comparative analysis of the current and potential role of legumes in Integrated Soil Fertility Management in southern Africa. Book chapter In: Bationo A, Waswa B, Okeyo JM, Maina JK, Mokwunye U (eds). Fighting poverty in sub-Saharan Africa: The multiple roles of legumes in Integrated Soil Fertility Management. Springer pp: 175-200.
8. Mpepereki S, Makonese F, Wollum AG (1997) Physiological characterization of indigenous rhizobia nodulating *Vigna unguiculata* in Zimbabwe soils. Symbiosis 22: 275-292.
9. Fageria NK, Barbosa Filho MP, Sntos AB (2008) Growth and zinc uptake and use efficiency in food crops. Commun Soil Sci Plant Anal 39: 2258-2269.
10. Hulse JH, Laing Pearson OE (1980) Sorghum and the millets: Their composition and Nutritive Value. Academic Press, London.
11. FAOSTAT (2009).
12. Kasasa P (1999) Biological nitrogen fixation by promiscuous modulating soyabean (*Glycine max* L. merr) varieties in communal area soil of Zimbabwe. M. Phil. thesis submitted to the Department of Soil Science and Agricultural Engineering, University of Zimbabwe, Mount Pleasant.
13. Rusinamhodzi L (2000) Effects of cotton-cowpea intercropping on crop yields and soil nutrient status under Zimbabwean rainfed conditions. MPhil thesis, University of Zimbabwe, Mount Pleasant.
14. Food and Agriculture Organization of the United Nations Natural Resources Management and Environment Department (2012) Potential impacts of climate change on food security in Mali. Rome, pp: 49.
15. McCaffrey D (2012) Amazing Tepary Beans.
16. Weil A (2015) Cooking with Legumes: Tepary Beans - Dr. Weil's Healthy Kitchen.
17. García-Gasca T, García-Cruz M, Hernandez-Rivera E, López-Matínez J, Castañeda-Cuevas AL, et al. (2012) Effects of Tepary bean (*Phaseolus acutifolius*) protease inhibitor and semipure lectin fractions on cancer cells. Nutr Cancer 64: 1269-1278.
18. Hart A (2012) Defeat Diabetes Month in April with tepary beans - *Sacramento vegan.*
19. Bogler D (2014) Descriptions and articles about the Tepary Bean (*Phaseolus acutifolius* as classified by Integrated Taxonomic Information System (ITIS)) - Encyclopedia of Life.
20. Zambre M, Van Montagu M, Angenon G, Terryn N (2006) Tepary bean (*Phaseolus acutifolius*). Methods Mol Biol 343: 407-414.
21. Tinsley AM, Scheerens JC, Alegbejo JO, Adan FH, Krumhar KC et al. (1985) Tepary beans (*Phaseolus acutifolius* var. *latifolius*): a potential food source for African and Middle Eastern cultures. Qualitas Plantarum Plant Foods for Human Nutrition 35: 87-101.
22. Stephens JM (2013) HS558/MV025: Bean, Tepary. *Phaseolus acutifolius* A. Gray.
23. Albala K (2007) Foods indigenous to the Western Hemisphere.
24. Shisanya CA (2005) Economic analysis of maize-tepary bean production using a soil fertility replenishment product (PREP-PAC) in semi-arid Eastern Kenya. J Food Agri Environ 3: 208-212.
25. Mogotsi K (2006) *Phaseolus acutifolias* A. Gray.
26. Jost C, Kyazze F, Naab J, Neelormi S, Kinyangi J, et al. (2015) Understanding gender dimensions of agriculture and climate change in small-holder farming communities. Climate Development 1-12.
27. CGIAR (2012) Leveraging legumes to combat poverty, hunger, malnutrition and environmental degradation.
28. IAC (2004) Realizing the promise and potential of African agriculture. Inter Academy Council.
29. González-Quijada MR, Alanís-Guzman MG, Serna- Saldivar SO (2003) Ebony (*Phitecellobium flexicaule* Benth) and proteins fractionation, solubilization, characterization and production of an isolate. Archivos Latinoamericanos de Nutrición 53: 84-89.
30. Bargout RN, Raizada MN (2013) Soil nutrient management in Haiti, pre-Columbus to the present day: lessons for future agricultural interventions. Agriculture and Food Security 2: 11.
31. Greenfingers J (2014) *Phaseolus acutifolius*: The Amazing Tepary Bean | Colorado Plateau Gardening and Horticulture.
32. Shisanya C (1998) The effect of nitrogen fertilizer and management on nodulation and growth of Legumes.
33. Tu J (2003) Some factors affecting the nodulation and nodule efficiency in soybeans infected by soybean Mosaic Virus.

34. Andrews D (2014) Tepary Bean, *Phaseolus acutifolius.* Arizona Wild Flowers. Pictures, Photos, Images, Descriptions, Information, Reviews.
35. Gary N (2010) Tepary bean crop ecology.
36. Constantino L (2009) Mediterranean Cooking in Alaska: Ingredient: Tepary Beans with Recipe for Tepary Bean and Vegetable Stew.
37. Penas (2011) Plant and Soil Sciences eLibrary.
38. Colorado State University Extension (2014) Plant Nutrition.
39. International Plant Nutrition Institute (2012) NSS-22 Amm Nit.pdf.
40. The fertilizer Institute (2014) Ammonium Nitrate Fact Sheet | TFI.
41. Fox J (2007) Legume-Rhizobium-Microbe Wiki.
42. Brkic` S (2004) Pea yield and its quality depending on inoculation, nitrogen and molybdenum fertilization.
43. Ministry of Science and Technology Development (2014) Inoculants a fertiliser substitute.
44. Ahmad R (2007) Improving crop harvest index-Newspaper-DAWN.COM.
45. FAO (2009) FAO-News Article: 1.02 billion people hungry Rome.
46. Food and Agriculture Organization (1999) A Fertilizer strategy for Zimbabwe. Food and Agriculture Organization of the United Nations and African Centre for Fertilizer Development, Rome. p: 96.

The Brazilian Nutritional Policy of Iodination of Culinary Salt to Control Iodine Deficiency in Population: From the Lack to the Excess

Rates SPM[1], Capanema FD[1], Albuquerque SR[1], Cordeiro ML[1], Laguardia S[1], Rocha DS[2] and Lamounier JA[3*]

[1]*College of Health and Human Ecology (FASEH), Alterosa Garden, Vespasian-MG, Brazil*

[2]*Federal University of Bahia, Campus Teixeira, Candeias, Victory of the Conquest, BA, Brazil*

[3]*School of Medicine, Federal University of Minas Gerais, Santa Efigenia, Belo Horizonte-MG, Brazil*

[*]**Corresponding author:** Lamounier JA, School of Medicine, Federal University of Minas Gerais, Santa Efigenia, Belo Horizonte-MG, Brazil
E-mail: jalamo@medicina.ufmg.br

Abstract

In the 1950's, Brazil adopted the iodination of the cooking salt to defeat chronic iodine deficiency diseases. The Federal government has been performing national inquiries periodically about the occurrence of endemic goiter in schools, adopting the urinary excretion of iodine and the thyroid volume as result indicators. The determination of the iodine concentration in the cooking salt has also been used as a determinant factor in these results analysis. This bibliographic review aims to present the actions taken by the Brazilian government in relation to iodine deficiency since the beginning of iodization policy of culinary salt in the 50's decade, the results achieved and the situation of excess iodine found in the Brazilian population at the present time. These measures systematically adopted by the Brazilian government, supported in laws, ordinances and ministry resolutions, have shown to be efficient instruments in the reduction of endemic goiter. Nowadays, the prevalence of goiter in the Brazilian population is between the parameters established by the World Health Organization, which means less than 5% of the population affected. Nevertheless, the last survey made by the Health Ministry highlighted an excessive ingestion of iodine, exposing the population to other health risks associated to this excess.

Keywords: Iodized salt; Urinary iodine; Hypothyroidism; Excess of iodine; Public health

Introduction

Iodine is an element essential to health, directly related to thyroid gland functioning, to adequate nervous system development and to general body growth [1]. Inadequate iodine ingestion is associated to several diseases identified as Iodine Chronic Deficiency Diseases (ICDD): Neonatal and adult hypothyroidism, multinodular goiter, iodine-induced hyperthyroidism, fertility decrease, fetal malformation, perinatal mortality, deaf-mutism and clinical variants of endemic cretinism [2,3].

Iodized salt for human consumption is considered the most effective measure to achieve appropriate iodine levels for populations. It is the universal strategy adopted in public health, without iodized salt some two billion people would have iodine deficiency, while the actual number is 700 million [4]. Populational programs of iodination of salt in every continent have significantly limited illnesses related to chronic iodine deficiency. However, there are still 266 million children and two billion adults living in the world with insufficient ingestion of iodine [5].

Data from the World Health Organization (WHO), referring to 130 countries, showed that 68% of all residences in the world have access to iodized salt and that 34% of them are in a country with more than adequate iodine ingestion or even excessive, among those countries is Brazil [5]. The Health Ministry has been developing periodic population inquiries to evaluate the impact of this intervention on the Brazilian population. This research has shown a decrease in the prevalence of endemic goiter from 20.7% in 1955 to 1.3% in 1994, proving the efficacy of the strategy to public health aims. A similar outcome was obtained in another study set in 2000, with prevalence of 1.4% showing control over the endemic in the country [3,6].

However 86.5% of the scholars involved in this study showed high levels of urinary iodine excretion, with urinary iodine above 300 mcg/L and half of these with numbers above 500 mcg/L, showing a new reality concerning excessive iodine consumption [3]. Iodine-induced hyperthyroidism, autoimmune chronic thyroiditis and secondary hypothyroidism are severe illnesses that can affect individuals exposed to an excessive amount of iodine [3].

This article aims to review literature concerning Brazilian strategy to fortify cooking salt with iodine to reduce endemic goiter in the country, its temporal evolution and the results achieved by the national program since its beginning. This article will also highlight the transition from deficiency to excess of corporal iodine and its side effects in the organism.

Methods

Bibliographic review of national and international publications in periodic indexed in the following database: National Library of Medicine (Medline, USA) and Literatura Latino-Americana e do Caribe em Ciências da Saúde (LILACS), during the time period between 1980 and 2014 comprising Portuguese, English and Spanish languages that approached the strategies of fortification of cooking salt with iodine recommended by the WHO and implemented in Brazil.

In the search strategy were included publications about the historical evolution of the actions and strategies of combat against iodine deficiency both in Brazil and globally The descriptors used were:

Goiter, iodine deficiency, iodine excess, urinary iodine, iodized salt, iodine-induced hyperthyroidism, hypothyroidism, autoimmune thyroid disease, isolated or as a combined form. It was selected 40 publications according to the inclusion criteria above. From these, eight publications were excluded for not showing direct relation to the main goal proposed in this article, being 32 publications remained to comprise this review.

History of iodation of salt to control endemic goiter in Brazil

Since the 1920's, most countries have been adapting in order to provide the necessary amount of iodine to their populations. Most countries adopt strategies to guarantee this control and eliminate endemic goiter as a public health issue. The universal iodination of cooking salt has shown to be the most simple and effective of all actions adopted to combat iodine deficiency illnesses [7]. WHO classifies goiter prevalence as severe when prevalence is above 30% in a population and moderate from 20 to 29.9%? Values under, between 5.0-19.9%, are considered as mild and communities with goiter prevalence of 4.9% and lower are considered null prevalence [4]. The Brazilian National Congress and the sanitary authorities have instituted legal mechanisms (Laws, ordinances and ministry resolutions) addressing chronic iodine deficiency in the country [3,8]. Table 1 presents the temporal evolution of goiter prevalence determined by populational inquiries from 1955 to 2000, highlighting the significant reduction of the illness observed in this period.

Reference	Year	Populatio n	Age (years)	Goiter prevalence (%)
National inquiry	1955	86.217	6–14	20.7
National inquiry	1974	42.752	7–14	14.1
National inquiry	1994	178.774	6–14	1.3
Thyromobil project	2000	2.013	6–14	1.4
Font: Knobel and Medeiros-Neto [3]				

Table 1: Populational based studies about endemic goiter in Brazil from 1955 to 2000.

In Brazil, since colonial time, there have been iodine deficiencies illnesses reported as an important cause of goiter in European originated populations, in blacks and mixed bloods, although in indigenous population this phenomenon was not discovered, likely related to eating factors of each population [6]. In 1953 there was the implementation of the first national program of salt iodination in endemic goiter areas of the country, with the addition of 10 mg/Kg of iodine in the culinary salt [3,9]. In 1955, the first national inquiry about goiter occurrence revealed a prevalence of 20.7% in the population [10,11].

In August 17th of 1956, the National Decree number 39,814 defined the endemic goiter areas, leading to an extension of salt iodination to the whole country. The Health Ministry became responsible for emphasizing the importance of iodized supplements [3,10]. In 1974, law number 6150 mandated 10 mg/kg of iodine in the salt for human consumption, transferred the expense of iodination to private initiative and required the states, territories and counties to supervise this initiative [3,10]. From 1974 to 1976, the Health Ministry/SUCAM (Superintendências de Campanhas de Saúde Pública) made the second national inquiry with 42,752 scholars from 7 to 14 years old, showing a goiter prevalence of 14.1% indicating a reduction of only 6.5% of this prevalence in 20 years [11]. Despite the proclamation of new laws and federal decrees, since 1980 Brazil has lived with the inefficiency of these regulatory documents due to the lack of control and supervision in the salt industry, which added to the drastic statistic of over 15 million Brazilians bearing endemic goiter [11].

From 1982 to 1992, researches interested in goiter endemia, salt industries representatives, Health Ministry's and Nutrition and Eating Institute's (NEIN) technicians, agreed to maintain the iodine concentration above 10 mg/kg of salt as a responsibility of the producers. The Health Ministry and the NEIN had the duty of creating a wide net of public laboratories to ensure the appropriate iodine concentration production. This movement established the decrease of goiter in scholars and overall improvement in health for the whole population being worldly recognized and cited as an example of success to be followed by other countries [3,10].

The third national inquiry made in 1994 with 178,774 scholars from 6 to 14 years showed a low prevalence of goiter (<5.0%) in most coastal states, compared to the presence of chronic iodine deficiency illness in states from northern and central regions of the country. This study highlighted the disparity in public health efforts targeted at eliminating iodine deficiency [12]. In 1995 the Health Ministry established the correct iodination of cooking salt with amounts of iodine between 40-60 mg/kg and authorized the potassium iodide supply to salt industries [3]. As NEIN was stopped in 1997, and the National Agency of Sanitary Surveillance (ANVISA) at the end of the 1990's, the boundaries of potassium iodide were liberated to 40-100 mg/kg of salt, exposing Brazilian to an elevated consumption of iodine from 1998 to 2003 [3].

In May and June of 2000, the Thyromobil Project in Brazil, adapted from the model developed in Europe and Latin America, ran 12,000 km from north to south of the country visiting 29 counties from eight states where there were the Sentinels Villages marking the iodine chronic deficiency in the 1995 inquiry [13]. In this project, concentration of the iodine in urinary samples was analyzed in a representative sample made of scholars from 6 to 14 from both genders, aside from the collect of a sample of consumed salt by these scholars to determine the concentration of iodine in the salt. The urinary excretion of iodine was the diagnostic indicator used to determine the nutritional state of iodine in the population, using the established references by WHO [3] according to Table 2.

The obtained results in the project were startling and showed 86.5% of scholars with excessive iodine levels in the urine, above 300 mcg/L, where in half of the researched showed levels above 500 mcg of iodine/L. In 5% of the scholars were detected levels of urinary iodine above 900 mcg/L. Such results show accordance with the fact that 50% of the samples of consumed salt in residences by the scholars showed concentrations of iodine above 60 mg/kg of salt [3,13].

Therefore, in 2003, ANVISA reduced again the levels of concentration of iodine in the salt for human consumption to 20-60 mg/kg of salt in an attempt to correct the situation of excess demonstrated with the nutritional iodine. Table 3 summarizes the fluctuations of iodine in the cooking salt according to the recommended concentrations in the regulatory governmental marks.

In 2006 the Health Ministry made a new national inquiry to collect data about the salt consumed in Brazilian residences, showing that 99% of these had the product for daily use with 95.7% of iodine in the cooking salt analyzed [15]. The lower proportions were in the rural areas of the north (90.4%) and of the center-west (91.4%). It concluded being necessary permanent actions of orientation e supervising in the steps of production and distribution of salt in the country.

Urinary iodine (µg/L)	Iodine ingestion	Iodine nutrition
<20	Insufficient	Severe iodine deficiency
20-49	Insufficient	Moderate iodine deficiency
50-99	Insufficient	Light iodine deficiency
100-199	Adequate	Great
200-299	More than adequate	Risk of iodine-induced hyperthyroidism in 5 to 10 years of introducing iodized salt with high levels of iodine
>300	Excessive	Risk of developing side effects (iodine-induced hyperthyroidism, chronic autoimmune thyroiditis)
Font: WHO [14]		

Table 2: Epidemiologic criteria to evaluate the adequate ingestion of iodine based on the median urinary concentration of iodine in scholars.

Year	Iodine concentration in salt
1953	10 mg/kg
1974	10 mg/kg
1994	40–60 mg/kg
1997	40–100 mg/kg
2003	20–60 mg/kg
Font: Adapted from Knobel and Medeiros-Neto [3]	

Table 3: Chronology of fluctuations of iodine concentration in salt–Brazil.

Excessive consumption of iodine and health risks

The insufficient ingestion of iodine or its excessive consumption can lead to illnesses of the thyroid [16]. Esteves [11] reaffirmed that the combined action of assessment of the thyroid volume, preferable by ultrasound, and the determination of urinary excretion of iodine of scholars consists in the best way to monitor the control of the endemic iodine deficiency [11]. Gandra [17] compared the concomitant prevalence of goiter in adults and children considering as vulnerable group scholars from 9 to 14 years old due to their prepubertal biophysiological characteristics related to growth, more prone to the effects both of deficiency and excess of iodine [17].

In Brazil, some studies have been done to better understand and control these problems. Nimer et al. [18] studied 280 students from two schools from fundamental education, one private and the other public, from the Ouro Preto (Minas Gerais State) county, dosing the urinary iodine concentration and the iodine concentration in cooking salt samples. The results showed consumption of cooking salt with levels of iodine below the recommendation in 89.9% in public schools and in 40.9% in private. Around 57.4% of students from public school showed urinary iodine compatible to light deficiency (35.6%), moderate (12.9%) and severe (8.9%). In the private school's students, 92.2% of them showed levels of urinary iodine among the recommended standard. The inadequate iodine concentration in salt consumed by the scholars contributes to a significant prevalence of iodine deficiency [18].

Pontes, Adan e Costa, in a study with individuals from 3 to 85 years determined the prevalence of thyroid diseases in the county of Cabaceiras (Paraíba State/Brazil). Group 1 was formed by 122 patients from rural areas of the state that made clinical control for diagnostic suspicion of thyroid disease and 88 healthy volunteers formed group 2. Most individuals (79%) were females. Both groups were submitted to serum dosages of TSH, T3, free T4 and antibody anti-microsomal research. Patients from the rural area submitted themselves to ultrasound of the thyroid gland and the ones from group 2, to palpation of the gland. The results found showed high prevalence of thyropathies in groups 1 and 2 (19.8% and 20.4% respectively) associated with genetic and environmental factors, pointing out to the need of epidemiological studies surrounding the excessive consumption of nutritional iodine [19].

A retrospective study of 43 children and adolescents from 1.1 to 17.6 years with Hashimoto thyroiditis (36 female and 7 male subjects) in the Unity of Pediatric Endocrinology of the Hospital das Clínicas/São Paulo University (São Paulo/Brazil) showed possible association between the stimulus to produce antibodies against thyroid components and the high ingestion of iodine, explaining the increase in thyroid autoimmune diseases frequency in the last few years [20].

Duarte et al. selected by random 844 scholars from both genders form 6 to 14 years from six regions of São Paulo state aiming to assess the thyroid volume by ultrasound exam and determine the urinary iodine. The echography of the thyroid showed a prevalence of 16% of goiter. It drew attention to the excessive urinary iodine excretion as 53% of the samples showed numbers above 300 mcg/L. The dosages of iodine in cooking salt showed an excessive iodine concentration in 47.4% of samples. Therefore, a likely increase in salt consumption with high levels of iodine contributed to the occurrence of iodine-induced hyperthyroidism as well as chronic autoimmune thyroiditis, therein this one predominant in females [21].

These effects can be shown in the study of Camargo et al. that evaluated the prevalence of chronic autoimmune thyroiditis, iodine-induced hypothyroidism, clinic and sub-clinical hyperthyroidism and goiter in 1085 subjects selected by random in the São Paulo metropolitan region of Brazil [22]. The female group prevailed with 62.5% of the subjects and the average age was between 24.7 and 81 years. In the male group (37.5%) the average age was between 55, 8 ± 12 years. Dosages of the iodine concentration were performed in urinary samples and in cooking salt. Despite the fact that iodine concentration in the cooking salt were included in the new official parameters (20-60 mg/kg of culinary salt), 45.6% of iodine urinary concentration were at excessive levels (above 300 mcg/L), therein greater than 400 mcg/L in 14.1%. The prevalences were: 3.3% of hyperthyroidism, 8.0% of hypothyroidism and 16.9% of chronic autoimmune thyroiditis [22]. This data, once more, supported the assumption that the excess of iodine consumption by the Brazilian from 1998 to 2003 may have contributed to the increase of these disturbs prevalence in subjects genetically predisposed.

Similar situation to the chronic autoimmune thyroiditis prevalence (Hashimoto's thyroiditis) in two regions of São Paulo Brazilian State:

attached area to the petrochemical pole of Capuava (409 subjects) and control area in São Bernardo do Campo (420 subjects). The prevalence of chronic autoimmune thyroiditis was proportionally elevated in both studied areas, not showing direct epidemiological connection to the proximity to petrochemical pole but probably connection to the elevated ingestion of nutritional iodine that the Brazilian population was submitted to from 1998 to 2003 [23].

Duarte et al. studied the iodine urinary excretion in 964 scholars from both genders in the state of São Paulo-Brazil, iodine-sufficient area. In 76.8% of researched students, the urinary iodine was above 300 mcg/L, with predominance in males. The ultrasound study in this population showed abnormalities in 13.1%; hemi agenesis in 0.5%, nodules in 0.2%, cists in 0.7% and hypo echogenicity in 11.7%. Authors of the study proposed the direct relation between the thyroid alterations and the excessive consumption of iodine [24].

Another cross-sectional study involving 300 students from three schools of different social economic levels from the Ribeirão Preto (São Paulo State/Brazil) county, being considered an iodine-sufficient area, analyzed the urinary iodine and the iodine concentration in cooking salt, as well as a thyroid ultrasound was evaluated in all participants. The iodine urinary excretion was above 300 mcg/L in 59.5% of samples. From the 300 children examined, 15.6% showed abnormalities of the thyroid in the ultrasound exam. Such results revealed that the thyroid gland alterations can be associated to the exposition to excessive amounts of iodine [25].

Furthermore, a regional study evaluated the iodine excretion in 145 students of two schools: One in the urban area and the other in the rural area of the county of Botucatu (São Paulo State/Brazil). At the same time, they dosed the iodine concentration in those children's residences. The results showed that 3.0% of students from the urban schools had urinary iodine below 100 mcg/L and 90.9% above 300 mcg/L. In the rural area group, 3.8% of scholars had some deficiency level of iodine and 60.0% had urinary iodine concentration above 300 mcg/L. As for the iodine concentration in cooking salt, in the urban residences 84.8% of the samples were between 20-60 mg/kg of salt and in the rural area, 59.5%. They came to the conclusion that the iodine deficiency in the population studied was controlled but showed a high prevalence of excessive urinary iodine excretion [26].

Carvalho et al. [27] collected casual samples of urine from 828 scholars form both genders from ages 4 to 13 years from eight schools in the city of São Paulo (Brazil) in order to determine iodine urinary excretion from these participants. Only 1.9% of the children and adolescents presented with urinary iodine values less than 100 mcg/L while 24.6% had urinary iodine between 100-200 mcg/L. Most students (67.1%) had urinary iodine above 300 mcg/L, a result that pointed to excessive consumption of iodine in this population [27].

In Novo Cruzeiro, in the semi-arid region of Minas Gerais State (Brazil), the prevalence of iodine deficiency was investigated in children from 7 to 71 months. A total of 475 children were allocated by probabilistic sampling stratified according to the iodine concentration in salt consumed by the family and urinary iodine excretion. Iodine excretion deficiency occurred in 34.4%, where 23.5% showed light deficiency, 5.9% moderate and 5.0% severe. Difference in the urinary iodine concentration was determined among urban and rural areas ($p<0.001$). Higher median concentrations of urinary iodine of 150.6 mcg/L were observed in the urban area versus 114.3 mcg/L in the rural area. Elevated deficiencies were observed among children who consumed salt with iodine amounts below the recommendation [28]. The borderline distribution of iodine associated to low levels of iodine in the salt suggested that greater standardization of iodation is needed between the urban and the rural areas.

In a recent study, Boasquevisque et al. determined the iodine concentration in 30 samples of urine and conducted an anatomic-pathological study of 55 thyroids from cadavers from the Forensic Medical Institute in the county of Vitória, Espírito Santo (ES) Brazilian State. Excessive urinary iodine (>300 mcg/L) was found in 96.7% of samples [29]. Histological findings compatible with thyroiditis were identified, which were likely related to the excess of iodine in the studied population and the higher incidence of inflammatory processes of the thyroid.

Final Considerations

Disorders coming from iodine deficiency and main causes of endemic goiter are still major public health issues affecting several regions in the world [4]. In 1993 WHO, UNICEF (United Nations Children's Fund) and the ICCIDD (International Council for Control of Iodine Deficiency Disorders) recommended the universal iodination of cooking salt as a more effective strategy to reach the elimination of iodine deficiency disorders, due to its ease of implementation e lower cost [30]. The American continent stands out worldwide for having reached optimal control of iodine deficiency, despite the cases of setbacks of some countries [6]. The iodination of cooking salt has shown to be an effective and low cost strategy to reduce this endemic.

From a global point of view, different strategies to defeat micronutrients deficiency have been adopted mostly in developing countries. The massive fortification of food from daily use has now been used in several regions of the world, although limited; progress has been attained in the struggle against iron, folic acid, zinc, vitamin A and iodine deficiencies [31].

Brazil has shown positive impact in reducing the prevalence rate of goiter, however there is also evidence of excessive ingest of iodine. This important epidemiological diagnosis draws attention to the need of improving the Brazilian National Program of Prevention and Control of Iodine Deficiency Disorders (Pró-iodo), aiming to monitor the iodine in salt for human consumption, by making a priority strategies of information, education, communication and permanent social mobilization [8,30].

In April 25th of 2013, the Brazilian Official Journal published the RDC 23/3013 with the new standards for iodine addition to salt for human consumption in the Brazilian territory. This decision was based upon the information from the Research of Familiar Budget (RFB-2011) showing that Brazilians consume an average of 10 g of salt per day. Therefore ANVISA started using the concentration of 15-45 mg of iodine per kilogram of salt in substitution to that of 20-60 mg of iodine per kilogram of salt [32].

Acknowledgements

This research was supported by Postgraduate Center of Medicine of the Federal University of Minas Gerais (UFMG) and by Faculdade da Saúde e Ecologia Humana (FASEH).

References

1. Delange F, de Benoist B, Pretell E, Dunn JT (2001) Iodine deficiency in the world: where do we stand at the turn of the century? Thyroid 11: 437-447.

2. Boyages SC (1993) Clinical review 49: Iodine deficiency disorders. J Clin Endocrinol Metab 77: 587-591.
3. Knobel M, Medeiros-Neto G (2004) [Disorders associated to chronic iodine deficiency]. Arq Bras Endocrinol Metabol 48: 53-61.
4. World Health Organization/United Nations Children's Fund/ International Council for the Control of Iodine Deficiency Disorders (2010) Assessment of elimination: a guide for programme managers (6th edn.), Geneve-Switzerland.
5. de Benoist B, McLean E, Andersson M, Rogers L (2008) Iodine deficiency in 2007: global progress since 2003. Food Nutr Bull 29: 195-202.
6. Medeiros-Neto G (1982) One hundred and eighty years of endemic goiter in Brazil. Arq Bras Endocrinol Metab 30: 226-231.
7. Dunn JT, Crutchfield HE, Gutekunst R, Dunn AD (1993) Two simple methods for measuring iodine in urine. Thyroid 3: 119-123.
8. Government of Brazil, Ministry of Health. Department of Health Care (2008) Technical and Operational Manual of the Pro-Iodine: National Programme for Prevention and Control of Iodine Deficiency Disorders by Brasília-DF.
9. Pontes AA, Rocha Ada M, Leite DF, Lessa Ada F, Adan LF (2009) Salt iodation in Brazil, a controversial subject. Arq Bras Endocrinol Metabol 53: 113-114.
10. Medeiros-Neto G (2009) Iodine nutrition in Brazil: where do we stand? Arq Bras Endocrinol Metabol 53: 470-474.
11. Esteves RZ, Kasamatsu TS, Kunii IS, Furuzawa GK, Vieira JG, et al. (2007) Development of a semi-automated method for measuring urinary iodine and its application in epidemiological studies in Brazilian schoolchildren. Arq Bras Endocrinol Metabol 51: 1477-1484.
12. Corrêa Filho H, Vieira JB, Silva YS, Coelho GE, Cavalcante Fdos A, et al. (2002) Endemic goiter prevalence survey in Brazilian schoolchildren 6 to 14 years old, 1994-1996. Rev Panam Salud Publica 12: 317-326.
13. Rossi AC, Tomimori E, Camargo R, Medeiros-Neto G (2001) Searching for iodine deficiency disorders in schoolchildren from Brazil: the Thyromobil project. Thyroid 11: 661-663.
14. World Health Organization (1994) Indicators for assessing Iodine Deficiency Disorders and their control through sal iodization. Micronutrient Series. Document. Geneve-Switzerland.
15. Ministry of Health, Brazilian Center for Analysis and Planning (2009) National Demographic and Health Children and Women-PNDS-2006. Brasília-DF, Brazil.
16. Teng W, Shan Z, Teng X, Guan H, Li Y, et al. (2006) Effect of iodine intake on thyroid diseases in China. N Engl J Med 354: 2783-2793.
17. Gandra YR (1984) Clinical evaluation of endemic goiter. Rev Saude Publica 18: 396-404.
18. Nimer M, Silva ME, de Oliveira JE (2002) Relationship between iodized salt and urinary iodine excretion in school children, Brazil. Rev Saude Publica 36: 500-504.
19. Pontes AAN, Adan LF, Costa ADM, Benicio AVL, Silva CRA, et al. (2002) Thyroid disease prevalence in a community in northeastern Brazil. Arq Bras Endocrinol Metabol 46: 544-549.
20. Szeliga DVM, Setian N, Passos L, Lima TMR, Kuperman H, et al.(2002) Hashimoto's thyroiditis in children and adolescents: a retrospective study of 43 cases. Arq Bras Endocrinol Metabol 46: 150-154.
21. Duarte GC, Tomimori EK, Boriolli RA, Ferreira JE, Catarino RM, et al. (2004) Echographic evaluation of the thyroid gland and urinary iodine concentration in school children from various regions of the State of São Paulo, Brazil. Arq Bras Endocrinol Metabol 48: 842-848.
22. Camargo RYA, Medeiros-Neto G, Tomimori KE, Neves SC, Rubio IGS, et al. (2008) Thyroid and the environment: exposure to excessive nutritional iodine increases the prevalence or thyroid disorders in São Paulo, Brasil. Eur J Endocrinol 159: 293-299.
23. Camargo RYA, Tomimori EK, Neves SC, Knobel M, Medeiros-Neto G (2006) Prevalence of chronic autoimune thyroiditis in the urban area neighboring a petrochemical complex and a control area in São Paulo, Brasil. Clinics 61: 307-312.
24. Duarte GC, Tomimori EK, de Camargo RY, Catarino RM, Ferreira JE, et al. (2009) Excessive iodine intake and ultrasonographic thyroid abnormalities in school children. J Pediatr Endocrinol Metab 22: 327-334.
25. Alves MLD, Duarte GC, Navarro AM, Tomimori EK (2010) Sonographic evaluation of thyroid, determination of urinary iodine and iodine concentration in table salt used by students from Ribeirão Preto, São Paulo, Brazil. Arq Bras Endocrinol Metab 54: 813-818.
26. Navarro AM, Oliveira LA, de Meirelles CJ, Costa TM (2010) Salt iodination and excessive iodine intake among schoolchildren. Arch Latinoam Nutr 60: 355-359.
27. Carvalho AL, Meirelles CJ, Oliveira LA, Costa TM, Navarro AM (2012) Excessive iodine intake in schoolchildren. Eur J Nutr 51: 557-562.
28. Macedo Mde S, Teixeira RA, Bonomo E, Silva CA, Silva ME, et al. (2012) Iodine deficiency and associated factors in infants and preschool children in an urban community in the semiarid region of Minas Gerais State, Brazil, 2008. Cad Saude Publica 28: 346-356.
29. Boasquevisque PC, Jarske RD, Dias CC, Quintaes IP, Santos MC, et al. (2013) Correlation between iodine urinary levels and pathological changes in thyroid glands. Arq Bras Endocrinol Metabol 57: 727-732.
30. Pretell EA, Delange F, Hostalek U, Corigliano S, Barreda L, et al. (2004) Iodine nutrition improves in Latin America. Thyroid 14: 590-599.
31. Berti C, Faber M, Smuts CM (2014) Prevention and control of micronutrient deficiencies in developing countries: current perspectives. Nutrition and Dietary Suplements 6: 41-57.
32. http://bvsms.saude.gov.br/bvs/saudelegis/anvisa/2013/res0023_23_04_2013.html

12

Effect of Wall Material on the Property of Gac Oil Spray-dried Power

Nguyen Thi Nhu Quynh[1], **Tran Chi Hai**[1], **Phan Van Man**[2*] **and Le Thanh Thanh**[3]

[1]*Ho Chi Minh City University of Food Industry, Ho Chi Minh City, Vietnam*

[2]*Faculty of Chemical and Food Technology, Ba Ria Vung Tau University, Vietnam*

[3]*Thu Dau Mot University, Binh Dương, Vietnam*

[*]**Corresponding author:** Phan Van Man, Faculty of Chemical and Food Technology, Ba Ria Vung Tau University, Vietnam, E-mail: nguyenphan05031987@gmail.com

Abstract

Gac fruit (*Momordica cochinchinensis*, Spreng) aril contains extraordinarily high levels of β-carotene, lycopene and unsaturated fatty acids, especially oleic and linoleic acids. These bioactive compounds have been proven to be beneficial to human health and are linked with a reduced risk of cardiovascular disease and cancers. There were previous researches which were carried out to encapsulate Gac oil using maltodextrin, whey protein and gum arabic. However, no reports have been found to study cyclodextrin and sodium caseinate as a carrier or encapsulating agent for producing Gac oil powder. The aim of this study using spray drying method was therefore to investigate the impacts of wall concentration on Gac oil microencapsulation. The data showed that 25% of maltodextrin (or cyclodextrin); ratio of maltodextrin (or cyclodextrin) and sodium caseinate of 0.6:1 resulted in high microencapsulation productivity. The figure of MEY, MEE and DY accounted for 92.4%, 66% and 70.3% respectively and higher than that of other samples. Gac powder is saffron color of turmeric, specific odor and completely dissolved in water. The moisture content reduced from 3.67% to 3.03% when increasing the rate of maltodextrin/ sodium casenate and cyclodextrin/sodium casenate, and more than 86% dissolved in water. Sodium casenate-cyclodextrin matrix as the wall material was effectively used for spray-drying encapsulation of Gac oil.

Keywords: Gac oil; Cyclodextrin; Sodium caseinate; Microencapsulation; Gac powder

Introduction

Gac (*Momordica cochinchinensis*, Spreng) is found throughout the region from Southern China to Northeastern Australia, including Thailand, Laos, Myanmar, Cambodia and Vietnam [1]. The aril of Gac fruit, 1-3 mm thick, covering black seeds, accounting for 25% of fruit weight, contains a significant amount of fatty acids, at 102 mg/g of edible portion [2]. According to Kubola et al. [1] gac aril has high concentration of oleic (29%), palmitic (32.3%) and linoleic acids (20.3%), of the total fatty acids in gac aril. Furthermore, the highest concentrations of β-carotene and lycopene are found in the fresh aril, at 101 μg/g and 380 μg/g, respectively [3].

Spray drying has been widely utilized for commercial production of dried fruits and vegetables due to economy, flexibility, and good quality of encapsulated products. Furthermore, it is a highly appropriate process for heat sensitive components such as carotenoids [4]. The encapsulation of fatty acids and carotenoids in plant materials has been reported by numerous studies. However, very little information is published on Gac oil encapsulation and no reports on spray drying using combinations of maltodextrin and sodium caseinate; or cyclodextrin and sodium caseinate as the carrier agents for producing Gac oil powder has been reported.

Maltodextrin is one of the supported material for spray drying owing to its beneficial role as a carrier or an encapsulating agent in increasing the stability of carotenoids. Cyclodextrins are cyclic oligosaccharides consisting of six α-cyclodextrin, seven β-cyclodextrin, eight γ-cyclodextrin or more glucopyranose units linked by α-(1,4) bonds. In food related application, cyclodextrins are also used to improve stability of flavor and/or oil which are being encapsulated for better retention and protection from various possible means of deterioration [5,6].

The aims of this research must be evaluated the effect of wall material formulation on encapsulation efficiency, encapsulation yield, physicochemical property, color characteristics and the changes in lycopene and β-carotene in Gac oil powder under storage condition.

Materials and Method

Wall and core material

Maltodextrin and cyclodextrin used as wall material were obtained from Qinhuangdao Lihua Starch Co., Ltd. Deionized water was employed in the preparation of all of the formulations. Core material used in this study was Gac oil, which was extracted by hexane according to a method described by Kubola et al. [1].

Preparation of the oil-in-water emulsions and spray drying conditions for Gac oil

Emulsions were prepared using a method from Kha et al. [7]. Aqueous stock solutions (500 mL) with different concentrations of wall materials with were prepared using a homogenizer (Wilmington, DE, USA) at 6000 rpm for 10 min. In the homogenizer, the solution samples were axially drawn into the dispersion head and then forced radially through the slots in the rotor/stator arrangement. The stock solutions were then kept at 4°C for at least 12 h to ensure complete hydration of proteins. Then these samples (about 500 mL) were spray-dried. The operating conditions of the spray drying were inlet air temperature of 180°C, and pressure of 2 bars, and the feed flow rate was about 400 mL/h.

Microencapsulation efficiencies (MEE) were determined based on the retention of Gac oil, β-carotene, and lycopene contents in the encapsulated powder as follows:

Formula	**15%**	**20%**	**25%**	**30%**	**0.2:1**	**0.4:1**	**0.6:1**	**0.8:1**	**1:1**
Gac oil (%)	15	15	15	15	15	15	15	15	15
Maltodextrin/Cyclodextrin (%)	15	20	25	30	20.83	17.86	15.62	13.89	12.5
Sodium Caseinate (%)	0	0	0	0	4.17	7.14	9.38	11.11	12.5

Table 1: Formulation of all concentration using for spry-drying.

$$MEE = \frac{Total\ Oil\ Content - Surface\ Oil\ Content}{Total\ Content} \times 100\%$$

$$MEY = \frac{Total\ Oil\ in\ Product}{Total\ Oil\ in\ Emulsification} \times 100\%$$

$$EY = \frac{Total\ Carotenoid\ in\ Product}{Total\ Carotenoid\ in\ Emulsification} \times 100\%$$

$$DY = \frac{Total\ Dry\ Weight\ in\ Product}{Total\ Dry\ weight\ in\ Emulsification} \times 100\%$$

The total oil content, surface oil, β-carotene, and lycopene content were determined described by Kha et al. [7].

Storage treatments for gac oil powder

Gac powder was stored at 55°C for 7 days. The color of Gac fruit powder sample was determined by using a Minolta Chroma Meter that calibrated with a white standard tile.

Water insolubility index (WII)-TCVN 6511:2007

Spray-dried Gac fruit powder (2.5 g) and (30 mL) were vigorously mixed in a 100 mL centrifuge tube, incubated in a 37°C water bath for 30 min and then centrifuged for 20 min at 10,000 rpm. The supernatant was carefully removed; distilled water was added and stirred again. Centrifuge this solution again and calculate the insoluble volume.

Moisture content

The moisture content (MC) of the samples was determined by drying at a temperature of 105°C in an oven until a constant weight was obtained.

Statistical analysis

The experiments were carried out in triplicate and results were presented as mean values with standard deviations. Different mean values were analyzed by analysis of variance (ANOVA) and least significant difference (LSD) using the software Stagraphics Centurion XV.

Result and Discussion

Effects of wall material on total carotenoid content and encapsulation efficiency

The effects of maltodextrin and cyclodextrin concentration on encapsulation and total carotenoid content (TCC) of Gac powder are presented in Figure 1, respectively. Results showed that higher MEE, MEY and DY were observed when increasing maltodextrin and cyclodextrin concentration.

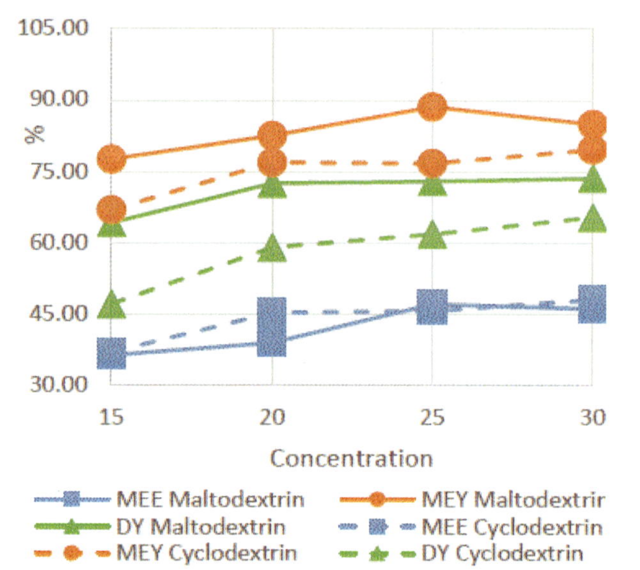

Figure 1: Effect of maltodextrin/cyclodextrin concentration on MEE, MEY and DY.

As maltodextrin concentration increased from 15-25%, MEE, MEY, DY enhanced 17%, 44% and 30%, respectively. However, no difference in MEE, MEY and DY between concentration of 25 and 30% was observed. A different trend was observed in study of Kha et al. [4], while maltodextrin concentration rose from 20 to 30%, there was no significant difference in encapsulation efficiency. For spay drying using cyclodextrin, MEE, MEY and DY raised 22%, 15% and 25%, respectively while cyclodextrin concentration increased from 15 to 20%, and no difference in MEE, MEY and DY between concentration of 20, 25 and 30% was observed.

As well as the MEE, carotenoid encapsulation yield (EY), which is one of the major parameters of the spray-drying operation. EY of encapsulated powder is presented in Figure 2. In general, the result showed that the highest EY was obtained when maltodextrin or cyclodextrin concentration of 25%. In addition, data also shows that the yield, which using cyclodextrin as supported material was higher than 5% in compared to using maltodextrin. However, maltodextrin or cyclodextrin alone could not effectively cover oil droplets because EY only increased nearly 25% in comparison with MEE increasing approximately 44%.

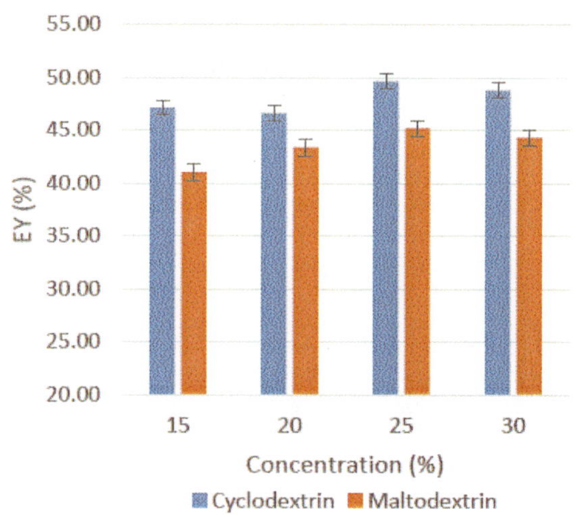

Figure 2: Effect of maltodextrin/cyclodextrin concentration on EY.

Results from Figure 3 showed that as increasing maltodextrin/ sodium caseinate ratio from 0.2/1 to 0.6/1 resulted in increasing MEE, MEY and DY from 48.05% to 66%, 59.44% to 70.31%, and 76.87% to 92.46% respectively. However, microencapsulation efficiency and microencapsulation yield were decreased when maltodextrin/sodium caseinate ratio exceeded 0.6/1. Dian et al. [6], Hogan et al. [8], Kobula and Siriamornpun [9] suggested that the higher protein load values observed at low oil/protein ratios may have conferred enhanced stability on emulsion oil droplets during atomization. It would appear also that the ability of sodium caseinate to effectively encapsulate soy oil at high oil/protein ratios is limited. A similar trend was obtained when we blended sodium caseinate with cyclodextrin but microencapsulation efficiency of carotenoid (Figure 4) were improved by 6% compared to mixture of sodium caseinate and maltodextrin.

Effects of wall material on physical property of Gac powder

The effects of wall materials on physicochemical property of Gac powder are showed in Table 1. Results showed that increasing maltodextrin or cyclodextrin concentration resulted in decreasing moisture content of samples. As maltodextrin concentration increased from 15 to 30% the moisture content of sample significantly reduced from 4.54 to 3.45%. Similarly, Abadio et al. [10], Grabowski et al. [11] reported that moisture content in pineapple juice powders, sweet potato puree powder. Similar trend was observed while increasing cyclodextrin from 15 to 30%. These findings could be explained by the fact that additional concentrations of maltodextrin resulted in an increase in feed solids and a reduction in total moisture for evaporation [4].

Moisture content of samples obtained at different ratio of maltodextrin (or cyclodextrin) and sodium caseinate also presented in Table 2. Statistical evaluation of results indicated that moisture content was not affected by ratio of support. However, when increasing the carriers support from 25 to 30%, water insolubility is lower than of the other samples (15%, 20%). According to Kha et al. [7], increasing carrier support lead to form thick and flexible firms, also increased coalescence. This phenomenon is similar to previous studies were carried out by Dian et al. [6]. The authors suggested that moisture content was not affected by the type of carriers, as well as the ratio of carriers/oil.

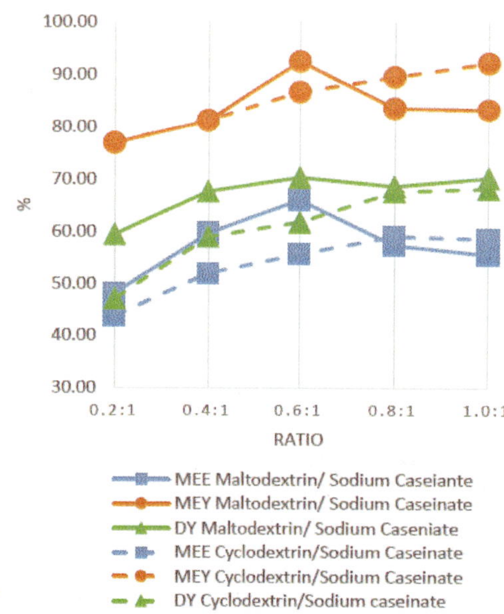

Figure 3: Effect of ratio of maltodextrin (cyclodextrin) and sodium caseinate on MEE, MEY and DY.

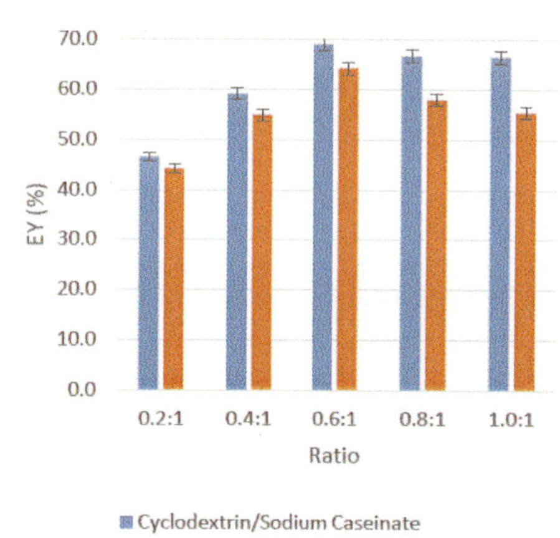

Figure 4: Effect of ratio of maltodextrin/cyclodextrin and sodium caseinate on EY.

In addition, it is important to improve the water solubility for ease of application in the food industry. In this study, water insolubility index (WII) <0.1 mL (at 50°C) indicated that Gac products microencapsulated by matrix of maltodextrin (or cyclodextrin) and sodium caseinate absolutely dissolved in water. The high solubility could be explained by the positive effects of between protein and carriers on the oil droplets containing carotenoids [7,12-22].

Wall material		Moisture content	Water insolubility index
Maltodextrin	15%	4.54 ± 0.05^{i}	$91.15\% \pm 0.04^{a}$
	20%	4.06 ± 0.13^{h}	$91.55\% \pm 0.03^{a}$
	25%	3.76 ± 0.15^{fg}	$90.15\% \pm 0.04^{b}$
	30%	3.45 ± 0.05^{bc}	$89.73\% \pm 0.03^{cb}$
Cyclodextrin	15%	3.43 ± 0.05^{i}	$90.24\% \pm 0.03^{b}$
	20%	3.86 ± 0.17^{gh}	$91.23\% \pm 0.03^{a}$
	25%	$3.67 \pm 0.15^{d\text{-}g}$	$89.15\% \pm 0.04^{bc}$
	30%	3.5 ± 0.05^{cd}	$89.73\% \pm 0.03^{bc}$
Sodium Caseinate/ Maltodextrin	0.2/1	$3.70 \pm 0.15^{d\text{-}g}$	$91.33\% \pm 0.01^{a}$
	0.4/1	$3.75 \pm 0.15^{e\text{-}g}$	$91.18\% \pm 0.06^{a}$
	0.6/1	$3.67 \pm 0.145^{d\text{-}g}$	$89.05\% \pm 0.04^{bc}$
	0.8/1	$3.55 \pm 0.10^{c\text{-}e}$	$87.03\% \pm 0.02^{d}$
	1/1	$3.6 \pm 0.12^{c\text{-}f}$	$86.30\% \pm 0.05^{d}$
Sodium Caseinate/ Cyclodextrin	0.2/1	$3.67 \pm 0.15^{d\text{-}g}$	$91.43\% \pm 0.02^{a}$
	0.4/1	3.45 ± 0.14^{bc}	$91.28\% \pm 0.03^{a}$
	0.6/1	3.27 ± 0.13^{b}	$89.45\% \pm 0.02^{bc}$
	0.8/1	3.28 ± 0.13^{b}	$88.13\% \pm 0.03^{d}$
	1/1	3.03 ± 0.12^{a}	$86.23\% \pm 0.02^{d}$

Table 2: Effects of wall material on physical property of Gac powder [a-i].

Conclusion

In conclusion, the effect of wall material on the property of Gac powder was investigated. Moisture content, colour characteristics, total carotenoid content, microencapsulation efficiency were significantly affected by maltodextrin (or cyclodextrin) concentration and ratio of maltodextrin (or cyclodextrin) and sodium caseinate. The ability of dissolved in water and the content of β-carotene and lycopene reduced insignificantly. Sodium casenate-cyclodextrin matrix as the wall material effectively protected β-carotene and lycopene from thermal degradation during storage.

References

1. Kubola J, Meeso N, Siriamornpun S (2013) Lycopene and beta carotene concentration in aril oil of gac (Momordica cochinchinensis Spreng) as influenced by aril-drying process and solvents extraction. Food Research International 50: 664-669.
2. Kha TC, Nguyen MH, Roach PD, Parks SE, Stathopoulos C (2013) Gac fruit: Nutrient and phytochemical composition, and options for processing. Food Reviews International 29: 92-106.
3. Hiromitsu A, Nguyen TMK, Noriko K, Kazue T, Nguyen VC (2002) Carotenoid pigments in Gac fruit (Momordica cochinchinensis Spreng). Biosci Biotechnol 66: 2479-2482.
4. Kha TC, Nguyen MH, Roach PD (2010) Effects of spray drying conditions on the physicochemical and antioxidant properties of the Gac (Momordica cochinchinensis) fruit aril powder. Journal of Food Engineering 98: 385-392.
5. Pinho E, Grootveld M, Soares G, Henriques M (2014) Cyclodextrins as encapsulation agents for plant bioactive compounds. Carbohydrate Polymers 101: 121-135.
6. Dian NLHM, Sudin M, Yusoff MSA (1996) Characteristic of Microencapsulated Palm Base-Oil as affected by Type of Wall Material. J Sci Food Agric 70: 422-426.
7. Kha TC, Nguyen MH, Roach PD, Stathopoulos CE (2014) Microencapsulation of Gac Oil by Spray Drying: Optimization of Wall Material Concentration and Oil Load Using Response Surface Methodology. Drying Technology 32: 385-397.
8. Hogan SA, McNamee BF, O'Riordan ED, O'Sullivan M (2001) Microencapsulation properties of sodium caseinate. J Agric Food Chem 49: 1934-1938.
9. Kubola J, Siriamornpun S (2011) Phytochemicals and antioxidant activity of different fruit fractions (peel, pulp, aril and seed) of Thai gac (Momordica cochinchinensis Spreng). Food Chem 127: 1138-1145.
10. Abadio FDB, Domingues AM, Borges SV, Oliveira VM (2004) Physical properties of powdered pineapple (Ananas comosus) juice: effect of maltodextrin concentration and atomization speed. Journal of Food Engineering 64: 285-287.
11. Grabowski JA, Truong VD, Daubert CR (2006) Spray-drying of amylase hydrolyzed sweet potato puree and physicochemical properties of powder. J Food Sci 71: 209-217.
12. Desobry SA, Netto FM, Labuza TP (1997) Comparison of spray-drying, drum-drying and freeze-drying forb-carotene encapsulation and preservation. J Food Sci 62: 1158-1162.
13. Dimitrios B (2006) Sources of natural phenolic antioxidants. Trends Food Sci Tech 17: 505-512.
14. Domınguez M, Nieto A, Marin JC, Keck AS, Jeffery E, et al. (2005) Antioxidants activities of extracts from Barkleyanthus salicifolius (Asteraceae) and Penstemon gentianoides (Scrophulariaceae). J Agric Food Chem 53: 5889-5895.
15. Geldart D, Abdullah EC, Hassanpour A, Nwoke LC, Wouters I (2006) Characterization of powder flowability using measurement of angle of repose. China Particuol 4:104-107.
16. Giusti MM, Wrolstad RE (2001) Current protocols in food analytical chemistry. John Wiley & Sons, New York, USA.
17. Kha TC, Nguyen MH, Roach PD, Stathopoulos CE (2013) Effects of Gac aril microwave processing conditions on oil extraction efficiency, and β-carotene and lycopene contents. Journal of Food Engineering 117: 486-491.
18. Kagami Y, Sugimura S, Fujishima N, Matsuda K, Kometani T, et al. (2003) Oxidative stability, structure and physical characteristics of microcapsules formed by spray drying of fish oil with protein wall materials. J Food Sci 68: 2248-2255.
19. Kim D, Lee C (2004) Comprehensive study on vitamin C equivalent antioxidant capacity (VCEAC) of various polyphenolics in scavenging a free radical and its structural relationship. Crit Rev Food Sci Nutr 44: 253-273.
20. Kagami Y, Sugimura S, Fujishima N, Matsuda K, Kometani T, et al. (2003) Oxidative stability, structure and physical characteristics of microcapsules formed by spray drying of fish oil with protein wall materials. J Food Sci 68: 2248-2255.
21. Labuza TP, Kaaname A, Chen Y (1985) Effect of temperature on the moisture sorption isotherms and water activity shift of two dehydrated foods. J Food Sci 50: 385-391.
22. Nguyen PM (2014) The changes of total Carotenoid content of GAC (Momordica cochinchinensis Spreng) powder product in accelerated temperature to the appropriate temperature and shelf-life of product storage. International Research Journal of Natural Sciences 2: 31-37.

13

Nutritional Status and its Associated Factors among School Adolescent Girls in Adama City, Central Ethiopia

Roba KT*, **Abdo M and Wakayo T**

College of Health and Medical Sciences, Haramaya University, Eastern Ethiopia, P.O.BOX 235, Harar, East Harargie 0000, Ethiopia

***Corresponding author:** Roba KT, College of Health and Medical Sciences, Haramaya University, Eastern Ethiopia, P.O.BOX 235, Harar, East Harargie 0000, Ethiopia, E-mail: kedir.t.roba@gmail.com

Abstract

Adolescence is a period of rapid growth and maturation in human development that demands extra nutrients and energy to support growth. Focusing on adolescents' nutrition, especially girls, provides a unique opportunity to break the intergenerational cycles of malnutrition. But, there is little information about nutritional status of school going adolescent girls in central Ethiopia.

Methods: Institutional based cross-sectional quantitative study was employed among school going adolescent girls in Adama city. Survey was conducted among 726 samples which were selected by using stratified cluster random sampling procedures. Data was entered into Epi Data and transferred to SPSS (version 16) for analysis. WHO Anthro plus software was used to calculate body mass index for age z-score and height for age z-score. Multivariable logistic regression was used to measure the association between the dependent variable and independent variables with 95% confidence interval.

Results: This study found that 21.3% of adolescent girls were underweighted, 3.3% were overweight, 1.0% was obese and 15.6% were stunted. Of the adolescents, 41.2% of them received minimum dietary diversity (MDD), but 73.0% of the underweighted adolescent's did not receive minimum dietary diversity in 24 h before the survey. The proportions of wasting, stunting and low dietary diversity were higher among subjects from government schools compared to those from private schools. The predictors of under-nutrition among adolescent girls were: being born from uneducated parents (father and mother), their fathers' occupation of being a merchant, adolescents with low dietary diversity, monotonous diet and adolescents attending government schools.

Conclusion: Malnutrition affects one out of five female adolescent in this community and was associated with poor dietary diversity and parent demography which demands appropriate health information disseminations to the target groups.

Keywords: Adolescent; Wasting; Thinness; Ethiopia

Introduction

Adolescence is the age between 10-19 years old, and it is the transition from dependent childhood to independent adulthood, that comprises 20% of the global population, and with approximately 80% of them live in developing countries [1,2]. This age is a stage of growth and development in the lifespan that needs adequate and proper quality food to meet the nutrient requirement for their physical, mental growth and development in addition to reproductive maturity [3].

Nutritional needs during adolescence are influenced mainly by the onset of puberty with its associated increased growth rate and changes in body composition and organ systems [4]. In this period adolescents gain 15% of their final adult height, 45% of increments in bone mass and 50% of adult weight is attained together with changes in body shape and composition [5-7].

Adolescents in all income and ethnic groups can be at risk for dietary excesses and deficiencies. Many boys and girls in developing countries enter adolescence undernourished, making them more vulnerable to disease and early death [8]. In addition, adolescents have a low rate of infection and chronic diseases compared to children under 5 years old and old age that makes them receive little attention, except reproductive health. Inadequate diet during this time can result in decreased learning ability, delayed sexual maturity, a lack of concentration, impaired school performance and slow growth. Pregnancy, lactation, physical activity and sports participation further increase nutrient requirements during this age [9]. Therefore, malnourished adolescent girls are at risk of being stunted mothers who are likely to suffer obstetric complications and to deliver low birth weight babies that could lead to intergenerational cycle of malnutrition. Thus, adequate nutrition and healthy eating habits at this age are foundations for good health in adulthood.

In Ethiopia, children and adolescent constitutes about 48% of Ethiopian population and about 25 percent of this age group is girls [10] but studies among this age group were insufficient. Few Studies in Ethiopia showed that under nutrition was common problem among adolescent girls. Of which, a study in the rural community of Tigray indicated that 25.5% and 58.3% of adolescent girls were stunted and thin respectively [11], 37.8% were wasting (thinness), 2.0% overweight and 0.4% had obesity [12]. Similarly, in Jimma, 53.2% were underweight [13], Hawassa, 12.9% were overweighed and 2.7% had obesity [14] but no study was reported among adolescent girls in

Adama city, the biggest city in south east Ethiopia. Therefore, this study aimed at identifying the level of malnutrition and associated factors among high school adolescent girls in Adama city, south eastern Ethiopia.

Materials and Method

Study area

This study was conducted in Adama city which is located 100 km away on eastern direction of Addis Ababa. This city is among the biggest cities in Ethiopia and the biggest in the Oromia region. The livelihoods of this city are predominantly trade followed by civil servants. This study was conducted in April 2015 GC among school going adolescent girls. The schools were categorized as private who are providing education by collecting fee from students and Government schools, provides educational services for free to all citizen by acquiring funding from government. No gender based schools were available in Adama city. There are five government and four private schools that render education for grade nine and above in Adama city.

This study employed quantitative institution based cross study design. The study populations were adolescent girls who were selected from four randomly selected schools. The sample size was determined using the formula for single population proportion with the assumption of 0.05% marginal error, 95% confidence interval (Za/2=1.96). Using on the prevalence (P) of 37.8% stunting in the study conducted in Tigray [12] (due to similarity of the population) and with design effect of 2, the final sample size was 726.

Sampling technique

A stratified cluster random sampling technique was used according to the following procedures. First the secondary schools grade 9 and grade 10 were identified by name and then the schools were stratified by ownership into government and non-government schools. Then, two government and two non-government schools were randomly selected by lottery method and sample size for each school was assigned based on proportionality to the number of adolescent girls in each school. Finally the study participants were selected by using Probability proportional to population size (PPS) from the total size in to grades 9 and 10. Then estimated sample size for each grade was distributed proportionally to each section and final samples were drawn using systematic random sampling method from student registry after identifying a list of female students. Adolescent girls suspected of pregnancy during screening, severe illness/history of admission to hospital in last months were excluded from the study.

Data collectors

Eight data collectors that have diplomas in nursing that monitor data collection filling and completeness of data on spot and provides necessary assistance for participants and two more supervisors with degrees who had experience of collecting similar data and were able speak the local language were recruited. Two days training was given to data collectors on how to approach the adolescent girls during data collections and pre-test was also conducted for standardization. After data collection each questionnaire was checked for completeness of information by immediate supervisors and the principal investigator.

Data collection

Data were collected using a structured, self-administered questionnaire under strict supervision of female supervisors and the overall quality control was conducted by the first author. The questionnaire was prepared based on the nutrition baseline survey report for the national nutrition program of Ethiopia, (Ethiopian Health and Nutrition Research Institute 2009/2010) and relevant literature. The questionnaire was pretested in similar setting out of sample schools and comments and suggestion identified in pretest was included in the final version. The questionnaire developed in English, was translated into Amharic and Afan Oromo language then back to English by another person to ensure consistency and contextualization.

Data collection tools were designing in logical sequenced and free of scientific terms and non-leading. The pre-test was conducted on 5% of the study population other than the selected schools in the town, but in schools other than study sites before the actual data collection begins and amendment was made on the questionnaires if necessary. Questionnaires were checked each day by principal investigator for any incompleteness and/or inconsistency and feedback was given every morning before commencement of the next day's work.

A household wealth index was calculated by principal component analysis based on household assets and housing quality was used as a proxy indicator for socioeconomic status of households. An absolute measure of household wealth (wealth index) used in this study is based on an earlier concept developed by Garenne and Hohmann [15], whereby the sum of dummy variables are created from information collected on housing quality (floor, walls, and roof material), availability of potable water in the compound and type of toilet facility, and ownership of household durable goods (e.g. bicycle, television, radio, motorcycle, telephone, cars, refrigerator, mattress, bed). These facilities or durable goods are often regarded as modern goods that have been shown to reflect household wealth. The scores were thus added up to give the proxy household wealth index. The index varied from 0 to 18. Similar classification was used in previous study [16].

Anthropometric data

Nutritional status of study participants was assessed based on the anthropometric measurements used to assess the physical development of adolescent girls. Height was measured once with a Portable Height Scale to the nearest 0.1 cm. The Body weight was measured using the platform (digital scale) weighing Scale (770 alpha; SECA, Hamburg, Germany) to the nearest 0.1 kg that has the capacity to measure 0-140 kg. Weight and height were measured by two different measurers and with any variation the final validations was made by supervisors immediately on site. The subjects were weighed with minimum of clothing. Body mass for age z-score was used to classify level of malnutrition in the study subjects and those who have less than -2 z-score were categorised as thin, between >-2 and <+1 as normal weight, overweight between +1 and <+2 and above +2 were categorized as obese (WHO, 2007). Having height for age z-score less than -2 was categorized as stunted [17].

Dietary diversity data were collected using a questionnaire developed by Food and nutrition technical assistance [18]. The questionnaire asked adolescents the types of food consumed in the home or outside the compound in the last 24 h. The information collected on dietary consumption was used to calculate the dietary diversity score (DDS) and additionally seven day food frequency was also noted to their household dietary diversity and regular access to food. The seven day food frequency was used to determine frequency of accessing to animals sources foods and phytates (that inhibits absorption of Iron and zinc from food). Each food group was counted only once resulting in a possible score of 0 to 9. The DDS was categorized into low/inadequate dietary diversity (<4 food groups), adequate dietary diversity (≥ 4 food groups) [19]. The recall was randomly made on week days or on weekend days, since weekends do not have any special significance in the context of our study. We took care not to include atypical days (local feasts or celebrations) in the recall.

The dependent variable was nutritional status of adolescent girls. The independent variables derived from socio-demographic and socioeconomic characteristics of the family, and dietary habits of the adolescents. The socio-demographic variables used in this study were age, sex, marital status, ethnicity and religion. The socio-economic variables were level of education of parents, type of last school attended, occupation, family size, income, water and sanitation. Adolescents were also asked about their lifestyles, source of income, pocket money, how spare time was spent in addition to their dietary diversity, meal pattern and habits of eating fast foods.

Data processing and analysis

Data were double entered into Epi Data 3.1 version and was checked for completeness and consistency, followed by data cleaning and editing. Then the data was analysed by using Statistical Package for Social Sciences, Version 16 (SPSS for Windows, SPSS Inc., and Chicago, IL, USA) software's and WHO Anthro Plus software for assessing growth of the adolescents was used [20]. Descriptive statistics using frequencies, proportions and correlation was used to present the study results. Odds ratio with 95% confidence interval was used for checking the strength of associations between dependent and independent variables. Bivariate analysis was used to identify candidate variables for multivariable logistic regression in determining factors associated with nutritional status and only variables with p-values <0.2 in bivariate analysis were entered into the final multivariable logistic regression model to adjust for confounders.

Ethical consideration

Prior to the commencement of the actual data collection process, the study proposal protocol was approved by Rift Valley University College Institutional Research Ethics Review Committee. Official letters of co-operation were written to all secondary school and concerned bodies in the city and to the schools. After getting permission from the schools, the principal investigator set dates and times of data collections with the school administrations. Students and their parents were notified and necessary explanations were also given about the purposes, procedure and all the confidentiality issues. Consent was collected from the parents of study subjects by sending letter to parent/guardians for each study subject less than 18 years old and oral assent was obtained from study subjects in the school. The respondents' confidentiality of information was assured by excluding names and identifiers from in the questionnaire and they were informed that they can refuse participation at any time.

Results

Socio-demographic characteristics of study participants

From calculated sample size of 726, 700 adolescent girls provided complete questionnaire making a response rate 97.2%. All of them were urban residents, 60.7% were from governmental schools and 56.3% of them were grade 9 students. Of the participants, 66.7% belonged to 15-19 years of age groups, 52.7 % of them were followers of Orthodox Christianity by religion (Table 1).

Variables	Categories	Number (n)	%
Age	15-17	236	34
	17-19	474	66
Religion	Muslim	229	33
	Orthodox	369	53
	Protestant	90	13
	Other	12	1.7
Grade	Grade 9	394	56
	Grade 10	306	44
Type of Schools	Private School	276	39
	Public School	424	61
Father Education	No formal Education	140	20
	Primary and Secondary	275	39
	Grade 12 and College	285	41
Mother Education	No formal Education	188	27
	Primary and secondary	302	43
	Grade 12 and College	210	30
Father occupation	Daily laborer	148	21
	Government	275	39
	Merchant	277	40
Mother occupation	House wife	163	23
	Government	261	37
	Merchant	276	39
Wealth Index	Poor	219	31
	Middle	264	38
	Rich	217	31

Table 1: Socio-demographic characteristics study participants in Adama city, south eastern Ethiopia, 2015.

Of the participants, 37.7% were among middle wealth class group while the rest were categorized among lower and upper class wealth index. Regarding the educational status parents, about 40.7% of their fathers attended some college/university while only 30% their mothers did so. As to the occupation of parents of the study subjects, 39.6% of the respondents' fathers were merchants and 39.3 % were government-employed (Table 1).

Diet/Dietary habit of school adolescent girls

Based on the 24 h dietary recalls the mean Dietary Diversity Score (DDS) was 4.2 (SD 2.01). The proportion of adolescents with minimum dietary diversity (at least consumed from four food groups out of nine food groups) was 41.2%. Among the participants, the all (100 %) of them consumed grains or other starchy roots and tubers (staples), followed by dark green vegetables (80.0%), others fruits and vegetables (79.3%) and legumes (66.7%). Consumption of animal source foods like, organ and flesh meat, dairy product and egg were relatively low (Table 2).

Food Type or Group	Categories	Frequency (n)	%
Grains or other starchy roots and tubers	Yes	700	100
Vitamin A rich fruits and vegetables	Yes	430	61
	No	270	39
Dark Green Leafy Vegetables	Yes	560	80
	No	140	20
Organ Meat	Yes	80	11
	No	620	89
Flesh foods	Yes	226	32
	No	474	68
Other fruits and vegetables	Yes	555	79
	No	145	21
Eggs	Yes	218	31
	No	482	69
Legumes and nuts	Yes	467	67
	No	233	33
Dairy products (milk, yogurt, cheese)	Yes	317	45
	No	383	55

Table 2: Adolescent's 24 h dietary diversity recall in Adama city, South Eastern Ethiopia 2015.

Food frequency of the study participants

A seven day food frequency questionnaire of major foods and beverages consumed by adolescents indicated that 73.3% of them consumed milk and milk products 1-2 times per week, 50% ate pasta/rice/bread/potatoes more than three times a week, but only 32.9% of the respondents reported they did not eat meat at least once per week (Table 3).

Nutritional status of the adolescent school girls

Under nutrition or thinness (BMI for age z score <-2) was observed among 21.3% respondents, while 3.3 % of them were overweight and 1.0% had obesity. Similarly 15.6% of the adolescents were stunted (have short stature for their age) (Table 4). Among 21.3% of adolescents with malnutrition, 59.1% and 42.5% of them were born from mothers and fathers who attended school respectively. Of the malnourished adolescents, 47% do not eat egg in weeks, 47.1% had monotonous diet pattern and only 26.8% of them took adequate dietary diversity as reported from 24 hrs before the survey (Table 5).

Consumption Frequency Food items		Frequency	%
Cereals	>3 times in a week	700	100
Pasta and rice	Never	66	9.4
	1-2 times/week	280	40
	>3 times	354	51
Milk and milk products	Never	11	1.6
	1-2 times/week	513	73
	>3times	176	25
Meat	Never	230	33
	1-2 times/week	277	40
	>3times	193	28
Egg	Never	239	34
	1-2 times/week	235	34
	>3 times	226	32
Sweets	Never	272	39
	1-2 times/wk	214	31
	>3 times	214	31
Cheese	Never	483	69
	1-2 times/week	141	20
	>3 times	76	11
Legumes	Never	222	32
	1-2 times/wk	295	42
	>3 times	183	26
Fast food	Never	324	46
	1-2 times/week	189	27
	>3 times	186	27

Table 3: Seven day food frequency of some food stuffs among school adolescent consumed in Adama city, South East of Ethiopia, 2015.

Variables	Total	Types of school		X^2 test (p-values)
	N (%)	Government	Private	
BMI for age z score				
<-2 z score (thin)	149 (21.3)	124	35	20.5 (<0.001)

>-2 to<0.99 (Normal)	521 (74.4)	297	214	1
1.00 to 1.99 (Overweight)	23 (3.3)	3	20	3.2 (0.07)
≥ +2 Obese	7 (1.0)	0 (0.0)	7	NA
Height for age z score				
<-2 z score (stunted)	109 (15.6)	81 (19.1)	25 (9)	0.7 (0.4)
≥ -2 (normal)	591 (84.4)	343 (80.9)	251 (91)	
Minimum Dietary Diversity				
Yes	289 (41.2)	195 (45.8)	94 (34.1)	9.4 (0.002)
No	411 (58.7)	231 (54.2)	182 (65.9)	

Table 4: Nutritional status of adolescent school girls in Adama City, South Eastern Ethiopia.

Factors associated with nutritional status of the school adolescents

Among socio-demographic and economic factors, age of mothers and fathers of adolescent girls, their households wealth index, religion, grade, , family income, were not significant at binary logistic regression (p values>0.2) and were removed from multivariable logistic regression models. Among dietary habits eating meat, cheese, fast foods predominantly diets eating vegetables and most other variables in seven day food frequency were not significant and then removed from further analyses. Finally, educational status of adolescent girls mothers and fathers, their fathers occupation, dietary diversity, frequency of eating egg, sweets and legumes in a week, perceptions of their dietary diversity, lifestyle's in their free time and types of schools they are attending fulfilled the criteria and were included in multivariable analysis.

In multivariable logistic regression analysis, adolescent girls' father and mother education level, occupation of their fathers, their DDS and pattern of meal diversity were significantly associated with under nutrition. Adolescent girls who were from an illiterate father were more likely to develop under nutrition (thinness) compared to those born from fathers of college level training (AOR=3.06, 95% CI=1.67-5.63). In addition, those adolescent girls from daily laborer fathers were twice more likely to be undernourished compared to those adolescent girls from merchant fathers (AOR=2.67, 95%, CI: 1.48-4.8). Adolescent girls who had low DDS were more likely to be thin (AOR: 2.1 95% CI: (1.54-3.89) than those adolescents with high DDS. Similarly, regarding meal diversity perception, those adolescent girls who perceived their diet was monotonous were more likely to develop wasting (AOR=2.52, 95%, CI=1.51-4.19) compared to those who had diversified food on daily bases. Adolescents from uneducated mothers and mothers who attended primary school were more likely to have undernourishment compared to mothers who attended some formal college training (Table 5).

Variables		**Nutritional Status**			
		Thin N (%)	**Normal N (%)**	**COR (95% CI)**	**AOR (95% CI)**
Mother education level	Illiterate	85 (57.1)	95 (18.2)	7.5 (4.3-13.6)	5.4 (4.71-9.1)*
	Primary	43 (28.9)	248 (47.6)	1.5 (0.82-2.7)	1.69 (0.91-3.17)*
	Secondary/College	21 (14.0)	178 (34.2)	1	
Father education level	Illiterate	44 (29.5)	78 (15.0)	3.2 (19-5.4)	3.06 (1.67-5.63)*
	Primary	63 (42.3)	206 (39.5)	1.73 (1.12-2.7)	2.40 (1.43-4.04)*
	Secondary/College	42 (28.2)	237 (45.5)	1	
Father occupation	Daily labor	53 (35.6)	97(18.6)	2.62 (1.59-4.3)	2.67 (1.48-4.8)*
	Government	54 (36.2)	222 (42.6)	1.16(0.73-1.87)	1.20 (0.74-2.05)
	Merchant	42 (28.3)	202 (38.8)	1	
DDS	Low	109 (73.1)	282 (54.1)	2.31 (1.5-3.5)	2.1 (1.54-3.89)*
	Adequate	40 (26.8)	239 (45.9)	1	
Sweets/week	Never	74 (49.7)	168 (32.2)	2.1 (1.3- 3.4)	1.24 (0.701-2.18)
	1-2 times/week	38 (25.5)	176 (33.8)	1.033 (0.3-1.7)	0.81(0.45-1.48)
	>3 times/week	37 (24.8)	177 (34.0)	1	
Legumes/week	Never	30 (20.1)	153 (29.4)	0.6 (0.36-1.0)	1.35 (0.74-2.47)
	1-2 times/week	54 (36.2)	167 (32.0)	0.99 (0.6-1.5)	1.42 (0.79-2.53)

	>3 times/week	65 (43.6)	201 (38.6)	1	
Pattern of eating diversified meal	Monotones diet	85 (57.1)	203 (39.0)	3.1 (1.7-5.5)	2.52 (1.51-4.19)*
	Sometimes	44 (29.5)	175 (34.0)	1.8(0.98-3.4)	1.8 (0.98-3.4)
	Always Different	20 (13.4)	143 (27.0)	1	
Free time practice	Watching TV/computer using	52 (35.0)	278 (53.4)	0.46 (0.31-0.70)	0.88 (0.49-1.58)
	Walking/sport	97 (65.1)	243 (46.6)	1	
Types of school	Private	35 (23.4)	214 (41.0)	1	
	Government	124 (83.2)	297 (57.0)	0.39 (0.25-0.60)	0.42 (0.21-0.75)*

Table 5: Determinant of nutritional status of school Adolescent girls in Adama city, South Eastern Ethiopia. NB: Adolescents who were overweight were removed from multivariate analysis. *percentage is calculated for column in this data.

Discussion

This study showed that 21.3% of the adolescents were underweight, 3.3% of them were overweight and 1.0% had obesity. Of the adolescents, 15.6% were stunted and 41.2% of them received minimum dietary diversity (MDD) recalled from a 24 h before the survey. The predictors of under-nutrition among adolescent girls were: adolescents from mothers and fathers who did not attend formal education, from daily laborer and government employee fathers, adolescents with low dietary diversity, and adolescents who perceived their diet was monotonous.

Problems related to nutrition have been identified as important concerns for public health in Ethiopia. Many studies have been carried out to identify the extent and consequence of malnutrition in different population groups. Thus, adolescents demonstrate the vulnerability of those who have not received appropriate attention to ensure that their nutritional needs are met. This study is important indicators for nutritional status of "tomorrow mothers" where all stakeholders should work hand in hand to cut the intergenerational cycle of malnutrition. It is worth to notices that this study is conducted in urban area where majority of the household have better exposure to health information and awareness through different media as well as the relative suffer of adolescent girls in city are assumed to be better than rural in fetching water, collecting fire wood and assisting families in farm activities. Therefore the magnitude of this study could be an indicative of public health importance of this study which may require different interventions.

This study revealed that prevalence of under-nutrition among adolescent students was 21.3% and this finding is lower than the study in Ambo (27.5%, [21], higher than study conducted in Addis Ababa city (13%) [22]. This might be due to the difference in socioeconomic background between the cities. Other studies in Ethiopia indicated that 37.8% were wasted in Tigray region [12]. These findings indicated that under-nutrition is a major public health problem in majority of Ethiopian communities including urban and rural adolescents. The differences in prevalence could be associated with the socio-demographic and economic characteristics of household.

The prevalence of overweight was 3.3%, which is another form of malnutrition that may be associated with nutritional transition among adolescents. The finding of this study is relatively low compared to the study conducted in Hawassa (12.9) [14], but higher than Mekelle (2%) [12], and Ambo (2.6) [21]. This finding can alert policy makers about the presence of double burden (under and over nutrition) in the same community. In addition, about 1.0% of adolescents were obese and this is lower compared to the findings from Ambo (1.7%) [21] and Addis (2.6) [22]. So, this study calls for a need to give health information about the impact of over nutrition in addition to teaching about endemic under-nutrition in Ethiopia. Among children with overweight and obesity, the majority of them were from private schools that may be associated with the welfare of the households and related reduced outdoor physical activities. The magnitude of overweight adolescents girls was higher among private school girls compared to government schools (p=0.07) and all of the obese adolescents were from private schools that could be due to the fact that private schools are mainly attended by students from better socioeconomic status.

The prevalence of stunting in this study was 15.6% which is due to a prolonged shortage of balanced meals, especially amongst children from poor families. This finding is similar to the study conducted in Babile, but higher than the previous study conducted among children in Adama (12.6%) [23] And Kersa district of eastern Ethiopia (8.9%) [24]. Similar to wasting, stunting is also relatively higher in government schools than in the private schools, even though the difference was not significant. It is know that short stature is associated is cephalopelvic disproportion and increased risk of maternal complications during child birth. In addition studies showed that stunted mothers will give birth of stunted child which indicate that international cycle of malnutrition. Studies showed that stunting was associated with delayed school entry, repetition and dropout rates, as well as decreased graduation rates from primary and secondary school, and lower school performance [25]. Similarly, early childhood stunting was associated with lower adult body-mass index (BMI) but higher risk of developing central adiposity [26].

The proportion of children, who received at least from four more food group out of nine, is 41.2%. This finding is lower than the study conducted in Bale zone (80.7%) [27] and chiro town (74.2%) [28], but higher than Libo Kemkem and Fogera Districts adolescents (5%) [29] and the study by Wassie et al. (15%) [30]. The current study revealed that adolescent girls with higher DDS were more likely to have normal BMI-for- age Z scores as compared to those having low DDS (Table 3). This is because when the IDDS is high, adolescents will get adequate energy and other important nutrients having role in growth and development. Even though the magnitude of adequate dietary diversity is varied across the regions, the proportion of adolescents with low dietary diversity is common in Ethiopia. This needs great attention to curb its long lasting consequences.

Dietary diversity has been used as proxy indicators for food quality and security [31], which may be due to its ability to capture consumption of both macro and micronutrients or a more balanced diet in the general sense without the need of measuring the quantity of food consumed, which may in turn be difficult in certain contexts. Malnutrition found in these school-aged adolescents living in Adama city is associated with a low DD together with other socio demographic factors of the household. In this study, we also found that 42.9% of adolescents expressed their diet as monotonous which is mainly based on low energy and low nutrient foods, such as cereals or tubers and is low in animal source foods. Of the children with wasting, 57.1% perceived that their diet is mostly monotonous. With regard to growth spurts in adolescents, even though the actual need of energy at this time may vary greatly with physical activity level, basal metabolic rate (BMR) and body composition, inadequate intake of energy leads to malnutrition. Studies also showed that meal pattern of the adolescent may follow pattern of their family as they grew up, they are influenced by their family feeding/dietary diversity behaviors [32].

Studies in Ethiopia indicated that food consumption patterns are very diverse and their food basket consists of a wide variety of grains and other staples, which are varied across agro-ecology, socioeconomic levels, and livelihood strategies [33] as well as affected by tradition of the societies and food preferences [34]. In addition, differences and inequalities in dietary diversity among urban and rural areas was reported previously [35,36].

This study found that adolescents of fathers from lower levels of education had a significantly higher risk of being underweight than those of fathers who attended above grade 12 or higher level of education. This finding is consistent with the study done in western Ethiopia [12]. This indicated that the educational attainment of the father could lead to a higher income and may imply a higher availability of food and household resources as well as being positively associated with higher nutritional awareness.

This study showed that being adolescents from mothers having non-formal education were significantly associated with under-nutrition. This study is in agreement with the study done in urban slums of Dibrugarh which showed that the prevalence of both stunting (41.80) and thinness (44.26%) was much higher among girls who came from families whose mothers were illiterate [37]. Similarly studies from different parties of the world indicted that maternal education are closely related to child health measured either by nutritional status or by infant and child mortality but the effect of father's education appears to be about one half that of mother's education [38,39].

Another striking finding of this study was that adolescents from private schools were less likely to acquire wasting compared to government school adolescents, which indicate that the causes of malnutrition are associated with household income. This difference is observed because most of the students going to private schools were from the families who are able to afford school fees while the government school is free of any charge. Another studies in Ethiopia indicated that higher prevalence of under nutrition among adolescents from lower family income or those adolescents born from lower income fathers was undernourished compared to counterparts [13].

A limitation of this study is that most of the data was collected from self-administered forms and therefore social desirability bias may be present. But during data collection adequate information was given to participants about the importance and confidentiality of information and were seat in separate chair and not able to see/read the response of each other's. Other limitation of this study was that this study was conducted in urban and do not generalize to rural adolescent girl population.

Conclusion

This study revealed that under-nutrition was relatively high among urban adolescent girls and adolescent's parent education, adolescent's meal pattern and dietary diversity were predictors of the observed under-nutrition. Recognizing the intergenerational effect of malnutrition and high prevalence of under-nutrition in the city, there is a clear need for carefully designing interventions that reduces the risks of malnutrition among adolescent girls in Adama city.

Acknowledgement

We would like to thank Rift Valley University for the financial support of this study. We would like to thanks the study participants, data collectors, data clerk, school directors and section leaders for their great contribution during our study.

References

1. WHO (2005) World Health Organization, Nutrition in adolescence-issues and challenges for the health sector: issues in adolescent health and development. Geneva: WHO.
2. Adams GR, Montemayor R, Gullotta TP (1989) Biology of adolescent behavior and development: Sage Publications, Inc.
3. Patanwar P, Sharma K (2013) Nutritional Status of Kurmi Adolescent Girls of Raipur City Chhattisgarh, India. Inter J Sci Res Pub 3: 172.
4. Stang J, Story M (2005) Guidelines for Adolescent Nutrition Services. 21.
5. Giuseppina D (2000) Nutrition in Adolescence. Pediatrics in Review shils ME, Olson JM, eds. Modern nutrition in health and disease. Philadelphia: Lea and Febiger, 1994: 759-769.
6. Spear BA (2002) Adolescent growth and development. J Am Diet Assoc 102: 23S-29S.
7. Rogol AD, Clark PA, Roemmich JN (2000) Growth and pubertal development in children and adolescents: effects of diet and physical activity. Am J Clin Nutr 72: 521S-8S.
8. Ransom EI, Elder LK (2003) Nutrition of women and adolescent girls: Why it matters.
9. Story M, Hermanson J (1990) Nutrient needs during adolescence and pregnancy. Nutrition management of the pregnant adolescent: A practical reference guide 21-28.
10. CSA (2007) Centeral statistics agency of Ethiopia, Addis Ababa.
11. Mulugeta A, Hagos F, Kruseman G, Linderhof V, Stoecker B, et al. (2010) Child malnutrition in Tigray, northern Ethiopia. East Afr Med J 87: 248-254.
12. Gebremariam H, Seid O, Assefa H (2015) Assessment of nutritional status and associated factors among school going adolescents of Mekelle City, Northern Ethiopia. Inter J Nutr Food Sci 4: 118-124.
13. Assefa H, Belachew T, Negash L (2013) Socioeconomic factors associated with underweight and stunting among adolescents of Jimma Zone, south west Ethiopia: a cross-sectional study. ISRN Public Health 2013.
14. Teshome T, Singh P, Moges D (2012) Prevalence and Associated Factors of Overweight and Obesity Among High School Adolescents in Urban Communities of Hawassa, Southern Ethiopia. Curr Res Nutr Food Sci Jour 1: 23-36.
15. Garenne M, Hohmann-Garenne S (2003) A wealth index to screen high-risk families: Application to Morocco. J Health, Popul Nutri 21: 235-242.
16. Saaka M, Osman SM (2013) Does household food insecurity affect the

nutritional status of preschool children aged 6-36 months? Inter J Popul Res.

17. De Onis M (2006) WHO child growth standards: Length/height-for-age, weight-for-age, weight-for-length, weight-for-height and body mass index-for-age: WHO.
18. WHO, UNICEF, USAID, FANTA, AED, et al. (2010) Indicators for assessing infant and young child feeding practices part 2: measurement. Geneva. The World Health Organization Department of Child and Adolescent Health and Development.
19. WHO (2008) Indicators for assessing infant and young child feeding practices: Conclusions of a consensus meeting held 6-8 November 2007 in Washington, DC, USA. Part 1: Definitions. Geneva: World Health Organization.
20. WHO (2009) World Health Organization, WHO AnthroPlus for personal computers manual: software for assessing growth of the World's Children and Adolescents. Geneva.
21. Yetubie M1, Haidar J, Kassa H, Fallon F (2010) Socioeconomic and Demographic Factors Affecting Body Mass Index of Adolescents Students Aged 10-19 in Ambo (a Rural Town) in Ethiopia. Int J Biomed Sci 6: 321-326.
22. Zeleke A (2010) Prevalence of childhood and adolescent overweight and obesity among elementary school students in Addis Ababa: double burden of malnutrition in Ethiopia. J Nutr Disorders Ther 5: 168
23. Belay G, Reji P, Erko B, Legesse M, Belay M (2011) Intestinal parasitic infections and malnutrition amongst first-cycle primary schoolchildren in Adama, Ethiopia. Afr J Pri Health Care Family Med 3: 5.
24. Mesfin F, Berhane Y (2015) Prevalence and associated factors of stunting among primary school children in eastern Ethiopia. Nutr Dietary Suppl 7: 61-68.
25. Daniels MC, Adair LS (2004) Growth in young Filipino children predicts schooling trajectories through high school. J Nutr 134: 1439-1446.
26. Schroeder DG, Martorell R, Flores R (1999) Infant and child growth and fatness and fat distribution in Guatemalan adults. Am J Epidemiol 149: 177-185.
27. Mohammed AY, Tefera TB (2015) Nutritional status and associated risk factors among adolescents girls in Agarfa High School, Bale Zone, Oromia Region, South East Ethiopia. Inter J Nutr Food Sci 4: 445-152.
28. Damie TD, Wondafrash M, Teklehaymanot AN (2015) Nutritional status and associated factors among school adolescent in Chiro Town, West Hararge, Ethiopia. Gaziantep Medical Journal 21: 32-42.
29. Herrador Z, Perez-Formigo J, Sordo L, Gadisa E, Moreno J, et al. (2015) Low dietary diversity and intake of animal source foods among school aged children in Libo Kemkem and Fogera Districts, Ethiopia. PLoS One 10: e0133435.
30. Wassie MM, Gete AA, Yesuf ME, Alene GD, Belay A, et al. (2015) Predictors of nutritional status of Ethiopian adolescent girls: A community based cross sectional study. BMC Nutrition 1: 1.
31. Allen LH (2003) Interventions for micronutrient deficiency control in developing countries: Past, present and future. J Nutr 133: 3875S-3878S.
32. Neumark-Sztainer D, Hannan PJ, Story M, Croll J, Perry C (2003) Family meal patterns: associations with socio-demographic characteristics and improved dietary intake among adolescents. J Am Diet Assoc 103: 317-322.
33. Berhane G, Paulos Z, Tafere K, Tamru S (2011) Food grain consumption and calorie intake patterns in Ethiopia. IFPRI Ethiopia Strategy Support Program II (ESSP II) Working Paper 23.
34. Alemayehu S, Dorosh P, Asrat S (2013) Crop production in Ethiopia: Regional patterns and trends. Food Agric Ethiop Prog Policy Chall 74: 53.
35. Dorosh P, Schmidt E (2010) The rural-urban transformation in Ethiopia. Citeseer.
36. Frehiwot F (2007) Food insecurity and its determinants in rural households in Amhara region.
37. Bhattacharyya H, Barua A (2013) Nutritional status and factors affecting nutrition among adolescent girls in urban slums of Dibrugarh, Assam. Natl J Community Med 4: 35-39.
38. Cochrane SH, Leslie J, O'Hara DJ (1982) Parental education and child health: Intra-country evidence. Health Policy Educ 2: 213-250.
39. Frost MB, Forste R, Haas DW (2005) Maternal education and child nutritional status in Bolivia: finding the links. Social Science and Medicine 60: 395-407.

14

Improved Prevalence of Anemia and Nutritional Status among Japanese Elderly Participants in the National Health and Nutritional Survey Japan, 2003-2009

Imai E, Nakade M, Kasaoka Tsuboyama and Takimoto H*

Department of Nutritional Epidemiology, National Institutes of Biomedical Innovation, Health and Nutrition, Tokyo, Japan

***Corresponding author:** Takimoto H, Department of Nutritional Epidemiology, National Institutes of Biomedical Innovation, Health and Nutrition, Toyama 1-23-1, Shinjuku-ku, Tokyo, Japan 162-8636, E-mail: thidemi@nih.go.jp

Abstract

Objectives: This study aimed 1) to examine the trends in the prevalence of anemia of the Japanese elderly population and 2) to evaluate the association between hemoglobin concentrations and diet and lifestyle factors, by using data from a population-based, nationwide cross-sectional survey in Japan, from 2003-2009.

Design: A cross-sectional nationally representative survey.

Setting: Japan.

Participants: A nationally representative sample of 10,606 community dwelling men (n=4656) and women (n=5950) aged 65 years and over.

Measurements: Information on anthropometry, dietary intake status, information on current medication, lifestyle habits, and blood biomarker measurements were obtained from the participants. Anemia was defined as hemoglobin concentrations <130 g/L in men and <120 g/L in women. Logistic regression analysis adjusted for subject age was applied to estimate the effect of survey year to anemia prevalence. Multiple regression analysis was applied to estimate the effect of survey year and clinical, dietary and lifestyle factors to hemoglobin values.

Results: Anemia prevalence was 19.3% in men and 21.7% in women. When adjusted for age, the prevalence of anemia significantly decreased by each survey year in both men (odds ratio: 0.933, 95% confidence interval: 0.899, 0.968, p<0.001) and women (odds ratio: 0.968, 95% confidence interval: 0.939, 0.999, p=0.040). The multivariate model explained 25% and 22% of the variance in hemoglobin values in men and women, respectively. In both men and women, each unit of increase in BMI, daily smoking, serum ferritin and albumin was positively associated to hemoglobin values, and age was negatively associated. After adjusting for all factors, hemoglobin values were estimated to increase 0.66 g/L per year in men, and 0.68 g/L per year in women.

Conclusion: Nutritional status of the Japanese elderly as observed by anemia prevalence and hemoglobin concentrations has improved in recent years.

Keywords: Elderly; Anemia; Hemoglobin; Medication

Introduction

The elderly population, defined as individuals aged ≥ 65 years, is rapidly increasing worldwide in numbers and proportions [1]. In Japan, which is one of the most rapidly ageing societies in the world, the proportion is estimated to increase from 22.8% in 2010 to 38.8% in 2050 [2]. The Japanese also enjoy longevity compared to other countries, with life expectancy of 19.08 years in men and 23.97 years in women at 65 years (http://www.mhlw.go.jp/toukei/saikin/hw/life/life13/index.html). It is an urgent public health issue to maintain health in later life, without disabilities or serious morbidities. Japan may serve as an ideal model of an ageing society, for other countries facing the same trend in the future.

Anemia is a common health problem in elderly populations and the prevalence of anemia is reported to increase with advancing age [3]. In the United States (US), anemia prevalence increases with advancing age after 50 years and rises to more than 20% at age ≥ 85 years [4,5]. In the community dwelling elderly Japanese population, the prevalence of anemia was reported to increase with age [6]. However, this study was not conducted in a nationally representative sample and limited the highest age category to ≤ 80 years. A previous study using the data on adult women in the National Health and Nutrition Survey of Japan (NHNS) from 1989-2003, showed that anemia was prevalent (25.3%-26.2%) among women aged 70 years and older [7]. Recently, studies have indicated anemia as one of the factors responsible for health decline among the elderly, such as increased risk in all-cause mortality [8-11], decline in cognitive function, dementia [12] and increased fracture risk [13].

In addition, anemia is not simply a natural consequence of the aging process. Anemia in the elderly may be the result of underlying chronic conditions and nutritional deficiencies of key nutrients, such as iron, folate, and vitamin B_{12}. Nearly one-thirds of elderly anemia cases are due to nutrient deficiencies, according to the US National Health and Nutrition Survey [4]. Very few studies have examined the anemia risk and nutrient intake in the elderly population, and these results are inconsistent. Meng et al. [14] examined anemia prevalence and nutrient intakes in Chinese elderly women, but did not describe the association between anemia prevalence and protein, iron, or vitamin C intake; while Thomson et al. [15] showed that low intake of protein, iron, vitamin B_{12}, folate or vitamin C were associated with greater risk of anemia in post-menopausal women. In order to promote a balanced diet in the elderly to prevent anemia, we need to identify dietary and life-style factors that are related to anemia risk. In the previous Japanese study [6], hemoglobin concentrations were reported to be higher in younger cohorts. The changes in diet and lifestyle may have a profound effect on the nutritional status of the Japanese elderly, and this should be examined in nationally representative samples, such as the NHNS.

The NHNS is an annual nationwide survey that covers approximately 5000 households in about 300 randomly selected census units defined by the Ministry of Health, Labor, and Welfare. It provides the largest available nationally representative sample with which to monitor dietary intakes, lifestyle factors, and selected biological indicators of Japanese people, including anthropometric measurements. The NHNS consists of three survey components, which are the household based dietary intake survey, the physical examination survey, and the lifestyle questionnaire survey on adults [16].

This study aimed 1) to examine the trends in the prevalence of anemia of the Japanese elderly population and 2) to evaluate the association between hemoglobin concentrations and diet and lifestyle factors, by using data from a population-based, nationwide cross-sectional survey in Japan.

Methods

Data source

We used the dataset from 2003-2009 NHNS, which were conducted by the Ministry of Health, Labor and Welfare, Japan. The present study was approved by the Ministry of Health, Labor and Welfare, Japan.

Subjects

A total of 70,037 individuals aged ≥ 1 year participated in the NHNS from 2003 to 2009, and among these, 17,589 subjects aged ≥ 65 were selected for analyses. As in the United Nations Report [1], we also chose 65 years as the cutoff in the present study. We excluded subjects who lacked height and weight measurements (n=2742), had not participated in the dietary survey (n=599), and lacked blood hemoglobin, blood ferritin and blood albumin data (n=3529) or had not participated in the lifestyle questionnaire survey related to smoking history, alcohol drinking and current exercise habits (n=112). The data from the remaining 10,606 subjects were selected for analyses in the present study.

Dietary assessment

A semi-weighed one-day household-based dietary record, with the approximate proportions by which family members shared each dish, was used to estimate nutrient and food intake. [16] The nutrient intake for each family member was estimated according to the Standard Tables of Food Composition in Japan, Fifth Revised and Enlarged Edition [17]. Energy and macronutrient intake estimated using this method highly correlated to the intake estimated using individualized diet records (Pearson's correlation coefficients; r=0.89-0.91) [18]. Further details regarding the methods used can be found elsewhere [19]. In the present study, intakes of energy, total protein, fat, carbohydrates, sodium, potassium, calcium, iron, vitamin B_{12}, folate, vitamin C, energy intake from cereals, and percent energy intake from cereals and 11 food groups (cereals, potatoes and starches, pulses, vegetables, fruits, fish and shellfish, meat, eggs, milk and milk products, fats, and beverages) were calculated.

Physical examinations and lifestyle characteristics

The subjects underwent measurements for height, body weight, and abdominal circumference in the physical examination survey. Body mass index (BMI) (kg/m^2) was calculated as body weight (kg) divided by the square of body height (m). Subjects also participated in the steps measurement using a standardized AS-200 pedometer (Yamasa Tokei Keiki Co., Tokyo) for a single day. Subjects also reported their current medication status regarding treatment of non-communicable disease. Current use of antihypertensives, antilipids, antiarrhythmics and antidiabetics/insulin was assessed throughout the survey period, and use of iron supplements was assessed only in 2008 and 2009. Current exercise habits were also assessed, and exercisers were defined as those reporting "exercising regularly for >30 min at a time, for >2 days/week, and for more than a year."

Through the lifestyle questionnaire, subjects reported their smoking history. Current smokers were those smoked daily. Frequency of current drinking was also assessed. The subjects chose either "never", "1-3 day(s)/month," "1-2 day(s)/week," "3-4 day/week," "5-6 day/week," or "daily" and current drinkers were categorized as those reporting daily drinking.

Blood sampling

Venous blood was drawn into the vacuum blood collection tube that contained EDTA and was drawn at least 4 h after the last meal, at the physical examination survey. Blood was allowed to clot at room temperature and centrifuged at 1,500 g for 10 min. Serum samples were divided into separate tubes and stored at -4C until delivered to the SRL. Inc. Blood hemoglobin was determined by the sodium lauryl sulfate (SLS)-hemoglobin method, and red blood cell count and hematocrit were determined by the sheath flow direct current (DC) detection method. Serum total protein was determined by the Biuret method, serum albumin by bromcresol purple method, and blood ferritin by chemiluminescent enzyme immunoassay. All analyses were performed by the SRL. Inc., (153 Komiya-cho, Hachioji, Tokyo, 192–0031 Japan).

Definitions of anemia

In this study, anemia was defined according to the WHO definition as hemoglobin concentrations <130 g/L in men and <120 g/L in women [20].

Statistical analysis

All analyses were separately performed for men and women. Results are expressed as means ± SD or medians for continuous variables, and proportions (%) for categorical variables. To assess the normality of the distribution of continuous variables, the Kolmogorov-Smirnov test was applied. For normally distributed variables such as blood hemoglobin and blood albumin concentrations, the student's t-test was applied to compare the results between anemic and non-anemic subjects. Blood ferritin concentration, energy, nutrients, and food intakes were skewed; therefore, the Mann-Whitney U test was used to examine these variables. Chi-square tests were applied to compare categorical variables between anemic and non-anemic subjects.

For continuous variables, the univariate regression analysis was applied, and for categorical variables, the logistic regression analysis was applied to examine the effect of survey year. Logistic regression analysis adjusted for subject age was applied to estimate the effect of survey year to anemia prevalence. The general linear regression analysis was applied to estimate the effect of survey year, clinical, dietary and lifestyle factors to hemoglobin values. Each selected variable was separately included in the general linear regression model (univariate model). In the next step, all variables were included in the model (multivariate model). The estimated changes in hemoglobin values for each unit of variable (estimate) and their standard errors, 95% confidence interval of estimate (lower and upper limits), standardized partial regression coefficients, t values, and generalized coefficients of determination statistics (R^2) were calculated. An R^2 for the multivariate model was shown separately for men and women.

For all analyses, two-tailed P values <0.05 were considered to indicate statistical significance. The SPSS software version 19.0 for Windows (SPSS Inc., Chicago, IL, USA) was used to perform all analyses.

Results

Physical characteristics, intake of energy and selected nutrients (/d), Intake of selected food groups (g/d), and blood biomarker values are summarized for men (Supplementary -Table 1) and women (Supplementary -Table 2). In both men and women, mean age (p<0.01) and height (p<0.05) of the subjects increased significantly over time. Mean body weight, waist circumference, and BMI significantly increased in men (all p<0.01), but mean BMI significantly decreased in women (p<0.05). Mean number of steps per day was also significantly decreased only in women (p<0.01). The trend in intake of energy, nutrients, and food groups differed between men and women. Changes in energy, protein, and calcium intakes were not significant in men, but decreased in women (all p<0.01). Intakes of sodium, iron, vitamin B_{12}, energy from cereals significantly decreased in both men and women (both p<0.01). Intakes of cereals significantly decreased (p<0.01) and intakes of vegetables and meat increased (both p<0.05) in both men and women. In women, intakes of fish/shellfish and milk/milk products significantly decreased (p<0.01), and intakes of beverages significantly increased (p<0.05). The trend for blood biomarker values was similar between men and women. Red cell count, hematocrit values, hemoglobin values, serum ferritin values significantly increased (all p<0.01), and serum total protein and albumin values decreased (both p<0.01).

Proportion of selected health status, blood biomarker status, medication and lifestyle habits of elderly men and women are summarized according to survey year in Table 1.

	Men									Women								
	2003	4	5	6	7	8	9	Total	P for trend	2003	4	5	6	7	8	9	Total	P for trend
N	722	559	632	654	624	803	662	4656		980	690	799	822	774	961	924	5950	
Age groups																		
65-69 years	34.8	32.7	32.3	30.7	30.4	31.6	33.2	32.3	0.339	35.4	34.8	35.0	31.8	29.7	30.0	30.5	32.4	<0.001
70-74 years	32	31.1	33.5	30.7	31.3	29.4	28.4	30.9	0.073	27.8	29.9	26.8	27.5	28.8	28.2	26.6	27.9	0.611
75-79 years	18.3	22.2	21.0	22.9	21.3	21.5	21.9	21.3	0.196	19.6	21.0	20.9	24.7	23.3	22.6	22.7	22.1	0.042
80-84 years	10.1	10.4	9.2	11.8	11.4	13.4	10.7	11.1	0.09	10.8	9.9	11.9	9.9	11.2	12.8	12.9	11.4	0.046
85 years+	4.8	3.6	4.0	3.8	5.6	4.0	5.7	4.5	0.305	6.4	4.5	5.4	6.2	7.1	6.5	7.3	6.2	0.1
Overweight (BMI>24.9)	24.8	29.7	29.3	28.7	33.3	28.4	29.8	29.0	0.054	31.4	29.7	30.2	28.7	29.1	27.7	26.6	29.0	0.33
Underweight (BMI<18.5)	8.2	6.3	3.8	5.4	4.5	3.7	3.6	5.0	<0.01	6.4	7.5	6.1	5.2	7.1	7.5	8.3	6.9	0.2
Anemia (hemoglobin <130 g/L for men, <120 g/L for women)	23.8	18.4	19.6	20.3	17.9	17.8	17.1	19.3	0.03	25.8	20.0	17.3	23.6	19.4	23.4	20.7	21.7	<0.01
Low serum albumin (<3.5 mg/L)	0.6	0.9	0.5	0.6	0.5	1.1	0.3	0.6	0.51	0.3	0.4	0.1	0.2	0.5	0.2	0.1	0.3	0.65
Low serum ferritin (<12 μg/L)	3.9	3.2	3.5	4.1	3.8	5.0	3.0	3.8	0.55	6.6	7.2	4.4	6.4	5.4	6.9	7.7	6.4	0.11

Currently using antihypertensives	39.9	40.8	43.7	40.2	42.3	46.2	46.1	42.9	0.058	41.4	44.6	42.1	42.8	46.8	47.6	49.4	45.0	<0.01
Currently using antilipids	14.0	11.8	10.8	9.5	13.8	12.1	15.2	12.5	0.026	21.0	21.4	23.8	22.3	22.9	24.8	26.3	23.3	0.094
Currently using antiarrhythmics	11.1	9.1	10.3	9.0	9.1	7.3	9.2	9.3	0.3	5.5	7.7	7.1	8.3	7.9	7.0	8.1	7.3	0.29
Currently using antidiabetics/insulin	9.7	10.6	10.5	9.9	12.7	10.6	12.3	10.9	0.52	5.9	6.0	7.0	8.0	7.1	8.0	7.8	7.2	0.39
Currently using iron supplements	-	-	-	-	-	1.5	1.8	-	0.63	-	-	-	-	-	1.5	2.1	-	0.32
Daily drinking	36.3	37.0	35.6	34.1	35.6	36.0	35.5	35.7	0.97	2.4	4.1	4.5	3.8	3.6	2.7	3.0	3.4	0.18
Daily smoking	64.4	64.4	62.2	48.6	52.6	61.1	57.6	58.8	<0.01	4.9	8.8	5.3	4.1	5.8	6.5	6.5	5.9	<0.01
Currently exercising	39.2	47.4	41.5	43.7	42.6	42.2	45.6	43	0.073	29.9	34.3	37.0	37.2	34.4	37.4	35.8	35.1	<0.01

Table 1: Proportion (%) of selected health status, blood biomarker status, medication and lifestyle habits of elderly men and women, 2003-2009, – unavailable.

The distribution of age groups did not change over time among men, but among women, the proportion of 65-69 years significantly decreased ($p<0.01$) and the proportion of both 75-79 and 80-84 years significantly increased ($p<0.01$). The proportion of underweight men significantly decreased ($p<0.01$), but not in women. The proportion of anemic subjects significantly decreased in both men and women ($p<0.01$). The proportion of men using anti-lipids increased, and women using antihypertensive increased (both $p<0.05$). The proportion of subjects smoking daily significantly decreased in men ($p<0.01$), but significantly increased in women ($p<0.01$). The proportion of women who were currently exercising significantly increased ($p<0.01$).

The characteristics of the anemic and non-anemic subjects are summarized in Table 2. Anemic subjects were significantly older, shorter, lighter, and had lower BMI compared to non-anemic subjects, among both men and women (all $p<0.01$). In men, anemic subjects had significantly lower intakes of energy and nutrients (all $p<0.01$) except vitamin C, however, percent energy intake from cereals was significantly higher ($p<0.01$). In women, anemic subjects had significantly lower intakes of energy and nutrients (all $p<0.01$), and their percent energy intake from cereals was also significantly higher ($p<0.01$). Regarding intakes of food groups, anemic men had significantly lower intakes of cereals, pulses, vegetables, fish/shellfish, meat, fats, and beverages (all $p<0.05$) compared to non-anemic men. In women, anemic subjects had significantly lower intakes of vegetables, fruits, fish /shellfish, meat, milk/milk products, fats, and beverages (all $p<0.01$) compared to non-anemic subjects. All of the blood biomarker values were significantly lower in anemic subjects (all $p<0.01$) compared to non-anemic subjects, among both men and women. The proportion of anemic men who were currently using anti-arrhythmics or anti-diabetics/insulin was significantly higher (both $p<0.01$) than non-anemic men, and the proportions of current daily drinking, daily smoking, and exercising were significantly lower (all $p<0.05$). The proportion of anemic women who were currently using anti-hypertensives or anti-arrhythmics was significantly higher (both $p<0.01$) than non-anemic women, and the proportions of current daily drinking, daily smoking, and exercising were significantly lower (all $p<0.05$).

Physical characteristics	Men					Women				
	Anemic (n=900)		Non-anemic (n=3756)		P value	Anemic (n=1289)		Non-anemic (n=4661)		P value
	Mean ± SD	Median	Mean ± SD	Median		Mean ± SD	Median	Mean ± SD	Median	
Age, years	76.0 ± 6.6	75	72.5 ± 5.5	72	<0.001	76.1 ± 6.8	76	72.8 ± 5.9	72	<0.001
Height*, cm	159.7 ± 6.4	160.1	161.7 ± 6.3	161.8	<0.001	146.2 ± 6.5	146.5	148.4 ± 5.9	148.5	<0.001
Weight*, cm	56.1 ± 8.8	55.5	62.3 ± 9.2	62	<0.001	47.9 ± 8.3	47	52 ± 8.3	51.3	<0.001
Abdominal circumference*, cm	81.8 ± 8.6	82	86.9 ± 8.2	87	<0.001	82.2 ± 10.3	82	85.7 ± 10.1	86	<0.001
BMI*	21.9 ± 3	21.9	23.8 ± 3	23.7	<0.001	22.4 ± 3.4	22.1	23.6 ± 3.5	23.3	<0.001
Number of steps(/d)	5333 ± 3981	4578	6128 ± 4069	5366	<0.001	4257 ± 3333	3509	5252 ± 3594	4631	<0.001
Intake of energy and selected nutrients(/d)										

Total energy, kcal	1980 ± 543	1924	2109 ± 552	2061	<0.001	1649 ± 438	1602	1718 ± 448	1687	<0.001
Total protein, g	72.7 ± 24.3	70.2	78.3 ± 24.6	76	<0.001	62.7 ± 21.2	60	66.9 ± 21.4	65.1	<0.001
Fat, g	45.7±21.3	42.8	49.8 ± 21.9	47.1	<0.001	39.8 ± 18.5	36.8	43.7 ± 19	41.5	<0.001
Carbohydrates, g	299 ± 89	289	306 ± 89	297	<0.001	255 ± 74	245	259 ± 72	252	<0.001
Sodium, mg	4766 ± 1917	4488	4912 ± 1960	4621	0.033	4234 ± 1711	4003	4337 ± 1730	4084	0.043
Potassium, mg	2669 ± 1032	2550	2794 ± 1003	2691	<0.001	2430 ± 930	2309	2621 ± 999	2507	<0.001
Calcium, mg	574 ± 299	513	603 ± 291	555	0.001	547 ± 300	499	591 ± 294	545	<0.001
Iron, mg	9.0 ± 3.4	8.6	9.4 ± 3.6	8.9	0.002	8.4 ± 5.4	7.7	8.7 ± 3.4	8.2	<0.001
Vitamin B_{12}, μg	8.3 ± 8.5	5.8	9.3 ± 10.1	6.4	0.004	6.6 ± 6.3	4.6	7.5 ± 7.5	5.3	<0.001
Folate, μg	373 ± 180	346	387 ± 183	359	0.014	345 ± 150	316	364 ± 159	343	<0.001
Vitamin C, mg	146.0 ± 143.5	115.7	152.2 ± 151.1	120.9	0.134	156.3 ± 208	117.6	171.2 ± 215.2	127.3	<0.001
Energy intake from cereals, kcal	876 ± 306	830	907 ± 320	865	0.003	699 ± 236	678	695 ± 231	672	<0.001
Percent energy intake from cereals, %	45.2 ± 12.7	44.6	43.7 ± 12.1	43	<0.001	43.3 ± 12.3	42.5	41.4 ± 11.7	40.6	<0.001
Intake of selected food groups, g/d										
Cereals	507.2 ± 188.8	479	524.8 ± 192.7	500.0	0.003	405 ± 146	390.0	398.9 ± 136.2	389.3	0.3
Potatoes and starches	75.1 ± 91.0	50.0	67.1 ± 79.6	46.7	0.149	66.3 ± 80.8	45.0	66.5 ± 79.7	45.0	0.957
Pulses	71.7 ± 82.8	50.0	76.1 ± 80.9	52.6	0.031	64.9 ± 70	48.0	70.7 ± 76.9	50.0	0.068
Vegetables	323.2 ± 192.2	289.0	341 ± 191	315.7	0.002	305.2 ± 175.8	274.3	325.1 ± 177.5	299.9	<0.001
Fruits	156.5 ± 159.8	120.0	162.4 ± 161.5	130.0	0.191	156.8 ± 154.2	130.0	180.9 ± 160.7	153.0	<0.001
Fish and shellfish	101.5 ± 86.8	85.0	112.5 ± 87.4	100.0	<0.001	83.1 ± 67	75.0	91.5 ± 71.8	81.3	<0.001
Meat	51.7 ± 56.3	40.0	61.3 ± 60.5	50.0	<0.001	41.2 ± 45.2	30.0	48 ± 49.8	38.4	<0.001
Eggs	34.8 ± 34.4	32.5	34.5 ± 33.4	34.0	0.869	30.8 ± 30.4	28.5	30.6 ± 31	25.5	0.766
Milk and milk products	104.4 ± 141.4	18.3	110.1 ± 134.8	41.2	0.068	103.7 ± 127.7	40.0	115.9 ± 131.7	84.0	0.001
Fats	7.5 ± 8.7	5.0	8 ± 8.9	5.7	0.03	6.2 ± 7.4	4.0	6.8 ± 7.5	4.8	0.002
Beverages	684.8 ± 524.4	600.0	780.8 ± 515.2	710	<0.001	593.8 ± 443.3	519.0	621.8 ± 421.5	577.0	0.003
Blood biomarkers										
Red cell count*, 10^4/mm^3	388 ± 41	390.0	462 ± 37	460	<0.001	375 ± 33	376	434 ± 31	431	<0.001
Hemoglobin*, g/L	119 ± 11	122.0	146 ± 10	145	<0.001	112 ± 8	114	13.2 ± 8	132	<0.001
Hematocrit*, %	38 ± 3.3	38.6	45.5 ± 3.2	45.3	<0.001	36.2 ± 2.6	36.5	42.1 ± 2.7	41.8	<0.001
Serum total protein, mg/L	7.3 ± 0.5	7.3	7.4 ± 0.5	7.4	<0.001	7.3 ± 0.5	7.3	7.5 ± 0.4	7.4	<0.001
Serum albumin, mg/L	4.2 ± 0.3	4.2	4.4 ± 0.3	4.4	<0.001	4.2 ± 0.3	4.2	4.4 ± 0.3	4.4	<0.001
Serum ferritin, μg/L	93.3 ± 152.9	56.0	124.9 ± 127.3	96.0	<0.001	62.6 ± 115.5	39.0	74.8 ± 61	61.0	<0.001
Medication and lifestyle habits (%)										
Currently using antihypertensives	45.3		42.3		0.097	48.5		44		0.004

Currently using antilipids	12.7		12.4		0.823	21.7		23.7		0.119
Currently using antiarrhythmics	13.1		8.4		<0.001	9.1		6.8		0.006
Currently using antidiabetics/insulin	13.3		10.3		0.008	7.5		7		0.549
Daily drinking	24.4		38.4		<0.001	2.5		3.6		0.044
Daily smoking	55.1		59.6		0.013	4.6		6.3		0.021
Currently exercising	38.4		44.1		0.002	29		36.8		<0.001

Table 2: General characteristics of anemic and non-anemic elderly in the National Health and Nutrition survey, Current exercisers were defined as those reporting "exercising regularly for >30 min at a time, for >2 days/week, and for more than a year." * T-tests for other continuous variables, Mann-Whitney's U-tests were applied, and for categorical variables, chi-square tests were applied.

The proportion of anemic subjects according to five-year age groups and survey year are shown in Figure 1 (A: men, B: women). According to the logistic regression analysis grouped by sex and five-year age groups, the odds ratio for anemia significantly decreased by each survey year in 75-79 years aged men (odds ratio: 0.904, 95% confidence interval: 0.840, 0.972, p=0.007), but not in other sex and age groups. When adjusted for age, the odds ratio for anemia significantly decreased by each survey year in both men (odds ratio: 0.933, 95% confidence interval: 0.899, 0.968, p<0.001) and women (odds ratio: 0.968, 95% confidence interval: 0.939, 0.999, p=0.040).

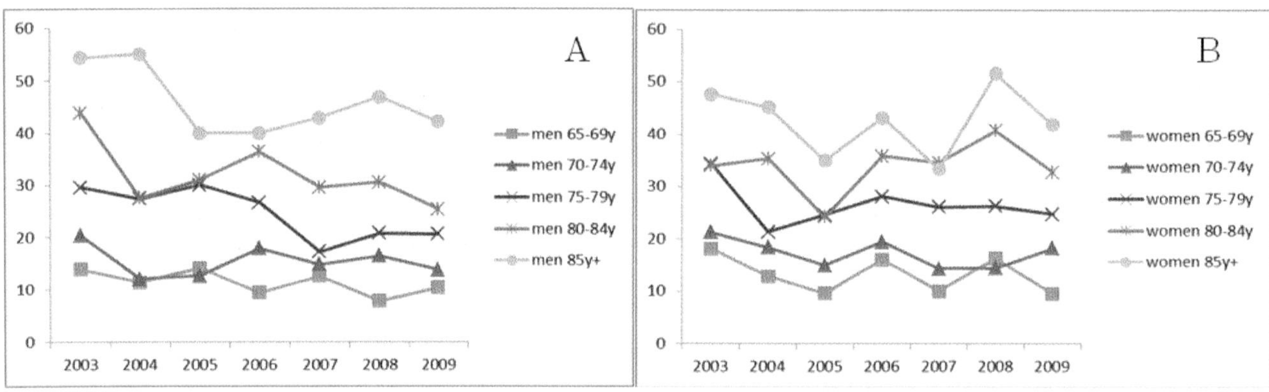

Figure 1: Proportion (%) of subjects with anemia among men (A) and women (B) in elderly subjects.

Table 3 shows the association between hemoglobin values and factors selected from results on Table 2, by using the univariate regression analysis. Since most of the dietary factors were influenced by the differences in energy intake between anemic and non-anemic subjects, percent energy from cereals was selected as the sole dietary factor.

Factors	Men							Women						
	Estimate	Standard error of estimate	95% CI of estimate	Standardized partial regression coefficient	t value	R^2	p value	Estimate	Standard error of estimate	95% CI of estimate	Standardized partial regression coefficient	t value	R^2	p value
Survey year (per year)	0.38	0.11	0.17, 0.59	0.052	3.54	0	<0.01	0.32	0.073	0.18, 0.47	0.056	4.36	0.003	<0.01
Age (per year)	-0.7	0.036	-0.77, -0.63	-0.276	-19.58	0	<0.01	-0.44	0.024	-0.49, -0.40	-0.235	-18.61	0.055	<0.01
BMI	0.13	0.068	1.19, 1.45	0.276	19.57	0	<0.01	0.76	0.042	0.67, 0.84	0.225	17.83	0.051	<0.01

Percent energy intake from cereals (per 10%)	-0.91	0.18	-0.13, -0.06	-0.074	-5.06	0	<0.01	-0.94	0.013	-0.12, -0.07	-0.09	-7.31	0.009	<0.01
Serum ferritin (per 10 μg/L)	0.17	0.016	0.14, 0.20	0.15	10.33	0	<0.00 1	0.21	0.002	0.17, 0.25	0.14	10.53	0.018	<0.001
Serum albumin (per mg/L)	18.97	0.72	17.56, 20.37	0.36	26.5	0	<0.00 1	15.43	0.53	14.38, 16.47	0.35	28.93	0.123	<0.001
Currently using anti-hypertensives	-0.99	0.44	-1.86, -0.12	-0.033	-2.23	0	0.026	0.31	0.31	-0.29, 0.91	0.013	1.01	0.0002	0.314
Currently using anti-arrhythmics	-3.36	0.75	-4.84, -1.88	-0.065	-4.45	0	<0.00 1	-1.52	0.59	-2.67, -0.37	-0.034	-2.59	0.001	0.01
Currently using antidiabetics/insulin (yes=1, no=0)	-2.02	0.7	-3.40, -0.64	-0.042	-2.87	0	0.004	-0.17	0.59	-1.33, 1.00	-0.004	-0.28	1.00E-05	0.779
Daily drinking (yes=1, no=0)	4.39	0.45	3.50, 5.28	0.141	9.7	0	<0.00 1	1.03	0.85	-0.63, 2.69	0.016	1.22	0.0002	0.224
Daily smoking (yes=1, no=0)	1.09	0.44	0.22, 1.96	0.036	2.45	0	0.014	1.09	0.44	0.22, 1.96	0.036	3.31	0.001	0.014
Currently exercising (yes=1, no=0)	1.41	0.44	0.54, 2.27	0.047	3.18	0	0.001	1.6	0.32	0.98, 2.23	0.065	5.02	<0.01	<0.001

Table 3: Estimation of hemoglobin values in elderly men and women, by univariate regression analysis.

All of the selected factors were significantly associated to hemoglobin values in men (all p<0.05). In women, current use of anti-hypertensives, anti-diabetics/insulin, and daily drinking habits were not significantly associated to hemoglobin values. The multivariate model (Table 4), explained 25% and 22% of the variance in hemoglobin values in men and women, respectively. In both men and women, each unit of increase in BMI, daily smoking, serum ferritin and albumin was positively associated to hemoglobin values, and age was negatively associated. In men, daily drinking was positively associated to hemoglobin values, and current use of anti-hypertensives and anti-diabetics/insulin were negatively associated. In women, current exercising was positively associated to hemoglobin values, and percent energy intake from cereals was negatively associated. After adjusting for all factors, hemoglobin values were estimated to increase 0.66 g/L per year in men, and 0.68 g/L per year in women.

Discussion

To our knowledge, this study is the first nationally representative cross-sectional study to evaluate the trends in nutritional status of community-dwelling elderly people [6,7,11]. In the current study, similar prevalence of anemia was observed in men (19.3%) and women (21.7%) compared to other developed countries. From the data on NHANES III, the prevalence of anemia in American elderly population aged ≥ 65 years was 11.0% in men and 10.2% in women [4]. In Europe, the prevalence of anemia was 15.2% in men and 13.6% in women (≥ 65 years) in Italy [21] and 23.4% in men and 19.3% in women (≥ 65 years) in Austria. [22] For Korean elderly population with median age of 70 years, the prevalence of anemia was 13.6%. [23] These previous reports [4,5,21-23] have not investigated the effect of nutrient intakes, although these differences may be influenced by dietary factors such as dietary iron intake and/or intake of iron supplements. In fact, iron intakes in the current study were much lower compared with those in the US [15]. We could not examine the effect of iron supplement use to hemoglobin values, because it was not assessed in 2003-2007. But we speculate that the influence of iron supplement use is negligible, given the low proportion of users in 2008 and 2009 (Table 1). Furthermore, better iron nutriture in Europe and the US has been largely attributed to increased dietary iron via fortified foods [24,25]. Also in the US, hemoglobin values in men and women have increased after the implementation of mandatory folic acid fortification policy [26]. However, Japan does not practice a food fortification policy, so the recent improvement in hemoglobin status in elderly Japanese may be due to the improvement of better dietary habits, such as observed by the yearly increase in intakes of vegetable and meat (Supplementary Tables 1 and 2).

Factors	Men							Women						
	Estimate	Standard error of estimate	95% CI of estimate	Standardized partial regression coefficient	t value	R^2	p value	Estimate	Standard error of estimate	95% CI of estimate	Standardized partial regression coefficient	t value	R^2	p value
Intercept	65.2	4.9	55.60, 74.80	-	13.31 5	0.25 1	<0.00 1	65.11	3.43	58.39, 71.84	-	18.97 4	0.22 1	<0.00 1

Survey year (per year)	0.66	0.1	0.47, 0.85	0.09	6.926	-	<0.001	0.68	0.07	0.55, 0.81	0.119	10.19	-	<0.001
Age (per year)	-0.33	0.03	-0.40, -0.26	-0.131	-9.567	-	<0.001	-0.25	0.02	-0.29, -0.20	-0.131	-10.607	-	<0.001
BMI	1.05	0.06	0.93, 1.18	0.22	16.58	-	<0.001	0.68	0.04	0.60, 0.76	0.202	16.944	-	<0.001
Percent energy intake from cereals (per 10%)	-0.01	0.02	-0.04, 0.02	-0.011	-0.8	-	0.424	-0.07	0.01	-0.09, -0.04	-0.065	-5.614	-	<0.001
Serum ferritin (per 10 μg/L)	0.1	0.01	0.0008, 0.0013	0.093	7.187	-	<0.001	0.002	0.0002	0.0012, 0.0019	0.098	8.449	-	<0.001
Serum albumin (per mg/L)	16.1	0.71	14.71, 17.49	0.307	22.731	-	<0.001	14.31	0.53	13.27, 15.35	0.326	27.021	-	<0.001
Currently using anti-hypertensives (yes=1, no=0)	-2.15	0.4	-2.93, -1.36	-0.071	-5.357	-	<0.001	-0.52	0.29	-1.10, 0.05	-0.022	-1.802	-	0.072
Currently using antiarrhythmics (yes=1, no=0)	-0.88	0.67	-2.19, 0.43	-0.017	-1.317	-	0.188	-0.36	0.53	-1.40, 0.68	-0.008	-0.685	-	0.493
Currently using antidiabetics/ insulin (yes=1, no=0)	-2.52	0.62	-3.73, -1.31	-0.052	-4.084	-	<0.001	-0.81	0.53	-1.86, 0.23	-0.018	-1.528	-	0.127
Daily drinking (yes=1, no=0)	3.54	0.41	2.73, 4.36	0.114	8.559	-	<0.001	0.4	0.76	-1.09, 1.88	0.006	0.523	-	0.601
Daily smoking (yes=1, no=0)	1.05	0.39	0.28, 1.81	0.035	2.686	-	0.007	2.26	0.58	1.13, 3.39	0.045	3.918	-	<0.001
Currently exercising (yes=1, no=0)	0.41	0.39	-0.35, 1.18	0.014	1.064	-	0.287	0.72	0.29	0.15, 1.28	0.029	2.487	-	0.013

Table 4: Estimation of hemoglobin values in elderly men and women, by multivariate regression analysis†, †All factors were forced into the model.

The strength of this study was our large population-based sample size. However, there were several limitations as well. First, nutrient and food intake data may not be representative of habitual dietary intake because they do not reveal day-to-day variations that would normally occur. Because the dietary survey was conducted on a single day, we could not examine the causal effects of individual food intakes to nutritional status. The only dietary factor applied was the percentage of energy from cereals (Table 4). As shown in Supplementary Tables 1 and 2, consumption of cereals (which is mainly rice in Japan), has been declining over time. But, mean percentage of energy from cereals was higher in anemic subjects compared to non-anemic subjects (Table 2). In other words, the higher the percentage of energy from cereals, the subjects are taking lower amount of foods that are rich in protein and fat, such as fish or meat. However, the negative effect of higher percentage of energy from cereals to hemoglobin value was observed only in women. Although the mean percentage of energy from cereals was higher in men (44.0 ± 12.2%) compared to women (41.8 ± 11.8%), the higher intake of fish and meat in men compared to women may have accounted to better iron status, as observed in the higher serum ferritin values in men (Supplementary Tables 1 and 2).

The results from the current study showed that current medication and life-style factors had different effects on hemoglobin values, in men and women. In men, current use of anti-hypertensives and anti-diabetics/insulin were negatively related to hemoglobin values. This was also consistent with previous reports [27,28]. Some types of anti-hypertensives cause hemodilution, hemolytic anemia, or suppress red cell production [27]. Long term metformin treatment for diabetes suppresses absorption of vitamin B_{12}, and may lead to anemia [28]. The reason why these relations were not observed in women is not clear, in spite of higher proportion of women taking anti-hypertensives. Detailed information on the types of medication was unavailable in the NHNS, so we could not examine whether this difference was due to gender, or due to differences in the types used in men and women. Both daily drinking and smoking were related to higher hemoglobin values in men. This was consistent with a previous study that examined the effect of smoking and drinking to hemoglobin values in adults [29]. In women, only positive relation with smoking was observed, probably due to the low proportion of daily drinkers. Current exercise habits were positively related to hemoglobin values only in women. Perhaps women who are able to keep exercising are already in good health, which is reflected in their higher hemoglobin values.

The current study demonstrated that hemoglobin values have improved over time in both men and women, after adjusting for selected factors. The background for this improvement could not be fully investigated through our present data. But we would like to note that the national action plan for health, the "Health Japan 21" project [30] which started in 2000, may have had an impact on health of elderly Japanese. In this project, the government set goals to increase the proportion of elderly who are physically active, i.e., those with exercise habits. This health policy may have contributed to improving general health in the elderly, resulting in increase in subjects with exercise habits and decrease in anemia (Table 1), reversing previous trends [7]. Further monitoring of the health status of community dwelling elderly should be conducted, in order to investigate the effect of national health policies.

Acknowledgement

This work was supported by Grant-in-Aid (H22-Junkankitou [Seishuu]-Shitei-015) from the Ministry of Health, Labor and Welfare, Health and Labor Sciences Research Grants, Japan.

References

1. United Nations, Department of Economic and Social Affairs, Population Division (2013). World Population Prospects: The 2012 Revision, Highlights and Advance Tables. Working Paper No. ESA/P/WP.228.
2. National Institute of Population and Social Security Research J (2013) Population projections for Japan. In Population Research Series. Tokyo.
3. Gaskell H, Derry S, Andrew Moore R, McQuay HJ (2008) Prevalence of anaemia in older persons: systematic review. BMC Geriatr 8: 1.
4. Guralnik JM, Eisenstaedt RS, Ferrucci L, Klein HG, Woodman RC (2004) Prevalence of anemia in persons 65 years and older in the United States: evidence for a high rate of unexplained anemia. Blood 104: 2263-2268.
5. Patel KV (2008) Epidemiology of anemia in older adults. Semin Hematol 45: 210-217.
6. Yamada M, Wong FL, Suzuki G; RERF's (Radiation Effects Research Foundation) Adult Health Study (2003) Longitudinal trends of hemoglobin levels in a Japanese population--RERF's Adult Health Study subjects. Eur J Haematol 70: 129-135.
7. Hayashi F, Yoshiike N, Yoshita K, Kawahara K (2008) Trends in the prevalence of anaemia in Japanese adult women, 1989-2003. Public Health Nutr 11: 252-257.
8. Go AS, Yang J, Ackerson LM, Lepper K, Robbins S, et al. (2006) Hemoglobin level, chronic kidney disease, and the risks of death and hospitalization in adults with chronic heart failure: the Anemia in Chronic Heart Failure: Outcomes and Resource Utilization (ANCHOR) Study. Circulation 113: 2713-2723.
9. Izaks GJ, Westendorp RG, Knook DL (1999) The definition of anemia in older persons. JAMA 281: 1714-1717.
10. Penninx BW, Pahor M, Woodman RC, Guralnik JM (2006) Anemia in old age is associated with increased mortality and hospitalization. J Gerontol A Biol Sci Med Sci 61: 474-479.
11. Zakai NA, Katz R, Hirsch C, Shlipak MG, Chaves PH, et al. (2005) A prospective study of anemia status, hemoglobin concentration, and mortality in an elderly cohort: the Cardiovascular Health Study. Arch Intern Med 165: 2214-2220.
12. Peters R, Burch L, Warner J, Beckett N, Poulter R, et al. (2008) Haemoglobin, anaemia, dementia and cognitive decline in the elderly, a systematic review. BMC Geriatr 8: 18.
13. Chen Z, Thomson CA, Aickin M, Nicholas JS, Van Wyck D, et al. (2010) The relationship between incidence of fractures and anemia in older multiethnic women. J Am Geriatr Soc 58: 2337-2344.
14. Meng L, Liu J, Zhang J, Wang C, Man Q, et al. (2009) Effect of dietary factors on anaemia among rural elderly women in south-west China: a case-control study. Public Health Nutr 12: 1540-1547.
15. Thomson CA, Stanaway JD, Neuhouser ML, Snetselaar LG, Stefanick ML, et al. (2011) Nutrient intake and anemia risk in the women's health initiative observational study. J Am Diet Assoc 111: 532-541.
16. Research Group for Health and Nutrition Information (2006) Ministry of Health, Labor, and Welfare: The 2003 report of the National Health and Nutrition Survey. In Dai-ichi Shuppan, Tokyo.
17. Council of Science and Technology; Ministry of Education, Sports, Science and Technology; the Government of Japan. (2005) Standard tables of food composition in Japan, the fifth revised and enlarged edition. Tokyo.
18. Iwaoka Fs, Yoshiike N, Date C, Shimada T, Tanaka H (2001) A validation study on a method to estimate nutrient intake by family members through a household-based food-weighing survey. J Nutr Sci Vitaminol (Tokyo) 47: 222-227.
19. Katanoda K, Matsumura Y (2002) National Nutrition Survey in Japan--its methodological transition and current findings. J Nutr Sci Vitaminol (Tokyo) 48: 423-432.
20. [No authors listed] (1968) Nutritional anaemias. Report of a WHO scientific group. World Health Organ Tech Rep Ser 405: 5-37.
21. Tettamanti M, Lucca U, Gandini F, Recchia A, Mosconi P, et al. (2010) Prevalence, incidence and types of mild anemia in the elderly: the "Health and Anemia" population-based study. Haematologica 95: 1849-1856.
22. Skjelbakken T, Langbakk B, Dahl IM, Løchen ML; Tromsø Study (2005) Haemoglobin and anaemia in a gender perspective: the Tromsø Study. Eur J Haematol 74: 381-388.
23. Choi CW, Lee J, Park KH, Yoon SY, Choi IK, et al. (2004) Prevalence and characteristics of anemia in the elderly: cross-sectional study of three urban Korean population samples. Am J Hematol 77: 26-30.
24. Ramakrishnan U, Yip R (2002) Experiences and challenges in industrialized countries: control of iron deficiency in industrialized countries. J Nutr 132: 820S-4S.
25. Hercberg S, Preziosi P, Galan P (2001) Iron deficiency in Europe. Public Health Nutr 4: 537-545.
26. Ganji V, Kafai MR (2009) Hemoglobin and hematocrit values are higher and prevalence of anemia is lower in the post-folic acid fortification period than in the pre-folic acid fortification period in US adults. Am J Clin Nutr 89: 363-371.
27. Sica DA, Mannino R (2007) Antihypertensive medications and anemia. J Clin Hypertens (Greenwich) 9: 723-727.
28. de Jager J, Kooy A, Lehert P, Wulffelé MG, van der Kolk J, et al. (2010) Long term treatment with metformin in patients with type 2 diabetes and risk of vitamin B-12 deficiency: randomised placebo controlled trial. BMJ 340: c2181.
29. Milman N, Pedersen AN (2009) Blood haemoglobin concentrations are higher in smokers and heavy alcohol consumers than in non-smokers and abstainers: should we adjust the reference range? Ann Hematol 88: 687-694.
30. "Health Japan 21" Steering Committee, "Health Japan 21" Planning Committee (2000) The National Action Plan for Health Promotion.

Meat in Modern Diet, Just as Bad as Sugar, Correlates with Worldwide Obesity: An Ecological Analysis

Wenpeng You[1*] **and Maciej Henneberg**[2]

[1]*Biological Anthropology and Comparative Anatomy Unit, The University of Adelaide, Adelaide, SA, Australia*

[2]*Institute of Evolutionary Medicine, University of Zurich, Switzerland*

***Corresponding author:** Wenpeng You, Biological Anthropology and Comparative Anatomy Unit, School of Medicine, The University of Adelaide, Adelaide, SA, Australia, E-mail: Wenpeng.you@adelaide.edu.au; wpyou@hotmail.com

Abstract

Background: The public have been educated that sugar intake should be minimized to avoid obesity, but no such recommendation regarding meat exists. We used FAO published comparable sugar and meat availability data to examine if they both contribute to obesity prevalence to the same extent.

Methods: Country-specific Body Mass Index (BMI) estimates of obesity and overweight were obtained. These were matched with country-specific per capita per day availability of major food groups (meat, sugar, starch crops, fibers, fats and fruits), total calories, per capita Gross Domestic Product (GDP PPP), urbanization and physical inactivity prevalence. Fisher's r-to-z transformation and Beta (B) range (B ± 2 Standard Errors) overlapping were used to test for potential differences between correlations and regressions results respectively. SPSS 22.0 was used for log-transformed data analysis.

Results: Pearson correlation showed that sugar and meat availability significantly correlated with obesity prevalence to the same extent (r=0.715, p<0.001 and r=0.685, p<0.001 respectively). These relationships remained in partial correlation analysis (r=0.359, p<0.001 and r=0.354, p<0.001 respectively) when controlling for calories availability, physical inactivity, urbanization and GDP PPP. Fisher's r-to-z transformation revealed no significant difference in Pearson correlation coefficients (z=-0.53, p=0.60), and partial correlation coefficients (z=-0.04, p=0.97) between sugar and meat availability with obesity prevalence.

Multiple linear regression analysis indicated that sugar and meat availability were the two most significant predictors of obesity prevalence in both Enter (B=0.455, SE=0.113, p<0.001 and B=0.381, SE=0.096, p<0.001, respectively) and Stepwise (B=0.464, SE=0.093, p<0.001 and B=0.433, SE=0.072, p<0.001, respectively) models. B ranges overlapping found in the Enter (0.289-0.573) and Stepwise (0.294-0.582) models showed sugar and meat availability correlated to obesity to the same extent with no statistically significant difference.

Conclusion: Sugar and meat availability comparably contribute to global obesity prevalence. Dietary guidelines should also advocate to minimize meat consumption to avoid obesity.

Keywords: Obesity; Sugar; Fructose; Meat; Meat protein; Fats; Insulin resistance; Energy surplus

Introduction

Obesity has been considered a major epidemic of the 21st century, and it has become a prelude to adverse health and premature death [1]. The World Health Organisation (WHO) estimates that obesity contributes significantly to the disease burdens of, among others, top causes of diseases, such as diabetes (44%), ischaemic heart disease (23%) and carcinogenesis (7-41%) [2]. Moreover, those considered overweight or obese have been subject to discrimination and prejudice [3].

Obesity and overweight are defined as abnormal or excessive fat accumulation that presents a risk to health. A crude measure of obesity is the body mass index (BMI). A person with a BMI of 30 kg/m^2 or more is generally considered obese. A person with a BMI equal to or more than 25 kg/m^2 is considered overweight (http://who.int/topics/obesity/en/).

Until the invention of food production in the Holocene, for several million years, human diet had relied on foods that could be found in natural environments. Since humans are unable to extract nutrition from cellulose, our food sources were limited to animals, fruits, nuts and tubers. This Palaeolithic diet contained large quantities of meat obtained through hunting [4] while it had fewer carbohydrates, especially simple carbohydrates. Besides large game that was hunted or scavenged, small vertebrates and invertebrates were gathered, and, where possible, fish were caught. Game meat does not contain much fat, so our metabolic system evolved to be efficient in using animal protein as a source of energy [5]. Deriving Acetyl CoA for use in the citric acid cycle from proteins is a complex process using a number of enzymes to obtain peptides, break them into separate amino acids and then deaminate those amino acids to obtain carbon skeletons-a source of pyruvates. Any pyruvates not used in the citric acid cycle to obtain energy can be converted via de novo lipogenesis into fats, and stored.

Obtaining pyruvates from carbohydrates is a simpler metabolic process, especially when simple carbohydrates that are easily breakable into glucose are consumed. Therefore, when simple carbohydrates are available in the diet they, soon after their ingestion and absorption, can be used to provide energy in the citric acid cycle while additional pyruvates coming later from protein digestion may be surplus to direct need for energy, and therefore converted into fat [6]. Sucrose, being a compound of glucose and fructose provides easily accessible energy from glucose while fructose is not easily digested. Since the introduction of agriculture, and especially from the time of industrialised food production, sucrose became readily available in large quantities. In traditional agricultural economies meat was expensive to produce and thus was consumed in small quantities, rather rarely. Mass animal husbandry lowered cost of meat production and now meat is readily available and regularly consumed in significant quantities in developed economies. Diet patterns have been extensively considered as the contributing factor to obesity. Sugar and meat are now two major food groups in our daily diet. The prevailing dogma is that we should limit or avoid sugar intake, and eat a moderate amount of meat, preferably lean meat since it is a source of essential aminoacids. This dogma is supported by various dietary or nutrition guidelines published by the authorities. Numerous studies have reported that meat [7] and added sugar (sugar in short hereafter) [8] food groups were in significant correlations to obesity and/or body weight increase. However, the majority of the studies could not single out total sugar or all meat consumption in our diet for the correlation analysis. One of the concrete evidences that sugar consumption was correlated to obesity is that sugar-sweetened beverages (SSBs) intake is associated with obesity prevalence [9]. Despite the correlations between sugar food and beverage products and obesity are controversial, SSBs has been mostly consistently correlated to obesity prevalence [8]. However, sugar consumed via beverage is only part of the dietary sugar intake, and other sugar products, such as confectionery and bakery products were not included in the study designs. Similarly, meat containing food groups rather than pure meat are considered, for example processed meat [10] instead of total meat intake [11] have been linked to obesity prevalence. Another issue with meat food group is that data used for study may not be able to exclude bias from other food components, which may have been linked to body weight increase. For instance, wheat consumption has been correlated to obesity [12,13], and meat food groups containing wheat products (frankfurter and sausage) could be associated with obesity and central obesity [11] because of their wheat content. Likewise, the correlation between SSBs and obesity prevalence may be biased with other obesity associated additives in SSBs, such as preservatives. Therefore, these research results may not present the whole picture of the correlation between obesity prevalence and sugar or meat consumption. Using these data may not allow us to explore and compare the correlations between obesity prevalence and total intake of sugar and meat accurately.

The Food and Agriculture Organization (FAO) Food Balance Sheet presents the comparative per capita availability of major food items during the reference period by country after combining sources of supply and its utilization in terms of nutrient value. This study aimed to use empirical, macro-level nutrient availability data at the country level to evaluate and compare, from a global perspective, the correlation levels of obesity prevalence to sugar and meat availability.

Materials and Methods

Data

The country specific data were collected for this study:

1) The WHO Global Health Observatory (GHO) data on estimated prevalence rates of obesity and overweight (percent of population aged 18^+ with BMI ≥ 30 and 25 kg/m^2 respectively) of the population aged 18+ by country were obtained for the year 2010 (http://www.who.int/gho/database/en/). We did not use the most recent version of body weight status in 2014 because of other key variables of interest (described below). From GHO, we also captured the estimated prevalence rate of physical inactivity for each country for the people aged 18^+. The estimated prevalence rate of physical inactivity is defined as percent of a given population attaining less than 150 minutes of moderate-intensity physical activity per week, or less than 75 minutes of vigorous-intensity physical activity per week, or equivalent.

2) The FAOSTAT Food Balance Sheet (FBS) data on major food group availability per capita per day of: i) Sugar (total sugar and sweeteners); ii) Total meat; iii) Starch crops (mixed cereals and starchy root); iv) Fibers (vegetables, treenuts and pulses); v) Fats (plant oils and animal fats) and vi) Fruits. We also extracted the per capita per day availability of grand total calories (calories in short hereafter) as one of the potential confounders of our data analysis. Unfortunately, FAOSTAT does not contain data allowing separation of processed meats from "pure meat". Because obesity develops after cumulative exposure to dietary risks (i.e., high intake of risk food groups today does not lead to immediate obesity, but a prolonged exposure to high intake of risk food type(s) is required [14-16]), we calculated the mean food availability per person per day over a 3-year period (2007-2009) in each of food categories to represent typical long-term exposure to each of these dietary components. The rationale for this decision is that studies have shown that three years is a practical period to develop metabolic syndrome leading to obesity after exposure to dietary risks. For instance, high intake of meat today does not lead to immediate obesity. Using the mean of three years of nutrients and food groups may also reduce the random errors during the data collection and calculation by FAO. The food items in each food groups were listed the Additional file 1: Food items in each food group.

3) The World Bank data on per capita GDP PPP (expressed in gross domestic product converted to international dollars using purchasing power parity rates) and country specific urbanization (the percent of population living in urban areas). Urbanization has been closely linked to human lifestyle change due to its process of modernization and industrialization.

How the above variables, such as food types (nutrients) and BMI were collected and how they lead to their robustness and to the subsequent validity of the current analysis have been described in details elsewhere [17,18].

WHO, FAO and the World Bank are intergovernmental organizations using specialized information relevant to their respective fields. Their professional personnel should have evaluated these data in consideration of their possible use, e.g. for scientific research and decision making, before they were published. Therefore, the data reporting is as free of bias and error as it can be with government statistics. This means that errors are reduced but some inaccuracies related to reporting quality may still be present in the data. Similar data from the same sources were recently used to analyse the relationships between nutrients and obesity [18,19] and diabetes [20-22] in a number of publications.

We obtained data for 170 countries after we matched the prevalence estimates of obesity and overweight to the year-and country-specific food groups and other variables. Each country was treated individually as the subject and all their availability for other variables information was analyzed. Data sources and summary statistics were further described in Additional file 2 Data descriptive summary and source.

For particular analyses, the number of countries included for variables may have differed somewhat because all information on other variables was not uniformly available for all countries due to unavailability from relevant UN agencies. All the data were extracted and saved in Microsoft Excel® for analysis.

Statistical analyses

It has been commonly believed that obesity is an affluence related medical condition [23], which is generally caused by eating too much (dietary) [24] and moving too little (lifestyle) [25]. Urbanization is a population shift from rural to urban areas. It causes changes in diet and exercise patterns of the population [26]. Therefore, in addition to the seven dietary predictors (availability of sugar, meat, fats, fruits, fibers, starch and calories), we also incorporated GDP PPP, urbanization and prevalence of physical inactivity for data analysis.

To assess the difference between relationships between obesity prevalence and availability of sugar and meat, the analysis proceeded in four steps.

Pearson correlation was used to evaluate the strength and direction of the associations between all variables.

2. Partial correlation of Pearson moment-product approach was used to find the relationship between obesity prevalence and each food group respectively while keeping calories availability, GDP PPP, physical inactivity and urbanization statistically constant. In order to show that meat and sugar availability contributed to obesity prevalence independent of each other, we controlled for availability of the other food groups (starch crops, fibers, fats and fruits) in addition to GDP PPP, urbanization, total calories availability, physical inactivity. Fisher's r-to-z transformation was performed to test significance of differences between correlation coefficients. The significance was reported when P-value was <0.01. We kept sugar and meat availability statistically constant respectively together with all the other variables to test if they were correlated to obesity prevalence significantly independent of each other in addition to all other variables.

3. Standard multiple linear regression (Enter) was conducted to describe the relationships between obesity prevalence and all independent variables, which include all the dietary, lifestyle and socioeconomic predictors. Standard multiple linear regression (Stepwise) was also performed to regress multiple variables while simultaneously retaining sugar and meat availability as the important predictors of obesity prevalence. Analysis results of multiple linear regression (Enter and Stepwise) model included both the indicative value of beta coefficient (B) and its standard error (SE). The actual B may fall into a range determined with its standard error. Therefore, we added twice the standard error (SE) to their respective B to obtain the upper bound of the range and subtracted two SEs from B to obtain the lower bound of the range. We compared the ranges of B's of obesity prevalence to sugar and meat availability to determine if the relationships were significantly different. If two B ranges have overlap, the difference between the B's would not be considered as significant. If there is no overlap, the difference would be considered significant.

4. We used scatter plots to explore and visualize the correlations between obesity and availability of sugar and meat. To compare the two relationships, we reversed x and y axes to allow the two correlations in one figure (chart).

Additional variables

We reassessed our models using overweight (BMI ≥ 25 kg/m^2 instead of obesity (BMI ≥ 30 kg/m^2) in case of sugar and meat availability as a late-stage predictor of obesity. The results were reported in tables aligning with those relationships between obesity prevalence and sugar and meat availability. To incorporate overweight data for analysis may allow us to reassure the quality of data which were used for this study.

SPSS v. 22 (SPSS Inc., Chicago Il USA) was used for data analysis. Prior to analysis data were log-transformed (natural logarithms) to bring their distributions close to normal.

Results

Pearson correlation analysis showed that both sugar and meat availability were significantly correlated with prevalence of obesity (r=0.715, p<0.001 and r=0.685, p<0.001, respectively) (Table 1). Spearman rho values were r=0.664 (p<0.001) and r=0.664 (p<0.001) respectively. Fisher's r-to-z transformation revealed no significant difference in Pearson correlations between sugar and meat availability with obesity (z=0.53, p=0.5961). The difference between two coefficients' values was negligible, indicating that both meat and sugar were related to obesity to the same extent.

When we controlled for availability of total calories, prevalence of physical inactivity, urbanization and GDP PPP in partial correlation analysis, sugar and meat availability were still in significant correlation with prevalence of obesity (r=0.359, p<0.001 and r=0.354, p<0.001, respectively) (Table 2). This indicates that it is not just the contribution of sugar and meat to the total caloric intake that relates to obesity, but specific contents of these two food groups that influence metabolic processes. Fisher's r-to-z transformation revealed no significant difference in partial correlations between sugar and meat availability with obesity prevalence based on the comparison of two correlations (z=0.04, p=0.9681). This means that both sugar and meat availability contributes to obesity to the same extent.

Table 2 also presented that fats availability was in strong and significant correlation (Pearson) with obesity prevalence (r=0.517, p<0.001), but the level of correlation was not retained in partial correlation analysis (r=0.057, p=0.537). Starch crops availability was in relative strong correlation with obesity prevalence, but this correlation almost disappeared in partial correlation analysis.

	BMI 30	BMI 25	Sugar	Meat	Fats	Fruits	Fibers	Starch crop	Calories	GDP	Urbanization	Physical Inactivity
BMI 30	1	0.931***	0.715***	0.685***	0.523***	0.477***	0.678***	-0.220**	0.619***	0.678***	0.497***	0.448**
BMI 25	-	1	0.776***	0.792***	0.644***	0.546***	0.806***	-0.290**	0.748***	0.798***	0.632***	0.458***
Sugar	-	-	1	0.718***	0.571***	0.470***	0.714***	-0.492***	0.650***	0.727***	0.529***	0.437***
Meat	-	-	-	1	0.614***	0.520***	0.826***	-0.431***	0.695***	0.831***	0.565***	0.406***
Fats	-	-	-	-	1	0.373***	0.696***	-0.223**	0.701***	0.684***	0.651***	0.300**
Fruits	-	-	-	-	-	1	0.565***	-0.215**	0.499***	0.560***	0.353***	0.230**
Fibers	-	-	-	-	-	-	1	-0.370***	0.779***	0.994***	0.625***	0.439***
Starch crop	-	-	-	-	-	-	-	1	-0.029	-0.394***	-0.150*	-0.425***
Calories	-	-	-	-	-	-	-	-	1	0.763**	0.643**	0.243**
GDP PPP	-	-	-	-	-	-	-	-	-	1	0.620***	0.437***
Urbanization	-	-	-	-	-	-	-	-	-	-	1	0.385***
Physical Inactivity	-	-	-	-	-	-	-	-	-	-	-	1
Numbers of countries included in the analysis range from 126 to 170. $^{*}p<0.05$; $^{**}p< 0.01$, $^{***}P< 0.001$												
BMI ≥ 30 and BMI ≥ 25 are percentages of defined population with a body mass index (BMI) of no less than 30 kg/m^2 and 25 kg/m^2 respectively												
Data sources: Dietary data from the FAO's FAOSTAT. BMI (≥ 30 and ≥ 25) and Physical Inactivity data from the WHO Global Health Observatory. GDP PPP and urbanization data from the World Bank												

Table 1: Pearson correlation matrix for all variables.

When we controlled for availability of fats, fruits, fibers and starch, prevalence of physical inactivity, total calories, urbanization and GDP PPP in partial correlation analysis, both sugar and meat availability were still in significant correlation with prevalence of obesity (r=0.431, p<0.001 and r=0.339, p<0.001, respectively) (Table 2). Fisher's r-to-z transformation did not show a significant difference in the correlations between obesity and sugar and meat availability (z=0.81, p=0.4179). Therefore, sugar and meat contributions to obesity are independent of the availability of other food groups.

Interestingly, meat and sugar availability significantly correlated with each other in Pearson correlation (r=0.718, p<0.001) analysis (Table 1) but this correlation disappeared in partial correlation analysis when we controlled for availability of fats, fruits, fibers and starch crops, calories, GDP, urbanization and physical inactivity prevalence. Partial correlation coefficient became very weak and insignificant (r=0.144, p=0.124, not indicated in Table 2). This means that sugar and meat availability may contribute to obesity prevalence independent of each other.

The further investigation on this independence showed that both sugar (r=0.375, p<0.001) and meat (r=0.308, p<0.001) availability were still significantly correlated to obesity prevalence when we respectively controlled for sugar and meat availability together with all the other variables (fats, fruits, fibers and starch crops, calories, GDP, urbanization and physical inactivity prevalence) for testing each other's relationship with obesity prevalence (Table 2). Fisher's r-to-z transformation did not show significant difference between these two independent relationships (z=0.57, p=0.2843).

Table 3 presented the results of multiple linear regression analyses to identify dietary, lifestyle and socioeconomic predictors of prevalence estimates of obesity and overweight. We found that both sugar and meat were the significant predicators of estimates of obesity (B=0.455, SE=0.113 and B=0.381, SE=0.096, respectively) at the same significance level of p<0.001. The B ranges between obesity prevalence and availability of sugar (0.229-0.681) and meat (0.189-0.573) overlapped each other greatly (0.229-0.573). This meant that meat availability was no different from sugar availability to predict the estimates of prevalence of obesity.

Table 4 indicated that sugar (B=0.464, SE=0.093, p<0.001) and meat (B=0.433, SE=0.072, p<0.001) availability stood out as the significant predictor of obesity prevalence simultaneously in stepwise multiple linear regression analyses. Two overlapping B ranges (0.294-0.582) indicated that there was no difference between sugar and meat availability to predict obesity prevalence.

One of the highlights in our data analysis with linear regression was that fats availability was a minor predictor of obesity prevalence in both Enter method (B=0.053, SE=0.095, p=0.565) (Table 3) and Stepwise method (fats availability was a removed variable) (Table 4).

	Pearson correlation				Partial Correlation										
Variable	n	BMI ≥ 30	BMI ≥ 25	df	BMI ≥ 30	BMI ≥ 25	df	BMI ≥ 30	BMI ≥ 25	df	BMI 30	BMI 25	df	BMI ≥ 30	BMI ≥ 25
Sugar	167	0.715***	0.776***	118	0.359***	0.372***	114	0.431***	0.399***	114	0.375***	0.363***	-	-	-
Meat	167	0.685***	0.792***	118	0.354***	0.418***	114	0.339***	0.370***	-	-	-	114	0.308***	0.341***
Fats	161	0.523***	0.644***	118	0.057	0.11	-	-	-	-	-	-	-	-	-
Fruits	167	0.477***	0.546***	118	0.112	0.159	-	-	-	-	-	-	-	-	-
Fibers	169	0.678***	0.806***	118	0.248**	0.269**	-	-	-	-	-	-	-	-	-
Starch crops	167	-0.220**	-0.290**	118	0.07	-0.036	-	-	-	-	-	-	-	-	-
Calories	167	0.619***	0.748***	-	-	-	-	-	-	-	-	-	-	-	-
GDP PPP	165	0.678***	0.798**	-	-	-	-	-	-	-	-	-	-	-	-
Urbanization	169	0.497***	0.632***	-	-	-	-	-	-	-	-	-	-	-	-
Physical Inactivity	131	0.448***	0.458***	-	-	-	-	-	-	-	-	-	-	-	-

*p<0.05, **P< 0.01, ***P< 0.001. -: Controlled variable

BMI ≥ 30 and BMI ≥ 25 are percentages of defined population with a body mass index (BMI) of no less than 30 kg/m2 and 25 kg/m2 respectively

Data sources: Dietary data from the FAO's FAOSTAT. BMI (≥ 30 and ≥ 25) and Physical Inactivity data from the WHO Global Health Observatory. GDP and urbanization data from the World Bank

Table 2: Pearson and partial correlation analysis of different food groups to prevalence estimates of obesity and overweight.

	Obesity prevalence (%)				Overweight prevalence (%)			
	Model 1 (Enter), R^2=0.656				Model 1 (Enter), R^2=0.823			
Predictors	B	SE	p	B range	B	SE	p	B range
Sugar	0.455	0.113	<0.001	0.229-0.681	0.315	0.066	<0.001	0.183-0.447
Meat	0.381	0.096	0.001	0.189-0.573	0.307	0.056	<0.001	0.195-0.419
Fats	0.053	0.095	0.565	-	0.056	0.055	0.391	-
Fruits	0.034	0.07	0.633	-	0.054	0.041	0.29	-
Fibers	-0.17	0.314	0.777	-	0.214	0.182	0.618	-
Starch crops	0.349	0.215	<0.001	-	0.164	0.124	0.008	-
GDP PPP	0.37	0.272	0.525	-	0.002	0.157	0.997	-
Urbanization	-0.04	0.119	0.635	-	0.054	0.069	0.368	-
Physical Inactivity	0.163	0.098	0.015	-	0.081	0.057	0.09	-
Calories	-0.147	0.544	0.233	-	0.069	0.315	0.434	-

B: Beta; SE: Std. Error; p: Sig.

BMI ≥ 30 and BMI ≥ 25 are percentages of defined population with a body mass index (BMI) of no less than 30 kg/m^2 and 25 kg/m^2 respectively

Data sources: Dietary data from the FAO's FAOSTAT. BMI (≥ 30 and ≥ 25) and Physical Inactivity data from the WHO Global Health Observatory. GDP and urbanization data from the World Bank

Table 3: Results of enter multiple linear regression analyses to identify dietary, lifestyle and socioeconomic predictors of prevalence estimates of overweight and obesity.

	Obesity prevalence (%)				**Overweight prevalence (%)**			
	Model 4 (Stepwise), Adjusted R^2=0.630				**Model 4(Stepwise), Adjusted R^2=0.802**			
Predictors	**B**	**SE**	**p**	**B Range**	**B**	**SE**	**p**	**B Range**
Sugar	0.464	0.093	<0.001	0.278-0.650	0.363	0.059	<0.001	0.245-0.481
Meat	0.438	0.072	<0.001	0.294-0.582	0.34	0.055	<0.001	0.230-0.450
Fats	-	-	-	-	-	-	-	-
Fruits	-	-	-	-	-	-	-	-
Fibers	-	-	-	-	0.359	0.034	<0.001	-
Starch crops	0.464	0.171	<0.001	-	0.187	0.097	<0.001	-
GDP PPP	-	-	-	-	-	-	-	-
Urbanization	-	-	-	-	-	-	-	-
Physical Inactivity	0.171	0.094	0.008	-	-	-	-	-
Calories	-	-	-	-	-	-	-	-
B: Beta; SE: Std. error; p: Sig.; -: Removed variable								
BMI ≥ 30 and BMI ≥ 25 are percentages of defined population with a body mass index (BMI) of no less than 30 kg/m^2 and 25 kg/m^2 respectively								
Data sources: Dietary data from the FAO's FAOSTAT. BMI (≥30 and ≥25 mean) and Physical Inactivity data from the WHO Global Health Observatory. GDP and urbanization data from the World Bank								

Table 4: Results of stepwise multiple linear regression analyses to identify dietary, lifestyle and socioeconomic predictors of prevalence estimates of overweight and obesity.

Figure 1 showed the unadjusted correlation between prevalence estimate of obesity and sugar and meat availability. The scatterplots are very similar. The relationships were noted to be best described by polynomial regression equations with strong correlation at very similar levels.

Our data analysis in different models showed the similar relationships between overweight prevalence and respective availability of sugar and meat when we substituted overweight prevalence for obesity prevalence. We did not describe the results in narrative form, but they were shown in Figure 2 and Tables 1-4, aligning with those with obesity prevalence.

Discussion

By examining the comparable per capita availability data of the sugar and meat for 170 countries we have shown that:

1. Sugar and meat consumptions may be two significant determinants of obesity prevalence.

2. The consumption of sugar and meat has statistically significant relations to obesity independent of the effect of other major food groups, socioeconomic and lifestyle factors.

3. Availability of sugar and meat availability are correlated to obesity prevalence independent of each other.

4. Statistically, there was no significant difference between sugar and meat relationship to global obesity prevalence at a population level.

Values of Pearson correlation coefficients may be influenced by non-homoscedasticity of distribution of correlated variables. We have tried to minimize such possibility by using logarithmically transformed data. Comparison of the values of Pearson correlation coefficients with Spearman rho values shows that effects of distributions are negligible. Thus, our partial correlation analysis produced acceptable results.

There is ample research on foods and diet patterns that contribute to body weight increase. Using the similar source of data, Siervo et al. reported that both meat and sugar availability were correlated to global obesity prevalence [18]. However, their study did not conduct in-depth investigation to compare the correlation levels of meat and sugar availability to obesity prevalence.

There are two similar mechanisms that may explain why sugar and meat availability contribute to obesity comparably.

1. Fructose and meat protein may produce energy surplus due to their slower digestion process.

Sucrose and high-fructose corn syrup (HFCS; 42% or 55% fructose) are two primarily consumed sugars, and they are very similar in their composition. HFCS is only consumed in the US, Canada, Japan, and some parts of Europe, while the rest of the world primarily consumes sucrose (50% fructose). Sucrose contains 50% fructose and 50% glucose. HFCS in common usage within the food industry comprises similar percentages (40-55%) of glucose and fructose, water and other carbohydrates which are readily hydrolysable polymers of glucose. Fructose, as the major component of sugar, is slow to absorb [27] and hard to assimilate and it can only be metabolized by the liver to have glycogen most of which may be converted into fat for storage [28-30].

Meat is mainly composed of protein, fat and water. The absolute energy value of meat is determined by the protein and fat content [31]. Because meat of domesticated animals contains relatively large amount of fat, a number of studies have considered meat consumption as a higher risk of obesity and waist circumference (WC) [11,32]. Studies have already shown that dietary fat may not be a major determinant of obesity [33,34]. Animal breeding and butchering techniques in modern agriculture have significantly reduced meat fat content and increased protein content in the past few decades, so dietary meat is much leaner than ever [35,36]. The macronutrient energy values are 9.0 kcal/g for fat, 4.0 kcal/g for protein and carbohydrates [37]. Therefore, meat is not high in "energy and fat content" because it contains less fat and higher meat protein due to modern agriculture techniques.

Despite energy value of protein is not high (4.0 kcal/g), it has been postulated to contribute to the development of obesity because it may only be digested later than fats and carbohydrates [17,38,39]. Modern agriculture has been bringing the cost of availability of carbohydrates rich crops, such as cereals and starchy roots, and fat (oil), such as rape and soy significantly down. Cheap carbohydrates and fats in a meal can easily supply enough energy to meet human needs. This may make the energy from slow digested protein a surplus and stored as fat [17,38,39]. This postulation was supported by our data analysis result (Table 2) with the changes of correlations between food groups (fats and starch crops correlated to obesity and prevalence in Pearson r correlation, but not in partial correlation) and obesity and overweight in Pearson and partial correlations. In modern diet, foods rich in carbohydrates and fats have been able to provide enough energy to meet human daily energy requirements, so meat protein has been postulated to produce energy surplus, thus contributing to obesity may support our hypothesis in this study [17].

Plant protein is always mixed with fiber which makes it difficult to digest. Therefore, meat protein as the major source of digestible protein may contribute to the "energy surplus" significantly.

2. Sugar and meat consumption may cause insulin resistance, a metabolic syndrome contributing to obesity.

Insulin is an anabolic hormone in human body. It encourages the synthesis of carbohydrate, fat and protein, inhibits the production of glucose by the liver [40]. Insulin also increases the storage of fat in fat cells and prevents fat cells from releasing fat for energy [41-44]. The cells in insulin resistance patient become "resistant" to insulin, and sugars in blood cannot enter cells for calories production [45-50], but are metabolized into glycogen in their liver, which may be forced by insulin to metabolise into fat [28,51] and accelerates body weight gain [52] independent of excessive energy intake [53]. Insulin resistance is a major underlying cause of excess weight and obesity [54,55].

Many studies showed that sugar consumption is linked to insulin resistance in both children and adults, especially when it is consumed in large amounts [45,46].

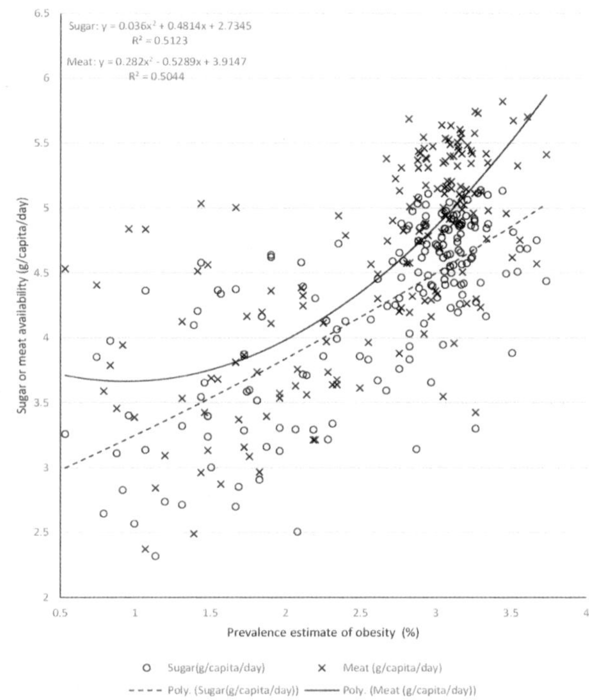

Figure 1: Polynomial correlation plot of obesity prevalence and sugar and meat availability.

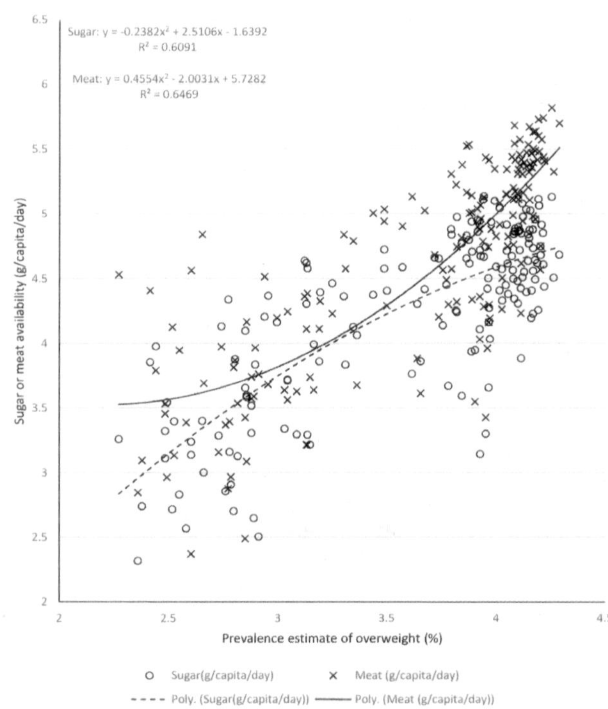

Figure 2: Polynomial correlation plot of overweight prevalence and sugar and meat availability.

High-dose fructose feeding can also cause insulin resistance in normal healthy human in as little as a week [56] and it can exacerbate insulin resistance in overweight and obese people [57].

Likewise, a number of studies have associated meat consumption as a risk factor for insulin resistance because: 1) Meat fat enhances intracellular lipid storage and impairs insulin metabolism [58,59]; 2) Heme iron from meat may damage pancreas cells [60,61] and 3) Meat sourced nitrites and sodium may impair the function of the pancreatic beta cells [62].

Leptin is a hormone made by adipose cells that helps to regulate energy balance by inhibiting hunger. A number of studies reported that sugar consumption was correlated to production of leptin, but the results were controversial [63,64].

The role of sugar consumption in the development of overweight and obesity has overly received scientific and policy attention. There are literally thousands of postings on the internet related to putative healthy diet guideline links between sugar and body obesity as well as insulin resistance. For instance, Morenga et al. [8] concluded that intake of sugar is a determinant of body weight after assessment of 6,557 relevant academic publications. Some authorities have taken action to limit young students' access to sugar products. Furthermore, taxation of sugar has been advocated or implemented in some countries/areas as a potential public health strategy to curb the obesity epidemic.

Meat, by contrast, has not been singled out as one of the worst dietary offenders. In terms of balanced diet components, what the public have been told overwhelmingly is that a moderate amount of meat (lean meat preferred) should be included in our daily diet as it contains essential protein and minerals. Although meat protein is nutritious and integral to our health, protein halo should not be prevailing. While recognizing that the evidence of harm to health against meat is statistically as strong as sugar, we should avoid the trap of waiting for absolute proof before allowing public health action to be taken. A survey of approximately 100,000 North American members of the Seventh Day Adventist Church [65] indicated that vegan members had the lowest BMI values, while mean BMI increased gradually with increasing amounts of animal protein consumed by lacto-ovo vegetarians, pesco-vegetarians and semi-vegetarians reaching the highest value in non-vegetarians.

A strength of this study is that we used comparable per capita availability data from 170 countries which enabled us to examine and compare relationships between obesity prevalence and different food groups (sugar and meat) at population level. However, there are several limitations in this study. Firstly, although we attempted to remove the potential confounding effects of variables such as GDP, caloric etc. by means of partial correlation analysis, some confounding factors may still influence correlations we found. Secondly, there may be some variables not included in our analysis that influence the correlation found in this study. It is however difficult to see what such variables may be. Thirdly, we could only use an international food group database that tracks the general market availability of different food types, not the actual human consumption. There are no direct measures of actual human consumption that can account for food wastage and provide precise measures of food consumption internationally. The database did not contain sufficient information to separate effects of "pure meat" from meat products that may contain other nutrients. Finally, the data analysed are calculated for per capita in each country, so we can only demonstrate a relationship between food group availability and obesity at a country level, which does not necessarily correspond to the same relationships holding true at the individual level. Prospective cohort studies are proposed to explore these associations further.

Conclusion

Both sugar and meat availability are correlated to obesity prevalence worldwide, and there is no significant difference between the levels of two correlations. Similar to the public campaign against excessive sugar consumption, considering the findings of adverse effects of meat on obesity and the environmental impact of meat production, the country authorities should also advise the public not to adopt a high-meat diet for long-term healthy weight management.

Declarations

Ethics approval and availability of data

All the data used in this study were freely downloaded from the United Nations (UN) agencies' websites. No ethical approval or written informed consent for participation was required.

Competing interests

The authors (WPY and MH) declare that there are no conflicts of interest, financial or otherwise, related to this paper.

Authors' contributions

MH conceived the idea for this study. WPY extracted the data. MH and WPY analysed and interpreted the data. WPY reviewed the literature and drafted the manuscript. WPY and MH edited and approved the manuscript for submission to the journal.

Acknowledgment

The authors express appreciation to the Statistics Department of FAO for the assistance in locating and defining the data.

Additional material

- Additional PDF 1 Food items in each food group
- Additional PDF 2 Data descriptive summary and source

References

1. Kanne WB, LeBauer EJ, Dawber TR, McNamara PM (1967) Relation of body weight to development of coronary heart disease. The Framingham study. Circulation 35: 734-744.
2. WHO (2009) Global health risks mortality and burden of disease attributable to selected major risks. World Health Organization, Geneva.

3. Puhl R, Brownell KD (2001) Bias, discrimination, and obesity. Obes Res 9: 788-805.
4. Thieme H (2005) The Lower Paleolithic art of hunting: The case of Schöningen 13 II–4, Lower Saxony, Germany. In: Gamble C, Parr M, editors. The hominid individual in context: archaeological investigations of Lower and Middle Paleolithic landscapes, locales and artefacts, London: Routeledge.
5. Henneberg M, Grantham J (2014) Obesity - a natural consequence of human evolution. Anthropological Review 77: 1-10.
6. Grantham JP, Staub K, Rühli FJ, Henneberg M (2014) Modern diet and metabolic variance--a recipe for disaster? Nutr J 13: 15.
7. Rouhani MH, Salehi-Abargouei A, Surkan PJ, Azadbakht L (2014) Is there a relationship between red or processed meat intake and obesity? A systematic review and meta-analysis of observational studies. Obes Rev 15: 740-748.
8. Te Morenga L, Mallard S, Mann J (2012) Dietary sugars and body weight: systematic review and meta-analyses of randomised controlled trials and cohort studies. BMJ 346: e7492.
9. Hu FB (2013) Resolved: there is sufficient scientific evidence that decreasing sugar-sweetened beverage consumption will reduce the prevalence of obesity and obesity-related diseases. Obesity reviews: an official journal of the International Association for the Study of Obesity14: 606-619.
10. Schulze MB, Fung TT, Manson JE, Willett WC, Hu FB (2006) Dietary patterns and changes in body weight in women. Obesity (Silver Spring) 14: 1444-1453.
11. Wang Y, Beydoun MA (2009) Meat consumption is associated with obesity and central obesity among US adults. Int J Obes (Lond) 33: 621-628.
12. You W, Henneberg M (2016) Cereal crops are not created equal: wheat consumption associated with obesity prevalence globally and regionally. AIMS Public Health 3: 313-328.
13. Koning F (2015) Adverse Effects of Wheat Gluten. Ann Nutr Metab 67: 8-14.
14. Davis B, Wansink B (2015) Fifty years of fat: news coverage of trends that predate obesity prevalence. BMC Public Health 15: 629.
15. den Engelsen C, Gorter KJ, Salomé PL, Rutten GE (2013) Development of metabolic syndrome components in adults with a healthy obese phenotype: a 3-year follow-up. Obesity (Silver Spring) 21: 1025-1030.
16. Trøseid M, Seljeflot I, Weiss TW, Klemsdal TO, Hjerkinn EM, et al. (2010) Arterial stiffness is independently associated with interleukin-18 and components of the metabolic syndrome. Atherosclerosis 209: 337-339.
17. You W, Henneberg M (2016) Meat consumption providing a surplus energy in modern diet contributes to obesity prevalence: an ecological analysis. BMC Nutrition 2: 22.
18. Siervo M, Montagnese C, Mathers JC, Soroka KR, Stephan BC, et al. (2014) Sugar consumption and global prevalence of obesity and hypertension: an ecological analysis. Public Health Nutr 17: 587-596.
19. Roccisano D, Henneberg M (2012) Soy consumption and obesity. Food and Nutrition Sciences 3: 260-266.
20. Basu S, Yoffe P, Hills N, Lustig RH (2013) The relationship of sugar to population-level diabetes prevalence: an econometric analysis of repeated cross-sectional data. PLoS One 8: e57873.
21. Basu S, Stuckler D, McKee M, Galea G (2013) Nutritional determinants of worldwide diabetes: an econometric study of food markets and diabetes prevalence in 173 countries. Public Health Nutrition 6: 1-8.
22. Weeratunga P, Jayasinghe S, Perera Y, Jayasena G, Jayasinghe S (2014) Per capita sugar consumption and prevalence of diabetes mellitus--global and regional associations. BMC Public Health 14: 186.
23. Giskes K, van Lenthe FJ, Turrell G, Kamphuis CB, Brug J, et al. (2008) Socioeconomic position at different stages of the life course and its influence on body weight and weight gain in adulthood: a longitudinal study with 13-year follow-up. Obesity (Silver Spring) 16: 1377-1381.
24. Nestle M (2003) Increasing portion sizes in American diets: More calories, more obesity. Journal of the American Dietetic Association 103: 39-40.
25. Berentzen T, Sørensen TI (2007) Physical inactivity, obesity and health. Scand J Med Sci Sports 17: 301-302.
26. Allender S, Foster C, Hutchinson L, Arambepola C (2008) Quantification of urbanization in relation to chronic diseases in developing countries: a systematic review. Journal of Urban Health: Bulletin of the New York Academy of Medicine 85: 938-951.
27. Sun SZ, Empie MW (2012) Fructose metabolism in humans - what isotopic tracer studies tell us. Nutr Metab (Lond) 9: 89.
28. Faeh D, Minehira K, Schwarz JM, Periasamy R, Park S, et al. (2005) Effect of fructose overfeeding and fish oil administration on hepatic de novo lipogenesis and insulin sensitivity in healthy men. Diabetes 54: 1907-1913.
29. Livesey G (2010) Fructose, Obesity, and Related Epidemiology. Critical Reviews in Food Science and Nutrition 50: 26-28.
30. Conlee RK, Lawler RM, Ross PE (1987) Effects of glucose or fructose feeding on glycogen repletion in muscle and liver after exercise or fasting. Ann Nutr Metab 31: 126-132.
31. Latham MC (1997) Human nutrition in the developing world Rome: Food and Agriculture Organization of the United Nations. FAO, Rome, Italy.
32. Rouhani MH, Salehi-Abargouei A, Surkan PJ, Azadbakht L (2014) Is there a relationship between red or processed meat intake and obesity? A systematic review and meta-analysis of observational studies. Obesity Reviews: An Official Journal of the International Association for the Study of Obesity 15: 740-748.
33. Willett WC, Leibel RL (2002) Dietary fat is not a major determinant of body fat. Am J Med 113: 47S-59S.
34. Melanson EL, Astrup A, Donahoo WT (2009) The relationship between dietary fat and fatty acid intake and body weight, diabetes, and the metabolic syndrome. Annals of Nutrition and Metabolism 55: 229-43.
35. Pearce KL, Norman HC, Hopkins DL (2010) The role of saltbush-based pasture systems for the production of high quality sheep and goat meat. Small Ruminant Research 91: 29-38.
36. Lawrie RA, Ledward DA. Lawrie's meat science. (7th Edn) Cambridge: Woodhead Publishing Limited.
37. FAO (2003) Food energy-methods of analysis and conversion factors Rome: Food and Agriculture Organization.
38. Grantham JP, Staub K, Rühli FJ, Henneberg M (2014) Modern diet and metabolic variance--a recipe for disaster? Nutr J 13: 15.
39. Henneberg M, Rühli FJ, Gruber P, Woitek U (2011) Alanine transaminase individual variation is a better marker than socio-cultural factors for body mass increase in healthy males. Food and Nutrition Sciences 2: 1054-1062.
40. Sonksen P, Sonksen J (2000) Insulin: understanding its action in health and disease. Br J Anaesth 85: 69-79.
41. Singh M, Shin YK, Yang X, Zehr B, Chakrabarti P, et al. (2015) 4E-BPs Control Fat Storage by Regulating the Expression of Egr1 and ATGL. J Biol Chem 290: 17331-17338.
42. Musselman LP, Fink JL, Ramachandran PV, Patterson BW, Okunade AL, et al. (2013) Role of fat body lipogenesis in protection against the effects of caloric overload in Drosophila. J Biol Chem 288: 8028-8042.
43. DiAngelo JR, Birnbaum MJ (2009) Regulation of fat cell mass by insulin in Drosophila melanogaster. Mol Cell Biol 29: 6341-6352.
44. Lee G, Park JH (2004) Hemolymph sugar homeostasis and starvation-induced hyperactivity affected by genetic manipulations of the adipokinetic hormone-encoding gene in Drosophila melanogaster. Genetics 167: 311-323.

45. Elliott SS, Keim NL, Stern JS, Teff K, Havel PJ (2002) Fructose, weight gain, and the insulin resistance syndrome (Abstract). American Journal of Clinical Nutrition 76: 911-922.
46. Basciano H, Federico L, Adeli K (2005) Fructose, insulin resistance, and metabolic dyslipidemia. Nutr Metab (Lond) 2: 5.
47. Dandona P, Aljada A, Bandyopadhyay A (2004) Inflammation: the link between insulin resistance, obesity and diabetes. Trends Immunol 25: 4-7.
48. Shoelson SE, Herrero L, Naaz A (2007) Obesity, inflammation, and insulin resistance. Gastroenterology 132: 2169-2180.
49. Hallfrisch J, Lazar F, Jorgensen C, Reiser S (1979) Insulin and glucose responses in rats fed sucrose or starch. Am J Clin Nutr 32: 787-793.
50. Hwang IS, Ho H, Hoffman BB, Reaven GM (1987) Fructose-induced insulin resistance and hypertension in rats. Hypertension 10: 512-516.
51. Stanhope KL, Schwarz JM, Havel PJ (2013) Adverse metabolic effects of dietary fructose: results from the recent epidemiological, clinical, and mechanistic studies. Current Opinion in Lipidology 24: 198-206.
52. Isganaitis E, Lustig RH (2005) Fast food, central nervous system insulin resistance, and obesity. Arterioscler Thromb Vasc Biol 25: 2451-2462.
53. Johnson RJ, Nakagawa T, Sanchez-Lozada LG, Shafiu M, Sundaram S, et al. (2013) Sugar, uric acid, and the etiology of diabetes and obesity. Diabetes 62: 3307-3315.
54. Grundy SM (1999) Hypertriglyceridemia, insulin resistance, and the metabolic syndrome. Am J Cardiol 83: 25F-29F.
55. Kahn SE, Hull RL, Utzschneider KM (2006) Mechanisms linking obesity to insulin resistance and type 2 diabetes. Nature 444: 840-846.
56. Beck-Nielsen H, Pedersen O, Lindskov HO (1980) Impaired cellular insulin binding and insulin sensitivity induced by high-fructose feeding in normal subjects. Am J Clin Nutr 33: 273-278.
57. Stanhope KL, Schwarz JM, Keim NL, Griffen SC, Bremer AA, et al. (2009) Consuming fructose-sweetened, not glucose-sweetened, beverages increases visceral adiposity and lipids and decreases insulin sensitivity in overweight/obese humans. The Journal of Clinical Investigation 119: 1322-1334.
58. Sparks LM, Xie H, Koza RA, Mynatt R, Bray GA, et al. (2005) A high- fat diet coordinately downregulates genes required for mitochondrial oxidative phosphorylation in skeletal muscle. Diabetes 54: 1926-1933.
59. Petersen KF, Dufour S, Befroy D, Garcia R, Shulman GI (2004) Impaired mitochondrial activity in the insulin-resistant offspring of patients with type 2 diabetes. N Engl J Med 350: 664-671.
60. Rajpathak SN, Crandall JP, Wylie-Rosett J, Kabat GC, Rohan TE, et al. (2009) The role of iron in type 2 diabetes in humans. Biochim Biophys Acta 1790: 671-681.
61. Hua NW, Stoohs RA, Facchini FS (2001) Low iron status and enhanced insulin sensitivity in lacto-ovo vegetarians. Br J Nutr 86: 515-519.
62. Pereira EC, Ferderbar S, Bertolami MC, Faludi AA, Monte O, et al. (2008) Biomarkers of oxidative stress and endothelial dysfunction in glucose intolerance and diabetes mellitus. Clin Biochem 41: 1454-1460.
63. Lana A, Rodríguez-Artalejo F, Lopez-Garcia E (2014) Consumption of sugar-sweetened beverages is positively related to insulin resistance and higher plasma leptin concentrations in men and nonoverweight women. J Nutr 144: 1099-1105.
64. Teff KL, Grudziak J, Townsend RR, Dunn TN, Grant RW, et al. (2009) Endocrine and metabolic effects of consuming fructose- and glucose-sweetened beverages with meals in obese men and women: influence of insulin resistance on plasma triglyceride responses. J Clin Endocrinol Metab 94: 1562-1569.
65. Tonstad S, Butler T, Yan R, Fraser GE (2009) Type of vegetarian diet, body weight, and prevalence of type 2 diabetes. Diabetes Care 32: 791.

16

Effect of Wood Charcoal Powder on Rate of Microbial Production of Lactic Acid in Dehulled and Undehulled *Vigna unguiculata* Pastes

Ibegbulem CO[1], Ene AC[1], Nwanpka P[2], Chikezie PC[2*] and Igwe CU[1]

[1]*Department of Biochemistry, Federal University of Technology, Owerri, Nigeria*

[2]*Department of Biochemistry, Imo State University, Owerri, Nigeria*

[*]**Corresponding author:** Chikezie PC, Department of Biochemistry, Imo State University, Owerri, Nigeria, E-mail: p_chikezie@yahoo.com

Abstract

Effect of Wood Charcoal Powder (WCP) on rate of microbial production of Lactic Acid (LA) in ground dehulled and an undehulled *Vigna unguiculata* (cowpea) paste was studied. The pastes were analysed for proximate compositions, energy values, tannin contents and microbial loads. Later, 4.0 g pastes were treated with incremental concentrations (0.03-0.05 g) of WCP diluted with 50 mL distilled water and fermented for 2 h at ambient temperature (29.5 ± 2.0°C). Results showed that decortication of cowpea significantly reduced ($p<0.05$) the crude protein, crude fibre, crude fat and tannin contents as well as energy value and microbial loads. Fermentation produced ethanol and LA. The WCP inhibited LA production in dehulled cowpea paste, whereas LA fermentation continued unhindered in Undehulled Cowpea Paste (UCP). A WCP-tannic acid-cellulose interaction study suggested that WCP interacted more with the fibre and tannin components of UCP thereby reducing the amount that would have bound the fermentative microorganisms. In conclusion, wood charcoal inhibited microbial production of lactic acid in ground dehulled cowpea paste.

Keywords: Cowpea; Decortication; Lactic acid; Microbial fermentation; Wood charcoal

Introduction

Vigna unguiculata (cowpea) is commonly consumed in developing countries, like Nigeria, as a source of plant protein [1]. The consumption of cowpea cuts across societal economic strata. It simply can be cooked whole with pepper, salt and palm oil. The paste of its dehulled form can be fried in hot edible oil into bean balls (*Akara* in Igbo and Yoruba) or wrapped in nylon, *Pandenus candelabrum* leaf, plastic container, aluminum foil or container and cooked into bean cake (*Moi-moi* in Igbo and Yoruba).

Microorganisms are ubiquitous. They degrade food materials producing organic acids, alcohols, toxins and other chemicals which impact off-flavour [2]. Food that is attractive and appealing can be transformed by microorganisms into a sour, fungus-covered or foul-smelling mass [3]. In order for food to serve its purpose, it must be protected from deterioration while being processed from its raw form to a consumable product. Food prepared from degraded raw materials is unappealing to the consumer and can lead to abandonment of the food and food wastage, downstream. Neta et al. [4] reported that sour taste results from low pH and the presence of organic acid(s); with the intensity of sourness being directly related to proton concentration and the number of molecules with at least one protonated carboxyl group.

Charcoal is an allotrope of carbon and forms covalent bonds with sulphur, oxygen and nitrogen. It is got by burning firewood in a limited amount of oxygen. Activated charcoal has been used in the management of chronic wounds [5], adsorption of verotoxin and verotoxin-producing *Escherichia coli* [6]. Wood charcoal adsorbs dyes [7] and gases [8]. Wood charcoal powder is traditionally used to clean dirt-coated teeth, glasses and mirrors because of its ability to adsorb dirt. A lump of wood charcoal is traditionally placed on pastes made from ground dehulled beans to prevent souring preparatory to processing into *Akara* or *Moi-moi*. This type of fermentation leads to food deterioration and/or spoilage because the taste of the final products is unacceptable to consumers. This study reports the effect of wood charcoal on the rate of microbial production of lactic acid in dehulled and undehulled cowpea pastes.

Materials and Methods

Collection of cowpea and wood charcoal

Cowpeas and dry wood charcoal used were purchased from Eke Ukwu market in Owerri Municipal Local Government Area, Imo State, Nigeria. The cowpeas were authenticated by Dr. F.N. Mbagwu, a taxonomist in the Department of Plant Science and Biotechnology, Imo State University, Owerri, Nigeria. Cowpea samples were deposited in the institution's herbarium with voucher number IMSUH 248.

Treatment of samples

A quantity (25.0 g) of apparently healthy cowpea seeds were put in each of two 500 mL capacity plastic bowels containing 150 mL of distilled water. The samples were soaked for 1 h and drained of water. One set was manually decocted, whereas the other set was left undehulled. The two sets of soaked bean samples were separately ground into pastes using the Thomas-Willey milling machine (ASTM D-3182; India) in 50.0 mL of distilled water. The dry wood charcoal was ground into powder using ceramic mortar and pestle.

Analyses of cowpea pastes

The proximate compositions and tannin contents of the ground bean pastes were determined using the methods of AOAC [9], energy content was determined as described by Codex Alimentarius [10], and FAO [11], and microbial analyses were carried out using the methods of UK SMI [12].

Fermentation study of cowpea pastes

A quantity (4.0 g) of each ground cowpea paste was weighed into four 50.0 mL capacity beakers. Ground charcoal was not put into the first beaker, but 0.03, 0.04 and 0.05 g of ground charcoal were added to the second, third and fourth beakers, respectively. The content of each beaker was diluted with 50.0 mL of distilled water and the beakers were allowed to ferment for 2 h at room temperature (29.5 ± 2.0°C). At the end of the fermentation period, each broth was mixed and filtered through a Whatman No. 24 filter paper. The presence of lactic acid and ethanol in the filtrates was detected as described by Mathotra [7], and Ibegbulem [13], respectively. The total acidity (as lactic acid) of the filtrate was determined using the method of Haddad et al. [14]. The rate of formation of lactic acid in the diluted paste for the 2 h study period was calculated as the ratio of lactic acid formed to time in minutes.

Tannic acid–charcoal–cellulose interaction study

Aliquots (10.0 mL each) of a 0.12% tannic acid solution were dispensed into three test tubes. To the first test tube, 0.04 g of charcoal was added. To the second test tube, 0.04 g of cellulose was added. To the third test tube, 0.04 g each of charcoal and cellulose were added. The content of each test tube was mixed thoroughly, allowed to stand at room temperature (29.5 ± 2.0°C) for 2 h and filtered using Whatman No. 24 filter paper. The tannic acid contents of the filtrates were determined using the methods of AOAC [9].

Statistical analysis

Data were analysed using percentage coefficient of variation and one-way analysis of variance (ANOVA) at 95% confidence limit where appropriate.

Results and Discussion

Dehulling or decortication of cowpea reduced its protein, mineral, crude fibre, energy and tannin contents (Table 1).

Parameter	Sample		Mean	SD	CV%
	Dehulled	Undehulled			
Crude protein (%)	5.81	7.58	6.69	0.88	13.23
Moisture (%)	72.55	69.94	71.25	1.3	1.82
Ash (%)	0.94	0.86	0.89	0.07	7.96
Crude fibre (%)	0.27	0.35	0.31	0.04	11.99
Crude fat (%)	0.36	0.8	0.58	0.22	37.65
Digestible carbohydrates (%)	20.07	20.53	20.3	0.23	1.13
Energy content (kcal/100 g)	107.84	121.04	114.44	6.6	5.77
Tannin (mg/100 g)	0.86	1.53	1.2	0.33	27.5
*wet-weight basis					

Table 1: Proximate composition, energy and tannin contents of dehulled and undehulled cowpea pastes*.

It suggests that when bean seeds are processed by soaking in water and decortication for the preparation of local delicacies like *Moi-moi* or *Akara*, some of their nutrients, fibre and polyphenols are lost. The loss of polyphenols was in agreement with the report of Ibegbulem et al. [15]. Tannins have been reported to reduce absorption of iron from the gastrointestinal tract [2], reduce digestibility because they bind and precipitate digestive enzymes, act as antioxidants because they scavenge free radical and have styptic and astringent properties [16] and inhibit microbial growth [3]. The crude protein, moisture, ash, crude fibre, crude fat and digestible carbohydrates contents of the raw, unsoaked cowpea seeds were found to be 29.48%, 7.81%, 3.27%, 1.72%, 4.68% and 53.04%, respectively; suggesting that is a carbohydrate-based food. Soaking the seeds in water markedly increased their moisture contents and decreased the other nutrients.

The concentrations of *Micrococcus* spp., *Escherichia coli, Staphylococcus* spp., *Bacillus* spp., *Streptococcus* spp. and *Lactobacillus* spp. isolated from the ground dehulled cowpea paste were significantly lower than those isolated from the ground undehulled cowpea paste (Table 2).

The seed coat seemed to have harboured much of the microorganisms. It suggests that decortications of beans prior to preparation of local delicacies like *Moi-moi* or *Akara*, causes loss of some of their naturally occurring microorganisms. Microbes found associated with cowpea include lactic acid bacteria such as *Lactobacillus casein, Lactobacillus leichmanni, Lactobacillus plantarum, Pediococcus pentosaceus* and *P. acidilactici* [17].

Lactic acid and ethanol were detected in the fermentation filtrates. This appears to suggest that the microbial modes of fermentation of the bean pastes may have included homolactic, heterolactic, and alcoholic fermentations. Majority of the microorganisms isolated from the pastes such as *Lactobacillus* spp., some *Bacillus* spp. and *Staphylococcus* spp. are lactic acid bacteria that can ferment glucose to lactic acid [3,17]. *E. coli* can ferment dextrose to acetic, formic and lactic acids [18] whereby pyruvate is first converted to format, then to carbon (IV) oxide and molecular hydrogen via formic acid fermentation, whereas Streptococcus can carry out mixed acid fermentation to produce ethanol, succinate, lactate and CO_2 [3]. *Micrococcus* spp. cannot ferment glucose [19,20]. However, of all the microorganisms isolated in this study, only the Bacillus spp. can hydrolyse starch [21].

Microorganism isolated	Microbial load of sample (cfu/mL)		Mean	SD	CV%
	Dehulled	Undehulled			
Micrococcus spp.	1.20×10^2	3.00×10^2	2.10×10^2	0.90×10^2	40.86
Escherichia coli	1.30×10^2	2.00×10^2	1.65×10^2	0.35×10^2	21.21
Staphylococcus spp.	1.00×10^2	2.00×10^2	1.50×10^2	0.50×10^2	33.33
Bacillus spp.	1.50×10^2	2.50×10^2	2.00×10^2	0.50×10^2	25
Streptococcus spp.	1.60×10^2	2.00×10^2	1.80×10^2	0.20×10^2	11.11
Lactobacillus spp.	1.60×10^2	2.50×10^2	2.05×10^2	0.45×10^2	21.95

Table 2: Microbial load of dehulled and undehulled cowpea pastes.

The rate of microbial production of lactic acid in the dehulled bean sample, devoid of wood charcoal powder, was significantly higher than that in its undehulled equivalent (Table 3).

Condition	Sample		Mean	SD	CV%
	Dehulled	Undehulled			
Without charcoal	4.17×10^{-3}	3.75×10^{-3}	3.96×10^{-3}	0.21×10^{-3}	5.3
With 0.03 g charcoal	4.50×10^{-3}	4.10×10^{-3}	4.30×10^{-3}	0.20×10^{-3}	4.65
With 0.04 g charcoal	5.25×10^{-3}	3.45×10^{-3}	4.35×10^{-3}	0.90×10^{-3}	20.69
With 0.05 g charcoal	3.85×10^{-3}	6.75×10^{-3}	5.30×10^{-3}	1.45×10^{-3}	27.36

Table 3: Rate of microbial production (g/100 mL/min) of lactic acid in dehulled and undehulled cowpea paste ferments.

Lactic acid production in the dehulled bean paste fermentation mixture increased but later decreased with increase in the concentration of wood charcoal powder unlike the undehulled bean paste fermentation mixture where lactic acid production increased consecutively with increase in the concentration of wood charcoal powder. Whereas rate of production of lactic acid in the undehulled bean paste fermentation mixture containing 0.04 g charcoal was not significantly higher than that of its dehulled equivalent, production of lactic acid in the undehulled bean paste fermentation mixture containing 0.05 g charcoal was significantly higher than that in its dehulled equivalent. Accordingly, the present study showed that at a critical wood charcoal concentration of 0.04 g, inhibition of fermentation of ground undehulled bean paste was lost but inhibition of fermentation was achieved in ground dehulled cowpea paste at 0.05 g wood charcoal powder.

The free tannic acid contents of the tannic acid–charcoal, tannic acid–cellulose and tannic acid–charcoal–cellulose solutions were significantly lower ($p<0.05$) than that of the benchmark tannic acid solution (Table 4). This seems to suggest that wood fibre can interact with both charcoal and plant pigments such as tannins.

The present study showed that increasing concentrations of wood charcoal powder did not inhibit the rate of fermentation of the undehulled bean pastes (Table 3). This may have been due to greater fibre–charcoal–phytochemical interactions in the undehulled bean, rather than charcoal–microorganism interaction. The undehulled bean paste contained more protein, fibre and oil than its dehulled equivalent (Table 1). Fibre bound wood charcoal and tannins (Table 4) thereby reducing the level of available charcoal that was supposed to adsorb the fermentative microorganisms. Adsorption of fermentative microorganisms by wood charcoal removes and makes them unavailable for fermentation [6]. This may explain its usage in medicine.

Solution	Tannic acid content (mg/100 mL)
Tannic acid	12.00 ± 0.00^a
Charcoal+tannic acid	9.40 ± 0.05^c
Cellulose+tannic acid	9.60 ± 0.49^c
Charcoal+cellulose+tannic acid	11.00 ± 0.37^b
*Values are mean ± SD of duplicate determinations. Values on the same column bearing different superscript letters are significantly different ($p<0.05$).	

Table 4: Free tannic acid content of solution.

Conclusion

The inhibition of fermentation in ground dehulled bean paste by wood charcoal may explain its traditional use to prevent the spoilage of ground bean pastes prior to processing them into bean balls or bean cake.

References

1. Phillips RD, McWatters KH, Chinnan MS, Hung YC, Beuchat LR, et al. (2003) Utilization of cowpea for human food. Field Crops Res 82: 193-213.
2. Wardlaw GM, Kessel MW (2002) Food safety (5th edn.). In: Perspective in Nutrition. Wardlaw GM, Kessel MW (eds.) McGraw-Hill, Boston pp: 745-788.
3. Prescott LM, Harley JP, Klein DA (2002) Microbiology (5th edn.). McGraw-Hill, Boston.
4. Neta ERC, Johanningsmeier SD, Drake MA, McFeeters RF (2007) A chemical basis for sour taste perception of acid solutions and fresh-pack dill pickles. J Food Sci 72: 352-359.
5. Kerihuel JC (2010) Effect of activated charcoal dressings on healing outcomes of chronic wounds. J Wound Care 19: 208-215.
6. Naka K, Watarai S, Inoue K, Kodama Y, Oguma K, et al. (2001) Adsorption effect of activated charcoal on enterohemorrhagic *Escherichia coli.* J Vet Med Sci 63: 281-285.
7. Mathotra VK (1989) Practical Biochemistry for Students (3rd edn.). Jaypee Brothers Medical, New Delhi, India.
8. Zakaria Z, George T (2011) The performance of commercial activated carbon absorbent for adsorbed natural gas storage. Int J Res Rev Appl Sci 9: 225-230.
9. Association of Official Analytical (AOAC) (2006) Official Methods of Analysis. (18th edition) Association of Official Analytical Chemists, Washington DC, USA.
10. Codex Alimentarius (2001) Codex Guidelines on Nutrition Labelling CAC/GL 2-1985. Codex Alimentarius Commission. Joint FAO/WHO Food Standards Programme. Food and Agricultural Organization of the United Nations/World Health Organization, Rome.
11. Food and Agricultural Organization (FAO) (2003) Food Energy-Methods of Analysis and Conversion Factors. Food and Nutrition Paper 77. Food and Agricultural Organization of the United Nations, Rome.
12. UK SMI (2015a) UK Standards for Microbiology Investigations. Public Health England.
13. Ibegbulem CO (2012) Nutritional effects of drinking terminalia iittoralis seem decoction. Int J Biochem Res Rev 2: 126-136.
14. Haddad PR, Sterns M, Warclaw J (1978) Analysis of wine–an undergraduate project. Edu Chem 15: 87-88.
15. Ibegbulem CO, Nwaogu LA, Iworie IL (2006) Effect of dehulling bean on volume of water drunk after its meal. J Agric Food Sci 4: 61-66.
16. Evans WC (2002) Trease and Evans Pharmacognosy (15th edn.). W.B. Saunders, Edinburgh.
17. Hedley CL (2001) Carbohydrates in Grain Legume Seeds: Improving Nutritional Quality and Agronomic Characteristics. CABI Publishing, NY, USA.
18. Frampton EW, Restaino L (1993) Methods for E. coli identification in food, water and clinical samples based on beta-glucuronidase detection. J Appl Bacteriol 74: 223-233.
19. Hugh R, Leifson E (1953) The taxonomic significance of fermentative versus oxidative metabolism of carbohydrates by various gram negative bacteria. J Bacteriol 66: 24-26.
20. UK Standards for Microbiology Investigations (2015b) Standard Units, Microbiology Services. UK Standards for Microbiology Investigations. Public Health England. Bacteriology Test Procedures Oxidation/ Fermentation of Glucose Test pp: 1-13.
21. Ibrahim SE, El Amin HB, Hassan EN, Sulieman AME (2012) Amylase production on solid state fermentation by *Bacillus* spp. Food Public Health 2: 30-35.

Effects of Alfalfa Saponins on Cholesterol Metabolism in Broilers

Ting Liu, Zhentian Li*, Tengfei Wang and Xiaoyan Zhu

College of Animal Science and Veterinary Medicine, Henan Agricultural University, Zhengzhou, PR China

***Corresponding author:** Zhentian Li, College of Animal Science and Veterinary Medicine, Henan Agricultural University, No. 95 Wenhua Road, Jinshui District, Zhengzhou, 450002, PR China, E-mail: lizhentian2006@126.com

Abstract

This experiment was conducted to evaluate the effect of different levels alfalfa saponins on cholesterol metabolism in broilers. A total of 320 Arbor Acres (AA) broilers of 1 day-old were randomly allotted to 4 treatments with five replicates in each treatment, and with 16 broilers in each replicate. The experiment last 49 days. During the stage from 0 to 3 weeks, broilers in the control group were fed basal diet and birds in the test groups were all fed the basal diets added with 0.02% alfalfa saponins. while from 4 to 7 weeks, birds in the test groups were fed the basal diets added with 0.04%, 0.08% and 0.12% alfalfa saponins, respectively. The results showed that: Supplemented 0.08% and 0.12% alfalfa saponins to broilers diets could significantly decrease cholesterol content of serum and liver ($P<0.05$), increased HDL-C content in serum and bile acids content in feces ($P<0.05$), highly decreased LDL-C content and HMG-CoAreductase mRNA abundance ($P<0.01$), implicating alfalfa saponins could block enterohepatic circulation of bile acids, thus supress the synthesis of cholesterol to some extent. 0.08% alfalfa saponins also could significantly reduce insulin content in serum ($P<0.05$). Added moderate alfalfa saponins to broilers feed could reduce TG content and Hydrocortisone content in serum to a certain extent, effectively improve cholesterol metabolism.

Keywords: Alfalfa saponins; Broilers; Cholesterol; Bile acids

Introduction

Hyperlipidemia is common worldwide, and is considered as a highly modifiable risk factor for coronary heart disease and peripheral artery diseases. Cardiovascular disease is a major cause of death worldwide, and is related to the level of cholesterol [1]. Increased serum low-density lipoprotein (LDL) level, can accelerate atherosclerosis. Limiting the intake of dietary cholesterol could be an effective approach to prevent Cardiovascular disease. People are advised to limit their intake of poultry products because of their high levels of cholesterol. Thus, lowering the content of cholesterol in poultry products is important to peoples health. In recent decades, increasing attention has been paid to new natural agents with lipid-reducing activity [2-4], and it may be an important way to lower the cholesterol level. Alfalfa (*Medicago sativa*) is used as a food additive in the USA, Russia, China and North Africa, for its high contents of vitamin and bioactive ingredients [5,6]. Saponins is extracted from *Medicago sativa* L., and its the main active component. Saponins is traditionally a natural surface-active glycosides. It is famous with forming a stable soap-like foam. In the meanwhile, as a natural alfalfa plants extractive, Alfalfa saponins have a variety of biological active fuctions, and played a positive role in lowering the cholesterol content [7-9]. A large number of research found that saponins could improve animal performance, increase antioxidant capacity, anti-tumor, reduce cholesterol, improve immunity and other useful biological functions [10-13]. Yu et al. [9] had fond that Saponins significantly reduced the level of TC and LDL-C in serum [9]. In view of the biological characteristics of alfalfa saponins, this experiment was conducted to determine the effects of different levels of alfalfa saponins on cholesterol metabolism in broilers, as well as provide the scientific basis in the application of broiler feed.

Materials and Methods

Experimental materials

Alfalfa saponin, extract by ethanol extraction from the alfalfa meal and macroporous resin column purified, was obtained from Bo Yan Biological Technology Co., Ltd. in Cangzhou City, Hebei Province. Alfalfa saponins was tested with Thin Layer Chromatography. The purity of alfalfa saponins tested by UV spectrophotometry was 20%.

Experimental birds and grouping

A total of 320 one-day-old Arbor Acres broilers (42 ± 2 g) were randomly divided into 4 treatments, with 5 replicates in each treatment, and with 16 broilers in each replicates, using the complete randomized blocks single factorial design. Feeding experiment was conducted from 2007-4-19 to 2007-6-6 in Erqi District Houzhai town of zhengzhou city.

Experimental diet and design

During the stage from 0 to 3 weeks, broilers in the control group were fed basal diet and birds in the test groups were all fed the basal diets added with 0.02% alfalfa saponins. while from 4 to 7 weeks, birds in the test groups were fed the basal diets added with 0.04%, 0.08% and 0.12% alfalfa saponins, respectively (Table 1).

Feeding and management

All broilers were fed in three-dimensional cages in accordance with routine immunization and disinfecting quarantine procedures. This experiment was carried out in strict accordance with the recommended AA broiler feeding and management manual. The temperature was set at 33 at the initiation of experimentationand lowered by 2-3°C each week thereafter, until a final temperature at

21-22 in the fourth weekend. From the initial daily 23 h, light gradually decreased to natural light. Maintain good ventilation. All broilers were free to feed and water.

Ingredient (%)	0-3 weeks	4-7 weeks
Corn	59.7	63
Soybean meal	32.5	28
Cottonseed meal	0	1.6
Fish meal	2	1
Soybean oil	1.5	2.5
Limestone	1.4	1.5
Phosphorous	1.4	1.2
Salt	0.3	0.3
DL-methionine	0.2	0.1
Premix	1	0.8
Nutrient level		
DE (MJ/kg)	12.2	12.59
CP	20.79	19.01
Lys	1.11	0.97
Met	0.54	0.41
Met + Cys	0.89	0.74
Ca	0.98	0.93

Note: Each kilogram of premix supplied such nutrients for the complete feed: V_A: 8000 IU; VD_3: 1500 IU; V_E: 30 IU; V_K: 2 mg; V_{B1}: 5 mg; V_{B2}: 8 mg; V_{B6}: 6 mg; V_{B12}: 1 mg; Nicotinic acid: 40 mg; Pantothenic acid: 20 mg; Folic Acid: 1 mg; Biotin: 0.4 mg; Choline chloride: 1500 mg; Composite trace elements: 1000 mg; Methionine: 2000 mg; Salinomycin: 60 mg. Calculated values for ME, Lys, Met, Analyzed values for others.

Table 1: Composition and nutrient levels in basal diet for broilers of different week age.

Sample collection

At 49 days of ageone broiler whose weight is similar to average weight was selected from each replicate. Blood samples were collected from heart and serum was separated by centrifugation at 3000 rpm and frozen at -70 for later analysis. 0.5 g liver of each broiler was homogenized in Phosphate Buffered Saline (PBS, pH 7.2) (0.25 g/mL) at 4 uC. The supernatant was then centrifuged at 4000, 4 for 10 min. The preparation was adjusted to indicated concentration and stored at -70 for later analysis of total cholesterol, as well as the abundance of HMG-CoA reductase and mRNA. At 47 days of age, Feces of each broiler were collected during the last 3 days experimental period and dried at 60. Feces were weighed and grinded into 0.5 mm diameter powder for bile acid concentrations analysis.

Parameters measured

Determination of serum indices: HITACHI 7170A automatic biochemical analyzer was used to detect total cholesterol (TC), Triglyceride (TG), high-density lipoprotein cholesterol (HDL-C), low-density lipoprotein cholesterol (LDL-C) Cortisol and insulin concentrations.

Determination of fecal total bile acid: Weigh faeces 0.5 g, added 5 mL distilled water, homogenized and centrifuged at 4,000 rpm for 10 min. Using Total Bile Acid Kit, TBA provided by BIOSINO BIO-TECHNOLOGY AND SCIENCE INC, the supernatant was examined with HITACHI 7170A automatic biochemical analyzer.

The identification of liver cholesterol concentrations and HMG-CoA reductase mRNA express production by RT-PCR HITACHI 7170A automatic biochemical analyzer was used to detect liver cholesterol concentrations. The method of Liver HMG-CoA reductase mRNA express production by RT-PCR, as follows:

Primer design and synthesis: According to the broiler (Gallus gallus) liver HMG-CoA reductase catalytic domain cDNA sequence (sequence number AB109635), β-actin sequence (serial number L08165) recorded by Gen-bank, we use Oligo 6.0 primer design software to design relevant sequence primer, and their primer are as follows:

HMG-CoA reductase primer sequence:

U 5'-CACTGGGTTTGGTTCTTGTT-3'

L 5'-GGATTCGGTCTCTGCTTGTT-3'

β-actin primer sequence:

U 5'-CAGAAAGACAGCTACGTTGG-3'

L 5'-TTCATAGATGGGCACAGTGTGG-3'

Primers above were synthesized by ThreeBoYuanZhi from Beijing Biotech Co., Ltd. PCR products of HMG-CoA reductase, β-actin were predicted at the lengths of 248 bp, 357 bp respectively.

Liver total RNA extraction: Total RNA was extracted Using one-step Trizol extraction reagent obtained from the Gene Technology Co., Ltd. Beijing Parkson, and the concentrations and purity were tested by GeneQuant pro from the Biochrom Ltd. Detecting A260 was used to calculated the concentration. The ratio of A260 and A280 determine the purity of RNA (1.8-2.0), while electrophoresis was used to detect the quality.

RT-PCR

Reverse transcription reaction: Fermentas (MBI) provided the M-MuLV kit for reverse transcription of total RNA, and changing the quantity of RNA to ensure the amount of RNA is at the same level in different group.

PCR: HMG-CoA reductase reaction program: 94°C initial denaturation for 5 min; 94 denaturation 30 s, 53 30 s, and then 72 extension for 1 min, 37 cycles, at last extension at 72°C for 10 min.

β-actin reaction program: 94°C intial denaturation for 5 min; 94°C denaturation 50 s, 54.5°C; 50 s, 72°C extension for 1 min, 37cycles; at last extension at 72°C for 10 min.

PCR products analysis: We take 7 μL HMG-CoA reductase PCR products and β-actin PCR products from the same sample, and 5 μL DNA marker, respectively. Using the agarose gel electrophoresis concentration of 2.5% and imaging system (AlphaImager) to get some camera shooting pictures. We use the PCR product ratio (IOD) of HMG-CoA reductase to β-actin to show the relative PCR products contents of HMG-CoA reductase.

Sequencing of HMG-CoA reductase PCR products: The selection of HMG-CoA reductase PCR products were purified and then send to Treasure biological engineering Co., Ltd. for sequencing.

Reaction System	Size
10 × PCR Buffer	2.5 μL
10 mM dNTP (2.5 mM)	3 μL
Forward Primer 20 μM	0.5 μL
Reverse Primer 20 μM	0.5 μL
Template DNA	1 μL
ddH_2O	17 μL
Total	25 μL

Statistical analysis

The statistical analysis was performed using the SAS 8.12 statistical program. A one-way ANOVA program was used to analyze the experimental data. Significant differences between treatment groups were further analyzed using Duncan's multiple range test (Duncan, 1955) and the results using "M ± SE". Differences were considered significant at P<0.05.

Results and Analysis

Effect of Different Levels of Alfalfa Saponin on Lipid Metabolism in Broiler

The serum TG, TC, HDL-C and LDL-C levels of different groups was described in Table 2. The TG content of broiler given 0.04%, 0.08% and 0.12% of alfalfa saponins was lower than the control groupP>0.05, and the TG content was decreased linearly with alfalfa saponins concentration (P>0.05). Likewise, with the addition of alfalfa saponins, serum TC levels decreased by sequence. But there was no significant difference between the 0.04% group and the control group (P>0.05), while the 0.08% and 0.12% group were significantly lower than the control group (P<0.05); Compared with the control group, serum HDL-C levels in each treatment increased, but no significant difference (P>0.05). Increasing with the addition of alfalfa saponins, the substance gradually increased. In contrast with serum HDL-C levels, serum LDL-C levels decreased compared with the control group, and 0.08% and 0.12% groups were significantly lower than the control group (P<0.01), while 0.04% group was no significant difference (P>0.05). Between three treatments, there were no significant diferrence P>0.05 on serum HDL-C levels except 0.12% group was lower than 0.04% group (P<0.05).

Effects of Different Alfalfa Saponins Levels on Hormone Levels and Total Fecal Bile Acid in Broilers

Serum Hydrocortisone and insulin levels were described in Table 3. The concentrations of serum Hydrocortisone in 3 treatments were highter than the control group, but the difference was not significant (P>0.05). On the contrary, Serum insulin levels in treatment groups were lower than the control group. Compared with the control group, there were significant difference (P<0.05) in 0.08% group, while 0.04%, 0.12% groups had no significant difference (P>0.05).

Addition	TG (mmol/L)	TC (mmol/L)	HDL-C (mmol/L)	LDL-C (mmol/L)
0	0.38 ± 0.08	3.99 ± 0.63^{a}	2.27 ± 0.30	1.15 ± 0.12^{Aa}
0.04	0.34 ± 0.03	3.55 ± 0.48^{ab}	2.31 ± 0.14	0.97 ± 0.14^{ABab}
0.08	0.30 ± 0.03	3.22 ± 0.24^{b}	2.38 ± 0.20	0.78 ± 0.30^{Bbc}
0.12	0.29 ± 0.03	3.13 ± 0.30^{b}	2.43 ± 0.34	0.68 ± 0.05^{Bc}

Note: Within the same row followed by different superscripts, a lower case letter means a significant difference (P<0.05), a capital letter means a highly significant difference (P<0.01).

Table 2: Contents of TGTCHDL-CLDL-C in serum [A,B,a-c].

Total fecal bile acid was described in Table 3. Total fecal bile acid of 0.04% group was similar with the control group, both had no significant difference, while the other two groups were significantly higher than the control group (P<0.05), and 0.12% group was significantly higher than the control group (P<0.01). Comparison between each treatment group, 0.12% group was significantly higher than 0.04% group (P<0.05).

Addition	Hydrocortisone (μg/dL)	Insulin (μIU/ML)	Total bile acid (μmol/L)
0	0.07 ± 0.01	0.57 ± 0.16^{a}	110.40 ± 2.55^{Bc}
0.04	0.09 ± 0.02	0.45 ± 0.15^{ab}	121.80 ± 11.41^{ABbc}
0.08	0.11 ± 0.04	0.22 ± 0.06^{b}	132.60 ± 2.45^{ABab}
0.12	0.08 ± 0.01	0.51 ± 0.10^{ab}	141.90 ± 7.13^{Aa}

Table 3: Contents of hormone in serum and total bile acid in soil [A,B,a-c].

Effects of Alfalfa Saponins On Liver Cholesterol and Hmg-CoA Reductase mRNA Abundance in Broilers

Effects of alfalfa saponins on liver HMG-CoA reductase mRNA expression products in broilers

Total RNA extraction results: The electrophoresis results of broiler liver HMG-CoA reductase mRNA RT-PCR products was shown in Figure 1. The ratio of A260 and A280 was used to determine the RNA purity (1.8-2.0).

RT-PCR and gel electrophoresis results: 2.5% agarose gel electrophoresis were used to test HMG-CoA reductase and β-actin RT-PCR products, and obtained two fragments close to 248 bp and 357 bp respectively, which were consistent with the expected results (Figure 2).

Sequencing: Compared with the GenBank nucleotide sequence of genes, it's homology was 98.56%.

Effect of adding alfalfa saponins on liver cholesterol contents and HMG-CoA reductase mRNA relative contents in broilers

Liver cholesterol contents and HMG-CoA reductase mRNA relative contents in broilers were described in Table 4. Compared with the control group, liver cholesterol contents and HMG-CoA reductase mRNA relative levels of 0.08% and 0.12% groups were significantly lower than the control group (P<0.05). Meanwhile, HMG-CoA reductase mRNA relative levels of 0.08% and 0.12% groups were significantly lower than the control group (P<0.01), while the 0.04% group had no significant difference, but lower than the control group. Comparison between each treatment, only liver HMG-CoA reductase mRNA relative contents of 0.08% group was significantly lower than the 0.04% group (P<0.01), while others were not significantly different (P>0.05).

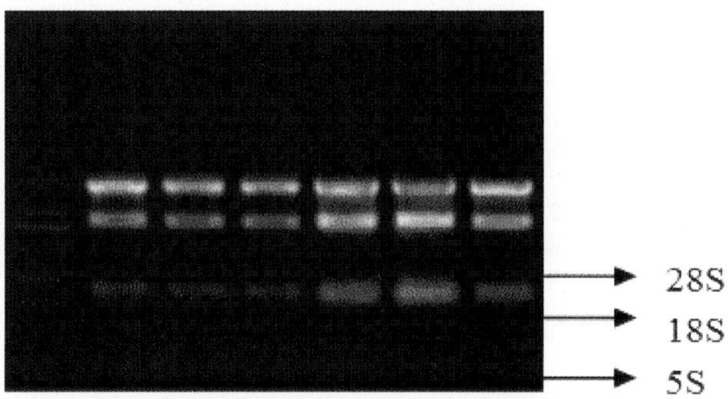

Figure 1: Agarose gel electrophoresis of the total RNA from broiler's liver.

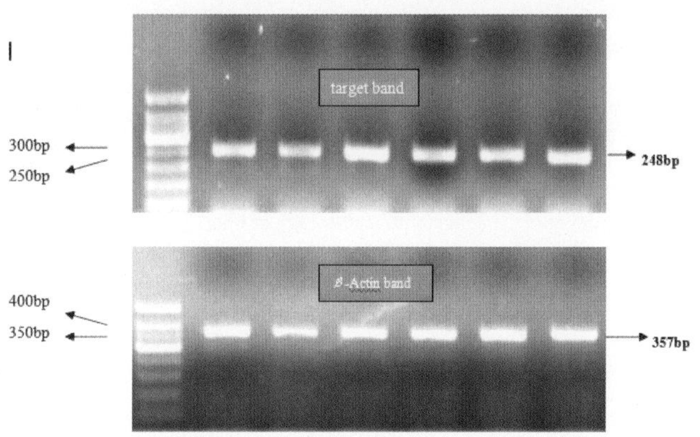

Figure 2: Gel electrophoresis analysis of the RT-PCR product.

Addition	Liver (nmol/L)	Relative contents of HMGR
0	377.50 ± 28.72^{a}	1.04 ± 0.09^{Aa}
0.04	353.33 ± 15.28^{ab}	0.95 ± 0.08^{ABab}
0.08	317.50 ± 10.61^{b}	0.71 ± 0.14^{Cc}
0.12	300.00 ± 40.00^{b}	0.80 ± 0.10^{BCbc}

Table 4: Contents of cholesterol in liver and relative contents of HMGR [A,B,a-c].

Discussion

Effect of alfalfa saponins on cholesterol metabolism in broilers

There are two main sources of cholesterol in broilers: One is the dietary supply, the other is its own synthesis. Most broiler feeds made of plant which Cholesterol intake is low. Therefore, cholesterol is almost synthesis by its own. The liver is the most active organ in which about 3/4 or more cholesterol is synthesized [14]. Cholesterol biosynthesis is a complex process. The substrate in cholesterol synthesis, acetyl CoA, can be converted to cholesterol through a series of multi-step enzymatic reaction intermediatesand HMG-CoA reductase is the rate-limiting enzyme of cholesterol synthesis. The activity of HMG-CoA reductase plays an important role on the regulation of cholesterol synthesis, That is phosphorylation by inactivation of the enzyme to reduce cholesterol synthesis. Hunger and satiation, cholesterol feedback regulation, hormones can regulate cholesterol synthesis. As we all know, hunger can inhibit the synthesis of cholesterol, but the cholesterol synthesis will increases when the intake of high sugar, high saturated fat diet. As for hepatic cholesterol synthesis of the cholesterol feedback inhibition is achieved by inhibiting the synthesis of HMG-CoA reductase. However, the regulation of hormones is more complex. Insulin-induced hepatic HMG-CoA reductase synthesis, Insulin can Induce hepatic synthesis of HMG-CoA reductase, However the cortisol and glucagon inhibit and decrease the activity of the enzyme, while thyroid hormone can increase the synthesis of the enzyme and promote the transition of cholesterol into the liver bile acid at the same time, and the effect of the latter is stronger than the former. Hepatic synthesis cholesterol and assemble most of the cholesterol (including exogenous and endogenous) in free into VLDL secreted into the blood, together with other lipid and apolipoprotein (ApoB, etc.) then utilized by other tissues and organs [14,15]. Liver is an important excretory organ of cholesterol, and almost all cholesterol are excreted by liver, except some from the intestinal mucosa. Liver bile acid formation is the most important way to reduce cholesterol, Primary bile acid of Cholesterol as the raw material is the main form of hepatic clearance of cholesterol, In addition, cholesterol can be converted into steroid hormones, vitamin D_3 and cholesterol ester [14].

Serum total cholesterol and low density lipoprotein cholesterol levels of adding 0.08% and 0.12% alfalfa saponins groups decreased significantly, while high density lipoprotein cholesterol contents was not significant effects, and Malinow MR had reported the similar result [16]. Yuan et al. [17] reported that adding with alfalfa saponins significantly decreased serum cholesterol and LDL cholesterol levels in rats [17]. Yu et al. [9] reported that the total alfalfa saponins significantly reduced the serum total cholesterol and LDL cholesterol in broilers [9], which were in agreement with the result of Ma [18]. These results are consistent with the current results. The mechanism of Alfalfa saponins reducing serum total cholesterol may be the formation of insoluble complexes of saponins combined with cholesterol, thus contributing to lower cholesterol levels. Low-density lipoprotein is the principle form of carring the endogenous cholesterol [14]. Alfalfa saponins can be combined with the endogenous cholesterol which is discharged by bile, thus preventing re-absorption of cholesterol [19]. It may be the reason that alfalfa saponins reduced serum low-density lipoprotein cholesterol but didn't effect serum high density lipoprotein cholesterol. The current result was that alfalfa saponins had not noticeable effect on serum triglyceride levels, and this is not consistent with the result Yu [19] reported. It is still need further study.

The liver HMG-CoA reductase mRNA expression levels of 0.08% and 0.12% alfalfa saponins groups were decreased by 31.73% and 23.08% ($P<0.01$) respectivelyeffectively reducing cholesterol synthesis in liver. 0.08% and 0.12% alfalfa saponins groups mRNA expression levels of HMG-CoA reductase in the liver decreased by 31.73% and 23.08% ($P<0.01$), respectively, which effectively reducing cholesterol synthesis in liver. The author speculated that alfalfa saponins may reduce liver HMG-CoA reductase mRNA abundance, thereby reducing cholesterol contents. This experiment showed that breast muscle, leg muscle and liver cholesterol levels significantly decreased in 0.08% and 0.12% alfalfa saponins groups. Wang et al. [20] also reported that fed with alfalfa extract, rat liver cholesterol was significantly decreased [20]. These results are consistent with the above, the mechanism may be that alfalfa saponins convert hepatic cholesterol into bile acids, thus contributing to the emission of cholesterol from the body, reducing the deposition of cholesterol in muscle. Result of serum hormone showed that serum insulin levels significantly reduced in 0.08% group, while no significant effect on cortisol levels. Compared with the other test groups, 0.12% alfalfa saponins group decreased cortisol, increased insulin contents, which may be caused by feedback inhibition of cholesterol synthesis. The mechanism of Alfalfa saponins reducing serum total cholesterol may be the formation of insoluble complexes of saponins combined with cholesterol, thus contributing to lower cholesterol levels. The mechanism may be that due to adding with 0.12% alfalfa saponins significantly reduced the hepatic cholesterol and serum cholesterol levels, thereby enhanced the HMGR (HMG-CoA reductase acid mono) activity, promoted the synthesis of hepatic cholesterol. Because of cortisol and insulin are effected by HMGR activity, high levels of alfalfa saponins have an effect on the levels of cortisol and insulin. Detection of fecal bile acid showed that addition of alfalfa saponins increased fecal bile acid excretion. Liu et al. [21] indicated that alfalfa saponins can affect or block the bile acid enterohepatic circulation, Bile acid in the body can not be converted to cholesterol but only discharged from the body by the intestinal tract [21]. These results are agreement with the current results.

Conclusions

Alfalfa saponin has a significant effect on total cholesterol and LDL cholesterol in broiler serum, and significantly reduced cholesterol levels in broiler breast muscle, leg muscle and liver. The addition of alfalfa saponins decreased the expression level of liver HMG-CoA reductase mRNA, reduced hepatic cholesterol synthesis effectively, and improved the excretion of feces bile acid in broiler. In conclusion, the broiler dietary supplemented with 0.08% alfalfa saponins can obtain the optimal performance.

Acknowledgement

This study was supported by China forage and grass research system (CARS-35-20) International science and technology cooperation research in Henan-015 (152102410030).

References

1. Larosa JH (1988) Third Report of the National Cholesterol Education Program (NCEP) Expert Panel on Detection, Evaluation, and Treatment of High Blood Cholesterol in Adults (Adult Treatment Panel III) final report. Circulation 106: 3143-3421.
2. Abidi P, Zhou Y, Jiang JD, Liu J (2005) Extracellular signal-regulated kinase-dependent stabilization of hepatic low-density lipoprotein receptor mrna by herbal medicine berberine. Arterioscler Thromb Vasc Biol 25: 2170-2176.
3. Choudhary MI, Naheed S, Jalil S, Alam JM, Atta-ur-Rahman (2005) Effects of ethanolic extract of iris germanica on lipid profile of rats fed on a high-fat diet. J Ethnopharmacol 98: 217-220.
4. Wu HY, Bei WJ, Guo J (2009) Chinese herbal medicine for the treatment of dyslipidemia. J Geriatr Cardiol 6: 119-125.
5. Barens DK, Sheaffer C (1995) Alfalfa. Agriculture 2: 205-216.
6. Cheeke PR (2000) Actual and Potential Applications of Yucca Schidigera, and Quillaja Saponaria, Saponins in Human and Animal Nutrition. Saponins in Food, Feedstuffs and Medicinal Plants. Springer, Netherlands 45: 241-254.
7. Malinow MR, Mclaughlin P, Papworth L, Stafford C, Kohler GO, et al. (1977) Effect of alfalfa saponins on intestinal cholesterol absorption in rats. Am J Clin Nutr 30: 2061-2067.
8. Malinow MR, Connor WE, Mclaughlin P, Stafford C, Lin DS, et al. (1981) Cholesterol and bile acid balance in macaca fascicularis. effects of alfalfa saponins. J Clin Invest 67: 156-162.
9. Yu CH, Xie G, He RR, Zhai YJ, Li YF, et al. (2011) Effects of a purified saponin mixture from alfalfa on plasma lipid metabolism in hyperlipidemic mice. J Health Sci 57: 401-405.
10. Gümüs̡ R, İMīK H (2012) Use of saponins as feed additive in animal nutrition. Atatürk Üniversitesi Veteriner Bilimleri Dergisi.
11. Chen PY, Wang JR, Lan-Li SU, Zhao YL, Zhu XF (2014) Research progress on separation of alfalfa saponins and its application in animal production. Chinese Journal of Animal Science.
12. Zhang Y (2006) The physical and chemical characters and biologicalfunctions of alfalfa glycoside. China Feed 4: 37-38.
13. Yin XZ, Tian LI, Wang X (2010) Study on anti-lipid peroxidative effects of soyasapogenols. Science and Technology of Food Industry 31: 143-145.
14. Zhou AR, Cha X (2000) Biochemistry. Beijing: people's medical publishing house pp: 130-377.
15. Sato K, Kamada T (2010) Regulation of bile acid, cholesterol, and fatty acid synthesis in chicken primary hepatocytes by different concentrations of t0901317, an agonist of liver x receptors. Comp Biochem Physiol A Mol Integr Physiol 158: 201-206.
16. Chen Y, Zhou Y, Chen Y, Hao W, Wei Q, et al. (2015) Advances in alfalfa saponin research. Journal of Henan Agricultural Sciences.
17. Yuan DD, Shi YH, Wang CZ, Guo R, Wang J (2013) Effect of alfalfa saponins on cholesterol metabolism and its molecular mechanisms. Acta Prataculturae Sinica 22: 294-301.
18. Ma Z (2014) Effects of diets added with alfalfa on production performance and nutrients digestibility in broiler breedei's. China Feed.
19. Yu YH (1990) Feed toxicology report of toxicology. Beijing: Agricultural Publishing House pp: 16-45.
20. Wang Y, Cheng QM, Cao WX, Xue hua HU, Jiang YM (2005) The effects of the extract mixture of alfalfa and perilla on lowering serum lipid, protecting liver and aortic wall in rats. Parenteral and Enteral Nutrition 12: 219-226.
21. Liu K, Yu S (1999) Effects of alfalfa saponin on rat cholesterol excretion and nitric oxide release from endothelial cells. Acta Academiae Medicinae Xuzhou 19: 442-444.

18

Nutritional Composition of Quail Meatballs and Quail Pickled Eggs

Bayomy HM[1], Rozan MA[1*] and Mohammed GM[2]

[1]*Department of Food Science and Technology, Damanhour University, Egypt*

[2]*Department of Nutrition and food Science, Tabuk University, KSA*

[*]**Corresponding author:** Rozan MA, Department of Food Science and Technology, Damanhour University, Egypt, E-mail: Mahmoud.abdelgalil@agr.dmu.edu.eg

Abstract

The aims of this study were to evaluate the acceptance of meatballs and pickled quail eggs, determine the nutritional composition of the quail pickled eggs and quail meatballs. Data indicate that quail meatballs and pickled quail eggs are an acceptable market product. The quail meatballs have 70.56% moisture content and 29.44% dry matter which include 7.78%, 12.98%, 7.10% and 2.48% in wet basis for total lipids, proteins, ash and carbohydrate, respectively. Total cholesterol content in quail meatballs was 0.087 g/100g. Regarding pickled quail eggs, the values of moisture, dry matter, total lipids, proteins, ash and carbohydrate are 53.32%, 46.68%, 20.09%, 20.38%, 4.70% and 1.51% in wet basis, respectively. Average of cholesterol content in pickled quail eggs is 2.06 g/100 g yolk. Total essential amino acids were 6.17 g/100 g protein in quail meatballs, while total non-essential amino acids were 5.87g/100g protein in quail meatballs. In pickled quail eggs the values of total essential amino acids and non-essential amino acids were 6.84 g/100g and 8.81 g/100g protein, respectively. Total saturated fatty acids (SFAs) in quail meatballs and quail pickled eggs are 26.37% and 37.52%, respectively. Total mono-unsaturated fatty acids and poly-unsaturated fatty acids contents in quail meatballs are 36.61% and 36.21, respectively, while these values for pickled quail eggs are 54.12% and 8.36%, respectively.

Keywords: Quail; Meatballs; Pickled egg; Nutritional composition

Introduction

Poultry meat and their products are consumed in large quantities and the consumption is growing all over the world [1]. Quail products have gained popularity in the last few years by consumers. Quail is belonging to the species *Coturnix coturnix japonica.* It was first domesticated in Japan as a source of both egg and meat after that quail distribution in the wild spreads over large areas of Asia, Europe and Africa, [2]. Quail meat is recommended for the low-fat diet because it contains low amount of fat and cholesterol especially thanks to its thin skin and low fat accumulation between its tissues [3]. Japanese quail meat may be taken into consideration in diet for prevention of heart diseases because of high C18:1 content. The ratio between PUFAs and SFAs was 0.43 in female quail meat and 0.40 in male quail meat. Both ratios are in accordance with the WHO recommendations. Quail eggs have a very interesting chemical composition, being rich in fat soluble vitamins and B-complex; in proteins, amino acids, macro and microelements, but are low in cholesterol [4], triglycerids and saturated fatty acids [5]. Quail eggs used to help treat tuberculosis, asthma, and even diabetes by Chinese. Also quail eggs can help prevent sufferer of liver, kidney or gallbladder stones, and remove these types of stones. Quail eggs have higher nutritional value than those offered by other eggs with they are rich sources of antioxidants, minerals, and vitamins, and give us a lot of nutrition than do other foods [6]. Because of its valuable chemical compositions, quail egg is considered to be a true universal panacea, placed 3rd in the Chinese natural medicine after snake venom and Ginseng [7,8]. The eggs of quail are used in the same manner as those of chickens. Because of their small size and attractive appearance quail eggs are often used for special purposes. Pickled quail eggs are a specialty. Pickles occupy an important place among processed foods. With the increasing popularity of quail *(Coturnix coturnix japonica),* there is a good scope for the utilization of small and tinted quail eggs in the form of pickle. Technological details pertaining to the manufacture of pickled quail eggs have been worked out with a view to offer such nutritious, ready-to-eat product to the consumers.

Quail meat is considered a delicacy. It can be fried or roasted, and many recipes have been developed. Meatballs are a popular meat product in Egypt. This includes products such as chicken meatballs, fish meatballs, beef meatballs; quail meat is also potential raw materials for meatballs production. According to [9] quail meat can be used for the manufacture of meatballs successfully by using different types of flour as an alternative to the use of other meats such as beef and chicken.

Egyptian consumer preferably eats chicken eggs. But quail eggs sold in the form much more restricted, commonly used in the ornamentation of cold dishes or snacks. In recent years, it has become spread the quail eggs consumed by the belief that these do not contain cholesterol or its content is irrelevant and greater value nutritious, belief that has been fueled to some extent by the producers themselves at the lack of information about their composition.

In developed countries continues to drive consumption chicken egg through the development of new egg products are used in various dishes, however quail egg by their different physical characteristics to chicken cannot be used for preparing the same egg products but can be exploited in other presentations. The objective of this work was to evaluate the acceptance of meatballs and pickled quail eggs. Determine the nutritional composition of the quail pickled eggs and quail meatballs.

Materials and Methods

Materials

Quail (*Coturnix coturnix japonica)* carcasses and eggs were collected from the National Center for Agricultural Research in Dokki, Egypt. Other materials were collected from local markets in Damanhour city, Egypt.

Methods

Preparation of Samples

Preparation of pickled quail eggs

According to Indian standard [10] fresh quail eggs stored at ambient temperature for at least 24 salts, for about 10 min at simmering temperature. After boiling, the eggs shall be cooled immediately in running tap water and peeled off manually. There shall be no pieces of egg shell or shell membrane adhering over the peeled eggs. Peeled eggs showing tom or rugged-looking albumen surface shall not be used for pickling. Pickling solution shall consist of vinegar and water (50: 50 vlv), 8% (w/v) common salt, and 2% (wlv) each spice mixture, onion (fresh and chopped), garlic and ginger. The solution shall be boiled for 10 min and then filtered using clean muslin cloth. Pickling solution shall be heated to 70 ± 2°C and poured onto the peeled eggs. Cover the peeled eggs with pickling solution. The pickled eggs shall be aged for 48 hours at ambient temperature in pre-sterilized glass container.

Preparation of meatballs

The quail carcasses were deboned mechanically. The mean carcass weights were 203.04±16.67 g. meatballs blend was prepared using the formula given by [11]. as follows: Meat 90% was mixed into house mincer, flour 3%, fresh onion 3% were peeled and minced before the addition, 2% salt and 2% spices. These ingredients were mixed together, divided to balls to formulate quail meatballs. Samples were freeze stored at -18±2°C. Meatballs cooked before analysis at 95°C for 5 min.

Sensory properties

The sensory properties of consumers were applied for the pickled quail eggs and meatballs. Sixty panelists evaluated the sensory attributes of the quail products. Panelists were given no time limit for the evaluation. Pickled quail eggs and meatballs were cut into small pieces and placed on a plastic plate. The attributes evaluated were color, flavor, texture and overall acceptability. For each sample, panelists scored their liking of these characteristics using a five-point hedonic scale (1 = dislike very much, 2 =dislike slightly, 3 = neither like nor dislike, 4 = like slightly, 5 = like very much) [12].

Analytical Methods

Chemical analysis

Moisture, protein, fat and ash contents were determined in accordance with standard AOAC methods of [13]. Protein determination involved a Kjeldahl assay (Nx6.25). Fat was determined extracting samples in a Folch apparatus using chloroform: Ethanol (2:1 v/v) as a solvent. Moisture was quantified by oven-drying 10 g samples at 100°C overnight. Ash was determined after incineration in a furnace at 500°C and carbohydrate content was calculated by computing the difference. Minerals (Ca; Na; P & Fe) contents were performed by the classical method of chemical analysis [13].

Total cholesterol content

It was determined by the method of Lieberman-Buchart [14].

Amino acid profile

The technique recommended by [15] for fractionation of amino acids was applied by Gas Liquid Chromatography (GLC).

Fatty acid methyl esters analyses

For fat content determination lipids were extracted from 10 g breast by the method described by [16,17]. Five mL chloroform/methanol (2:1 v/v) solution was added to sample and shook thoroughly by vortex for 3 min. One mL of 0.9% NaCl was added to mix and shake again. The chloroform phase containing lipids were collected. Lipid extracts were converted to fatty acid methyl esters as described by [17]. It was prepared after alkaline hydrolysis following procedures. Briefly, lipid extract was mixed with 0.5N 2mL methanolic NaOH and held at 100°C for 10 min. This solution was cooled to room temperature and mixed with 2mL of (14% Boron tri fluoride, 86% Methanol). Then after, solution obtained by adding BF_3 was incubated at 100°C for 2 min and cooled dawn to again room temperature. 1mL n-heptane was added to final solution and thoroughly mixed by vortex for 3min and reheated to 100°C for 1min. Final solution was cooled down to room temperature and centrifuged at 300 rpm for 5 min. Upper layer (heptane phase) was transferred to glass tube for the GC analysis. The final concentration of the Fatty acid methyl esters analyses was approximately 7mg/mL in heptane.

Statistical analysis

The obtained data were statistically analyzed by routine statistical methods by means ± standard deviation of Microsoft Excel software.

Results and Discussion

Sensory properties

Sensory properties was conducted to measure the organoleptic properties of organic, which include color, taste, smell, texture and general acceptance of both meatballs quail and pickled quail eggs. General precautions to taste tests have been taken. Evaluation of sensory properties of quail meatballs and pickled eggs are shown in Table (1). In general, the assessment of panelists indicates moderate likeability, may be due to the fact that the panelists were not very familiar with meatballs made from quail meat. Regarding to pickled product, the data indicate that pickled quail eggs are an acceptable market product.

Data of chemical composition for quail meatballs and pickled quail eggs are presented in Table 2. Results demonstrated that quail meatballs have 70.56% moisture content and 29.44% dry matter which include 7.78%, 12.98%, 7.10% and 2.48% in wet basis for total lipids, proteins, ash and carbohydrate, respectively. These results are agreed with results produced by [9]. They found that quail meatballs have value of 65.94% moisture, 13.53(% wet basis) protein, 10.59 (% wet basis) fat, 2.30(% wet basis) ash and 7.63(% wet basis) carbohydrates. According to [18] the proximate analysis values of quail meatballs are not so different with those of meatballs made from chicken which prepared by [18]. They found that chicken meatballs have 64.33-71.81%, 9.94-15.96 (% wet basis), 4.26-14.00(% wet basis), 1.92-2.82(% wet basis) and 5.54-20.85(% wet basis) for moisture, protein, fat, ash and carbohydrate content, respectively.

Properties	Meatball Quail	Pickled quail egg
Colour	4.7 ± 0.23	4.2 ± 0.51
Taste	4.5 ± 0.35	4.5 ± 0.35
Odour	5.0 ± 0.37	4.0 ± 0.65
Flavour	4.3 ± 0.27	4.3 ± 0.45
Texture	4.3 ± 0.17	4.1 ± 0. 65
Overall acceptability	4.5 ± 0.24	4.2 ± 0.45
The value ± standard deviation (SD)		

Table 1: Sensory properties of quail meatballs and pickled quail egg.

Chemical composition

Chemical composition (g/100 g DW)	Quail meatballs	Pickled quail eggs
Moisture	70.56 ± 2.04	53.32 ± 1.74
Dry matter	29.44 ± 1.63	46.68 ± 0.86
Total lipids	7.78 ± 0.68	20.09 ± 0.85
Cholesterol	0.087 ± 0.005	2.06 ± 0.56 g/100 g yolk
Proteins	12.98 ± 1.03	20.38 ± 2.03
Carbohydrate	6.10 ± 0.74	1.51 ± 0.04
Ash	2.48 ± 0.22	4.70 ± 0.33
Na (mg/kg)	1425.23 ± 21.67	1058.96 ± 7.97
P (mg/kg)	3838.79 ± 18.31	955.19 ± 6.55
Ca (mg/kg)	1448.60 ± 8.08	613.21 ± 1.27
Fe (mg/kg)	36.028 ± 0.17	22.476 ± 0.68
All values are means of triplicate determinations ± standard deviation (SD). DW: Dry Weight; TC: Total Carbohydrates		

Table 2: Chemical composition of quail meatballs and pickled quail egg (g/100 g in wet basis).

According to the results of [19], quail meatballs in Malaysian markets have higher protein content and lower carbohydrate content than various kinds of commercial chicken meatballs, who reported protein and carbohydrate contents ranging from 12.83-13.71% and 5.23-8.25%, respectively. Total cholesterol content in quail meatballs was 0.087 g/100g. This value is agreed with that reported by [20] who found that cholesterol content in quail carcass was 0.097 and 0.094 g/100g for male and female, respectively. It is clear that quail meatballs have high minerals content this may be due to the mixing of soft bone with flesh of quail when manufacturing.

With regard to pickled quail eggs, Table 2 indicated that the values of moisture, dry matter, total lipids, proteins, ash and carbohydrate are 53.32%, 46.68%, 20.09%, 20.38%, 4.70% and 1.51% in wet basis, respectively. Average of cholesterol content in pickled quail eggs is 2.06 g/100 g yolk. [21] found that the proximal composition of quail eggs with a protein content of 13.6 ± 2.1%, total lipids of 12.59 ± 2.2 and 1.13± 0.33% cholesterol in wet basis. [22] reported that the quail eggs have 1.06, 4.01, 9.89, 12.7, and 72.25 g /100g for ash, carbohydrate, fat, protein and moisture, respectively. Tunsaringkarn et al. indicated that the quail egg yolk has a 1.21 ± 0.07 g of cholesterol per 100 g of yolk [23]. According to Bragagnalo et al. [24] the highest cholesterol content was observed in ostrich and duck eggs, whereas the lowest in [23] compared the cholesterol content of Brazilian chicken and quail eggs. They found that the cholesterol level between chicken and quail eggs in terms of yolk were not significant difference. Opposite results were presented by Kaźmierska et al. [25], who reported higher cholesterol content in quail egg yolk (13.6 mg/g) compared to Tunsaringkarn et al. [23].

Amino acids content

Amino acid composition is one of the most important factors to determine the quality of food protein. In general, high protein food is also high in contents of amino acids including eight which are essential in human nutrition: lysine, valine, leucine, isoleucine, threonine, tryptophan, methionine and phenylalanine [26]. Analysis of amino acids (g/100g sample) in quail meatballs and pickled quail eggs are recorded in Table 3.

Essential amino acids were 6.17 g/100 g sample this value equals 47.5% from protein in quail meatballs. Among the essential amino acids lysine has the greatest value (1.63%) of amino acids. lysine is assists in calcium absorption, required for growth and bone development in children, and assists in maintaining the correct nitrogen balance in the body, as well as maintaining lean body mass. Lysine is also needed to produce antibodies, enzymes, collagen formation, hormones, as well as repair of tissue [27]. While total non-essential amino acids was 5.87g/100g sample in quail meatballs. In pickled quail eggs, total essential amino acids and total non- essential amino acids were 6.84 g/100g sample and 8.81 g/100g sample, respectively. The greatest value of amino acids refers to leucine as essential amino acid. Leucine is a branched chain amino acid along with valine and isoleucine. It is beneficial and functional to protein structure for 60-70% in human body, and blood sugar level regulation which maintains a balance of insulin and glucose [28]. It proposed as a promising pharmaconutrient in the prevention and treatment of sarcopenia and/or type 2 diabetes [29]. The "ideal" protein should contain the following concentrations of essential amino acids: lysine – 5.5%, leucine – 7%, isoleucine – 4%, valine – 5%, methionine + cysteine – 3.5%, threonine – 4%, phenylalanine + tyrosine – 6% as reported in FAO/WHO specialists in 1973 [30].

Fatty acids composition

Quail is the good source of both saturated and unsaturated fatty acids. In our studies, we found that quail meatballs and pickled quail eggs used in study contain saturated and unsaturated fatty acids. As shown in Table (4), Palmitic acid (C14:0) is present in higher number in saturated fatty acids with values of up to 20.48% and 28.11% for quail meatballs and pickled quail eggs, respectively. It is similar with results reported by [31]. They found that Palmitic acid (C16:0) was the major fatty acid, followed by stearic acid (C18:0) in female and male quail meats. Myristic acid was in very low concentration in comparison to palmitic and stearic acid. Sum of saturated fatty acids (Σ SFA) in quail meatballs and quail pickled eggs are 26.37% and 37.52%, respectively. Saturated fatty acids play important role in different biological functions like source of metabolic energy and in cell membrane structure formation. Whereas Oleic (C18:1) is present in highest value in all fatty acids. Sum of mono unsaturated fatty acids (Σ MUFA) and Sum of poly unsaturated fatty acids (Σ PUFA) in quail meatballs are 36.61% and 36.21, respectively. While Σ MUFA and Σ PUFA values for pickled quail eggs are 54.12% and 8.36%, respectively. These data are similar with that reported by [32]. He found that Σ MUFA and Σ PUFA values for egg in Pharaoh Japanese quail are 51.3 % and 9.9%, respectively. Generally, bird's meat is relatively rich in the essential Ω-3 α-linolenic fatty acid (C18:3). Our results for α-linolenic acid content in quail meatballs and pickled quail eggs are 23.6% and 5.36%, respectively and higher than to those of [33] who reported that content of α-linolenic acid was 1.74% in chicken meat. The α-linolenic acid content in the meat of the different duck populations varies in a wider range – 0.8-1.62% [34].

Amino acids	Quail meatballs	Pickled quail eggs
Essential amino acids		
Lysine	1.63 ± 0.41	1.36 ± 0.16
	1.63 ± 0.41	1.36 ± 0.16
Methionine	0.48 ± 0.08	0.78 ± 0.03
Leucine	0.89 ± 0.17	1.47 ± 0.09
Isoleucine	0.97 ± 0.03	0.77 ± 0.02
Phenylalanine	0.94 ± 0.08	0.81 ± 0.08
Threonine	0.47 ± 0.24	0.71 ± 0.03
Valine	0.79 ± 0.16	0.94 ± 0.12
Σ essential amino acids	6.17	6.84
Non-essential amino acids		
Cysteine	0.12 ± 0.01	0.83 ± 0.06
Tyrosine	0.43 ± 0.06	0.51 ± 0.04
Histidine	0.62 ± 0.11	0.47 ± 0.02
Arginine	0.51 ± 0.09	0.47 ± 0.04
Glycine	0.64 ± 0.15	0.51 ± 0.07
Glutamic acids	1.02 ± 0.28	2.02 ± 0.04
Serine	0.38 ± 0.06	1.41 ± 0.07
Alanine	0.59 ± 0.13	0.73 ± 0.05
Proline	0.51 ± 0.03	0.60 ± 0.07
Asparatic acids	1.05 ± 0.06	1.26 ± 0.03
Σ Non-essential amino acids	5.87	8.81

All values are means of triplicate determinations ± standard deviation (SD)

Table 3: Amino acids content in quail meatballs and pickled quail eggs %.

Sample Fatty acid	Quail meatballs	Pickled quail eggs
Myristic (C14:0)	0.95 ± 0.06	0.79 ± 0.07
Myristoleic (C14:1)	1.15 ± 0.06	6.29 ± 0.51
Palmitic (C16:0)	20.42 ± 0.34	28.11 ± 0.62
Palmitoleic (C16:1)	0.46 ± 0.03	2.60 ± 0.04
Stearic (C18:0)	5.00 ± 0.08	8.62 ± 0.11
Oleic (C18:1)	35.80 ± 0.74	45.23 ± 0.65
Linoleic (C18:2)	23.62 ± 0.05	5.36 ± 0.04
γ-Linolenic (C18:3)	3.16 ± 0.02	2.27 ± 0.13
Eicosapentaenoic acid (C20:5)	9.43 ± 0.28	0.73 ± 0.07
Σ SFA	26.37	37.52
Σ MUFA	36.61	54.12
Σ PUFA	36.21	8.36

All values are means of triplicate determinations ± standard deviation (SD)

Table 4: Fatty acid content (%) of quail meatballs and pickled quail eggs (%) from total lipids.

Wolaszyn et al. [35] reported that Quail eggs have lower content of polyunsaturated fatty acid (25.1%) than chicken eggs (31.3%) and higher concentration of monounsaturated fatty acid in yolk (45%) compared to chicken eggs (39.1%). The total concentration of saturated fatty acid in yolk was similar in both species.

Conclusion

Quail meatballs and pickled quail eggs are an acceptable market product, have a very interesting chemical composition. Quail meatballs have high concentration of protein content, lower carbohydrate content and high minerals content. Sum of essential amino acids in quail meatballs was 6.17 g/100 g sample this value equals 47.5% from protein, while in pickled quail eggs total essential amino acids and was 6.84 g/100g sample which represents 33.56% from protein content in pickled egg. Sum of saturated fatty acids (Σ SFA) in quail meatballs and quail pickled eggs are 26.37% and 37.52%, respectively. So we should transfer knowledge to people for good nutrient benefits of quail eggs as good nutritional foods and may be the alternative resolving problem of people in some or all nutritional nutrients necessary for human health in developing countries.

Acknowledgements

The authors gratefully acknowledge National Center for Agricultural Research in Dokki, Egypt for providing necessary facilities for the successful completion of this research work.

References

1. Mielnik MB, Aaby K, Rolfsen K, Ellekjær MR, Nilsson A (2002) Quality of comminuted sausages formulated from mechanically deboned poultry meat. Meat Sci 61: 73-84.
2. Mizutani M (2003) The Japanese Quail. Laboratory Animal Research Station, Nippon Institute for Biological Science, Kobuchizawa, Yamanashi, Japan.
3. Alarslan OF (2006) Modern quail manufacturing and basic nutrition principles.
4. Teuşan A, Prelipcean A, Teuşan V (2011) Research regarding the structure, chemical composition and caloricity of quail eggs (Coturnix coturnix japonica), deposited at the beginning phase of lying.
5. Vacaru-Opriş I (2002) Poultry treaty. Publisher Ceres: Bucharest.
6. Lalwani P (2011) Quail Egg Nutrition.
7. Polen T, Erman V (2007) Tips about raising quail, Rev. Collection Farm Publishing World press: Timisoara.
8. Teuşan (Prelipcean) Anca (2010) Contributions to the knowledge qualities hatching quail eggs (Coturnix coturnix japonica) and embryonic development in this species.
9. Ikhlas B, Huda N, Noryati I (2011) Chemical composition and physicochemical properties of meatballs prepared from mechanically deboned quail meat using various types of flour. Int J Poult Sci 10: 30-37.
10. Indian Standard (1988) Poultry Products-Pickled Quail Eggs.
11. Youssef MH (1972) Meat Cooling, Storage, Preservation and Industry. Agriculture Ministry, General Management for Veterinary Laboratories and Researches.
12. Hoang DN (2008) Sensory evaluation of food. Ho Chi Minh City University of technology Press. Ho Chi Minh City (in Vietnamese).
13. AOAC (2002) Official Methods of Analysis of the Association of Official Analytical Chemists (14th Rew edn.). Washington, DC, USA.
14. Carmo BM (2005) Lipid Extraction and Cholesterol Quantification: A Simple Protocol. Journal Chemical Education 82: 103-104.
15. Mabbott AG (1990) Qualitative amino acid analysis of small peptide by GC/MS. J Chem Educ 67: 441-445.
16. Folch JM, Lees M, Stanley GHS (1957) A simple method for the isolation and purification of total lipids from animal tissues. J Biol Chem 226: 497-509.
17. AOAC (1995) Official Methods of Analysis of the Association of Official Analytical Chemists (16th edn.). Washington, DC, USA.
18. Huda N, Yap HS, Yong LH (2009) Proximate composition, color, textural profile of Malaysian chicken balls. Pak J Nutr 8: 1555-1558.
19. Huda N, Shen YH, Huey YL, Ahmad R, Mardiah A (2010) Evaluation of physico-chemical properties of Malaysian commercial beef meatballs. Am J Food Tech 5: 13-21.
20. Genchev A, Mihaylova G, Ribarski S, Pavlov A, Kabakchiev M (2008) Meat quality and composition in Japanese quails. Trakia J Sci 6: 72-82.
21. Fernando GS, Aideé HU (2011) Sensory evaluation of pickled quail eggs and nutritional composition. Veterinary Journal Magazine.
22. Tunsaringkarn T, Tungjaroenchai W, Siriwong W (2012) Nutrient benefits of quail (Coturnix Coturnix Japonica) Eggs. Ann Food Sci Technol 13: 122-131.
23. Bragagnalo N, Rodriguez-Amaya DB (2003) Comparison of the cholesterol content of Brazilian chicken and quail eggs. J Food Comp Anal 16: 147-153.
24. Kaźmierska M, Jarosz B, Korzeniowska M, Trziszka T, Dobrzański Z (2005) Comparative analysis of fatty acid profile and cholesterol content of egg yolks of different bird species. Pol J Food Nutr Sci 55: 69-73.
25. Sinanoglou VJ, Strati IF, Miniadis-Meimaroglou S (2011) Lipid, fatty acid and carotenoid content of edible egg yolks from avian species: A comparative study. Food Chem 124: 971-977.
26. Kim BH, Lee HS, Jang YA, Lee JY, Cho YJ, et al. (2009) Development of amino acid composition database for Korean foods. J Food Comp Anal 22: 44-45.
27. Vitalhealthzone (2007) Lysine amino acid.
28. Khan S (2012) Leucine Structure.
29. Van Loon LJ (2012) Leucine as a pharmaconutrient in health and disease. 15: 71-77.
30. Ribarova F, Shishkov S, Baklova I (1987) Amino acid content of the Bulgarian foodstuffs.
31. Gecgel U, Yilmaz I, Gurcan EK, Karasu S, Dulger GC (2015) Comparison of fatty acid composition between female and male japanese quail meats. J Chem 2015: 1-8
32. Genchev A (2012) Quality and composition of Japanese quail eggs (Coturnix japonica). 10: 91-101.
33. Rondia P, Delmotte C, Maene D, Blecker C, Toussaint JF, et al. (2003) Effect of the inclusion time of extruded linseed supplementation before slaughter on n-3 fatty acids enrichment of chicken meat. Proceeding of the XVIth European Symposium on the Quality of Poultry Meat, Saint-Brieuc, France.
34. Wolaszyn J, Ksiazkiewicz J, Orkusz A, Skrabka-Blotnicka T, Biernat J, et al. (2003) Fatty acid profile of lipids from duck muscles of three polish conservative flocks. Proceeding of the XVIth European Symposium on the Quality of Poultry Meat, 23-26 September 2003, Saint-Brieuc, France.
35. Polat ES, Citil OB, Garip M (2013) Fatty acid composition of yolk of nine poultry species kept in their natural environment. Anim Sci Pap Rep 31: 363-368.

Effect of Nutrition Education and Dietary Modification on the Health Status of Kindergarten Children

Debnath M* **and Agrawal S**

[1]*Sports Authority of India, Netaji Subash Eastern Centre, Salt Lake, Kolkata, India*

[2]*Department of Food and Nutrition, Bajbaj College, Kolkata, India*

***Corresponding author:** Debnath M, Research Fellow, Sports Authority of India, Netaji Subash Eastern Centre, Salt Lake, Kolkata, India, E-mail: monalisadebnath1108@gmail.com

Abstract

Objective: To assess the effect of nutrition education and dietary modification on the health and nutritional status of kindergarten children.

Study design: A prospective case-control study was executed on 104 kindergarten children bifurcated 50 cases and 54 controls. Intervention: After anthropometrically segregating the KG children of both the groups, first primary data including socio-demographic, clinical and dietary assessments were noted using observation and interview method. Later, 45 minutes of nutrition education and dietary modification workshop 5 days a week were intervened among the cases of group A for a month whereas the controls were kept on casual daily routine. After one month of follow-up, the second primary data including the anthropometric and dietary changes among both the groups were noted and compared with the initial findings.

Analysis: Obtained results were statistically analyzed using paired T test.

Result: Number of cases taking optimal nutritional intake increased by 74% after the trial period of one month. There was a significant increase in the anthropometric status of the cases particularly height and chest circumference whereas no remarkable increase has been noted among the controls.

Conclusion: Nutrition education and optimal dietary changes showed improved health status of the kindergarten children in comparison to the controls which can further up-regulate their growth and development. Main outcome measure: Providing nutrition education to students at a young age would be beneficial for improving their nutritional status for lifelong.

Keywords: Health; Nutrition; Malnutrition; Nutrition education; Dietary modi ication

Introduction

Kindergarten years are considered as a pivotal phase for growth and development of the children that affects future learning as well as physical, mental and emotional health persisting throughout life [1-3]. A child being highly sensitive and least protected from the adverse living circumstances, is found more susceptible to diseased conditions and morbidity [4-6]. Hence, it is very important to build a strong health profile right from early years of life through adequate dietary intervention and addressing good food habits which will serve throughout protecting the body from broad spectrum of health hazards [7].

Health is affected by many predisposing factors, including-gender, family size, socio-economic status, residential condition, parental education, working status, nutritional knowledge of mothers, food availability, physical activity, social environment etc. [8]. Parental education is one of the important factors relating to childhood nutrition [9].

Fathers being the main earner and decision maker of the family, their higher education play an important role in ensuring better nutritional status of the children [10]. Physical activity (PA) is a reliable factor for the modulation of health status as the frequency or time incorporated in it is associated with number of positive mental and physical health outcomes and prevents weight gain among children as well [11-15].

Altered nutritional uptake or deviation from the standardized dietary allowances may lead to health disturbances, commonly termed as malnutrition which includes both obesity and under nutrition. There has been notable increase in the prevalence of overweight and obesity in the developing countries [16]. It is observed that approximately 10% of the schools going children are overweight as an outcome of unhealthy dietary habits that may further leave detrimental effects on their health status [17,18].

This further contributes to early onset of diseases of adulthood such as Type 2 Diabetes, arterial hypertension etc. [19]. Inadequate maternal and child caring practices, food insecurity and unhealthy environment are also the underlying causes aggravating the condition [20]. Malnutrition on the other hand has long-lasting effects on children's health and therefore should be properly checked through nutritionally adequate diets and optimal eating pattern [21].

Anthropometric assessments commonly introduced for determining the nutritional status of a child include height, weight, body mass index (BMI), head circumference (HC), chest circumference (CC), mid-upper arm circumference (MUAC), skinfold thickness etc. [22]. Weight for height is considered as the most appropriate and reliable indicator of growth as it reflects wasting that may persist as a result of malnutrition or other predisposing factors like diarrhea, malaria etc. [23]. MUAC is often used as an efficient indicator of nutritional status as it is influenced by recurrent change in weight. The key dependent variable is BMI, increase of which denotes obesity whereas starving body denotes malnutrition [24].

Nutrition education is attracting ample of interest and concern for curbing health problems during childhood, but it is yet to be incorporated in the school curriculum nationwide [25]. Our study was executed with an objective to assess the effect of nutrition education on the nutritional intake and health status of kindergarten children.

Method and Materials

To obtain a homogenous group of children for the case-control study, two branches of the school-Sri Aurobindo institution, Barrackpore, West Bengal were selected. Following random sampling method, a gross total of 104 kindergarten children of age range of 3-6 years were enrolled as study subjects for the research work for a study period of 2 months. Following the inclusion and exclusion criteria as mentioned in the study protocol (Figure 1), 50 KG children from the main branch termed as group A and 54 KG children from the supporting branch termed as group B were treated as cases and controls respectively. Inclusion criteria constituted children of the respective age range, regular comers to the school while exclusion criteria included child with any serious health problem or suffering from chronic disease, not able to attend regular classes and physically/ mentally handicapped.

The study protocol was checked and approved for standardization and authentication before further proceedings. The questionnaire to be filled was standardized by the authorities of the Department, BRSN College (WBSU). Parents of all the subjects were required to submit a written informed consent and a pre-formed questionnaire including socio-demographic information were needed to be filled by them prior to participation.

All 104 KG students of both the groups were assessed anthropometrically to segregate the samples into healthy and malnourished ones following WHO scaling. Observation and interview method were followed using a semi-structured questionnaire containing all the concerned parameters to be noted viz. socio-demographic status, anthropometric assessment, dietary assessment and visible clinical symptoms. Following the rating of socio-economic status in accordance to Kuppuswami's scale, children of both the groups were further categorized under low, high or middle classes. For anthropometric assessment, height, weight, mid-upper arm circumference (MUAC), head circumference and chest circumference of the kindergarten children were noted, belonging to both the case (group A) and control (group B) categories.

Body weight was measured using portable weighing machine, height using an anthropometer; and MUAC, head circumference and chest circumference using a measuring tape. Dietary assessment was done using interview scheduled questionnaire following dietary recall method. Visible clinical symptoms or health problems were noted among the children. After collection of the primary data, nutrition education and dietary modification were intervened among group A whereas; rest 54 KG students of group B were kept as control. The nutrition education program was continued for a month consisting of 45 min nutrition education class five days a week.

The nutritional education program was executed in accordance to provide children with information on diet and nutrition, with the aim of forming healthy dietary habits. The information was taught using learning-through play teaching methods, including posters, demo models, placards, games, group games and children's stories. Concerned care and priorities was given to the children's interaction, interest and participation during trial period, with an aim to establish a distinctive and dynamic educational process. Every child in the case group was provided with an individual dietary recommendation for daily food intake in accordance to RDA and even distribution of five food groups in their platter. Children were observed under strict supervision during the nutrition education session. After a month of follow-up, the kindergarten students were assessed to note the anthropometric and dietary differences in the cases (group A) and controls (group B). After data collection, the results expressed as mean ± SD were statistically analyzed using paired t test and the effect of nutrition program on health status of cases to that controls were drawn eventually.

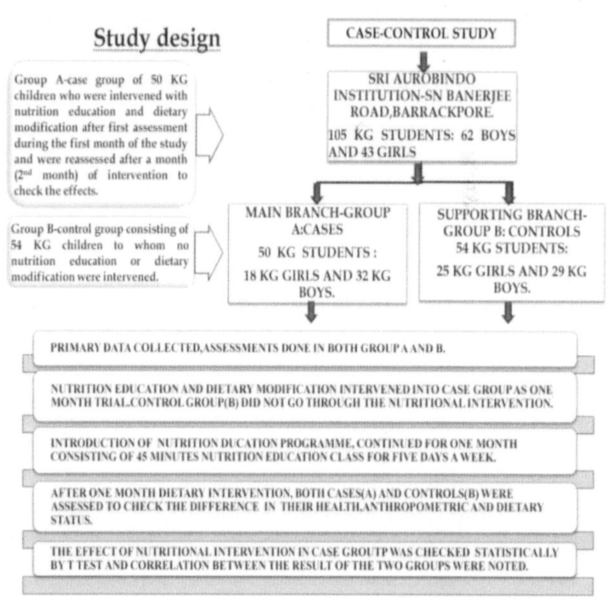

Figure 1: Study protocol.

Result

The segregation of the study population through random sampling method resulted in case groups with 50 kindergarten children-18 girls and 32 boys; and control groups with 54 kindergarten children-25 girls and 29 boys, all belonging to the age range of 3-6 years with no severe occurrence of diseases or deformity as followed by the inclusion and exclusion criteria's. As mentioned in Table 1, Kuppuswami's scaling was used for the categorization of children according to the socioeconomic class which depicted that maximum child of group A belonged to upper middle class whereas moreover equal proportion of children of group B belonged to upper and upper middle class groups.

Table 2 shows the frequency of physical activity (PA) performed by the children of case and control groups. The time incorporated into PA was observed to be elevated among the case groups after nutrition education session. After the trial period about 80% of the children were found to do regular physical activity in the form of outdoor games or co-curricular activities as performed in schools whereas, the time spent by the control groups before and after the study period was same as no knowledge about physical education was delivered to them.

Group			**Upper Class**		**Upper Middle Class**		**Lower Middle Class**	
			No. of Students	**Percentage (%)**	**No. of Students**	**Percentage (%)**	**No. of Students**	**Percentage (%)**
A (n=50)	**Male**	**Female**	16	32	24	48	10	20
	32	18						
B (n=54)	29	25	23	43	21	39	10	18

Table 1: Categorization of students according to the scoring of Kuppuswami's scale.

Group A (n=50)									
Gender	**Month**	**Daily**		**Alternate Days**		**Weekends**		**Seldom**	
		No. of Students	**Percentage (%)**	**No. of Students**	**Percentage (%)**	**No. of Students**	**Percentage (%)**	**No. of Students**	**Percentage (%)**
Male (n=32)	1st	3	9.37	5	15.63	11	34.38	13	40.63
	2nd	16	50	7	21.88	6	18.75	3	9.38
Female (n=18)	1st	2	11.12	2	11.12	8	44.45	6	33.34
	2nd	8	44.45	5	27.78	3	16.67	2	11.12
Group B (n=54)									
Gender	**Month**	**Daily**		**Alternate Days**		**Weekends**		**Seldom**	
		No. of Students	**Percentage (%)**	**No. of Students**	**Percentage (%)**	**No. of Students**	**Percentage (%)**	**No. of Students**	**Percentage (%)**
Male (n=29)	1st	6	20.69	5	17.24	8	27.58	10	34.48
	2nd	6	20.69	5	17.24	8	27.58	10	34.48
Female (n=25)	1st	4	16	2	8	11	44	8	32
	2nd	4	16	2	8	11	44	8	32

Table 2: Categorization of students according to the frequency of physical activity performed.

Group A (n=50)							
Gender		**Near about RDA**		**Less than RDA**		**More than RDA**	
		No. of Students	**Percentage (%)**	**No. of Students**	**Percentage (%)**	**No. of Students**	**Percentage (%)**
Male (n=32)	Before	15	46.87	11	34.37	6	18.75
	After	23	71.87	5	15.63	4	12.5
Female (n=18)	Before	9	50	5	27.78	4	22.23
	After	13	72.23	2	11.12	3	16.67
Group B (n=54)							

Gender	Month	Near about RDA		Less than RDA		More than RDA	
		No. of Students	Percentage (%)	No. of Students	Percentage (%)	No. of Students	Percentage (%)
Male (n=29)	Before	14	48.27	10	34.48	5	17.24
	After	12	41.38	13	44.83	4	13.79
Female (n=25)	Before	11	44	7	28	7	28
	After	9	36	7	28	9	36

Table 3: Categorization of students according to their daily calorie consumption.

Table 3 shows the daily calorie consumption by the cases and controls. It was found that merely 47% of the cases were taking optimal calorie intake daily, which hiked up to 72% after nutrition education session. Children taking less and more than the RDA nearly reduced to half whereas, among the controls there was no such significant increase in the number of children taking optimal dietary intake after the study period.

Tables 4 and 5 reveal the assessments of anthropometric status of the cases. The mean height before intervention was 100.74 ± 5.64 cm which increased to 102.26 ± 5.62 cm (P value <0.05***) after the follow up. The BMI as observed before and after the nutrition education session falls on normal range as provided by WHO. The head circumference before (49.20 ± 1.23) and after (49.80 ± 1.16) nutrition intervention have revealed significant improvement (P value <0.05***). There was remarkable net increase in 0.22 cm in the chest circumference after the session (P value <0.05***).

Tables 6 and 7 shows the anthropometric assessments of the controls evaluated prior and later to the trial period. It was found that no such significant improvement was noticed in the anthropometric parameters. Previously done research studies have evaluated better improvement in Weight-for-age to that of height-for-age through nutrition education [26]. On contrary Sneha et al. documented significant difference in the height after nutrition education program along with marginal difference in weight and BMI [27].

Anthropometric Parameters Assessed among Cases (group A, n=50)			Mean ± SD	Std. Error Mean (SEM)	Correlation
Pair 1	Height (cm)	Before	100.74 ± 5.64	0.79	0.991
		After	102.26 ± 5.62	0.79	
Pair 2	Weight (Kg)	Before	15.70 ± 3.00	0.42	0.978
		After	16.61 ± 3.11	0.44	
Pair 3	Body Mass Index (BMI, Kg/m)	Before	15.43 ± 2.38	0.33	0.967
		After	15.82 ± 2.41	0.34	
Pair 4	Head Circumference (HC, cm)	Before	49.20 ± 1.23	0.17	0.874
		After	49.80 ± 1.16	0.16	
Pair 5	Chest Circumference (CC, cm)	Before	52.26 ± 3.26	0.46	0.964
		After	53.48 ± 3.54	0.50	
Pair 6	Mid-Upper Arm Circumference (MUAC, cm)	Before	15.72 ± 1.77	0.25	0.887
		After	17.18 ± 1.63	0.23	

Table 4: Comparison of anthropometric status of case group before and after nutrition education and dietary modification.

Anthropometric Parameters Assessed among Cases (Group A, n=50)		Paired Differences						
		Mean ± SD	Std. Error Mean	95% Confidence Interval of the Difference		t test (two-tailed)	Df	Significance Level (P value)
				Lower	Upper			
Pair 1	Height: Before-After	-1.52 ± 0.74	0.10	-1.7328	-1.3072	-14.35	49	P value <0.05***
Pair 2	Weight: Before-After	-0.912 ± 0.65	0.09	-1.0989	-0.7251	-9.8	49	P value <0.05***

Pair 3	BMI: Before-After	-0.38 ± 0.61	0.08	-0.5624	-0.21	-4.4	49	P value <0.05***
Pair 4	Head Circumference: Before-After	-0.60 ± 0.60	0.08	-0.7723	-0.4278	-7	49	P value <0.05***
Pair 5	Chest Circumference: Before-After	-1.22 ± 0.95	0.13	-1.4926	-0.9474	-8.99	49	P value <0.05***
Pair 6	MUAC: Before-After	-1.46 ± 0.81	0.11	-1.6929	-1.2271	-12.59	49	P value <0.05***
Values are expressed as mean ± SD, *=P value <0.0, **=P value <0.001, ***P value <0.0001 (at 95% confidence interval), t=Paired t test, two tailed, p<0.05=Significant								

Table 5: Comparative analysis of the anthropometric status of the case group before and after nutrition education and dietary modification using paired t test.

Anthropometric Parameters Assessed among Controls (Group B, n=54)			Mean ± SD	Std. Error Mean (SEM)	Correlation
Pair 1	Height (cm)	Before	108.49 ± 7.76	1.05	0.995
		After	109.49 ± 7.73	1.05	
Pair 2	Weight (Kg)	Before	17.96 ± 3.99	0.54	0.986
		After	18.67 ± 4.13	0.56	
Pair 3	Body Mass Index (BMI, Kg/m^2)	Before	15.17 ± 1.91	0.26	0.920
		After	15.49 ± 1.95	0.26	
Pair 4	Head Circumference (HC, cm)	Before	49.50 ± 1.71	0.23	0.948
		After	49.78 ± 1.58	0.21	
Pair 5	Chest Circumference (CC, cm)	Before	49.50 ± 1.71	0.23	0.948
		After	49.781.58	0.21	
Pair 6	Mid-Upper Arm Circumference (MUAC, cm)	Before	16.09 ± 1.87	0.25	0.953
		After	17.59 ± 1.81	0.24	
Values are expressed as mean ± SD, *=P value <0.0, **=P value <0.001, ***P value <0.0001 (at 95% confidence interval), t=Paired t test, two tailed, p<0.05=Significant					

Table 6: Comparison of anthropometric status of control group before and after nutrition education and dietary modification.

Anthropometric Parameters Assessed among Controls (Group B, n=54)		Paired Differences						
		Mean ± SD	Std. Error Mean	95% Confidence Interval of the Difference		t test (Two-tailed)	Df	Significance level (P value)
				Lower	Upper			
Pair 1	Height: Before-After	-1.00 ± 0.75	0.10	-1.2071	-0.7929	-9.687	53	P value <0.05***
Pair 2	Weight: Before-After	-0.70 ± 0.68	0.09	-0.8921	-0.519	-7.587	53	P value <0.05***
Pair 3	BMI: Before-After	-0.32 ± 0.77	0.10	-0.537	-0.1148	-3.097	53	P value <0.05**
Pair 4	Head Circumference: Before-After	-0.28 ± 0.54	0.07	-0.4361	-0.138	-3.863	53	P value <0.05***
Pair 5	Chest Circumference: Before-After	-0.28 ± 0.54	0.07	-0.4361	-0.138	-3.863	53	P value <0.05***

Pair 6	MUAC: Before-After	-1.50 ± 0.56	0.07	-1.6546	-1.3454	-19.463	53	P value <0.05***
Values are expressed as mean ± SD, *=P value <0.0, **=P value <0.001, ***P value <0.0001 (at 95% confidence interval), t=Paired t test, two tailed, p<0.05=Significant								

Table 7: Comparative analysis of the anthropometric status of the control group before and after nutrition education and dietary modification using paired t test.

Final Anthropometric Reading Taken at 2nd Month of Study (Equal Variances Not Assumed)	t test for Equality of Means						
	t test (Two-tailed)	Df	Sig. Level (P value)	Mean Difference	Std. Error Difference	95% Confidence Interval of the Difference	
						Lower	Upper
Final height	-5.481	96.687	0.000	-7.23074	1.31929	-9.84927	-4.61221
Final weight	-2.883	98.017	0.005	-2.06022	0.71463	-3.47839	-0.64206
Final BMI	0.751	94.486	0.454	0.32547	0.43328	-0.53476	1.18569
Final HC	0.048	96.883	0.962	0.01296	0.27146	-0.52581	0.55174
Final CC	6.770	66.823	0.000	3.69296	0.54549	2.60411	4.78182
Final MUAC	-1.219	101.918	0.226	-0.41259	0.33850	-1.08400	0.25882

Table 8: Statistical analysis to compare the anthropometric results of case and control groups using t test.

Discussion

It was found that one month trial of dietary modification and nutrition intervention among the case group had a positive effect on the health condition and nutrition profile in comparison to that of the control group. These improvements in the quality of nutrition despite of short duration interventional process have been highlighted by other researchers too [28]. It was observed that prescribing RDA to the children shifted the underweight ones to the normal groups within a month. Alike our results, previously done research have also observed significant increase in the number of meals taken per day [29]. The consumption of junk food was curbed to the threshold levels by giving nutrition education and personalized daily dietary intake format to every children of the case group. Children were observed to have more hygiene concerns with neat and clean attire during the second assessments done after the one month trial period. Similar results to that of our study have been obtained by several researchers mentioning significant reduction in the number of subjects who were underweight and wasted after intervention program. An evidential increase in the Levels of serum proteins, calcium and Vitamin D after intervention has also been notified by many [30]. An experimental study done by Ayesha et al. came up with a primary outcome of decreased severity of wasting and changes in the feeding habits as well [29].

There was no change found in the control group concerning the anthropometric and dietary status as assessed after the interventional period of month signifying the reason being no dietary modification or nutrition education was implemented on them. The numbers of subjects under the normal, overweight and underweight category were the same during the second assessment as before. There was no increase in the frequencies PA among them. It has been found that very few kindergarten children engage in physical activities daily whereas the current PA guidelines recommends 180 min of PA per day [30,31]. The meal frequency, dietary pattern, calorie consumption, frequency of milk consumption, distribution of other food groups in their diet remained unaltered during the second month of evaluation.

Understanding the feeding attitudes and behavior of children is important in terms of child health. Environmental factors play an important role in children's dietary profiles and parents should receive guidance on what foods should be given at home [32]. For nutrition programs to be successful, it is essential to have adequate time, adequate knowledge transfer, appropriate resources, and suitable educational materials and teacher training [33]. School Environment, social and physical environments including schools' can directly and indirectly affect health beliefs and behaviors [34]. Many studies introduced previously reveals that dietary habits opted by the children after nutrition education along with subjecting them to psycho-educational games and conducting summer camps have seem to enhance their nutritional profile [35-44]. On contrary, many nutrition research works have found no significant differences in the dietary habits of the children before and after the nutritional intervention program [45-52].

Conclusion

There comes a broad inference with the result of the study in accordance to the dietary modification being made and nutrition education being delivered to the case group keeping the controls as a constant. As found in the literature, use of information that is developmentally appropriate impacts the subjects' ability to gain knowledge and skills needed for implementation of behavior change. Helping subjects to increase their nutrition knowledge better enables them to adopt and follow the Dietary Guidelines, improving overall health and promoting academic achievement. Reinforcement of the lessons presented is important to help the children make informed choices about foods and nutrition. Incorporating nutrition lessons into the school curricula would provide increased knowledge about healthful choices for the students. Providing nutrition education to students at a young age would be beneficial in helping the students make lifelong changes.

Implications for Research and Practice

The results as obtained can be utilized further for extensive research to analysis how varied nutritional intervention can affect the overall growth and development of the kindergarten children and the study can be extended to a discrete level so as to observe the effect of individual nutrient modification on specific body function.

References

1. Hertzman C (2013) The significance of early childhood adversity. Paediatr Child Health 18: 127-128.
2. Boivin M, Hertzman C (2014) Early childhood development: adverse experiences and developmental health. Royal Society of Canada. Canadian Academy of Health Sciences Expert Panel pp: 267-272.
3. McCain MN, Mustard JF, Mc Cuaig K (2013) Early years study: making decisions, taking action. Margaret & Wallace McCain Family Foundation pp: 122-126.
4. McCain MN, Mustard JF, Shanker S (2013) Council for Early; Early years study 2: putting science into action. Child Dev pp: 146-148.
5. Marmot M (2011) Fair London. Strategic review of health inequalities in England post-2010. Available Society, Healthy Lives pp: 98-102.
6. Shonkoff JP, Garner AS (2012) Committee on Psychosocial Aspects of Child and Family Health; Committee on Early Childhood, Adoption, and Dependent Care; Section on Developmental and Behavioral Pediatrics (2012) The lifelong effects of early childhood adversity and toxic stress. Pediatrics 129: e232-e246.
7. Marmot M, Friel S, Bell R, Houweling TAJ, Taylor S (2008) Closing the gap in a generation: health equity through action on the social determinants of health. Commission on Social Determinants of Health 372: 66-69.
8. Mahgoub SEO, Nnyepi M, Bandeke T (2006) Factors affecting prevalence of malnutrition among children under three years of age in Botswana. Afr J Food Agric Nutr Dev 6: 15.
9. Rahman M, Mostofa G, Nasrin SO (2009) Nutritional status among children aged 24-59 months in rural Bangladesh: an assessment measured by BMI index. Internet J Biol Anthropol 3: 10.
10. Rayhan MI, Khan MSH (2006) Factors causing malnutrition among under five children in Bangladesh. Pak J Nutr 5: 558-562.
11. Timmons BW, Leblanc AG, Carson V, Connor Gorber S, Dillman C, et al. (2012) Systematic review of physical activity and health in the early years (aged 0–4 years). Appl Physiol Nutr Metab 37: 773-792.
12. Timmons BW, Naylor PJ, Pfeiffer KA (2007) Physical activity for preschool children–how much and how? Can J Public Health 2: S122-S134.
13. Reilly JJ, Jackson DM, Montgomery C, Kelly LA, Slater C, et al. (2004) Total energy expenditure and physical activity in young Scottish children: mixed longitudinal study. Lancet 363: 211-212.
14. Jones RA, Hinkley T, Okely AD, Salmon J (2013) Tracking physical activity and sedentary behavior in childhood: a systematic review. Am J Prev Med 44: 651-658.
15. Hills AP, Andersen LB, Byrne NM (2011) Physical activity and obesity in children. Br J Sports Med 45: 866-870.
16. Lobstein T, Frelut ML (2003) Prevalence of overweight among children in Europe. Obes Rev 4: 195-200.
17. Wang Y, Monteiro C, Popkin BM (2002) Trends of obesity and underweight in older children and adolescents in the United States, Brazil, China, and Russia. Am J Clin Nutr 75: 971-977.
18. Lobstein T, Baur L, Uauy R (2004) Obesity in children and young people: a crisis in public health. Obes Rev 5: 4-85.
19. Falcão-Gomes RC, Coelho AA, Schimitz BA (2006) Evaluation studies of the characterization of the food intake of preschool. Rev Nutr 19: 713-727.
20. UNICEF (1998) The state of the world's children. Focus on nutrition. Oxford University Press, New York.
21. Schroeder DG (2001) Nutrition and health in developing countries. In: Semba RD, Bloem MW (eds.) Humana Press, Totowa, New Jersey, USA.
22. WHO (1995) Physical status: the use and interpretation of anthropometry. Report of a WHO Expert Committee. World Health Organ Tech Rep Ser 854: 1-452.
23. De Onis M (2001) Child growth and development. Humana Press Inc. Totowa, New Jersey pp: 71-91.
24. Ludwig DS (2007) Childhood obesity–the shape of things to come. N Engl J Med 357: 2325-2327.
25. Perez-Escamilla R, Haldeman L, Gray S (2002) Assessment of nutrition education needs in an urban school district in Connecticut: Establishing priorities through research. J Amer Dietetic Assoc 102: 559-562.
26. Walsh CM, Dannhauser A (2002) The impact of a nutrition education programme on the anthropometric nutritional status of low-income children in South Africa. Public Health Nutr 5: 3-9.
27. Prakash AS, Rupali S (2015) Effect of Nutrition Education Program on Anthropometric Measurements of Adolescent Girls (16-19 Years). IJAR 5: 217-219.
28. Fernandes PS, Bernardo CDO, Campos RMMB, de Vasconcelos FDAG (2009) Evaluating the effect of nutritional education on the prevalence of overweight/obesity and on foods eaten at primary schools. J Pediatr (Rio J) 85: 315-321.
29. Zahid KA, Ghazala R, Haneen Q, Salma HB (2013) A Nutrition Education Intervention to Combat Undernutrition: Experience from a Developing Country. Human Development Programme 2013: 1-7.
30. Sloney S, Sonika S (2015) Impact of nutrition counselling on the anthropometric and biochemical profile of lactose intolerant children. Int J Food Sci Nutr 4: 198-202.
31. Hinkley T, Salmon J, Okely AD, Crawford D, Hesketh K (2012) Preschoolers' physical activity, screen time, and compliance with recommendations. Med Sci Sports Exerc 44: 458-465.
32. Tremblay MS, Leblanc AG, Carson V, Choquette L, Connor Gorber S, et al. (2012) Canadian Physical Activity Guidelines for the Early Years (aged 0–4 years). Appl Physiol Nutr Metab 37: 345-356.
33. Fox MK, Reidy K, Novak T, Ziegler P (2006) Sources of energy and nutrients in the diets of infants and toddlers. J Am Diet Assoc 106: S28-S42.
34. Story M, Mays RW, Bishop DB, Perry CL, Taylor G, et al. (2000) 5-a-day Power Plus: process evaluation of a multicomponent elementary school program to increase fruit and vegetable consumption. Health Educ Behav 27: 187-200.
35. Bauer KW, Yang YW, Austin SB (2004) "How can we stay healthy when you're throwing all of this in front of us?" Findings from focus groups and interviews in middle schools on environmental influences on nutrition and physical activity. Health Educ Behav 31: 34-46.
36. Baranowski T, Baranowski J, Cullen KW, Marsh T, Islam N, et al. (2003) Squire's Quest! Dietary outcome evaluation of a multimedia game. Am J Prev Med 24: 52-61.
37. Cullen KW, Watson K, Baranowski T, Baranowski JH, Zakeri I (2005) Squire's Quest: intervention changes occurred at lunch and snack meals. Appetite 45: 148-151.
38. Horne PJ, Tapper K, Lowe CF, Hardman CA, Jackson MC, et al. (2004) Increasing children's fruit and vegetable consumption: a peer-modelling and rewards-based intervention. Eur J Clin Nutr 58: 1649-1660.
39. Mangunkusumo RT, Brug J, de Koning HJ, van der Lei J, Raat H (2007) School-based internet-tailored fruit and vegetable education combined with brief counselling increases children's awareness of intake levels. Public Health Nutr 10: 273-279.

40. Baranowski T, Baranowski J, Thompson D, Buday R, Jago R, et al. (2011) Video game play, child diet, and physical activity behavior change a randomized clinical trial. Am J Prev Med 40: 33-38.

41. DeBar L, Dickerson J, Clarke G, Stevens V, Ritenbaugh C, et al. (2009) Using a website to build community and enhance outcomes in a group, multi-component intervention promoting healthy diet and exercise in adolescents. J Pediatr Psychol 34: 539-550.

42. DeBar LL, Ritenbaugh C, Aickin M, DeBar LL, Rittenbaugh C, et al. (2016) Youth: A health plan-based lifestyle intervention increases bone mineral density in adolescent girls. Arch Pediatr Adolesc Med 160: 1269-1276.

43. Haerens L, Deforche B, Maes L, Cardon G, Stevens V, et al. (2006) Evaluation of a 2-year physical activity and healthy eating intervention in middle school children. Health Educ Res 21: 911-921.

44. Haerens L, Deforche B, Maes L, Brug J, Vandelanotte C, et al. (2007) A computer-tailored dietary fat intake intervention for adolescents: results of a randomized controlled trial. Ann Behav Med 34: 253-262.

45. Williamson DA, Martin PD, White MA, Newton R, Walden H, et al. (2005) Efficacy of an internet-based behavioural weight loss program for overweight adolescent African-American girls. Eat Weight Disord 10: 193-203.

46. Bannon K, Schwartz MB (2006) Impact of nutrition messages on children's food choice: pilot study. Appetite 46: 124-129.

47. Haire-Joshu D, Nanney MS, Elliott M, Davey C, Caito N, et al. (2010) The use of mentoring programs to improve energy balance behaviors in high-risk children. Obesity (Silver Spring) 1: S75-S83.

48. Moore JB, Pawloski LR, Goldberg P, Kyeung MO, Stoehr A, et al. (2009) Childhood obesity study: a pilot study of the effect of the nutrition education program Color My Pyramid. J Sch Nurs 25: 230-239.

49. Pempek TA, Calvert SL (2009) Tipping the balance: use of advergames to promote consumption of nutritious foods and beverages by low-income African American children. Arch Pediatr Adolesc Med 163: 633-637.

50. Thompson D, Baranowski T, Cullen K, Watson K, Liu Y, et al. (2008) Food, fun, and fitness internet program for girls: Pilot evaluation of an e-Health youth obesity prevention program examining predictors of obesity. Prev Med 47: 494-497.

51. Casazza K, Ciccazzo M (2007) The method of delivery of nutrition and physical activity information may play a role in eliciting behavior changes in adolescents. Eat Behav 8: 73-82.

52. Long JD, Stevens KR (2004) Using technology to promote self-efficacy for healthy eating in adolescents. J Nurs Scholarsh 36: 134-139.

Nutrients Compositions and Phytochemical Contents of Edible Parts of *Chrysophyllum albidum* Fruit

Ibrahim HO[1,4*], Osilesi O[1], Adebawo OO[2], Onajobi FD[1], Karigidi KO[3] and Muhammad LB[4]

[1]*Department of Biochemistry, Babcock University, Ilishan-Remo, Ogun State, Nigeria*

[2]*Department of Biochemistry, Olabisi Onabanjo University, Ikenne, Ogun State, Nigeria*

[3]*Department of Chemical Sciences, Ondo State University of Science and Technology, Okitipupa, Nigeria*

[4]*Department of Science Laboratory Technology, Federal Polytechnic, Offa, Kwara State, Nigeria*

[*]**Corresponding author:** Ibrahim HO, Department of Biochemistry, Babcock University, Ilishan-Remo, Ogun State; Present Address: Department of Science Laboratory Technology, Federal Polytechnic, Offa, Kwara State, Nigeria, E-mail: ibrahimho234@gmail.com

Abstract

Background: Fruits and fruit products are important part of food and contribute significantly to the food security of the society especially in terms of vitamins and micronutrients.

Objectives: To investigate the nutrient composition and phytochemical contents of the lyophilized-edible parts of *Chrysophyllum albidum* fruit.

Methods: The edible parts (fruit-pulp, fruit-skin and seed-shell pericarp) of *C. albidum* were separated, lyophilized and pulverized into powdered. The edible parts were evaluated for phytochemicals constituents, proximate, fibers, sugars, starch and mineral elements using standard methods.

Results: The fruit-skin in comparison with the fruit-pulp and seed shell pericarp had the highest proximate (except for crude fat, crude protein, carbohydrate and moisture); fiber fractions (except lignin), starch, minerals (except for chloride and iron) and phytochemical (except for alkaloids, tannin and vitamin C) values. Fruit-pulp had the highest lignin (3.16 ± 0.07%), iron (7.66 ± 0.02 mg/100 g) and sugar (except arabinose) contents. Seed shell pericarp had the highest chloride (81.28 ± 0.56 mg/100 g), alkaloids (25.80 ± 0.51%), tannin (10.19 ± 0.12%) and vitamin C (0.12 ± 0.01%) contents. Results are significantly ($p<0.05$) different between samples for sugar, starch, fat, calcium, magnesium, potassium, chloride, alkaloid, tannin and flavonoid contents. The Gas chromatography/Mass spectrometry analysis of n-hexane extract of the edible parts showed the presence of diverse phytochemicals which are mainly of antioxidants and fatty acid origins.

Conclusion: The study established that the fruit-skin contained more essential nutrients composition than other samples investigated and with moderate bioactive compounds of diverse purposes.

Keywords: Nutrients; *Chrysophyllum albidum*; Proximate; Minerals; Gas chromatography; Mass spectrometry

Introduction

Fruits have been shown to be one of the best sources of dietary fiber with lots of vitamins especially C, E and A as well as minerals. Frequent consumption of fruits and vegetables has been associated with a lowered risk of diabetes, hypertension, coronary heart disease, cancer, and stroke [1,2]. Fruits give carbohydrates in the form of soluble sugars, cellulose and starch [3] and serve as source of nutrient, appetizer and supplement for food in a world faced with problem of food scarcity.

Chrysophyllum albidum (Linn), also known as African star apple, belongs to the family *Sapotaceae*, is primarily a forest tree species (Figure 1a) with its natural occurrences in diverse ecozones in Uganda, Nigeria and Niger Republic [4]. The fruit (Figure 1b) is seasonal (December-April) and has immense economic potential, especially following the report that jams obtained from the fruit-pulp could compete with raspberry jams and jellies [5] while the oil from the seed has been used for diverse purposes [6]. In Nigeria, *C. albidum* is known as "agbalumo" in South Western Nigeria and "udara" in South Eastern Nigeria. Its rich sources of natural antioxidants have been established to promote health by acting against oxidative stress related diseases such as diabetics, cancer and coronary heart diseases [7].

The fruit-pulp has been reported to contain significant amount of ascorbic acid [8], vitamins, iron and food flavors [9], fat [10,11], carbohydrate and mineral elements [8,10-13]. The fruit-peel has been shown to be a rich source of fiber and mineral [10,14] while the seed shell pericarp has been reported to be a good source of carbohydrate and minerals [15]. The fruits are not only consumed fresh but also used to produce stewed fruit, marmalade, syrup and several types of soft drinks [16].

Proximate and nutrient analysis of edible fruits and vegetables plays a crucial role in assessing their nutritional significance [17,18]. Freeze-drying method is a drying technique considered appropriate for the preservation of nutritional values of the dehydrated products due to the absence of liquid water and the low temperatures required in the process [19].

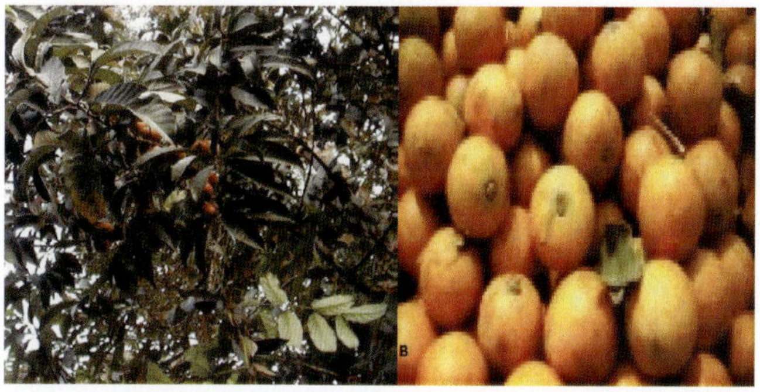

Figure 1: *Chrysophyllum albidum* tree (A) and fruits (B) [17].

In spite of wide application of *C. albidum* plant and its great potential as good sources of fiber and carbohydrate, information on the fiber fractions and sugar contents of its edible parts seems to be scanty in the available literature has not been fully investigated. This study was designed to evaluate the nutritional and phytochemical contents of the edible parts (seed shell pericarp, fruit pulp and fruit-skin) of *C. albidum* fruit. The results of this study may provide useful information on its nutritional potential and contribution to nutrient intake of the nation. It may also create public awareness of its utilization when in season.

Materials and Methods

Plant materials

The fresh fruits of *C. albidum* were purchased in Moniya market, Akinyele Local Government Area of Oyo State, South-Western Nigeria. The fruit was identified and authenticated in the herbarium unit of Botany Department, University of Ibadan, Oyo State, Nigeria where a voucher specimen was deposited with the voucher registration No. UIH/2016/22502.

Preparation of plant materials

The fresh ripe fruit of *C. albidum* was separated, washed, weighed and its fruit-pulp, fruit-skin and seed-shell pericarp (samples) removed and cut into small pieces. The samples were lyophilized for 54 h using Lyophilizer, Millorock Bench-Top Freeze Dryer, and Germany. Lyophilized samples were stored at -20°C until further use.

Extraction of plant materials

The lyophilized samples (fruit-pulp, fruit-skin and seed-shell pericarp) of *C. albidum* fruit were pulverized into powder using Thomas-Wiley laboratory mill (model 4) before being extracted. A portion of one hundred grams (100 g) each of the pulverized sample was suspended in 800 ml of n-hexane for 48 hrs using cold maceration methods with intermittent shaking [20]. The crude extract was filtered first with cotton wool followed by Whatman No. 1 filter paper (1 mm mesh size), concentrated in a rotary evaporator at 40°C and dried to completion in water bath at 35°C. The crude extract was kept in sealed containers and refrigerated at 2-4°C for GC-MS analysis.

Qualitative phytochemical screening

Preliminary qualitative phytochemical screening of the samples was determined using the methods [21-23].

Quantitative Phytochemical Determination

Determination of Tannin

Tannin content of the samples was determined based on the modified vanillin-HCI menthanol method as described by Noha et al. [24]. The principle is that tannins are usually extracted using aqueous organic solvents, mainly methanol and acetone. Vanillin reacts with proantocyandins and leucoanthocyanidins or catechins in the presence of HCI giving rise to a bright red color.

Procedure:

Serial dilution of 1 mg/ml solution A (0.05, 0.1, 0.3, 0.4, 0.5) ml was mixed with 3 ml of 1% vanillin prepared in methanol and 1.5 ml of HCI and made up to a total volume of 5 ml using distilled water. About 0.2 g of the ground sample was placed in a small conical flask. Then 10 ml of 1% concentrated HCI in Methanol was added. The flask was capped, shaken continuously for 20 min and the content was further centrifuged at 2500 rpm for 5 min. About 1.0 ml of the supernatant was pipetted into a test tube containing 5 ml of Vanillin–HCI reagent (solution A). Absorbance at 450 nm was read on spectrophotometer after 20 min of incubation at 30°C. A standard curve was prepared expressing the result as tannic acid equivalent as follow:

$$Tannin(\%) = C \times \frac{10}{200} \times 100$$

Where C=Concentration corresponding to the optical density; 10=Volume of the extract (ml)=Sample weight (mg).

Determination of Saponin

Saponin content determination was carried out according to the procedure described by Okwu and Josiah [25]. 5 g of the sample was dispersed in 50 ml of 20% v/v ethanol prepared in distilled water. The suspension was heated over hot water bath for 4 h with continuous stirring at 55°C. The mixture was filtered and the residue re-extracted with another 50 ml of 20% ethanol. The combined extracts were reduced to 20 ml in a hot water bath. The concentrated solution obtained was shaken vigorously with 10 ml of diethyl ether in a 250 ml separating funnel; the aqueous layer was collected while the ether layer was discarded. The purification process was repeated twice. Twenty milliliters but-1-ol was added to the filtrate and washed twice with 10 ml of 5% w/v aqueous sodium chlorine. The mixture heated to evaporation on hot water bath and later oven dried at 40°C to a constant weight. The percentage saponins content of the sample was calculated using this formula:

$$\%Saponin = \frac{weight\ of\ final\ filtrate}{weight\ of\ sample} \times 100$$

Determination of alkaloids

This was done by the alkaline precipitation gravimetric method described by Harborne [23]. One gram of the sample was dispersed into 10 ml of 10% acetic acid solution in ethanol to form a ratio of 1:10 (10%). The mixture was shaken and then allowed to stand for 4 h before it was filtered. The filtrate was concentrated to one quarter of its original volume on hot plate and treated with drop wise addition of conc. aqueous NH_4OH until the alkaloid was precipitated. A pre-weighed filter paper was used to receive the precipitate, washed with 1% ammonia solution, dried in an oven at 60°C for 30 min, transferred into desiccators to cool; rewashed and dried until a constant weight was obtained. The constant weight was recorded and alkaloid content was determined by weight difference of the filter paper and expressed as a percentage of the sample analyzed.

$$\%Alkaloids = \frac{w_1 - w_2}{w_0} \times 100$$

Where WO=Sample weight in g; W1=Weight of filter paper +precipitate.

W2=weight of filter paper only.

Determination of flavonoids

This was determined according to the method of Harborne [23]. 5 g of the sample was boiled in 50 ml of 2 M HCl solution for 30 min under reflux. It was allowed to cool and then filtered. About 2 ml of the filterate was treated with 2 ml ethyl acetate starting with a drop. The flavonoid precipitated was recovered by filtration using weighed filter paper. The resulting weight difference gave the weight of flavonoid in the sample.

Determination of vitamin C

Vitamin C content was determined by UV-spectrophotometry as described by Rahman et al. [26]. One gram (1g) each of sample was weighed into test tubes. 1 mm ascorbic acid stock was pipetted into a separate test tube as a standard. 1 mm Trichloreacetic Acid (TCA) solution was placed in another test tube to serve as blank. Ten millilitre TCA solutions were added to the sample tubes. 1 mm Dinitrophenyl Hydrazine-Thiourea-Copper Sulphate (DTCS) reagent was added to all the tubes and caped. The tubes were incubated in a water bath at 37°C for 3 hrs. They was removed from the water bath and chilled for 10 min in an ice bath while shaking slowly and 2 ml of cold 12 M H_2SO_4 was added to all the test tubes. The spectrophotometer was adjusted with the blank to read zero absorbance at 520 nm. The absorbance of standard and test samples was also read. The result was calculated as follows:

$$Vitamin\ C\ (mg/100g) = \frac{Absorbance\ of\ test\ samples \times Concentration\ of\ standard}{Absorbance\ of\ standard \times Weight\ of\ sample}$$

Proximate Composition

Moisture, ash and crude fibre contents of the samples were determined by the AOAC [27] methods. The micro-Kjeldahl method was used for the determination of crude protein (N × 6.25) using the methods of AOAC [27]. Crude lipid contents were determined by the continuous soxhlet lipid extraction method was determined by the method of AOAC [27]; the carbohydrate content was estimated by difference [28].

Characterization of carbohydrate content

The characterization of carbohydrate content of the samples was done with HPLC using the method described by Prapasri and Kunchit [29].

Determination of mineral content

Sodium (Na) and potassium were determined by the flame emission photometer using the AOAC [27], Phosphorus (P) was determined by vanadomolybdate colorimetric method, Calcium (Ca), Magnesium (Mg), Iron (Fe), zinc (Zn), manganese (Mn), chromium (Cr) and copper (Cu) were determined using Atomic Absorption Spectrophotometer (AAS) [30] and Chloride by Mohr's Method [31]. All values were expressed in mg/100 g.

Starch and fiber fractions determination

The total starch was determined by the method of McCleary et al. [32]. The Neutral Detergent Fibre (NDF), Acid Detergent Fraction (ADF), hemicellulose, cellulose and lignin were determined using fiber analyzer [33]. Pectin was determined by nitric acid extraction method and percentage content was calculated by non-enzymatic gravimetric method [34].

Gas chromatography-mass spectrometry (GC-MS) analysis

The GC-MS analysis of n-hexane extract of the samples were carried out using a Perkin-Elmer GC Clarus 500 system and Gas chromatograph interfaced to a Mass spectrometer (GC-MS) equipped with an Elite-I, fused silica capillary column (30 × 0.25 mm 1 D × 1 μMdf, composed of 100% Dimethyl poly siloxane). For GC-MS detection, an electron ionization system with ionization energy of 70 eV was used. Helium gas (99.999%) was used as the carrier gas at constant flow rate 1ml/min and an injection volume of 2 μl was employed (Split ratio of 10:1) injector temperature -250°C; ion-source temperature 280°C. The oven temperature was programmed from 110°C (Isothermal for 2 min.) with an increase of 10°C/min to 200°C then 5°C/min. to 280°C/min, ending with a 9 min. isothermal at 280°C. Mass spectra were taken at 70 eV; a scan interval of 0.5 s and fragments from 40 to 550 Da. Total GC running time was 36 minutes.

Identification of components

Interpretation on mass spectrum GC-MS was conducted using the database of National Institute Standard and Technology (NIST) having more than 62,000 patterns. The spectral of the unknown component were compared with the spectral of the known components stored in the NIST library. The possible names, molecular weights and structures of the components of the test materials were thus ascertained [35].

Statistical Analysis

Data were expressed as mean ± SEM for triplicate determinations (n=3). Comparisons of the data were performed by analysis of variance (ANOVA) followed by Least Significant Difference (LSD) post hoc test at 5% ($p<0.05$) probability.

Results

Qualitative phytochemical

Preliminary phytochemical investigation (Table 1) of the crude edible parts of *Chrysophyllum albidum* fruit revealed the presence of alkaloids, tannins, saponins, flavonoids and terpenoids in all the edible parts of *C. albidum*. Cardiac glycosides was found to be absent in the fruit-skin while phlobatannin was also found to be absent in both seed shell pericarp and fruit-skin of *C. albidum*.

Parameters	Seed shell pericarp	Fruit pulp	Fruit skin
Alkaloid	+ + +	+ + +	+ + +
Tannin	+ +	+ +	+ +
Saponin	+	+	+
Flavonoid	+ + +	+ + +	+ + +
Terpenoid	+ + +	+ + +	+ + +
Phlobatannin	-	+	-
Cardiac glycoside	+	+	-

(+): Presence (trace amount), (++): Presence (moderately concentrated), (+++): Presence (highly concentrated), (-): Absent

Table 1: Phytochemical screening of the edible parts of freeze dried *Chrysophyllum albidum* fruit.

Quantitative phytochemicals

The quantitative phytochemical values of *C. albidum* edible parts are shown in Table 2. Seed shell pericarp had the highest contents of Alkaloid, Tannins and vitamin C. while the Fruit skin had the highest content of Saponin and Flavonoid. Data obtained between samples with the exception of Vitamin C are significantly ($P<0.05$) different.

Parameters (%)	Seed shell pericarp	Fruit pulp	Fruit skin
Alkaloid	$25.80^a \pm 0.51$	$14.60^b \pm 0.16$	$12.22^c \pm 0.10$
Tannin	$10.19^a \pm 0.12$	$7.49^c \pm 0.12$	$8.18^b \pm 0.07$
Saponin	$0.09^b \pm 0.01$	$0.07^b \pm 0.02$	$0.41^a \pm 0.02$
Flavonoid	$15.11^b \pm 0.07$	$11.24^c \pm 0.15$	$17.23^a \pm 0.09$
Vitamin C (mg/100g)	$0.12^a \pm 0.01$	$0.10^{a,b} \pm 0.01$	$0.09^b \pm 0.01$

Results are the mean ± SE value of triplicate determinations. Means followed by different alphabet within the row are significantly ($P<0.05$) different while those with the same alphabet within the row are not significantly ($P>0.05$) different.

Table 2: Quantitative phytochemical constituents of the freeze dried edible parts of *Chrysophyllum albidum* fruit.

Proximate composition and starch content

Data on proximate composition and starch content are presented in Table 3. The seed shell pericarp had the highest crude protein, crude fat and energy contents; fruit-pulp had the highest moisture and carbohydrate contents while fruit skin had the highest ash, crude fibre, total dry weight and starch contents. The values are significantly different ($p<0.05$) across samples (with the exception of ash, crude protein and carbohydrate).

Fiber, sugar and mineral contents: The Fiber fractions are presented in Figure 2. The fruit skin had the highest contents of Acid Detergent Fraction (ADF), Neutral Detergent Fiber (NDF), cellulose, hemicelluloses and pectin while the fruit pulp had the highest contents of lignin. Values are significantly ($p<0.05$) different across samples except pectin where $P>0.05$. The sugar contents of *C. albidum* fruit showed that the seed shell pericarp had the highest contents of the sugar studied except arabinose while the fruit skin had the highest content of arabinose and lowest contents of other sugar studied (Table 4). The mineral contents *C. albidum* fruit (Tables 5 and 6) showed that the fruit skin had the highest contents of the mineral elements studied except chloride and iron while the highest chloride and iron contents were found in the seed shell pericarp and fruit pulp respectively. Values are significantly ($P<0.05$) different across samples except for copper.

Results are expressed as the mean ± SE value of triplicate determinations. All values are significantly different ($P<0.05$) with the exception of pectin and hemicelluloses (between seed shell pericarp and fruit pulp).

GC-MS analysis

The GC-MS identified compounds and their reported bioactivity in the n-hexane extract of the edible parts of *C. albidum* with percentage of purity ≥70% is presented in Table 7. The identified compounds are of fatty acids, fatty acid derivatives and aromatic origin. The studies showed that they are rich in phytochemicals of diverse nutritional and biological significance. Result of n-hexane extract of *C. albidum* seed shell pericarp showed that it contained 6 compounds, 1 of these compounds is known to exhibit both antioxidant and hypocholesterolemic activities; and 1 compound is known to exhibit hypolipidemic activity while 2 compounds of unknown bioactivity were also detected.

The n-hexane extract of *C. albidum* fruit-pulp contained 23 compounds, 3 of these compounds are known to exhibit both antioxidant and hypocholesterolemic activities; 1 compound exhibits both anti-inflammatory and hypocholesterolemic activities; 1 compound exhibits hypolipidemic activity; and 1 compound exhibits only anti-inflammatory activity while 10 compounds of unknown bioactivity were also detected. The n-hexane extract of *C. albidum* fruit-skin contained 10 compounds, 3 of these compounds are known to exhibit both antioxidant and hypocholesterolemic activities, 1 compound exhibits anti-inflammatory, antioxidant and hypocholesterolemic activities, and 1 compound exhibits both anti-inflammatory and hypocholesterolemic activities; while 4 compounds of unknown bioactivity were also detected.

Parameters (%)	Seed shell pericarp	Fruit pulp	Fruit skin
Moisture	$5.63^b \pm 0.24$	$7.76^a \pm 0.15$	$4.80^c \pm 0.15$
Ash	$2.36^b \pm 0.07$	$2.29^b \pm 0.04$	$3.27^a \pm 0.13$
Crude Protein	$8.66^a \pm 0.19$	$7.31^b \pm 0.46$	$6.91^b \pm 0.48$
Fat	$8.07^a \pm 0.13$	$6.97^b \pm 0.51$	$4.68^c \pm 0.23$
Crude Fiber	$10.06^b \pm 0.14$	$9.21^c \pm 0.19$	$15.57^a \pm 0.25$
Carbohydrate	$65.22^a \pm 0.61$	$66.45^a \pm 0.65$	$64.70^a \pm 0.21$
TDW	$94.37^a \pm 0.22$	$92.24^b \pm 0.15$	$95.20^a \pm 0.31$
Gross Energy (kj/100 g)	$1537.91^a \pm 7.23$	$1494.74^b \pm 5.52$	$1373.31^c \pm 5.10$
Starch	$20.86^b \pm 0.22$	$13.13^c \pm 0.12$	$29.15^a \pm 0.11$

Results are the mean ± SE value of triplicate determinations. Means followed by different alphabet within the row are significantly ($P<0.05$) different while those with the same alphabet within the row are not significantly ($P>0.05$) different. TDW: Total Dry Weight.

Table 3: Proximate Composition of the freeze dried edible parts of *Chrysophyllum albidum* fruit.

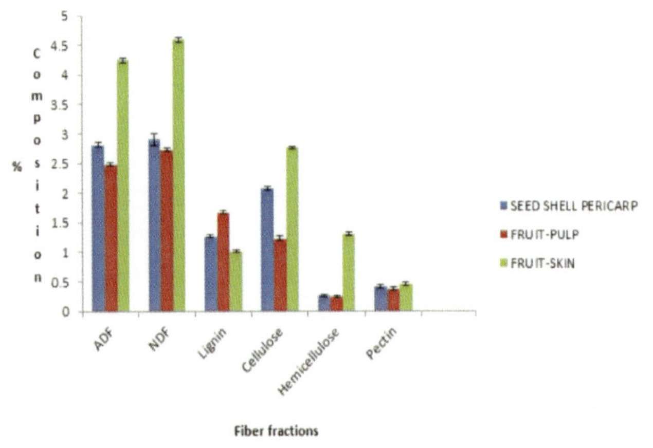

Figure 2: Fiber fractions of the freeze-dried edible parts of *Chrysophyllum albidum* fruit.

ADF: Acid Detergent Fraction; NDF: Neutral Detergent Fiber.

Sample/Parameters (mg/100 g dry wt)	Glucose	Fructose	Arabinose	Sucrose
Seed Shell Pericarp	8133.61^{b} ± 20.50	14146.98^{b} ± 32.55	3523.06^{b} ± 14.84	1095.66^{b} ± 14.05
Fruit Pulp	13937.01^{a} ± 20.40	16574.10^{a} ± 35.77	3294.55^{c} ± 12.10	8236.61^{a} ± 21.89
Fruit Skin	7764.02^{c} ± 11.45	10880.41^{c} ± 7.33	4854.79^{a} ± 12.40	67.27^{c} ± 0.08
Results are the mean ± SE value of triplicate determinations. Means followed by different alphabet within the row are significantly (P<0.05) different while those with the same alphabet within the row are not significantly (P>0.05) different.				

Table 4: Sugar contents of the edible parts of *Chrysophyllum albidum* fruit.

Parameters (mg/100 g dry wt)	Seed Shell Pericarp	Fruit Pulp	Fruit Skin
Na	28.26^{c} ± 0.02	31.03^{b} ± 0.09	34.00^{a} ± 0.71
K	532.08^{b} ± 33.71	268.00^{c} ± 0.55	585.75^{a} ± 0.78
Mg	122.41^{c} ± 0.20	135.00^{b} ± 1.80	144.25^{a} ± 1.02
Ca	212.50^{b} ± 0.51	100.00^{c} ± 5.51	258.25^{a} ± 6.86
Cl	81.28^{a} ± 0.56	24.74^{c} ± 0.43	70.68^{b} ± 0.40
P	12.04^{b} ± 0.00	10.03^{b} ± 0.00	30.22^{a} ± 0.01
Results are the mean ± SE value of triplicate determinations. Means followed by different alphabet within the row are significantly (P<0.05) different while those with the same alphabet within the row are not significantly (P>0.05) different.			

Table 5: Macro elements content of the edible parts of freeze dried *Chrysophyllum albidum* fruit.

Parameters (mg/100 g dry wt)	Seed Shell Pericarp	Fruit Pulp	Fruit Skin
Fe	3.48^{b} ± 0.17	7.66^{a} ± 0.02	3.37^{b} ± 0.15
Zn	0.12^{b} ± 0.02	0.57^{a} ± 0.04	ND
Mn	0.23^{c} ± 0.03	0.45^{b} ± 0.02	2.25^{a} ± 0.06
Cr	ND	0.25 ± 0.02	ND
Cu	0.36^{a} ± 0.02	0.44^{a} ± 0.04	0.55^{a} ± 0.05
Results are the mean ± SE value of triplicate determinations. Means followed by different alphabet within the row are significantly (P<0.05) different while those with the same alphabet within the row are not significantly (P>0.05) different. ND: Not Detected.			

Table 6: Micro elements content of the edible parts of freeze dried *Chrysophyllum albidum* fruit.

Sample type	Compound name	Retention time	Compound Nature	Activity*
Seed shell pericarp	Pentadecanoic acid	13.793	Fatty acid	Antimicrobial
	n-Hexadecanoic acid	15.727	Fatty acid	Antioxidant Hypocholesterolemic
	Trans-13-Octadecenoic acid	16.934	Trans Monoenoic Fatty acid	#
	6-Octadecenoic acid	17.003	Petroselinic acid	#
	Cis-Vaccenic acid	17.804	Monoenoic Fatty acid	Hypolipidemic
	Octadecanoic acid	18.044	Fatty acid	Antifungal, antitumor

Fruit pulp	Naphthalene	6.217	Bicyclic Aromatic Hydrocarbon	Anti-inflammatory, Antimicrobial
	Tetradecane	8.860	Alkane	Antifungal, Antibacterial
	Undecanoic acid, 10-methyl-methyl ester	10.434	Fatty acid ester	#
	9-Ecosene	11.246	Alkene	#
	Hexadecane	11.327	Alkane	#
	Benzene(1-propyloctyl)-	11.939	Aromatic compound	#
	Methyl tetradecanoate	12.757	Myristic acid ester	Antioxidant, Hypocholesterolemic
	Benzene(1-pentylheptyl)	12.866	Aromatic compound	#
	Benzene(1-butyloctyl)	12.923	Aromatic compound	#
	Benzene(1-propylnonyl)	13.060	Aromatic compound	#
	Benzene(1-ethyldecyl)	13.306	Aromatic compound	#
	Trifluoroacetoxy hexadecane	13.490	Fluoro compound	Antifungal
	Octadecane	13.558	Alkane	#
	Hexadecanoic acid, methyl ester	14.863	Palmitic acid methyl ester	Antioxidant, Hypocholesterolemic
	Hexadecanoic acid ethyl ester	15.521	Palmitic acid ethyl ester	Antioxidant, Hypocholesterolemic
	Eicosane	15.572	Alkane	Antifungal, Antitumor
	9,12-Octadecadienoic acid-methyl ester	16.516	Linoleic acid methyl ester	Anti-inflammatory, Hypocholesterolemic
	11-Octadecenoic acid, methyl ester	16.562	Vaccenic acid methyl ester	Hypolipidemic
	Octadecanoic acid, methyl ester	16.774	Stearic acid methyl ester	Antifungal, Antimicrobial
	Cyclohexene,4-(4-ethylcyclohexyl)	17.123	Cyclo Hydrocarbon	#
	Octacosyl trifluoroacetate	17.369	Fluoro Compound	Antimicrobial
	Docosane	17.421	Alkane	Antibacterial
	Sulfurous acid, Octadecyl-2-propyl ester	19.103	Sulfurous compound	Antimicrobial
Fruit skin	Hexadecane	11.332	Alkane	#
	Methyltetradecanoate	12.757	Myristic acid ester	Antioxidant, Hypocholestero-lemic
	1-octadecene	13.489	Alkene	#
	Octadecane	13.558	Alkane	#
	Hexadecanoic acid methyl ester	14.863	Palmitic acid methyl ester	Antioxidant, Hypocholestero-lemic
	3-Eicosene	15.521	Alkene	#
	Eicosane	15.578	Alkane	Antifungal, antitumo
	9,12-octadecadienenoic acid, methyl ester	16.522	Linoleic acid methyl ester	Anti-inflammatory, Hypocholesterolemic
	9-Octadecenoic acid, methyl ester	16.568	Oleic acid methyl ester	Antioxidant, Hypocholestero-lemic
	Octadecanoic acid, methyl ester	16.780	Stearic acid methyl ester	Antioxidant, Hypocholestero-lemic

Table 7: Phytochemicals of n-hexane extract of freeze dried edible parts of *Chrysophyllum albidum* Fruit.

Discussion

The health promoting properties of plant-based foods have largely been attributed to their wide range of phytochemicals [36-38]. The presence of flavonoids, alkaloids, terpenoid, tannins and saponin in the edible parts of *C. albidum* fruit agreed with the reports of Egharevba et al. [39] who reported the presence of phenols, glycosides, terpenoids in the leaf; flavonoids, saponins, steroids and alkaloids in the leaf and seed of *Chrysophyllum albidum* methanol extract. This work is also in line with the findings of Imaga and Urua [40] who showed that ethanol and aqueous extracts of *Chrysophyllum albidum* fruit contain tannins, phenols, flavonoids, cardiac glycosides, terpenoids, reducing sugar and phlobatannins while saponins, steroids and alkaloid were reported to be present only in the aqueous extract and anthraquinone found to be absent in both extracts. These metabolites are of great importance in phytomedicines development [21].

Flavonoids and Tannins in fruits are important sources of natural antioxidants that are preferred over synthetic ones as they are less toxic [41]. Flavonoids scavenge free radicals produced by Reactive Oxygen Species (ROS) thereby preventing diseases caused by oxidative stress. Alkaloids have anti-inflammatory property [42] while saponins exhibit hypocholesterolemic property through the formation of insoluble complexes with cholesterol and consequently slowing down its absorption [43]. The freeze dried edible parts of *C. albidum* upon quantification by colorimetric methods were found to be rich in alkaloids, tannins and flavonoids with moderate amount of saponin. This indicates that the edible parts of *C. albidum* fruit might possess antioxidant, anti-inflammatory and hypocholesterolemic properties.

There is a growing awareness in correlating the phytochemical components and their biological activities [44]. The GC-MS analysis of n-hexane extract of edible parts of *C. albidum* fruit showed the presence of various bioactive compounds. In terms of biological activity six of the compounds possess both antioxidant and hypocholesterolemic properties. These compounds are n-hexadecanoic acid; methyl tetradecanoate; hexadecanoic acid, methyl ester; hexadecanoic acid, ethyl ester; 9-octadecenoic acid, methyl ester and octadecanoic acid, methyl ester. Three compounds (cis-vaccenic (11–octadecenoic) acid; 11–octadecenoic acid, methyl ester and 9, 12-Octadecadienoic acid, methyl ester) possess only hypocholesterolemic property.

Daily diet has an important role in human health and healthy diet means getting enough of the essential nutrients needed daily by the body. Proximate and nutrient analysis of edible fruit and vegetables play a crucial role in assessing their nutritional significance. The obtained moisture contents are lower than the values reported for this fruit seed shell pericarp by Ewansiha et al. [15]; pulp by Ukana et al. [14]; Bello and Henry [16] and skin (peel) by Bello and Henry [16]. The observed low moisture content could be due to the shielding effect of the freeze drying method over air drying method on the samples against rehydration by relative humidity in air [45]. This result is in line with the findings of Abiodun et al. [46] who reported that freeze drying method is the most appropriate method to reduce moisture content of *Ocimum gratissimum* and *O. basillicum*. The moisture content of any food material is a measure of the life span of the food. It indicates how long a food material can be stored without becoming mouldy [47]. Hook et al. [48] reported that the moisture level of a food influence the texture and the more ordered the endosperm structure, the lower the rate of moisture content. This indicates that freeze dried samples could be stored for long period without becoming mouldy.

The obtained ash contents are in close range with the findings of Amusa et al. [6]; Ureigho [13]; Christopher and Dosunmu [11]; Ewansiha et al. [15] and Ukana et al. [14]. Ash content indicates the amount of inorganic matter and oxides present in the sample. It is the determinant factor of the mineral constituents in the sample [17]. Proteins are class of nitrogenous compound that consist of large molecule composed of one or more long chain of amino acid. The obtained protein values are higher compared to the values reported for this fruit by Amusa et al. [6]; Ewansiha et al. [15] and Ukana et al. [14].

However, the observed crude fat values agreed with the reports of Christopher and Dosunmu [11]; Ewansiha et al. [15] and Ukana et al. [14] for this fruit. Fat provide an excellent source of energy, enhance transport of fat soluble vitamins, insulate and protect internal tissues and contribute to vital cell process. However, it is strongly believed that excess of saturated fatty acids are responsible for a tendency to coronary thrombosis and aortic atheroma in men while high level of poly unsaturated fatty acids are important in lowering blood cholesterol level.

The obtained crude fiber content are higher than the values reported for this fruit by Amusa et al. [6]; Ewansiha et al. [15]; Bello and Henry [16]. These variations could be due to different methods of drying effects. This result is in line with the findings of Adejumo [49] who reported significant effects of different drying methods on crude fiber content of tomato powder and Oni et al. [45] who showed an increasing effect of drying methods on the crude fiber contents of different vegetables in the order of freeze drying>Air drying>Sun drying>Oven drying. Fiber decreases the absorption of cholesterol from the gut, delays the digestion and conversion of starch to simple sugars, and also functions in the protection against cardiovascular disease, colorectal cancer and obesity [50]. The fiber-like substances particularly the gums and pectin when ingested with a diet have been reported to reduce postprandial blood glucose levels [51,52]. Feeding of xanthan gum to diabetic subjects have been shown to lower fasting and postload serum glucose levels and total plasma cholesterol [53]. Daily soluble fiber intake of 5–10 g from a variety of sources has been found to reduce serum cholesterol by 5–10% [51]. This implies that the fruit-skin with the highest fiber fractions could be effectively utilized in the management of diabetes mellitus, colorectal cancers and weight reduction in the obese individuals. However, the fruit-skin will take longer time to chew because of its fiber-rich contents.

The obtained carbohydrate contents are consistent with the reports of Christopher and Dosunmu [11]; Ewansiha et al. [15] and Ukana et al. [14] for this fruit. Polysaccharides such as starch have low glycemic index and thus effective in the control of postprandial blood glucose levels. The observed high starch content in the *C. albidum* fruit skin suggests that the fruit skin could reduce glycemic response when ingested with carbohydrate diet. However, the low caloric value of the fruit skin may be a disadvantage for its suitability for consumption as a snack by the athletes.

There is evidence for a direct, independent link between sugar exposure and diabetes and increased access to sugar may explain part of the association between urbanisation and increased risk of type 2 diabetes [54]. The high content of arabinose and low content of fructose in the fruit skin have beneficial effects. Diet high in fructose has been reported to promote energy imbalance, obesity [55]; glucose intolerance, insulin resistance, hyperlipidaemia [56] and total cholesterol/HDL-cholesterol ratio which are known to be high-risk factors for development of cardiovascular diseases [57]. Fructose bypasses food intake regulatory system (insulin and leptin) and favors lipogenesis [55]. This implies that the high fructose content of the fruit pulp may be a disadvantage for its suitability for consumption as a snack by the obese.

Studies using animal model and clinical trials have shown that L-arabinose supplemented diet could effectively reduce postprandial blood glucose level by uncompetitive inhibition of intestinal sucrose [58,59]. This implies that the fruit skin might possess ability to suppress glycaemic response when taken with carbohydrate diet.

Minerals are critical in the regulation of a number of cell membrane, permeability, muscles contraction, heart function, blood clothing, protein and red blood synthesis [60,61]. These essential minerals are important components of the daily diet. The high contents of potassium, magnesium, calcium, phosphorus, sodium, manganese and copper in the fruit skin, chloride content in the seed shell pericarp and iron content in the fruit pulp is an indication that the edible parts of *C. albidum* fruit can supply some essential minerals needed for healthy life.

Calcium, magnesium, manganese and copper have been shown to have stimulatory effect on the pancreas leading to enhanced insulin secretion and ß-cell proliferation, thus contributing to improved glucose disposal [62]. This suggests that the fruit skin with the highest contents of calcium, magnesium, manganese and copper could contribute to the control of hyperglycaemic cases through the enhancement of insulin secretion.

Conclusion

As a result of the phytochemicals and essential nutrients in the form of soluble and insoluble fibers, starch, arabinose and mineral elements found in the fruit skin of *C. albidum* in comparison with the seed shell pericarp and fruit pulp, it can be deduced that the fruit skin of *C. albidum* has a great potential in contributing to the healthy growth and as supplementation in food industries.

Recommendations

Further studies are required to elucidate the antioxidant, hypocholesterolemic, hypolipidemic and hypoglycemic potentials of *C. albidum* edible parts.

Acknowledgement

This research was supported in part by grant provided by the Education Trust Fund (ETF) of the Federal Government of Nigeria. The authors declare that there are no conflicts of interest.

References

1. Southon S (2000) Increased fruit and vegetable consumption within the EU: Potential health benefits. Food Res Intl 33: 211-217.
2. Wargovich MJ (2000) Anticancer properties of fruits and vegetables. Hort Sci 35: 573-575.
3. Nahar N, Rahaman S, Mosiihuzzaman M (1990) Analysis of carbohydrates in seven edible fruits of Bangladesh. J Sci Food Agr 5: 185-192.
4. Bada SO (1997) Preliminary Information on the Ecology of *Chrysophillum albidum* G. Don, in West and Central Africa. In: Proceedings of a National workshop on the potentials of the star apply in Nigeria. Denton.
5. Okafor JC (1975) The place of wild (uncultivated) fruits arid vegetables in the Nigerian diet. Proceedings, Recommendations and Papers of the First National Seminar on Fruits and Vegetables. Ibadan Nigeria, pp: 153-154.
6. Amusa NA, Ashaye OA , Oladapo MO (2003) Biodeterioration of African star apple (*Chrysphylum albidum*) in storage and the effect on its food value. Afr J Biotechnol 2: 56-59.
7. Burits M, Bucar F (2000) Antioxidant activity of *Nigella sativa* essential oil. Phytother Res 14: 323-328.
8. Adepoju O, Adeniji TPO (2012) Nutrient composition and micronutrient potential of three wildly grown varieties of African star apple (*Chrysophyllum albidum*) from Nigeria. Afr J Food Sci 6: 344-351
9. Adisa SA (2000) Vitamin C, protein and mineral content of African apple (*Chrysophillum albidum*) in proceedings of the 18th Annual Conference of NIST, pp: 141-146.
10. Ige MM, Gbadamosi SO (2007) Chemical Composition and Physical Properties of African Star Apple (*Chrysophyllum albidum*). ASSET Int J 7: 37-42.
11. Christopher EA, Dosunmu MI (2011) Chemical Evaluation of Proximate Composition, Ascorbic Acid and Anti-Nutrients Content of African Star Apple (*Chrysophyllum afrcanum*) Fruit. IJRRAS 9: 17-46.
12. Edem DO, Eka OU, Ifon ET (1984) Chemical evaluation of the value of the fruit of African Star apple (*Chrysophyllum albidum*). Food Chem 14: 303-311.
13. Ureigho UN (2010) Nutrient Values of *Chrysophyllum albidum* Linn African Star Apple as a Domestic Income Plantation Species. Afr Res 4: 50-56.
14. Ukana DA, Aniekan EA, Godwin NE (2012) Evaluation of proximate compositions and mineral elements in the star apple peel, pulp and seed. J Basic Appl Sci Res 2: 4839-4843.
15. Ewansiha CI, Asia IO, Ekebafe LO, Jatto OE, Okodugha G (2011) Proximate and Mineral Composition of Seed Shell Pericap of *Chrysophyllum albidum*. Pac J Sci Technol 12: 363-365.
16. Bello FA, Henry AA (2015) Storage Effects and the Postharvest Quality of African Star Apple Fruits (*Chrysophyllum africanum*) Under Ambient Conditions. A J Food Sci Technol 6: 35-43.
17. Orwa C, Mutua A, Kindt R, Jamnadass R, Anthony S (2009) Agrofores tree Database:a tree reference and selection guide version.
18. Pandey M, Abidi AB, Singh S, Singh RP (2006) Nutritional Evaluation of Leafy Vegetable Paratha. J Hum Ecol 19: 155-156.
19. Marques LG, Ferreira MC, Freire JT (2007) Freeze-drying of acerola (*Malpighia glabra* L.). Chemical Engineering and Processing 46: 451-457
20. Ncube NS, Afolayan AJ, Okoh AI (2008) Assessment techniques of antimicrobial properties of natural compounds of plant origin: current methods and future trends. A J Biotechnol 7: 1797-1806.
21. Sofowora A (1993) Medicinal Plants and Traditional Medicine in Africa (2nd edn.) Spectrum Books Limited, Ibadan, Nigeria pp: 1-153.
22. Trease GE, Evans WC (2002) Pharmacognosy (15th edn.). Saunders pp: 214-393.
23. Harborne JB (1973) Phytochemical Methods A guide to modern techniques of plant analysis. London. New York. Chapman and Hall.
24. Noah A, Mohammed IA, Mohamed A, Elfsdil EB (2011) Nutritional Evaluation of Sorghum flour (*Sorghum bicolor* L. Moench) during processing of Injera. World Academy of Science, Engineering and Technology 75: 86-112.
25. Okwu DE, Josiah C (2006) Evaluation of the chemical composition of two Nigerian Medicinal plants. A J Biotechnol 5: 357-361.
26. Rahman MM, Khan MMR, Hosain MM (2007) Analysis of Vitamin C (ascorbic acid) Contents in Various Fruits and Vegetables by UV-spectrophotometry. Bangladesh J Sci Ind Res 42: 417-424.
27. AOAC (Association of Official Analytical Chemists) (2000) Official Methods of Analysis International (17th edn.). AOAC, Washington, DC, USA.
28. McDonald P, Edwards RA, Greenhalgh JFD (1973) Animal nutrition. T & A Constable Ltd., Edinburgh, pp: 2-5.

29. Prapasri P, Kunchit J (2011) ASEAN Manual of Food Analysis (1st edn.). In: Tee ES, Julia K, Graham C, Rafael RF (eds.) Institute of Nutrition, Mahidol University, Thailand. pp: 27-32.
30. Onwuka GI (2005) Food analysis and instrumentation theory and practice. Napthali prints. Lagos.
31. Kraemer EO, Stamm AJ (1924) Mohr's Method for the Determination of Silver and Halogens in other than Neutral Solutions. J Am Chem Soc 46: 2707-2709.
32. McCleary BV, Solah V, Gibson TS (1994) Quantitative measurement of total starch in cereal flours and products. J Cereal Sci 20: 51-58.
33. Anderson JM, Ingram J (1989) Tropical Soil Biology and Fertility: A Handbook of Methods. Wallingford, UK: CAB International.
34. Abhijit C, Subhajit R (2011) Development of a Process for the Extraction of Pectin from Citrus Fruit Wastes viz. Lime peel, Spent guava extract, Apple pomace etc. Internet Journal of Food Safety 13: 391-397.
35. Sathyaprabha G, Kumaravel S, Panneerselvam A (2011) Bioactive Compounds Identification of Pleurotus platypus and Pleurotus eous by GC-MS. Adv Appl Sci Res 2: 51.
36. Duke JA (1992) Database of Biologically Active Phytochemicals and Their Activity. Boca Raton, Fla: CRC Press, pp: 183-191.
37. Duke JA (2013) Phytochemical and Ethnobotanical Databases.
38. Arshad HR, Salah MA, Habeeb Al, Ali YB, Sauda S, et al. (2014) Therapeutic effects of date fruits (*Phoenix dactylifera*) in the prevention of diseases via modulation of anti-inflammatory, anti-oxidant and anti-tumour activity. Int J Clin Exp Med 7: 483-491.
39. Egharevba HO, Ibrahim JA, Nduaguba GA, Kunle OF (2015) Phytochemical, proximate pharmacognosy analyses and thin layer chromatography of *Chrysophyllum albidum* seed. Ew J Herb Chem Pharmacol Res 1: 6-12.
40. Imaga NOA, Urua EE (2013) Chemical and antioxidant evaluation of star apple fruit (*Chrysophyllum albidum*) crude extracts. Planta Med. Congress Abstract pp: 79-83.
41. Ifeson BOT, Fashakin JF, Ebosele F, Oyerinde AS (2013) Antioxidant and antimicrobial properties of selected plant leaves. Eur J Med Plants 3: 465-473.
42. Kuras M, Pilarski R, Nowakowska J, Zobel A, Brzost K, et al. (2009) Effect of alkaloid-free and alkaloid-rich preparations from Uncaria tomentosa bark on mitotic activity and chromosome morphology evaluated by Allium test. J Ethnopharmacol 121: 140-147.
43. Aletor VA (1993) Allelochemicals in plant foods and feedingstuffs: 1. Nutritional, biochemical and physiopathological aspects in animal production. Vet Hum Toxicol 35: 57-67.
44. Robertson DG (2005) Metabonomics in toxicology: a review. Toxicol Sci 85: 809-822.
45. Oni MO, Ogungbite OC, Akindele AK (2015) The Effect of Different Drying Methods on some common Nigerian Edible Botanicals. Int J Adv Res Botany (IJARB) 1: 15-22.
46. Abiodun AR, Aletor O, Aladesanwa RD (2012) The influence of freeze and sun-drying on the nutrient and the anti-nutrient constituents of scent and basil leaves. Int J Chem 22: 197-205.
47. Fellows PJ (2000) Food Processing Technology: Principles and Practice. Wood Head Publishing in Food Science, Technology and Nutrition pp: 22-28.
48. Hook SCW, Rone GT, Fearn T (1982) The Conditioning of wheat moisture content on the milling performance of UK wheat with reference to wheat texture. J Sci Food Agric 32: 655-662.
49. Adejumo BA (2012) Effect of Drying Methods and Pre-treatment on some Physicochemical Quality attributes of Tomato Powder. Int J Innov Res Dev 1: 50-58.
50. Spiller GA (2001) Dietary fiber in prevention and treatment of disease. In: Spiller GA (ed.), CRC handbook of dietary fiber in human nutrition. Washington: CRC Press LLC, pp: 363-431.
51. Jenkins DJ, Wolever TM, Leeds AR, Gassull MA, Haisman P, et al. (1978) Dietary fibres, fibre analogues, and glucose tolerance: importance of viscosity. Br Med J 1: 1392-1394.
52. Ou S, Kwok K, Li Y, Fu L (2001) *In vitro* study of possible role of dietary fiber in lowering postprandial serum glucose. J Agric Food Chem 49: 1026-1029.
53. Osilesi O, Trout DL, Glover EE, Harper SM, Koh ET, et al. (1985) Use of xanthan gum in dietary management of diabetes mellitus. Am J Clin Nutr 42: 597-603.
54. Basu S, Stuckler D, McKee M, Galea G (2013) Nutritional determinants of worldwide diabetes: an econometric study of food markets and diabetes prevalence in 173 countries. Public Health Nutr 16: 179-186.
55. Teff KL, Elliott SS, Tschop M (2004) Dietary Fructose Reduces Circulating Insulin and Leptin, Attenuates Postprandial Suppression of Ghrelin, and Increases Triglycerides in Women. J Clin Endocrinol Metab 89: 2963-2972.
56. Thorburn AW, Crapo PA, Beltz WF, Wallace P, Witztum JL, et al. (1989) Lipid metabolism in non-insulin-dependent diabetes: effects of long term treatment with fructose-supplemented mixed meals. Am J Clin Nutr 50: 1015-1022.
57. UK Prospective Diabetes Study Group (1998) Intensive blood-glucose control with sulphonylureas or insulin compared with conventional treatment and risk of complications in patients with type 2 diabetes (UKPDS 33) Lancet 352: 837-853.
58. Seri K, Sanai K, Matsuo N, Kawakubo K, Xue C, et al. (1996) L-arabinose selectively inhibits intestinal sucrase in an uncompetitive manner and suppresses glycemic response after sucrose ingestion in animals. Metabolism 45: 1368-1374.
59. Preuss HG, Echard B, Bagchi D, Stohs S, (2007) Inhibition by natural dietary substances of gastrointestinal absorption of starch and sucrose in rats and pigs: 1. Acute studies. Int J Med Sci 4: 196-202.
60. Hendricks DG (2002) Mineral analysis by traditional methods. In: Introduction to the Chemical Analysis of Food. CBS, New Delhi, India, pp: 123-130.
61. Aremu MO, Olonisakin A, Otene IW, Atolaiye BO (2005) Mineral content of some agricultural products grown in the middle belt of Nigeria. Oriental Journal of Chemistry 21: 419-425.
62. Mohamed B, Abderrahim Z, Hassane M, Abdelhafid T, Abdelkhalaeq L (2006) Medicinal plants with potential antidiabetic activity-A review of ten years of herbal medicine research (1990-2000). Int J Diabetes Metabol 14: 1-25.

Nutritional Characterization of Selected Fodder Species in Abol and Lare Districts of Gambella Region, Ethiopia

Emana Megersa[1*], Ashenafi Mengistu[2] and Getahun Asebe[3]

[1]*Department of Animal Science, Gambella Agricultural, Technical and Vocational Training College, Ethiopia*

[2]*Department of Tropical Animal Production and Health, College of Veterinary Medicine and Agriculture, Addis Ababa University, Ethiopia*

[3]*Department of Animal Science, College of Agriculture and Natural Resource, Gambella University, Ethiopia*

[*]**Corresponding author:** Megersa M, Department of Animal Science, Gambella Agricultural, Technical and Vocational Training College, Ethiopia
E-mail: emana2004@yahoo.com

Abstract

In Ethiopia the commonly identified feed resource are natural pasture, crop residue, improved pasture and forages, agro-industrial by-products, other by-products like food and vegetable refusal, of which the first two contribute the largest share. This research was done with the objective of nutritional characterization of selected forage species in two districts of Gambella regional state Lare and Abol, Southwest Ethiopia. The study was done using a formal survey, focus group discussions and field observations followed by sample collection, chemical analysis and *In vitro* Dry Matter Digestibility (IVDMD) of selected grass and browse species. Purposive sampling was employed to select 90 Households (HHs) having livestock. Four grasses and 10 browses species were collected during November to December 2013 and their nutritive values were evaluated. The average Crude Protein (CP) was 11.51% for the grasses and 13.16% for the browses, respectively. The average neutral detergent fibre (NDF) content was 75.37% for grasses and 56.43% for browse species whereas the IVDMD of grasses and browses were 64.45% and 59.3%, respectively. The selected grasses and browse species were good potential as livestock feed in the area and is recommended if further analysis in more species and study sites in the area.

Keywords: Browse; Grass; Nutritive value; Digestibility

Introduction

Livestock feed resources in Ethiopia includes natural pasture, crop residue, improved pasture and forages, agro-industrial by-products, other by-products like food and vegetable refusal, of which the first two contribute the largest share [1]. Natural pastures are naturally occurring grasses, legumes, herbs, shrubs and tree foliage that are used as animal feed [2]. These natural pastures comprise the largest feed resources, the contribution of which is estimated at 80-85% in Ethiopia [3]. Grass and browse species of communal grazing lands of sub-Saharan Africa are important sources of feed for smallholder ruminant production systems [4]. Livestock grazing is the predominant form of land use in pastoral areas which receive less than 600-700 mm annual rainfall. Natural pastures are decreasing from time to time and gradually disappearing due to rapidly increasing human population and expansion of cropland [2]. Studies report that overgrazing might also have been the main factor for the decline in the composition and diversity of plant species over a long period of time [5,6].

As a major source of animal feeds in Africa, fodder trees and shrubs are highly valued by farmers [7]. They play a significant role in arid areas where moisture is inadequate [8]. Pastoralists depend heavily on woody plants for multiple uses [9]. These forage species contain appreciable amounts of nutrients that are deficient in other feed resources such as grasses during dry periods. They have deep root systems enabling the extraction of water and nutrients from deep in the soil profile [10]. Most browse plants have high crude protein content, ranging from 10 to more than 25% on a dry matter basis [11]. This reliable protein resource can be used to develop a sustainable feeding system and increase livestock productivity [12].

Gambella region is endowed with diverse species of grasses and browses [13]. Gelayenew et al. [14] indicated in natural pasture was the dominant feed resources during the wet season. Crop residue and browse forage species play a significant role during the dry season. The major livestock production constraints in the study area were disease and parasite (67%) followed by feed shortage (50%) and water scarcity (46%).

This biodiversity is of a substantial potential to support local livestock production and serve as candidate source of germplasm for further research aimed at improving livestock production elsewhere in the country. This requires a systematic documentation of information on chemical characterization of common feed resources. Thus, the objective of this piece of work was to characterize some common fodder species in terms of their nutritive value.

Materials and Methods

Description of the study area

The study was carried out at Abol and Lare districts of the Gambella People's Regional State (GPNRS). Abol district is one of the districts in Anuak zone having a total land area of 3,118.79 km^2 where 20% of it is covered by forest. The total human population of the district is 10,590 with 2595 households. The district is found at an elevation of 400-600 masl bordered on the south by Abobo and on the west by Itang districts and on the north and east by Oromia Regional State [15].

Lare district is part of the Nuer zone which covers a total land area of 685.17 km^2 a human population size of 31,406 and 5,432 households. It is found at an elevation of 300-400 masl and bordering on south and east by Anuak zone, on west by Baro River, which separates Jikawo, and on north by Jikawo River which separates from south Sudan. The terrain in Lare consists of marshes and grasslands [15]. The study districts were an annual rainfall varying from 900 to 1,500 mm. The absolute maximum temperature occurs in mid-March and is about 45°C and the absolute minimum temperature occurs in December and is 10.3°C [13].

Study design

The study involved questionnaire surveys, field visits and observation, focus group discussions and key informant interviews with the main objectives of chemical characterization of selected/common fodder species.

Sampling procedures and determination of sample size

The districts were selected randomly from the low lands of Gambella from which three peasant associations (PAs) were also selected randomly from each of the districts. Those districts and PAs that have security problems were excluded. The sample size was determined according to Arsham [16] with the formula of $n=0.25/SE^2$, where SE=5.27% and at confidence interval of 5%. Accordingly, a total of ninety (90) households (HHs) were purposively selected, 30 from Abol and 60 from Lare districts distributed based on the principle of sample proportional size, were involved in the study. The sampling frame comprised only of those households with livestock.

Data Collection

Method of data collection

Closed and open ended questionnaires were prepared and used for data collection through field visits, group discussions and key informant interviews. During the assessment, discussions were held with pertinent experts and secondary data were collected from the Agriculture Office of the districts. In addition to the closed and open-ended questionnaires, informal discussions were held with a group of households in each of the PAs and with development agents working in the localities. Enumerators were recruited and trained to administer the pretested questionnaires. The researcher was also involved in supervising the processes and the actual data collection which extended from November to December 2013.

Sampling of feeds and preparation of samples

During the focus group discussions, the available feed resources were listed and common forages (grasses, and browses) were ranked according to animal preference and availability as livestock feed at each of the PAs in the districts. For plant identification, the common prioritized forage samples were collected from the study sites. Information on local name of plant, plant morphology and photographs of the plant samples were also taken during the field work to facilitate identification which was done at the Addis Ababa University's herbarium.

For chemical analysis of the browse species the sample was hand plucked with a mix of all edible parts(leaves, fine stems and pods) and a composite sample of three kilogram on fresh bases from ten and above plant was taken from each species when available along peasant associations (Pas) while for grass samples two quadrants (1 × 1 m) were made around river bank in PA that were river border when available and harvested at about 5 cm above the ground and after harvest other species of the forages were separated. Grass and browse samples of same species were pooled over the PAs and one sub-sample of 0.5 kg representing the specific species was taken for nutritional quality analysis. The materials analyzed included four grass and ten browse species.

Fresh samples with high moisture content were weighed with suspended beam balance and then partial sun dried to reduce the moisture content to a safe level for storage until it was brought to Holleta Research Center's animal nutrition laboratory for oven-drying at 135°C for 2 h and ground to pass through 1 mm sieve for chemical analysis and *in vitro* digestibility. The ground samples were kept in air-tight containers until used for analysis.

Chemical analyses of the feed sample

Chemical analyses and *in vitro* dry matter digestibility of collected forage samples were determined using standard analytical methods. Dry matter and ash contents of feed samples were determined according to the procedures of AOAC [17]. The organic matter (OM) content was obtained as 100 minus ash content of the sample. Nitrogen (N) content was determined by Kjeldahl method and crude protein (CP) was calculated as N × 6.25 [17]. The neutral detergent fibre (NDF), acid detergent fibre (ADF) and acid detergent lignin (ADL) were determined according to Van Soest et al. [18]. Hemicellulose was determined by subtracting ADF from NDF. The method of Tilley and Terry [19] as modified by Van Soest and Robertson [20] was used to determine *in vitro* DM digestibility (IVDMD). The analyses were done at Holetta Agricultural Research Center animal nutrition laboratory.

Data management and analysis

The collected data were organized, summarized and analysed with the help of Statistical Package for the Social Sciences [21]. Chemical composition and IVDMD of major browse and grass forages were determined using descriptive statistics.

Results

Available feed resources and their distribution overtime

As ranked during focus group discussions the predominant livestock feed resources in the area were grasses followed by browse plants (Table 1). Grasses are the most preferred feed resources by cattle in the area where as browses are the main feeds of goats and mostly used for cattle during dry period. These browse plants in addition to feed for livestock and food for human consumption they are also used for construction purpose, fire wood and traditional medicines. Crop residues (stovers of maize and sorghum) were also in the list of important feed resources in those areas which practice crop cultivation. Other important feed resources include 'Atela' the by product from local brewing beverages. However, in the area there was no practice of conserving feed resources (hay and silages), planting of improved forages, using of agro by-products and storing of crop residues.

Feed resources	Availability by percentage	Time of Availability
Grasses	100	May to October
Browse species	63.3	Year round
Crop residues	32.2	September
Others ('Atela')	3.3	At the time when available

Table 1: Feed resources and their time of availability listed in their rank of importance.

Seasonal variation in feed quality and quantity is one of the most important constraints that limit livestock productivity in the area. For instance, in the area feed shortage was occurring due to flood during rainy season and drought during dry period. Plenty of grasses are available for about six months starting from May to December (Table 1). The browse plants were evergreen and available year round but mainly browsed in the dry season at the time when the growth of grasses and other herbaceous plants is severely affected. Feeds were abundant during the rainy season in the district except in areas affected by flood.

Chemical composition and *in vitro* dry matter digestibility of selected grass and browse species

During the focus group discussions, the available feed resources were listed and common forages (grasses, and browses) were ranked according to animal preference and availability as livestock feed in the districts. The materials analysed included four grass and ten browse species and site of collection indicated (Table 2).

Scientific name	Vernacular name	Forage category		Site of collection	
		Grass	Browse	Abol	Lare
Pennistetum sp.	*Pon/Mono*	X	-	-	X
Pennisetum unssetm (Nees.) Benth	*Bor/Ubo*	X	-	-	X
Eustachys paspaloids (Vahl.)Lanza&Pahei	*Wath/Agada*	X	-	X	-
Cynodon sp.	*Moth/Teli*	X	-	X	-
Senna sp.	*Wak/Akano*	-	X	X	-
Combretum Molle	*Jijat*	-	X	X	-
Anogeissus leiocarpus (DC.) Guill. & Perr	*Math*	-	X	X	-
Gardenia volensii K. Schum.	*Gari*	-	X	X	-
Landolphia Buchannanii (Hall. f.)Stap. f.	*Yewafmeshila*	-	X	X	-
Grewia tenax (Forssk.) Fiori	*Pori*	-	X	-	X
Maerua angolensis DC	*Neti/Anido*	-	X	-	X
Ziziphus abyssinica	*Bow/Lang*	-	X	X	-
Tamarindus indica L.	*Roka/Kuat/Choa*	-	X	X	X
Medicago plymorpha L. *(shrub legume)*	-	-	X	X	-

Table 2: Common fodder species sampled for laboratory analysis and the sites of collection.

Chemical composition and *in vitro* dry matter digestibility of selected grass species

The chemical composition and *in vitro* dry matter digestibility (IVDMD) of selected grass species are shown in Table 3. The chemical composition showed wide variation among the four grass species. The DM content of *Pennistetum unssetum* (95.85%) was the highest in the grasses. Among the grass species, the ash content in *Pennistetum* sp. (14.58%) was the highest and the lowest was in the *Cynodon* sp. (8.04%). Crude protein (CP) content varied from 8.95% in *Cynodon* sp. to 14% in the *Pennistetum* sp. The average NDF content of the four grass species was 75.37 ± 2.20 with range of 72.45% in *E. paspaloids* to 77.79% in *Cynodon* sp. The ADF content of *Pennistetum* Sp. (54.99%) was the highest whereas the lowest was observed in *P. unssetum* (42.33%) with the average group value of 48.53 ± 5.33. The mean ADL percentage reported was 10.20 ± 3.22 with the range of 7.03% in *P. unssetum* and 12.99% in *Cynodon* sp. In case of hemicelluloses *Pennistetum* sp. (20. 70%) was the lowest but highest in *P. unssetum* (33.23%). The average IVDMD contents of the four grass species under the study were 64.40 ± 3.97 with the range of 69.08% in *P. unssetum* to 66.13% in *E. paspaloids.*

Grass species	DM	OM	Ash	CP	NDF	ADF	ADL	Hem.	IVDMD
Pennistetum sp.	95.79	85.42	14.58	14.00	75.69	54.99	12.96	20.70	60.22
Pennisetum unssetm	95.85	89.62	10.38	12.00	75.56	42.33	7.03	33.23	69.08
Eustachyspaspaloidsi	95.14	87.20	12.80	11.10	72.45	46.84	7.83	25.61	66.13
Cynodon sp.	94.42	91.69	8.04	8.95	77.79	49.97	12.99	27.82	62.17
	93.3	88.55	11.45	11.51	75.37	48.53	10.2	21.2	64.4
Mean ± SD	± 0.66	± 2.85	± 2.85	± 2.09	± 2.20	± 5.33	± 3.22	± 11.13	± 3.97

Table 3: Chemical composition and *in-vitro* organic matter digestibility of selected grass species from Abol and Lare districts of Gambella by percentages.

Chemical composition and *in vitro* dry matter digestibility (IVDMD) of selected browse species

The chemical composition and IVDMD of different browse species of the districts are shown in Table 4. There were differences in nutrient contents between the ten browse species. Among the browse species the average DM content was 93.53 ± 0.97 with the range of 92.13% in *G. volensii* to 94.99% in *C. molle*. In *M. plymorpha* L. the ash content (15%) was the highest but the OM (76.36%) and ADL (7.50%) contents were the lowest. The average CP content of the species were 13.16 ± 4.17 and ranged from 8.05% in *Z. abyssinica* to 19.66% and 19.91% in *Senna* sp. and *M. plymorpha* L., respectively. The average NDF content were 56.43 ± 13.48 with the range of 43.49% in *A. leiocarpus* to 87.01% in *G. tenax*. The average content of hemicelluloses was 18.95 ± 12.25 ranged from 10.39% in *C. molle* to 52.63% in *G. tenax*. The average ADF and ADL content of the browse plants were 37.49 ± 7.9 and 9.82 ± 1.12 and their ranges were 30.43% in *A. leiocarpus* to 56.38% in *G. volensii* for ADF and 7.50% in *M. plymorpha* L. to 11.67% in *G. volensii* for ADL, respectively. The averages IVDMD of the species were 59.30 ± 6.06 with the range of 50.98% in *C. molle* to 68.86% in *Senna sp.*

Browse species	DM	OM	Ash	CP	NDF	ADF	ADL	Hem.	IVDMD
Senna sp.	93.03	89.85	10.15	19.66	44.21	32.58	8.73	11.63	68.86
Combretum Molle	94.99	93.99	6.01	16.00	52.44	42.05	10.69	10.39	50.98
Anogeissus leiocarpus	93.13	92.04	7.96	11.17	43.49	30.43	10.34	13.06	63.34
Gardenia volensii.	92.13	91.93	8.07	10.68	73.22	56.38	11.67	16.84	63.57
Landolphia buchannanii.	93.77	90.44	9.56	13.99	52.40	32.19	9.94	20.21	64.56
Grewia tenax	93.60	90.54	9.46	9.26	87.01	34.38	10.06	52.63	59.43
Maerua angolensis	94.34	90.96	9.04	9.64	54.07	37.25	10.04	16.82	54.97
Ziziphus abyssinica	92.46	87.11	12.89	8.50	49.99	31.98	9.54	18.01	51.07
Tamarindus indica	94.84	92.10	8.06	12.77	55.79	43.26	9.70	12.53	55.1
Medicago polymorpha	92.89	76.36	15.00	19.91	51.70	34.36	7.50	17.33	61.12
	93.52	89.52	9.62	13.16	56.43	37.49	9.82	18.95	59.30
Mean ± SD	± 0.97	± 4.96	± 2.60	± 4.17	± 13.48	± 7.9	± 1.12	± 12.25	± 6.06

Table 4: Chemical composition and *in vitro* dry matter digestibility of selected browses from Abol and Lare districts, Gambella by percentages.

Discussion

Available feed resources and their distribution overtime

Feed resources available in the area were natural pastures which includes grasses and browse species. These feed resources were highly depending up on climate or seasons that agree with report of Mohamed-Saleem and Abate [22] and Gelayenew et al. [14]. Seasonal variations in feed quality and quantity is the main limitation to animal production and cause fluctuation in productivity throughout the year, particularly in the dry and flooding seasons during which feed is scant and poor in nutritive value which consistence with the report of Alemayehu and Sissay [1].

The use of browse plants in addition to feeds and food they have been used for different purposes that agrees with report of Gemedo-Dalle et al. [23] and Teshome et al. [9]. Being perennial plants, fodder plants are not susceptible to sudden climatic changes and continue to maintain their green leaves longer into the dry season and known to produce high quality fodder even during drought years when grasses and other annual forages are dry and long gone due to their deep root systems which agrees with report of Coppock [24] and Eshetu [8]. However, no farmers climb up fodder plants to lop down for their livestock except very few farmers when they face critical problems similar with the report of Yeshitila [25].

Chemical composition and *in vitro* dry matter digestibility of selected grass and browse species

The average dry matter for the samples analyzed was 95.30 for grasses and 93.52% for browses, respectively, which is similar to the one reported by Beyene et al. [26] in Assosa Zone where the figures were 94.86% and 95.4% for grass and browse, respectively. This small variation could be attributed to the different times at which plants were collected, differences in species of plants, stage of harvest as reported by Gworgwor et al. [27]. The average ash content of the samples was 11.45% and 9.62% for grass and browse, respectively. This result is in consistence with the result reported by Aster et al. [28], in Borana range land 12.23% for grasses and 8.34% for browse and similarly Beyene et al. [26] reported 13% for grasses and 9% for browse. Gworgwor et al. [27] argued that differences in the ash content of the forage plants might be attributed to differences in soils and species.

The average Crude Protein (CP) of the samples was 11.51% for the grasses and 13.16% for the browse, respectively. These values were above the critical value of 7.5% reported to be required for optimal rumen function [29]. The CP for the grasses was higher and for the browse lower than that reported by Aster et al. [28] the values was 8.22% for grasses and 15.18% for browse, respectively. The variation in CP content may be attributed to different stage of harvest and seasons [30]. However, the CP of the grasses is consistent with the result of Shenkute [31], who reported that the CP content for most of immature grasses ranged from 7.2-20.2% of DM, whereas for matured grasses ranged from 5.6-11.5% of DM. The relatively high CP values in the forage studied appeared satisfactory for animal production since they exceeded the minimum protein requirement of 10-12% [32] for ruminants. On the other hand Norton [33] has reported CP level required to support lactation and growth to be 15%. This indicates that supplementation is imperatives for highly productive animals.

The average NDF content of the samples was 75.37% for grasses and 56.43% for browse species, respectively. The NDF contents of the grasses lie above the critical value of 60% which was reported to result in decreased voluntary feed intake, feed conversion efficiency and longer rumination time [34]. According to Singh and Oosting [35] if the roughage contains above 65% NDF, it is considered as poor quality feed. Moreover, Norton [33] indicated that the NDF content that ranged from 67% to 78% to be high enough to limit DM intake and digestibility, yet the study by Nyamangara and Ndlovu [36] with goats on natural vegetation with NDF contents of between 59% and 79%, indicates that this cell wall component in the foliage should be adequately degraded. Higher NDF in browse comparing with result of Aster et al. [28] 34.14% and Beyene et al. [26] 33.29 is attributed in the sampling procedures where fine stems and dry pod were included which have higher lignin contents than leaves and hence high NDF. This makes them less digestible.

The IVDMD of grasses and browses were 64.45% and 59.3%, respectively. Mugerwa et al. [37] has reported that the digestibility values greater than 65% indicate good nutritive value and values below these level results in reduced in take due to lowered digestibility. So the digestibility of the browse species was lower than the threshold level indicated. Since digestibility were affected by many factors, the lower digestibility of browse plants were attributed by lignification's of the high proportion of the fine stem and dry pod in the feed analysed. However, according to Youngquist et al. [38] the digestibility level needed for maintenance of cattle in the tropics is 45%.

Conclusion

The region as whole is endowed with diverse species of grasses and browse plants covering a vast area of land. During the main rainy season, availability of feed is not a problem in the area. However, feed shortage is prevalent during the dry period and times of flood affecting livestock production and productivity. At times of feed shortage, no practice of supplementing livestock by conserving feed resources (hay and silage) or improved forages or crop residues was observed. However, they move livestock around the riverbank during dry period and flat areas during flooding. From the results of this study, it has been observed that the browse and grass species evaluated have good potential as livestock feed.

Acknowledgments

The authors would like to acknowledge Gambella ATVET College and Addis Ababa University for financial support, Holleta Agricultural Research center for logistic and laboratory facility. The authors would like to thank staff members of Lare and Abol Woreda Agriculture and Rural Development Office and those farmers participated in this study for their hospitality and genuine approach throughout the study period without whom, complete data collection would have been impossible. The authors also would like to thank Dr. Diriba Geleti and Dr. Ermias T/tsedik, for their valuable professional support.

Authors Contribution

E.M., A.M. and G.A. conceived and designed the study; E.M. performed the experiments; A.M. analysed the data; E.M. and G.A. intensively involved in the data collection and wrote the paper.

Conflict of Interest

The authors declare no conflict of interest. The funding sponsors had no role in the design of the study; in the collection, analyses, or interpretation of data; in the writing of the manuscript, or in the decision to publish the results.

References

1. Alemayehu M, Sissay A (2003) Integrated Livestock Development Project (ILDP). Livestock Feed Resources Survey. North Gondar, Ethiopia pp: 75-82.
2. Adugna T (2007) Feed Resources for Producing Export Quality Meat and Livestok in Ethiopia. Ethiopia Sanitary and Phytosanitary Standards and Livestock and Meat Marketing Program (SPS-LMM) managed by Texas Agricultural Experiment Station (TAES) of Texas A & M University System.
3. Alemayehu M (1998) The Borana and the 1991-92 drought: A rangeland and livestock resource study. Institute of Sustainable Development, Addis Ababa, Ethiopia pp: 102-110.
4. Dicko MS, Sikena LK (1991) Fodder trees and shrubs in range and farming systems in dry tropical Africa. In: Speedy A, Pugliese PL (eds.) (2000) Legume Trees and other Fodder Trees as Protein Sources for Livestock. FAO, Rome, Italy pp: 27-41.
5. Alemayehu M (2006) Range Management for East Africa: Concepts and Practices, Sponsored by RPSUD and Printed by A.A.U Printed Press. Addis Ababa, Ethiopia.
6. Amaha K (2006) Characterization of rangeland resources and dynamics of the pastoral production system in the Somali region of Eastern Ethiopia. PhD Thesis. University of the Free State, Bloemfontein, South Africa p: 417.
7. Luseba D, Vander Merwe D (2006) Ethnoveterinary medicine practices among Tsongs speaking people of South Africa. Onderstepoort Journal of Research 73: 115-122.
8. Eshete G (2002) An assessment of feed resources, their management and impact on Livestock productivity in the Ginchi watershed area. MSc Thesis, Alemaya University, Ethiopia p: 171.
9. Teshome A, Abule E, Lisanework N (2012) Evaluation of woody vegetation in the rangeland of Southeast Ethiopia. Int Res J Agri Sci Soil Sci 2: 113-126.
10. Terefe A, Solomon M, Lisanework N (2008) Management and utilization of browse species as livestock feed in semi-arid district of North Ethiopia. Livestock Research for Rural Development.
11. Moleele NM (1998) Encroacher woody plant browses as feed for cattle. Cattle diet composition for three seasons at Olifants Drift, south-east Botswana. Journal of Arid Environments 40: 255-268.
12. Chepape RM, Mbatha KR, Luseba D (2011) Local use and knowledge validation of fodder trees and shrubs browsed by livestock in Bushbuckridge area, South Africa. Tshwane University of Technology Private Bag X680, Pretoria 0001, South Africa.
13. Hailemariam B, Mulugeta TS, Ali J, Galua K, Riek W, et al. (2011) Action plan of adaptation to climatic change. Gambella, Ethiopia.
14. Gelayenew B, Nurfeta A, Assefa G, Asebe G (2016) Assessment of Livestock Feed Resources in the Farming Systems of Mixed and Shifting Cultivation, Gambella Regional State, Southwestern Ethiopia. Global Journal of Science Frontier Research: D Agriculture and Veterinary.
15. CSA (2007) Agricultural sample survey. Livestock and Livestock characteristics, Central Statistical Authority (CSA) Bulletin 2: 123.
16. Arsham H (2007) Sample Size Determination. Merrick School of Business University of Baltimore, Charles at Mount Royal, Baltimore, Maryland, USA.
17. Thiex N, Novotny L, Crawford A (2012) Determination of ash in animal feed: AOAC official method 942.05 revisited. J AOAC Int 95: 1392-1397.
18. Van Soest PJ, Robertson JB, Lewis BA (1991) Methods for dietary fiber, Neutral detergent fiber and non-starch polysaccharides in relation to animal nutrition. J Dairy Sci 74: 3587-3597.
19. Tilley JMA, Terry RA (1963) A two-stage technique for the *in vitro* digestion of forage crops. Journal of British Grassland Society 18: 104-111.

20. Van Soest PJ, Robertson JB (1985) Analysis of forage and fibrous foods. A laboratory manual for Animal science. Cornell University, Ithaca, NY, USA.
21. SPSS (2003) Statistical procedures for social sciences (SPSS) INC, Chicago, USA.
22. Mohamed-Saleem MA, Abate T (1995) Feed Improvement to Support Intensification of Ruminant Production Systems in the Ethiopian Highlands. In: Proceedings of the 3rd National Conference of the Ethiopian Society of Animal Production, Addis Ababa, Ethiopia pp: 27-29.
23. Gemedo-Dalle T, Maass BL, Isselstein J (2006) Rangeland condition and trend in the semi-arid Borana lowlands, southern Oromia, Ethiopia. Afr J R Forage Sci 23: 49-58.
24. Coppock DL (1994) The Borana plateau of southern Ethiopia: Synthesis of pastoral Research development and change 1980-1991. International Livestock Center for Africa (ILCA), Addis Ababa, Ethiopia.
25. Yeshitila AM (2008) Assessment of Livestock Feed Resources Utilization in Alaba Woreda, Southern Ethiopia. Msc Thesis, Haramaya University, Ethiopia.
26. Beyene T, Teshome N, Ayana A (2010) Effects of farming systems on floristic composition, yield and nutrient content of forages at the natural pasture of Assosa zone (Western Ethiopia). Tropical and Subtropical Agro-Ecosystems pp: 583-592.
27. Gworgwor ZA, Mbahi TF, Mbaya YP (2006) Semi-arid trees and shrub fodders as livestock feed in North Eastern Nigeria: A Review. Nigeria J Agr 8: 263-271.
28. Aster A, Adugna T, Oystein H, Tormod A, Lars OE (2012) Seasonal Variation in Nutritive Value of some Browse and Grass species in Borana Rangeland, South Ethiopia. Tropical and Subtropical Agroecosystems 15: 261-271.
29. Van Soest PJ (1982) Nutritional Ecology of the Ruminants. O and B books, Corvallis, Oregon, USA pp: 33-184.
30. Gworgwor ZA, Kibon A, Mbahi TF (2006) Assessment of the nutritive values of somesemi arid browse plants. Nigerian Journal of Tropical Agriculture 8: 246-254.
31. Shenkute T (1972) Nutritional value of Some Tropical Grass Species Compared to Some Temperate Grass Species. PhD Thesis, Cornell Univ. Ithaca, NY, USA.
32. ARC (1985) The nutrient requirements of ruminant livestock. Agriculture Research Center (ARC). Common wealth Agricultural Bureaux, Farnham Royal, UK.
33. Norton BW (1982) Difference between species in forages quality. In: Hacker JB (ed.) Proceedings of international Symposium held at St. Luica, Queensland, Australia 24 to 28 September 1981. Nutritional limits to animal production from pastures. Commonwealth Agriculture Bureau, UK.
34. Reed JA, Goe MR (1989) Estimating the Nutritive Value of Cereal Crop Residues: Implications for developing feeding standards for draught animals. ILCA. Bulletin No. 4 ILCA, Addis Ababa, Ethopia.
35. Singh GP, Oosting SJ (1992) A model for describing the energy value of straws. Indian Dairyman XLI pp: 322-327.
36. Nyamangara ME, Ndlovu LR (1995) Feeding behaviour, feed intake, chemicals and botanical composition of the diet of indigenous goats rose on natural vegetation in a semiarid region of Zimbabwe. J Agr Sci 124: 455-461.
37. Mugerwa JS, Christianson JA, Ochetin S (1973) Grazing behavior of exotic dairy cattle in Uganda. East Afr Agri Fores J 19: 1-11.
38. Youngquist JB, Carter DC, Clegg MD (1990) Grain and forage yield and Stover quality of sorghum and millet in low rainfall environments. Exp Agr 26: 279-286.

Phenolic Acid, Flavonoids and Antioxidant Activity of Common Brown Beans (*Phaseolus vulgaris* L.) before and after Cooking

Karina Huber, Priscila Brigide*, Eloá Bolis Bretas and Solange Guidolin Canniatti-Brazaca

Food and Nutrition Department, Luiz de Queiroz College of Agriculture, University of São Paulo, Brazil

Corresponding author: Priscila Brigide, Agri-Food Industry, Food and Nutrition Department, Luiz de Queiroz College of Agriculture, University of São Paulo, Avenida Pádua Dias, 11 CP 9, CEP 13418-900 Piracicaba, SP, Brazil, E-mail: pbrigide@hotmail.com

Abstract

This study aimed to evaluate the impact of thermal processing and soaking on the profiles and contents of phenolic compounds in brown beans, as well as their antioxidant activity. We evaluated the antioxidant activity of extracts and the contents of phenolic acids and flavonoids by high-performance liquid chromatography (HPLC). With the exception of chlorogenic acid, the contents of all of the other phenolic acids were increased by cooking. Kaempferol was only detected in samples treated by soaking followed by cooking. Catechin and kaempferol-3-glucoside were found in all of the brown bean extracts. Cooking, with or without soaking, caused significant increases in the concentrations of quercetin and quercetin-3-glucoside only. The effect of the heat treatment increased the antioxidant activity and the concentrations of the phenolic compounds evaluated.

Keywords: 2,2-diphenyl-1-picrylhydrazyl (DPPH); 2,2'-azino-bis (ABTS); Polyphenols; Bioactive compounds; Thermal processing

Introduction

Similar to other legumes, beans possess large contents of bioactive compounds such as polyphenols [1]. These compounds are secondary metabolites in plants and are widely known for their antioxidant capacities. Polyphenols therefore play an important role in reducing the risk of cardiovascular disease, diabetes, some cancers, and Alzheimer and Parkinson's diseases [2]. The antioxidant activity of beans is due mainly to the reducing properties of polyphenols, which play an important role in the neutralisation or sequestration of free radicals and in the chelation of transition metals, acting against both the initiation and propagation of oxidative processes. The intermediates formed by the action of phenolic antioxidants are relatively stable due to the resonance of the aromatic rings in the structures of these substances [3].

Common beans possess antioxidant activity due to the presence of phenolic acids and flavonoids, mainly tannins [4].

It is known that the phenolic acids most commonly found in raw and cooked beans are gallic acid, vanillic, p-coumaric, ferulic, sinapic and chlorogenic acids and that they have great importance as precursors for the synthesis of other phenolic compounds in plants [3,5].

Flavonoids share a common structure consisting of two aromatic rings that are linked through three carbons, forming an oxygenated heterocycle. They are divided into six subclasses, depending on the type of heterocycle formed: Flavonols, flavones, isoflavones, flavanones, anthocyanidins and flavanols (catechin and proanthocyanidin). The main flavonoid representatives are quercetin and kaempferol in glycosylated forms. In raw and cooked beans, the main flavonoid representatives are catechin, kaempferol, quercetin, myricetin and procyanidins [3,5].

To improve the nutritional quality of beans, peeling, soaking, cooking and germination methods are used. Therefore, the present study aimed to evaluate the impact of cooking preceded by soaking and cooking without soaking on the profiles and contents of phenolic acids and flavonoids, as well as the antioxidant activity of brown beans.

Materials and Methods

Samples of the common bean (*Phaseolus vulgaris* L.) BRS9435-cometa cultivar (brown) were analysed raw and after thermal processing.

The beans were stored at refrigerator temperature (4°C) before the measurements and then they were ground and sieved. The beans intended for use as cooked samples were divided into two treatments: Treatment 1 involved soaking the beans for 10 h in distilled water, followed by an exchange of the water and then cooking in an autoclave at 121°C for 10 min; Treatment 2 involved cooking the beans in an autoclave at 121°C for 10 min. After cooking, the samples were lyophilised and stored at −26°C. Milling of the cooked beans was performed at the time of the analyses and under the same conditions as the raw samples (Treatment 3).

The polyphenol extraction was performed according to Cardador-Martínez et al. [6]. Five extractions were performed for each treatment.

The extracted material was separated into six fractions (A, B, C, D, E and F) using open column chromatography under vacuum according to the methodology proposed by Aparicio-Fernandez, Manzo-Bonilla, and Loarca-Piña [7]. Lyophilised extract in 0.5 g quantities was diluted in 1 mL of methanol and poured into an open column over silica gel (Sigma Aldrich, 13% $CaSO_4$). The reagents were added as shown in Figure 1 and the fractions were collected after each passage.

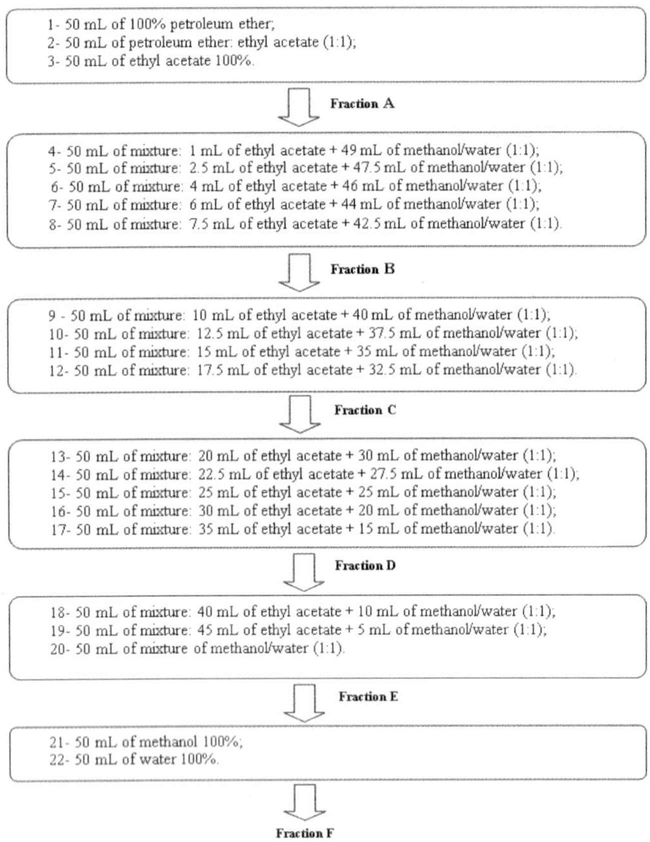

Figure 1: Polyphenol separation into six fractions (A-F) using open column chromatography under vacuum.

After the recovery of each fraction (except for fraction A which was discarded as a lipid-removal and column-cleaning fraction), the mixtures were placed in a flask to evaporate the solvents in a rotary evaporator. The fractions FB, FC, FD and FF were lyophilised for further analysis; however, Fraction FE did not generate sufficient phenolic compounds for analysis.

To measure antioxidant activity via 1,1-diphenyl-2-pycrylhydrazyl (DPPH) Sigma Chemical Co., we used the methodology proposed by Brand-Williams, Cuvier, and Berset [8]. The results were expressed in milligrams of 6-hydroxy-2,5,7,8-tetramethylchroman-2-carboxylic acid (Trolox) Sigma Chemical Co. equivalent antioxidant capacity (TEAC) g^{-1} of the extract. We used the 2,2-azino-bis(3-ethylbenzothiazoline-6-sulfonic acid) diammonium salt (ABTS) Sigma Chemical Co. method proposed by Re et al. [9], Van Den Berg et al. [10] and Arts et al. [11], with modifications' to determine the antioxidant activity. The results were expressed in mg of Trolox-equivalent antioxidant capacity (TEAC) g^{-1} of extract.

To identify and quantify the phenolic acids, free phenolic acids were separated by high-performance liquid chromatography (HPLC) according to Xu and Chang [12], with modifications. A Shimadzu model 20 A, equipped with a UV detector (270 and 325 nm) was used. A Zorbax ODS Stablebond-C18 (Agilent Technology), 4.6 × 250 mm, 5 mm analytical column was used for the separation, at 40°C. The mobile phases used were A, 0.1% trifluoroacetic acid solution in water; B, 100% methanol and an isocratic gradient that include 20% phase A and 80% phase B with flow rates of 1.0 mL min^{-1}.

To identify the HPLC peaks, one stock solution (1 mg mL^{-1}) of each phenolic acid profile was individually prepared and diluted. These dilute solutions were injected (20 μL) separately, duplicating the conditions described above. The peak areas and their retention times were used to compare, identify and quantify these phenolic acids in the samples injected afterwards.

To prepare the stock solutions, 10 mg of each phenolic acid was dissolved in 10 mL of 80% methanol and then diluted in 80% methanol in the following solutions: 0.5, 1, 2.5, 5, 10 and 25 μg mL^{-1} of vanillic acid; 10, 25, 50 and 100 μg mL^{-1} of chlorogenic acid; 1, 2.5, 5, 10, 25, 50 and 100 μg mL^{-1} of sinapic acid and 1, 5, 10, 25 and 50 μg mL^{-1} of gallic acid. The content of each phenolic acid was expressed in micrograms per gram of extract (μg g^{-1}).

The chromatographic system and methodology used for the separation of flavonoids were the same as those used for the phenolic acids analysis. The oven temperature was 34°C. The mobile phases used were A, 0.1% acetic acid solution in water and B, 0.1% acetic acid in acetonitrile in the following concentration gradients and flow rates: 1.0 mL min^{-1} with 15% phase B and 85% phase A during the first 5 min; 1.5 mL min^{-1} with an increase in phase B to 29% and a reduction in phase A to 71% from 5 to 23 min; 1.0 mL min^{-1} with an increase in phase B to 35% and a reduction in phase A to 65% from 23 to 44 min; 1.0 mL min^{-1} with an increase in phase B to 50% and a reduction in phase A to 50% from 44 to 46 min and 1.0 mL min^{-1} with a reduction in phase B to 15% and an increase in phase A to 85% from 46 to 48 min.

To identify the HPLC peaks, a stock solution (1 mg mL^{-1}) of each phenolic acid profile was individually prepared and then diluted. These dilute solutions were injected (20 μL) separately and in duplicate under the conditions described above. The peak areas and their retention times were used to compare, identify and quantify these phenolic compounds in the subsequently injected extracts.

To prepare the stock solution, 10 mg of each flavonoid was dissolved in 10 mL of 80% methanol and then diluted in 80% methanol in the following concentrations: 5, 10, 25 and 50 μg mL^{-1} of catechin; 25, 50, 100 and 250 μg mL^{-1} of quercetin; 2.5, 5, 10, 25 and 50 μg mL^{-1} of kaempferol-3-glucoside; 10, 25, 50 and 100 μg mL^{-1} of kaempferol 3-O-rutinoside; 10, 25, 50 and 100 μg mL^{-1} of kaempferol and 10, 25, 50 and 100 μg mL^{-1} of quercetin-3-glucoside. The content of each flavonoid was expressed as micrograms per gram of extract (μg g^{-1}).

The statistical design was completely randomised. Analyses of the antioxidant activity were performed in duplicate, with two replicates for each extract and fraction and the identification and quantification analyses of the phenolic acids and flavonoids were performed in duplicate, with two replicates only for crude extracts of polyphenols. The results were analysed by the Tukey test at 5% probability.

Results

Some differences between the two methods can be observed. According to the DPPH method, both cooking processes resulted in higher antioxidant activity in the cooked beans compared to the extracts of the raw beans. For crude extracts of the beans, the results of DPPH ranged from 2.96 to 14.04 mg TEAC g^{-1} extract.

	DPPH			ABTS		
	Raw	**Cooked**	**Cooked and soaked**	**Raw**	**Cooked**	**Cooked and soaked**
Crude extract	8.73 ± 0.6[a]B[b]	12.65 ± 0.3A	13.74 ± 0.1A	22.30 ± 2.3A	29.51 ± 4.6A	20.28 ± 0.9B
Fraction FB	4.48 ± 0.5B	7.13 ± 0.1A	4.82 ± 0.2B	34.96 ± 21.2A	11.57 ± 0.1A	20.96 ± 0.8A
Fraction FC	6.05 ± 0.3A	6.25 ± 1.0A	7.26 ± 0.2A	46.70 ± 3.1A	29.31 ± 2.3B	19.72 ± 1.8B
Fraction FD	4.48 ± 3.3A	3.28 ± 1.3A	3.41 ± 0.1A	20.15 ± 0.5A	13.06 ± 0.2B	11.42 ± 1.0B
Fraction FF	0.53 ± 0.3A	0.87 ± 0.3A	1.37 ± 0.1A	13.48 ± 1.1A	15.57 ± 1.6A	10.92 ± 2.5A

[a]Means of two replicates ± standard deviation; [b]Means with different uppercase letters (s) in the horizontal direction (s) indicate that the fractions differ significantly ($p \leq 0.05$). FB, FC, FD, and FF: polyphenol fractions obtained by open column chromatography under vacuum.

Table 1: Antioxidant activity (mg TEAC g^{-1} of extract) of crude extracts and fractions of polyphenols from brown raw, cooked and cooked and soaked beans as measured by the DPPH and ABTS methods.

In the ABTS assays, the extracts ranged from 13.70 and 29.51 mg TEAC g^{-1} extract. Table 1 shows the antioxidant activity values according to the DPPH and ABTS methods.

The levels of phenolic acids present in the crude extract are shown in Table 2. It was found for phenolic acids that all extracts evaluated have the gallic acid ranged from 2203.55 to 3693.39 μg g^{-1} extracts of the beans, chlorogenic from 1272.04 to 4430,26 μg g^{-1} extracts of the beans, vanillic from 377.49 to 1404.45 μg g^{-1} extracts of the beans and sinapic from 88.52 to 382.37 μg g^{-1} extracts of the beans, and the first two were found at higher levels.

	Raw	**Cooked**	**Cooked and soaked**
Vanillic acid	498.17 ± 2.0[a]C[b]	779.83 ± 21.4A	563.97 ± 1.6B
Gallic acid	2872.37 ± 5.5C	3693.39 ± 44.2A	3510.18 ± 59.5B
Chlorogenic acid	3139.81 ± 6.3A	1812.56 ± 2.8B	1552.49 ± 5.3C
Sinapic acid	140.19 ± 8.3C	258.71 ± 3.9A	194.17 ± 1.2B

[a]Means of two replicates ± standard deviation; [b]Means with different uppercase letters (s) in the horizontal direction(s) indicate that the phenolic acid contents differ significantly ($p \leq 0.05$).

Table 2: Phenolic acids (μg g^{-1} extract) in crude extracts from raw, cooked and cooked and soaked brown beans.

Table 3 shows the results regarding the phenolic acid fractions of the crude extracts. All of fractions FC were indentified whith high level the phenolic acid. Table 4 shows the results of the analyses of the flavonoids in the crude bean polyphenol extracts. Almost all flavonoids were detected in almost all samples, except for kaempferol (0-311.20 μg g^{-1} of extract), wich was only detected in soaked and cooked samples. For extracts from white beans, flavonoids found in highest concentrations were catechin (547.33 μg g^{-1} of extract) and kaempferol-3-rutinoside 327.68 μg g^{-1} of extract; brown beans extracts showed mostly catechin 1886.61 μg g^{-1} of extract and kaempferol-3-glucoside 1690.77 μg g^{-1} of extract, and in extracts of black beans, mainly catechin 986.12 μg g^{-1} of extract, kaempferol-3-glucoside 307.60 μg g^{-1} of extract and quercetin-3-glucoside 343.65 μg g^{-1} of extract.

	Raw	**Cooked**	**Cooked and soaked**
Vanillic acid			
FB	783.74 ± 2.1[a]A[b]	-	1136.23 ± 8.7A
FC	768.06 ± 0.8A	628.71 ± 0.8A	688.81 ± 18.3A
FF	-	69.18 ± 2.7A	-
Gallic acid			
FB	3494.27 ± 3.8A	-	6475.18 ± 76.8A
FC	4530.60 ± 6.7A	3100.71 ± 1.7	4766.28 ± 42.6A
FF	-	Nd	-
Chlorogenic acid			
FB	1595.09 ± 0.3A	-	2050.96 ±1.2A
FC	2833.63 ± 3.4A	1325.83 ± 2.1	1994.51 ± 4.6A
FF	-	Nd	-
Sinapic acid			
FB	173.40 ± 2.1A	-	346.12 ± 18.1A
FC	195.73 ± 2.6A	148.87 ± 0.5A	156.61 ± 6.4A
FF	-	47.12 ± 0.4A	-

[a]Means of two replicates ± standard deviation; [b]Means with different uppercase letters in the horizontal direction and in the vertical direction for the same treatment differ significantly ($p \leq 0.05$) according to the means test. FB, FC and FF: fractions of polyphenols obtained by open column chromatography under vacuum that had higher antioxidant activities. Two fractions were used for each treatment. Nd: Not detected.

Table 3: Phenolic acid (μg g^{-1} of extract) fractions of polyphenols from raw, cooked and cooked-and-soaked brown beans.

	Raw	Cooked	Cooked and soaked
Kaempferol	0.00 ± 0.00[a]B[b]	0.00 ± 0.00B	127.41 ± 10.29A
Kaempferol-3-glucoside	1098.62 ± 37.57B	1690.77 ± 16.71A	1136.59 ± 24.50B
Kaempferol-3-rutinoside	13.62 ± 0.83C	69.78 ± 13.41B	176.81 ± 1.36A
Catechin	1105.77 ± 112.37B	1886.61 ± 73.03A	1428.83 ± 36.50B
Quercetin	9.58 ± 2.03A	10.67 ± 4.03A	12.14 ± 1.22A
Quercetin-3-glucoside	23.07 ± 5.54A	33.70 ± 9.58A	12.81 ± 5.44A

[a]Means of two replicates ± standard deviation; [b]Means with uppercase different letters(s) in the horizontal direction(s) differ significantly (p ≤ 0.05).

Table 4: Flavonoids (μg g^{-1} of extract) in crude extracts of polyphenols from raw, cooked and cooked-and-soaked brown beans.

The results for the flavonoid fractions in crude beans extracts are presented in Table 5. The highest level were for soaked and cooked beans.

Discussion

Some differences between the two methods can be observed. According to the DPPH method, both cooking processes resulted in higher antioxidant activity in the cooked beans compared to the extracts of the raw beans. Similar results were also reported in the study of Rocha-Guzmán et al. [4], who concluded that cooked beans removed of free radicals at a higher rate compared to raw beans. This increase in antioxidant potential after heat treatment with or without soaking may be due to the concentration of phenolic compounds in the cooking broth, which facilitates their extraction. In the work of Xu and Chang [12], the ability of the compounds scavenge free radicals as measured by DPPH was reduced by 28-36% in boiled beans under pressure compared to raw beans and reduced by 23-31% compared to beans that were soaked before cooking.

In the ABTS assays, the extracts and fractions from the raw beans did not have the lowest results. In the FC and FD fractions, cooking promoted a decrease in antioxidant activity, with or without soaking, compared to the extract of the same raw bean. Xu and Chang [12] attributed this decrease in antioxidant activity after thermal treatment to the possibility that chemical transformations, decomposition of phenolic compounds, formation of complexes between polyphenols and proteins and solubilisation of water-soluble antioxidants in the discarded soaking water occurred.

Although both results of the ABTS and the DPPH that the evaluated antioxidant has the ability to donate hydrogen, a comparative study of the FRAP, ORAC, DPPH and ABTS methodologies by Fernandez-Panchon et al. [13] indicated that the sensitivity of the ABTS radicals was lower compared to the DPPH radical following heat processing.

With the DPPH method, the antioxidant activities of the extracts were higher than those found for fractions. This is possibly due to synergy between all of the antioxidant compounds that were present in the crude extract, while no such synergy was possible in the isolated fractions. However, in the ABTS assays, the extracts did not did not contain higher fractions.

	Raw	Cooked	Cooked and soaked
Kaempferol			
FB	0.00	-	427.50[a] ± 0.41A[b]
FC	0.00	0.00	173.61 ± 5.35A
FF	-	0.00	-
Kaempferol-3-glucoside			
FB	1564.37 ± 0.35A	-	1813.33 ± 15.25A
FC	1888.64 ± 1.65A	1416.16 ± 4.56	1269.96 ± 22.53A
FF	-	Nd	-
Kaempferol-3-rutinoside			
FB	18.33 ± 0.02A	-	8.40 ± 1.29
FC	19.78 ± 0.06A	71.17 ± 2.97	Nd
FF	-	Nd	-
Catechin			
FB	1057.41 ± 1.43A	-	1097.99 ± 3.03A
FC	1594.51 ± 3.96A	1501.24 ± 168.31A	1466.67 ± 4.22A
FF	-	44.27 ± 0.37B	-
Quercetin			
FB	8.19 ± 0.04B	-	15.40 ± 0.64
FC	12.49 ± 6.72A	Nd	Nd
FF	-	10.76 ± 0.40	-
Quercetin-3-glucoside			
FB	9.46 ± 0.44A	-	16.48 ± 0.93A
FC	7.55 ± 0.20A	20.39 ± 0.06	19.28 ± 2.65A
FF	-	Nd	-

[a]Means of two replicates ±standard deviation; [b]Means with uppercase letters (s) that are different(s) in the vertical direction differ significantly (p ≤ 0.05) according to the means test. FB, FC and FF: the fractions of these polyphenols that were obtained by open column chromatography under vacuum had higher antioxidant activities. Two fractions were used for each treatment. Nd: Not detected.

Table 5: Flavonoid (μg g^{-1} of extract) fractions of polyphenols from raw, cooked, and cooked-and-soaked brown beans.

Using both methods, the fraction obtained with a more polar solvent (FF) had the lowest values of Trolox-equivalent antioxidant capacity. The polarity of the compounds in brown beans may affect their extraction from the feedstock [14]. Depending on the polarity of the solvent, more of one or another phenolic compound may be present in food and thus affect the antioxidant capacity of the extract.

Overall, the crude extracts showed similar antioxidant activities in relation to their respective fractions. The same finding was reported in the study by Beninger and Hosfield [14], who explained their results by noting that the flavonoids present in the crude extract were further concentrated in the extracts; this concentration may have been primarily responsible for the observed antioxidant activity.

In all of the samples analysed, gallic and chlorogenic acids were found to have the highest contents. These findings regarding beans have also been reported in the literature. The contents measured in this study are higher than those in other studies due to the units in which these data are expressed (per gram of extract in this study vs. per gram of food in others). Xu and Chang [5] reported contents of 89.64 and 32.93 μg of gallic acid g^{-1} in black bean that were raw and cooked under pressure for 10 min, respectively, and 226.1 and 89.9 μg of chlorogenic acid g^{-1} in black bean that were raw and cooked under pressure for 10 min, respectively. However, Luthria and Pastor-Corrales [15] evaluated 15 types of beans and detected only p-coumaric, sinapic and ferulic acids, the last showing the highest concentration. Ranilla et al. [16] detected chlorogenic acid in only three of twenty-eight cultivars analysed (between 2.8 and 5.6 mg 100 g^{-1}).

It was observed that cooking significantly increases the concentration of vanillic acid. By contrast, Diaz-Batalla et al. [1] found lower levels of vanillic acid in cooked beans than in raw beans for the 14 analysed cultivars. Aguilera et al. [17] found no vanillic acid in cooked beans, with or without soaking and found 10.71 μg g^{-1} in raw beans. This phenolic acid has the following desirable activities: antihelminthic activity, the prevention of sickle erythrocytes and the suppression of liver fibrosis in chronic liver diseases [5,18].

Similarly, higher concentrations of gallic acid were found in the extracts of cooked beans. Xu and Chang [5], however, reported contents of 83.17 μg g^{-1} in raw beans and 38.16μg g^{-1} in cooked brown beans; both of these values are well below those reported here and indicate an effect of cooking on the content of this specific phenolic acid that is the opposite of that reported here. We note that recent studies report that gallic acid, in addition to its antioxidant properties, has the following biological effects: antineoplastic and bacteriostatic activity, repression of brain tumours, antitumor properties, induction of apoptosis in prostate carcinoma cells, antiangiogenic activity, inhibition of disaccharidases in the intestinal brush border of mammals and induction of apoptosis or necrosis of cancer cells [18]. Therefore, the consumption of beans is highly beneficial, as high contents of gallic were measured in the extracts that were analysed.

Large amounts of chlorogenic acid were measured in the extracts of raw beans. The action of this compound in the prevention of Alzheimer's disease via a reduction in apoptosis induced by amyloid-β cells. Additionally, chlorogenic acid displays anticholinesterase, anti-inflammatory and antioxidant activities. The phenolic compound can be easily oxidised via polyphenol oxidases leading to its interaction with NH_2 groups of proteins and amino acids, resulting in reducing the nutritional value of foods. The acid in question increases homocysteine levels in human plasma, which constitutes a risk factor for the onset of cardiovascular disease [18].

Regarding sinapic acid, the highest levels were found in extracts of cooked beans without soaking. In a study by Espinosa-Alonso et al. [19] sinapic acid as found at a concentration equal to 22.4 mg Kg^{-1} of different coloured beans. Campos-Vega et al. [2] reported that antioxidant activity is the main biological activity provided by sinapic acid.

We analysed the two fractions that had the highest antioxidant activity according to the DPPH and ABTS methods and these fractions varied according to the beans and treatment. Therefore, tests of the averages of duplicates that were injected into the chromatograph were performed.

In general, heat treatment increased the antioxidant activities and the concentrations of phenolic compounds evaluated. This finding is important because raw beans have antinutritional factors and should therefore be cooked before they are consumed. Soaking, on the other hand, had variable effects in each of the analyses.

Table 3 shows the results regarding the phenolic acid fractions of the crude extracts. We analysed the two fractions that had the highest antioxidant activity according to the DPPH and ABTS methods and these fractions varied according to the beans and treatment. Therefore, tests of the averages of duplicates that were injected into the chromatograph were performed.

In general, heat treatment increased the antioxidant activities and the concentrations of phenolic compounds evaluated. This finding is important because raw beans have antinutritional factors and should therefore be cooked before they are consumed. Soaking, on the other hand, had variable effects in each of the analyses.

It is observed that some phenolic acids were not present in either fraction evaluated. It must then be the case that the significant antioxidant activity of these fractions was due to other, unidentified materials present in the extracts evaluated.

The phenolic acids that were found in the highest concentrations were gallic and chlorogenic acid. Among the various phenolic compound fractions that were evaluated, the FB and FC fractions had higher scores compared to the FF, although many of the fractions did not differ significantly. This finding corroborates the results from the DPPH and ABTS methods, which indicated that the FF fraction had lower antioxidant activity and the results regarding the polarity of acids that were evaluated and solvents used in the fractionation. It is known that the phenolic acids quantified herein are typically polar.

The literature reports that chlorogenic, gallic and sinapic acid have high antioxidant activities and that the activity of vanillic acid is lower [20]. Thus, it is concluded that, due to the large fractions of chlorogenic and gallic acid measured in the extracts of the beans evaluated here, brown beans have high potential as antioxidants, as confirmed by the results of the DPPH and ABTS assays.

Table 4 shows the results of the analyses of the flavonoids in the crude bean polyphenol extracts. Most of the flavonoids examined were detected in almost all of the samples, except for the kaempferol, which was only detected in the soaked and cooked samples. However, in a study by Diaz-Batalla et al. [1], kaempferol was present at higher concentrations in raw beans (average of 52.3 μg g^{-1} of bean) compared to cooked beans (average of 27.2 μg g^{-1} of bean). Likewise, in a work by Amarowicz and Pegg [3], cooking promoted a reduction of this flavonoid by 5-71%. Romani et al. [21], who assessed the levels of various flavonoids in Italians beans, did not detect even trace amounts of quercetin-3-glucoside and this flavonoid as not detected in the extracts evaluated in this study either.

We mainly found catechin and kaempferol-3-glucoside flavonoids. Ranilla et al. [16] detected quercetin and kaempferol in brown beans and Lin et al. [22] detected kaempferol-3-glucoside. It is known that kaempferol is associated with a reduced risk of developing cancer and that kaempferol-3-glucoside possesses anticancer properties and neuroprotective properties against diseases such as Parkinson's and Alzheimer's [2,18].

It was expected that higher concentrations of catechin would be detected because catechin is a type of procyanidin and is the main flavonoid present in beans [23]. However, Xu and Chang [5] did not detect this compound in raw or cooked brown beans.

Based on the data in Table 4, it is observed that, for all flavonoids, when there was a significant difference among the extracts from raw and cooked beans, the former always exhibited inferior results. The effect of soaking varies for each compound evaluated; however, the effect of this process on the increases in the concentrations of kaempferol and kaempferol-3-rutinoside was clear. These results are contrary to published reports claiming that cooking and soaking have a negative impact on flavonoid concentrations [1,5,17].

It is also notable that quercetin and quercetin-3-glucoside were not influenced by cooking, with or without soaking. Amarowicz and Peggy [3], however, found that the concentration of quercetin was reduced by 12-65% after the beans were cooked and Díaz-Batalla et al. [1] found mean values of 10.9 µg of quercetina g^{-1} in raw beans and 6.5 µg of quercetina g^{-1} in cooked beans. It is reported in the literature that quercetin has various effects in the prevention and treatment of some types of cancer, in the reversal of cognitive deficits and the inhibition of H_2O_2 and histamine generation [2,18].

It was expected that higher concentrations of catechin would be detected because catechin is a type of procyanidin and is the main flavonoid present in beans [23]. However, Xu and Chang [5] did not detect this compound in raw or cooked brown beans.

Based on the data in Table 4, it is observed that, for all flavonoids, when there was a significant difference among the extracts from raw and cooked beans, the former always exhibited inferior results. The effect of soaking varies for each compound evaluated; however, the effect of this process on the increases in the concentrations of kaempferol and kaempferol-3-rutinoside was clear. These results are contrary to published reports claiming that cooking and soaking have a negative impact on flavonoid concentrations [1,5,17].

It is also notable that quercetin and quercetin-3-glucoside were not influenced by cooking, with or without soaking. Amarowicz and Peggy [3], however, found that the concentration of quercetin was reduced by 12 to 65% after the beans were cooked and Díaz-Batalla et al. [1] found mean values of 10.9 µg of quercetina g^{-1} in raw beans and 6.5 µg of quercetina g^{-1} in cooked beans. It is reported in the literature that quercetin has various effects in the prevention and treatment of some types of cancer, in the reversal of cognitive deficits and the inhibition of H_2O_2 and histamine generation [2,18].

The results for the flavonoid fractions in crude beans extracts are presented in Table 5. It is noted that many of the fractions did not contain one or more of the phenolic compounds analysed; additionally, the behaviour of the kaempferol was similar to that observed for other polyphenols and this compound was present only in extracts of cooked and soaked beans.

Aparicio-Fernandez et al. [7] performed fractionations similar to those in this study, but they used methanol extracts of black beans. They detected kaempferol-3-glucoside, quercetin-3-glucoside and myricetin glycosylated only in the FB fraction, at ratios of 5.8, 4.1 and 6.7 respectively. These authors note that the presence of glycosylated myricetin in these beans was unexpected and has been rarely documented for these beans.

Catechin was the only flavonoid that was found in all of the analysed extract fractions; the fact that this compound belongs to the procyanidin group, which is present in virtually all beans, further explains this observation. A study by Aguilera et al. [17] reported concentrations of catechin in macerated raw and cooked beans of 142.58 µg g^{-1} and 76.25 µg g^{-1}, respectively; these results are very similar to those obtained in this study (Table 5). It is known that catechin assists in the reduction of cholesterol absorption in the intestine and in the inhibition of LDL cholesterol oxidation [2].

Virtually all of the flavonoids analysed occurred in lower concentrations in the FF fraction relative to the fraction analysed for the same treatment. This observation leads to the conclusion that most of these phenolic compounds were not extracted or were extracted in small amounts by the solvent used in each fraction.

Although Beninger and Hosflied [14] indicated that flavonoids exist mainly in the glycosylated form, the fractions evaluated in this study also contained the aglycone flavonoid.

The occurrence, in significant quantities, of almost every flavonoid analysed (especially after cooking, which reflects how beans are most commonly prepared for consumption) confirms the importance of including beans daily as part of a healthy diet that is rich in bioactive compounds because all of the analysed flavonoids demonstrate free radical scavenging activity and other biological effects, which were described above [2,18].

Brown beans contain all of the flavonoids and phenolic acids analysed in this study, making their consumption highly beneficial due to the rich variety of physiological activities that phenolic compounds exert.

Acknowledgment

The authors are thankful to the rice and beans department of the Brazilian agricultural company EMBRAPA for donating the beans and FAPESP for granting the scholarship and research funding process number 2009/14924-4.

References

1. Díaz-Batalla L, Widholm JM, Fahey-Junior GC, Castaño-Tostado E, Paredes-López O (2006) Chemical components with health implications in wild and cultivated mexican common bean seeds (*Phaseolus vulgaris* L.). J Agric Food Chem 54: 2045-2052.
2. Campos-Vega R, Loarca-Piña G, Oomah BD (2010) Minor components of pulses and their potential impact on human health. Food Res Intern 43: 461-482.
3. Amarowicz R, Pegg RB (2008) Legumes as a source of natural antioxidants. Eur J Lipid Sci Technol 110: 865-878.
4. Rocha-Guzmán NE, Annete H, González-Laredo RF, Ibarra-Pérez FJ, Zambrano-Galván, G, et al. (2007) Antioxidant and antimutagenic activity of phenolic compounds in three different colour groups of common bean cultivars (*Phaseolus vulgaris).* Food Chem 103: 521-527.
5. Xu BJ, Chang SKC (2009) Total phenolic, phenolic acid, anthocyanin, flavan-3-ol, and flavonol profiles and antioxidant properties of pinto and black beans (*Phaseolus vulgaris* L.) as affected by thermal processing. J Agric Food Chem 57: 4754-4764.
6. Cardador-Martínez A, Aalbores A, Bah M, Calderón-Salinas V, Castaño-Tostado E, et al. (2006) Relationship among antimutagenic, antioxidant and enzymatic activities of methanolic extract from common beans (*Phaseolus vulgaris* L.). Plant Foods Hum Nutr 61: 161-168.
7. Aparicio-Fernandez X, Manzo-Bonilla L, Loarca-Piña G (2005) Comparison of antimutagenic activity of phenolic compounds in newly

harvested and stored common beans *Phaseolus vulgaris* against aflatoxin B1. J Food Sci 70: 73-78.

8. Brand-Williams W, Cuvier ME, Berset C (1995) Use of a free radical method to evaluate antioxidant activity. LWT- Food Sci Tech 28: 25-30.
9. Re R, Pellegrini N, Proteggente A, Pannala A, Yang M, et al. (1999) Antioxidant activity applying na improved ABST radical cation decolorization assay. Free Radic Biol Med 26: 1231-1237.
10. Van Den Berg R, Haenen GRMM, Van Den Berg H, Bast A (1999) Applicability of an improved Trolox equivalent antioxidant capacity (TEAC) assay for evaluation of antioxidant capacity measurements of mixtures. Food Chem 66: 511-517.
11. Arts MJTJ, Dallinga JS, Voss HP, Haenen GRMM, Bast A (2004) A new approach to assess the total antioxidant capacity using the TEAC assay. Food Chem 88: 567-570.
12. Xu BJ, Chang SKC (2008) Total phenolic content and antioxidant properties of eclipse black beans (*Phaseolus vulgaris* L.) as affected by processing methods. J Food Sci 73: 19-27.
13. Fernandez-Panchon MS, Villano D, Troncoso AM, Garcia-Parrilla MC (2008) Antioxidant activity of phenolic compounds: from in vitro results to in vivo evidence. Crit Rev Food Sci Nutr 48: 649-671.
14. Beninger CW, Hosfield GL (2003) Antioxidant activity of extracts, condensed tannin fractions and pure flavonoids from *Phaseolus vulgaris* L. seed coat color genotypes. J Agric Food Chem 51: 7879-7883.
15. Luthria DL, Pastor-Corrales MA (2006) Phenolic acids content of fifteen dry edible bean (*Phaseolus vulgaris* L.) varieties. J Food Comp Anal 19: 205-211.
16. Ranilla LG, Genovese MI, Lajolo FM (2007) Polyphenols and antioxidant capacity of seed coat and cotyledon from Brazilian and Peruvian bean cultivars (*Phaseolus vulgaris* L.). J Agric Food Chem 55: 90-98.
17. Aguilera Y, Estrella I, Benitez V, Esteban RM, Martín-Cabrejas MA (2011) Bioactive phenolic compounds and functional properties of dehydrated bean flours. Food Res Intern 44: 774-780.
18. Rauter AP, Dias C, Martins A, Branco I, Neng NR, et al. (2012) Non-toxic *Salvia sclareoides* Brot. Extracts as a source of functional food ingredients: phenolic profile, antioxidant activity and príon binding properties. Food Chem 132: 1930-1935.
19. Espinosa-Alonso LG, Lygin A, Widholm JM, Valverde ME, Paredes-Lopez O (2006) Polyphenols in Wild and Weedy Mexican Common Beans (*Phaseolus vulgaris* L.). J Agric Food Chem 54: 4436-4444.
20. Aaby K, Hvattum E, Skrede G (2004) Analysis of flavonoids and other phenolic compounds using high-performance liquid chromatography with colorimetric array detection: relationship to antioxidant activity. J Agric Food Chem 52: 4595-4603.
21. Romani A, Vignolini P, Galardi C, Mulinacci N, Benedettelli S, et al. (2004) Germplasm characterization of zolfino landraces (*Phaseolus vulgaris* L.) by flavonoid content. J Agric Food Chem 52: 3838-3842.
22. Lin LZ, Harnly JM, Pastor-Corrales MS, Luthria DL (2008) The polyphenolic profiles of common bean (*Phaseolus vulgaris* L.). Food Chem 107: 399-410.
23. Kosinska A, Karamac M, Penkacik K, Urbalewicz A, Amarowicz R (2011) Interactions between tannins and proteins isolated from broad bean seeds (*Vicia faba* Major) yield soluble and non-soluble complexes. Eur Food Res Technol 233: 213-222.

23

The Concept of Cyclical Nutritional Therapy for Hair Growth which can be Applied for Wellness

Rajendrasingh Rajput*

Hair Transplant Surgeon, Member ISHRS, IAT, and AHRS, India

***Corresponding author:** Rajendrasingh Rajput, Hair Restore, Hair Transplant Surgeon, Member ISHRS, IAT, and AHRS, India, E-mail: drrajeshrajput@gmail.com

Abstract

Hair growth can be achieved by fighting hair loss with medications or by strengthening the hair roots with nutrients. Caution as excess vitamin A, vitamin E, omega 3 cause hair loss instead of hair growth. Supplements are considered harmless and consumed without thinking of interactions or overdose. Therapeutic doses of vitamins to treat disease are high, however preventive or prophylactic dose for wellness are low. Antioxidants improve health by neutralizing Reactive oxygen species, but ROS have important role in infection control and phagocytosis. Overuse of antioxidants interferes with protective mechanisms. High doses of one nutrient affect the absorption and efficiency of others. Administered together, vitamin C can destroy vitamin B12. Iron and calcium reduce the absorption of one another. High vitamin C, increases sodium & reduces potassium levels. Nutrients are also synergistic. Vitamin E regenerates Beta carotene. Vitamin C regenerates vitamin E. Toxic effects of Beta carotene break down products are reduced by alpha tocopherol, N acetyl cysteine and vitamin C. Single deficiency causes multiple inefficiencies. Inappropriate combinations and nutrient overdose are easily possible with rising use of multivitamins and fortified foods. Nutrient deficiencies are compensated by autophagy and also prevail as subclinical deficiencies making them difficult to detect on laboratory tests. To utilize nutrients without interaction and overdose we have proposed the use of different synergistic nutrients on different days of the week, repeating in a three day cycle. The concept was initiated for achieving consistent hair growth as published earlier. It can be applied to a set of nutrients identified for various other indications like geriatrics, pediatrics, growing teens, athletes, body builders, women's health, cardiac patients, diabetics, athletes, bariatric surgery etc. ensuring low dose, low cost, and optimum benefit nutrient program allowing the body to assimilate and utilize each nutrient, without wastage or overdose.

Keywords: Hair growth; Hair loss; Cyclical nutritional therapy

Introduction

Hair growth can be achieved by fighting hair loss with anti-androgens, enzyme blockers and medications with potential side effects. Or by strengthening the hair roots with the right choice of antioxidants, minerals, vitamins, and amino acids and promoting hair growth. However, excess use of antioxidants, vitamin A, vitamin E, omega 3 can cause hair loss instead of hair growth [1-4]. Hair growth achieved through a combination of nutrients delivers wellness, good health and hair growth without the possibility of side effects from the use of hair loss medications. In this article we are attempting to share the approach for selective use of nutrient combinations and avoiding nutrient interactions to achieve hair growth. A similar approach of selective synergistic combinations can be applied for general wellness. Loss of hair, deterioration of health and creating a breeding ground for diseases, have common risk factors like smoking, pollution, stress, lack of sleep, sedentary lifestyle, poor nutrition, obesity, exposure to chemicals, insecticides, fertilizers, artificial preservatives, taste makers in processed foods etc. People find it easy to create a false protection through self-perceived benefits from unrestricted use of vitamins and supplements rather than changing their habits or lifestyle. The general perception that vitamins and supplements promote health has encouraged people to feel that more multivitamins and more supplements of all kinds is equivalent to more health [5]. Today we are in an era of abuse and overuse of vitamins which are being consumed as a celebration of your own free will. People consume supplements randomly without inquiring in to the rationale or true benefits of such practice [5]. As a general assumption it is perceived that use of supplements will prevent illness, give more energy, improve health and make people feel better [5,6]. Such thinking is driven by advertising and promotion [5]. Rising trend of vitamin and supplement consumption has been noted in several studies and national surveys [5-9].

Commonly people consume antioxidants, iron, calcium, zinc, selenium, omega 3, omega 6, amino acids, B-complex, Beta carotene, vitamin C, vitamin D, vitamin E and health promoting herbal preparations. These nutrients have interactions which may reduce the absorption, bioavailability and efficiency of one another. On the other hand, synergistic combinations of the nutrients can also be used to improve the efficiency and benefit from the nutrients.

Supplement manufacturers do not need to study interactions with other nutrients or drugs as is mandatory for the more regulated pharmaceutical industry [5,6]. It is our responsibility to guide the end users about adequate dosage, optimum efficacy, prevention of overdose, interactions, avoid unnecessary wastage and overuse of vitamins and nutrients. There was a time when vitamin supplements were recommended to patients in convalescence to aid in recovery from sickness or disease. But today supplements are required for a regular, day to day healthy living and we must provide the best understanding for the rationale and the basis for these various recommendations.

Food Cannot Provide Complete Nutrition

There are many studies to conclude that routine diets are short of meeting the complete nutritional requirement of an individual. The study by Misner [10] compared diets of men and women, athletes and sedentary workers with computer analysis by Harris Benedict formula comparing energy expense against micronutrient requirement, age and BMI. Seven minerals and ten vitamins were evaluated. All these minerals and vitamins through the food were short of meeting the nutritional requirement in all individuals in the study. Therefore supplements are necessary. The same paper mentions a statement by experts in the 1936 Nutritional Congress. It was then said in 1936 that ' food was no more nutritious as it was in their prior generations, when our forefathers enjoyed good health just by selecting the right foods to eat' [10]. What was said eight decades ago remains true even today.

American Dietetic Association [10,11] does not follow RDA which is recommended daily allowance but mentions much lower RDI which is recommended daily intake for prevention of any disease being caused due to nutritional deficiency. RDI aims at preventing overdose. However, all these standards are decided by group of experts after review of benefits reported in the scientific literature and not by any laboratory studies or experiments or investigations. The benefits and side effects from use of supplements are scarcely reported, not providing the required basis to derive the best advice [12,13]. As is the prevalent, permitted practice, using multivitamins with 30-100% added overages (to compensate for losses), along with self-selected individual nutrients and routine consumption of fortified foods and easily lead to unaccounted overuse and overdose [14-16].

Loss of nutritive value of foods

The problem of deriving nutrition from food is compounded by the fact that the nutritive value of the agricultural produce from the farms itself is falling down due to changes in the soil, use of pesticides, fertilizers and fast growing crops which do not assimilate enough nutrients or develop resistance to natural variations in soil and climate as when growing in the wild [17-20]. Studies have been done on vegetables, fruits [17], milk meat and cheese [18]. Reporting Loss of 49% sodium, 16% of their potassium, 24% magnesium, 46% calcium, 27% Iron and 76% copper content. In contrast the use of NPK fertilizers has led to 9% rise in Phosphorous [19]. Over 80-90% of the content in farm products and grains being carbohydrate, the high yield concentrates on more carbohydrate content and loses on phytochemicals, vitamins, and minerals contents as a tradeoff [19]. These Researchers have expressed concern that replenishment of nutrient depleted soils and wind, water erosion are harming agriculture. Nutrient mining and leaching is exacerbated by use of fertilizers [21]. Nutrient exhaustion, over cultivation, lack of return of organic matter to the soil and deforestation are leading to this global phenomenon [21]. Loss of nutrients in the soil estimated in the year 2000 was reported to be 75% in developing countries, 14% in developed countries, and 11% in least developed countries [21]. Artificially grown foods do not gain the properties of the wild and do not deliver the desired benefits for wellness.

Nutrients and supplement are not always beneficial to health

By the end of the 19th century, researchers established the role of oxidative stress is pathogenesis of various diseases, synthetic vitamin A, vitamin C, vitamin E and Beta carotene were manufactured and widely promoted for wellness and as adjunct therapy. These were recommended with random round off figures, in high doses, as every day, regular intake for healthy living. Recent studies on various supplements of all kinds, have found limited benefits in prevention of disease and made it clear that the aim of healthy living with use of supplements is not always achieved [22-26].

Excess use of antioxidants compromises important body functions

You cannot achieve more health by using more antioxidants and neutralizing all the free radicals and metabolic toxins in the body. Study by Salganik points out that free radicals, the ROS (Reactive Oxygen Species) are required for their important role in body defence mechanisms, infection control, phagocytosis and apoptosis of cancer cells [27]. Bacteria and cancer cells are killed in the body by creating a sudden flood of ROS [28,29]. ROS oxidizes hydrophobic toxins, steroids, drugs to hydrophilic compounds which then can be easily transferred out of the cells, achieving detoxification [30,31]. ROS are a part of metabolic processes for prostaglandin synthesis, hydroxylation of proline, lysine and oxidation of xanthine [27,30]. Overuse of antioxidants and neutralizing functions of the ROS and can interfere with the well-being of a person [31,32].

Excess iron and minerals reverse the conversion of super oxides

Superoxides in the body are converted to less reactive hydrogen peroxide, by Superoxide Dismutase (SOD). A person having regular iron and multimineral supplements triggers Fenton reaction between metallic iron or copper ions with the reduced form, hydrogen peroxide, generating more reactive hydroxyl ions and reversing the benefit from conversion of super oxides and peroxides [27,32-34]. Therefore high doses of iron and mineral supplements should be avoided to ensure the benefit of antioxidants.

Excess use of vitamins leads to interactions and reverses the benefits

Rutkowski and Grzegorczyk reviewed adverse effects of vitamins [5]. Labelling under the category of dietary supplements creates a delightful and harmless meaning to the use of vitamins, minerals unknowingly leading to easy abuse and overuse. Vitamin A, E and C, are commonly promoted as co therapy with various treatments and as general source of beauty and wellness [5].

Excess vitamin A can lead to aplastic anemia, hair loss, dry skin, rashes, raised Erythrocyte Sedimentation Rate (ESR), and interfere with blood coagulation [5]. Synthetic retinoids can impair liver functions [5]. Vitamin A has been found to damage bone and increase incidence of hip fractures at just marginally higher doses without signs of hypervitaminosis [35-37]. Excess β-carotene which is an effective antioxidant at low partial pressure of oxygen (pO_2) as in peripheral tissues becomes pro oxidant at high pO_2 as in lungs even leading to DNA (Deoxyribonucleic acid) damage [38-41]. Regular supplements of β-carotene could not protect patients with lung asbestosis. β-carotene increased the incidence of lung cancer in smokers by 18% and caused intra cerebral hemorrhage in alcoholics [38,42,43]. Vitamin A stores are depleted with high intake of vitamin E [41].

High intake of vitamin C causes electrolyte imbalance increasing sodium levels and reducing potassium in the blood [43]. When administered together vitamin C can destroy vitamin B12 [44,45].

High doses of vitamin C inhibit enzymes ceruloplasmin and superoxide dismutase (Cu, Zn-SOD) due to interference of vitamin C with copper absorption [46]. High doses of vitamin C in glucose-6-phosphate dehydrogenase (G-6-PD) and vitamin B12 deficiency can cause haemolysis of the erythrocytes [43,18] and damage pancreatic β-cells, similar to that known with drug alloxan [47-49]. Vitamin C taken at night can lead to difficulty in falling asleep due to its stimulant effect [50]. High doses of vitamin C lead to tolerance and dependency, sudden withdrawal causes scurvy like state of deficiency, gradual tapering is advised [18,51,52].

Excess vitamin E antagonizes vitamin K, reduces platelet aggregation, promoting anti-coagulant activity [41], it also interferes with generation of beneficial ROS flood used for killing of the infective phagocytosis agents engulfed by granulocytes [53-55]. Vitamin E in high doses becomes pro oxidant [56,57]. With high doses of minerals and easy availability of iron and copper ions vitamin E encourages generation of ROS [47,58,59]. Meta-analysis of 135,000 people taking vitamin E 400 IU or higher per day for over one year showed increased risk, instead of health benefit [43].

Favorable or synergistic nutrient interactions

Vitamin E regenerates the Beta carotene utilized for antioxidant activity and also preserves the activity of vitamin A [50,57,60,61]. Vitamin C regenerates vitamin E consumed for reduction of peroxide and peroxyl radicals [62-65]. Vitamin C neutralizes the xenobiotics leading to formation of ROS helping in detoxification [66]. Vitamin A and Beta carotene in the diet make the non heam iron soluble at pH 6 neutralizing inhibition due to chelation by phytates, polyphenols and iron inhibitors in food to improve iron absorption more than three times [67].

Under oxidative stress, Beta carotene cleavage products generate aldehydes and epoxides which impair the function of the mitochondrial respiratory chain, creating a genotoxic effect and promoting inflammation, especially on prolonged use. These toxic effects are known to be reduced with concomitant use of other antioxidants, alpha tocopherol, N acetyl cysteine and vitamin C [68-71]. Vitamin C is known to improve iron absorption by preventing the formation of insoluble iron complexes with tannins and phytates. Vitamin C also converts ferric iron to ferrous form which is the required form for absorption by the intestinal mucosal cells [72].

Higher doses do not lead to higher benefits

The preceding information so far has tried to present the view that overdose of vitamins or supplements should be avoided and synergistic combinations can enhance efficiency with prevention of toxicity and undesired side effects. Especially because people tend to use supplements for a long time. We should now see if the rationale is applicable to the commonly used iron and calcium, minerals as well. The amount of iron absorbed depends on the gradient across the gut lumen and the blood. Iron is absorbed better in a relatively low iron states rather than in presence of good circulating levels [73,74]. Higher iron content in the meal or recurrent high doses of iron supplements lead to low absorption [75-77]. Iron absorption is regulated at the mucosal level depending on the deficiency status and the iron load in the food [77,78]. The intestinal mucosal cells or enterocytes are equipped to down regulate iron absorption in response to daily exposure to high intake of iron [78,79]. Since iron and calcium are the oldest and most popular mineral supplements, there are studies done as early as 1958 to show that iron supplements administered once in three days (or twice a week) are more efficient for absorption and utilization, than providing iron every day [80]. The mucosal cells need to renew and regain their ability for iron transport with a three day gap [80,81]. High iron levels are not always desirable. High iron leads to formation of pro oxidative, harmful, hydroxyl ions, through Fenton reaction [82]. Thus excess iron should be avoided and there is a rationale for a once in three days low dose recommendation [80].

Presence of Iron and calcium together reduce the absorption of one another [83]. Calcium absorption also depends on the calcium load and the relative deficiency in an individual [84,85]. High concentration of extracellular iron leads to a concomitant buildup of calcium ions, leading to premature apoptosis and cell death [86]. Higher bioavailability of nutrients is not necessarily better. When there is a combination of all minerals together, administered in multivitamin, multimineral formulations, the individual minerals compete with each other for absorption. Levels of zinc, magnesium, calcium, selenium, iron, affect the absorption of each other [87].

Even after absorption of the nutrients the metabolic systems have a rate limiting capability of utilizing the nutrients. High doses of Folic acid cannot be utilized well due to limited metabolic capacity of the cells for reduction and methylation of folic acid to its active form [88]. High doses of vitamin C not only reduce further absorption of vitamin C, but also become pro oxidant in behavior [5,89]. We decided to follow the thought of providing low but effective dosage in preference over high doses of nutrients, leading to poor absorption, incomplete utilization or the risk of reversing the benefits due to continuous, repeated, daily doses or uncontrolled high doses. The thought has led to a low dose once in three days Cyclical Nutrition Therapy.

The concept of Low dose once in three days Cyclical Nutritional Therapy

The conclusion derived from the studies, nutritional and our experience of similar approach in achieving wellness along with hair growth has lead us to believe in some new concepts of administering nutritional supplements as enlisted below:

- Nutritional supplements are required for healthy living as food alone cannot meet all the requirements.
- One single nutrient cannot function effectively. A balance of micronutrients, vitamins, minerals is required for optimum function, without an excess of any single nutrient.
- We should not encourage multivitamin, multimineral supplements as these would compete for uptake, exceed the metabolic capability for activation, reduce the absorption of nutrients, limit the bio availability, efficiency and utilization of each other, resulting in compromised outcome, reversal of benefits, no benefits or harmful conversion of behaviour to pro oxidation.
- Nutrients administered in intermittent doses can have better absorption than being repeated every day. Such approach will maintain a low gradient in circulation which favours more efficient absorption and complete utilization. The intermittent gap of three days allows time for the cells and systems to regenerate. It prevents wastage, avoids overuse, making the therapy efficient and cost effective.
- Nutrients can be administered in synergistic combinations that favour one another and do not adversely interfere with the metabolism of one another.

- Large amount of money is spent by clients in an attempt to derive health benefits from seemingly harmless use of supplements. It is our responsibility to make them aware of the best options preventing overuse and abuse of nutrients.
- RDA and RDI are guidelines decide by a review committee with the best intention of delivering wellness. These are not concurred by scientific or metabolic experiments or studies. The guidelines are updated and revised as per new reports, changing lifestyles and regular feedbacks.

In order to reduce the dosage, improve the efficiency, have broad spectrum coverage to include required vitamins, minerals, amino acids, fatty acids, coenzymes and supportive nutrients we have created a comprehensive approach of using different nutrient combinations on different days of the week. Six nutrient combinations are utilized as two per day over a three day cycle. Monday-Antioxidant and Calcium with Vitamin D. Tuesday-Iron, Folic acid, Vitamin C and Omega 3. Wednesday-Essential Amino acids, B-complex and Biotin. The same cycle repeats on Thursday, Friday, and Saturday. Sunday is break for detoxification. There is also an option where additional supplements can be added on Sunday if required (Table 1). Our program was created for hair regrowth. However, the hair regrowth has been achieved by improving general wellness of the patients and creating a nutrition balanced, toxin free environment for all the cells in the body to divide and grow. In our clinic we have been delivering wellness and good health leading to hair growth for past 19 years. The clinical benefit, compliance, efficacy of this program would comprise an elaborate report. These have been published clinical observations and benefits under various indications [1-4,90-92]. The clinical observations are reported here. Detail experimental and laboratory studies to document the benefits from low dose nutritional combinations would be required to corroborate the benefits and study other relevant aspects of the new approach. The program has received safety clearance and approval from regulatory health authorities from Australia, USA and Canada.

Monday & Thursday	Antioxidant, Calcium, Vitamin D3
Tuesday & Friday	Iron, Folic Acid, Vitamin C, Omega 3
Wednesday & Saturday	Essential Amino acids, B-Complex, Biotin
Sunday–no medicines	Detox on Sunday OR add extra a dose of another nutrient as per individual status if required
Provides ten different nutrient combinations that are synergistic with each other over three days preventing overdose and inter nutrient interaction.	

Table 1: Cyclical Nutrient Therapy two supplement per day in a 3–days cycles.

Patients who are on this program have reported general health benefits like raise in iron and calcium levels, better energy levels, no fatigue, mental alertness, correction of thyroid function, no more nagging aches and pains in the body, waking up feeling fresh in the morning, good sleep, some rare patients also had weight gain.

A similar set of vitamins, minerals and essential nutritional supplements can be identified for geriatrics, pediatrics, growing teens, women's health, cardiac patients, diabetics, athletes, bariatric surgery and patients with special gastric or intestinal needs. We can make synergistic combination for individual conditions. Make sure the combinations do not counter the efficiency of one another and spread these nutritional supplements over a similar three day cycle for optimum coverage of all essential nutrients and consistent benefit.

We would like to address the concern of weather an evidence of clinical deficiency detected by laboratory tests is required to be established before recommending nutritional supplements?

Why existing nutrient deficiencies cannot be detected on routine laboratory tests?

The Nobel Prize for Medicine in year 2016 was awarded to the Yoshinori Oshumi from Japan for his work on Autophagy. When the cells in our body experience lack of nutrients the process of autophagy triggers programmed breakdown of intracellular organelles in order to retrieve required nutrients, amino acids, minerals from the cells [93,94]. Autophagy is one step before apoptosis. Nutritional deficiencies are masked and compensated back to normal levels by retrieving nutrients and preserving circulating levels, through autophagy. Deficiencies are thus compensated and cannot be detected in the laboratory tests. You do not have to wait for clinically detectable nutritional deficiencies to develop before administering the low dose supplements. Therefore, though high dose supplements are not indicated, the low dose once in three days nutritional supplements can be advised, for patients having hair loss or clinical signs of fatigue, continuous stress, low immunity, borderline lower margins of nutrients on tests results, these patients shall benefit before they suffer or display frank nutritional deficiencies. This approach can be safely advised to patients who intend to have supplements only to maintain good health. We can prevent such fitness conscious users from overuse and known or unknown long term effects from indiscriminate use, self-determined or unguided use of supplements. In our experience the moment you provide these minimal corrections the patients show dramatic benefits in all aspects of good health. Correction of severe nutritional deficiencies is often difficult but prevention with low dose once in three days cycle is safe, easy and effective. Nutrients have two kinds of dosage. The dose given to a person suffering from deficiency disorder like scurvy or rickets is very high. This is a therapeutic dose or a treatment dose but the dose required for prevention of deficiency is a prophylactic dose which can be as low as possible [95], for promoting wellness.

Subclinical deficiencies

Researchers around the world have expressed concern over subclinical deficiencies [96] which are another type of nutritionally compromised states that are not clinically detectable. Covert malnutrition or subclinical deficiencies are a state where the metabolism and biological system of an individual has adjusted, reset and adapted to continue functioning under sub optimal lower levels of nutrients without clinical signs of failure. Certain ethnic communities are known to have reduces height, low body mass and stunted growth due to endemic deficiencies.

We regard the subclinical deficiencies as a status of compensated failure, where the failure is masked, until there is a demand or need for complete functional capacity. Vitamin C 10 mg per day is enough to prevent scurvy [95]. The deficiency will manifest only when there is requirement for wound healing [95]. The prevalence of such covert deficiencies is more than our perception of this rising problem [95,96]. In a surprising report, healthy donors certified to be fit and selected for blood donation after due screening with laboratory tests were been found to have subclinical iron deficiencies [97]. All the body systems are interrelated; covert deficiencies that become apparent in one element affect other body systems as well and are associated with multiple undetected deficiencies. Hypothyroidism known to result from iodine deficiency has been reported to be associated with subclinical deficiencies of vitamin A, vitamin D, iron and selenium [98-101]. Subclinical deficiencies have been reported to affect the thyroid pituitary axis [102]. Therefore we require a low dose but long term, comprehensive nutritional supplement program rather than a selective, short term, immediate, single nutrient correction approach. In one of the studies, covert deficiencies due to inadequate diet in athletes did not manifest as these were adequately compensated by their use of nutritional supplements.

Conclusion

Nutritional deficiencies are on the rise becoming more common than we can realize. The deficiencies are multi nutrient, multi vitamin and multi mineral in nature and not limited to single individual nutrients. Administering too many nutrients together leads to reduced absorption and reduced efficiency from inter nutrient interactions. Nutritional supplements also need to be continued for a long time. Excess use of any single nutrient turns out to be ineffective as a balance of all micro nutrients in the body is essential to ensure wellness. High dose nutritional supplements can become ineffective and also reverses the benefits. A low dose once in three day nutritional cycle has been suggested with synergistic combinations which reduces dosage, improves efficiency, brings down total cost of the therapy, provides comprehensive coverage of all required supplements and is safe for long term use. We have used this approach successfully for hair loss management and achieving new hair growth. We suggest similar approach can be planned for geriatrics, paediatrics, growing teens, athletes, body builders, women's health, cardiac patients, diabetics, athletes, bariatric surgery and patients with special gastric or intestinal needs. Cyclical nutritional therapy is a new way to look at safe, comprehensive nutritional supplementation avoiding nutrient interactions and improving efficiency without overdose. The unique approach can applied to more clinical conditions and tailored to meet the demand for promotion of wellness at various levels.

References

1. NIH State-of-the-Science Panel (2006) National Institutes of Health State-of the- science conference statement: multivitamin/mineral supplements and chronic disease prevention. Ann Intern Med 145: 364-371.
2. Rutkowski M, Grzegorczyk K (2012) Adverse effects of antioxidative vitamins. Int J Occup Med Environ Health 25: 105-121.
3. RadimerK, Bindewald B, Hughes J, Ervin B, Swanson C, et al. (2004) Dietary supplement use by US adults: data from the National Healthand Nutrition Examination Survey, 1999-2000. Am J Epidemiol 160: 339-349.
4. Timbo BB, Ross MP, McCarthy PV, Lin CT (2006) Dietary supplements in a national survey: Prevalence of use and reports of adverse events. J Am Diet Assoc 106: 1966-1974.
5. Misner B (2006) Food alone may not provide sufficient micronutrients for preventing deficiency. J Int Soc Sports Nutr 3: 51-55.
6. American Dietetic Association (2005) Position of the American Dietetic Association: fortification and nutritional supplements. J Am Diet Assoc 105: 1300-1311.
7. Woo JJ (2007) Adverse event monitoring and multivitamin-multimineral dietary supplements. Am J Clin Nutr 85: 323S-324S.
8. Mulholland CA, Benford OJ (2007) What is known about the safety of multivitamin-multimineral supplements for the generally healthy population? Theoretical basis for harm. Am J Clin Nutr 85: 18S-22S.
9. http://www.food.gov.uk/multimedia/pdfs/vitmin2003.pdf
10. http://www.consumerlab.com/results/multivit.asp
11. Feifer AH, Fleshner NE, Klotz L (2002) Analytical accuracy and reliability of commonly used nutritional supplements in prostate disease. J Urol 168: 150-154.
12. Veatch AE, Anne-Marie Mayer B (1997) Historical changes in the mineral content of fruits and vegetables. Br Food J 99: 207-211.
13. Thomas D (2003) A study on the mineral depletion of the foods available to us as a nation over the period 1940 to 1991. Nutr Health 17: 85-115.
14. Davis DR, Epp MD, Riordan HD (2004) Changes in USDA food composition data for 43 garden crops, 1950 to 1999. J Am Coll Nutr 23: 669-682.
15. White PJ, Broadley MR (2005) Historical variation in the mineral composition of edible horticultural products. J Horti Sci Biotechnol 80: 660-667.
16. Davis DR (2006) Commentary on 'Historical variation in the mineral composition of edible horticultural products'. J Horti Sci Biotechnol 81: 553-554.
17. Swami HM, Thakur JS, Bhatia SP (2007) Impact of mass supplementation of vitamin A. Indian J Pediatr 74: 443-447.
18. Assouline S, Miller WH (2006) High-dose vitamin C therapy: renewed hope or false promise? CMAJ 174: 956-957.
19. Scientific Committee on Food (SCF) (2003) Opinion of the Scientific Committee on Food on the tolerable upper intake level of vitamin E. Brussels: Commission of the European Communities.
20. Scientific Committee on Food (SCF) (2000) Opinion of the Scientific Committee on Food on the tolerable upper intake level of beta-carotene. Brussels: Commission of the European Communities.
21. Herbert V (1999) Underreporting of dietary supplements to health-care providers does great harm. Mayo Clin Proc 74: 531-532.
22. Salganik RI (2001) The benefits and hazards of antioxidants: controlling apoptosis and other protective mechanisms in cancer patients and the human population. J Am Coll Nutr 20: 464S-472S.
23. Babior BM (1978) Oxygen-dependent microbial killing by phagocytes. N Engl J Med 298: 721-725.
24. Rossi F, Zatti M (1980) Biochemical aspects of phagocytosis in polymorphonuclear leucocytes. NADH and NADPH oxidation by the granules of resting and phagocytizing cells. Experientia 20: 21-27.
25. Halliwell B, Cutteridge JMC (1999) Free radicals in biology and medicine. Oxford: Oxford University Press 1: 331-332.
26. Ghosh MK, Mukhopadhyay M, Chatterjee IB (NADPH-initiated P450-dependent free-iron-dependent microsomal lipid peroxidation: specific prevention by ascorbic acid. Mol Cell Biochem 166: 35-44.
27. Cedro K, Klosiewicz-Wasek B, Wasek W (1994) Inhibitory effect of vitamins C and E on the oxygen free radical production in human polymorphonuclear leucocytes. Eur J Clin Invest 24: 316-319.
28. Halliwell B (1996) Antioxidants in human health and diseases. Ann Rev Nutr 20: 2261-2266.
29. Halliwell B (2000) The antioxidant paradox. Lancet 355: 1179-1180.
30. Feskanich D, Singh V, Willett WC, Colditz GA (2002) Vitamin A intake and hip fractures among postmenopausal women. JAMA 287: 47-54.
31. Michaëlsson K, Lithell H, Vessby B, Melhus H (2003) Serum retinol levels and the risk of fracture. N Engl J Med 348: 287-294.
32. Melhus H, Michaëlsson K, Kindmark A, Bergström R, Holmberg L, et al. (1998) Excessive dietary intake of vitamin A is associated with reduced bone mineral density and increased risk for hip fracture. Ann Intern Med 129: 770-778.
33. Bendich A (2004) What have we learned about the biological actions of beta-carotene? J Nutr 134: 125S-130S.
34. Rutkowski M, Grzegorczyk K (2002) What should be known nowadays about ß-carotene and other carotenoids? Farm Pol 58: 97-105.

35. Tanumihardjo SA (2002) Factors influencing the conversion of carotenoids to retinol: bioavailability to bioconversion to bioefficacy. Int J Vitam Nutr Res 72: 40-45.
36. Young AJ, Lowe GM (2001) Antioxidant and prooxidant properties of carotenoids. Arch Biochem Biophys 385: 20-27.
37. Tanvetyanon T, Bepler G (2008) Beta-carotene in multivitamins and the possible risk of lung cancer among smokers versus former smokers: a meta-analysis and evaluation of national brands. Cancer 113: 150-177.
38. Mayne ST, Redlich CA, Cullen MR (1998) Dietary vitamin A and prevalence of bronchial metaplasia in asbestos-exposed workers. Am J Clin Nutr 68: 630-635.
39. Reuter HD (2004) Vitamins. In: Aronson JK (ed.) Side effects of drugs. Annual 27. Amsterdam: Elsevier BV pp: 405-413.
40. Rogovik AL, Vohra S, Goldman RD (2010) Safety considerations and potential interactions of vitamins: should vitamins be considered drugs? Ann Pharmacother 44: 311-324.
41. Halliwell B (1999) Establishing the significance and optimal intake of dietary antioxidants: the biomarker concept. Nutr Rev 57: 104-113.
42. Stargrove MB, Treasure J, McKee DL (2008) Herb, nutrient, and drug interactions: clinical implications and therapeutic strategies. St. Louis: Mosby Elsevier.
43. Rutkowski M, Grzegorczyk K (1999) Vitamins with antioxidant action: a general characterisation. Part III: Vitamin C. Farm Pol 55: 74-79.
44. Halliwell B (1999) Vitamin C: poison, prophylactic or panacea? Trends Biochem Sci 24: 255-259.
45. Auer BL, Auer D, Rodgers AL (1998) Relative hyperoxaluria, crystalluria and haematuria after megadose ingestion of vitamin C. Eur J Clin Invest 28: 695-700.
46. Coates PM, Blackman MR, Cragg GM, Levine M, Moss J, et al. (2005) Encyclopedia of dietary supplements. Marcel Dekker. New York.
47. Hamrick I, Counts SH (2008) Vitamin and mineral supplements. Prim Care 35: 729-747.
48. Reuter HD (2004) Vitamins In: Aronson JK, editor. Side effects of drugs. Annual 27. Amsterdam: Elsevier BV pp: 405-413.
49. Temple BR (2004) Vitamin toxicity. In: Dart RC, editor. Medical toxicology. Philadelphia: Lippincott Williams and Wilkins pp: 1017-1024.
50. Rutkowski M, Grzegorczyk K, Chojnacki J, Kedziora J (2006) Antioxidative properties of vitamin E as a new approach to its applications in therapy. Pol Merkur Lekarski 20: 609-614.
51. Rota S, McWilliam NA, Baglin TP, Byrne CD (1998) Atherogenic lipoproteins support assembly of the prothrombinase complex and thrombin generation: modulation by oxidation and vitamin E. Blood 91: 508-515.
52. Pearson P, Lewis SA, Britton J, Young IS, Fogarty A (2006) The pro-oxidant activity of high-dose vitamin E supplements in vivo. Bio Drugs 20: 271-273.
53. Expert Group on Vitamins and Minerals (2003) Risk assessments. In: Safe upper levels for vitamins and minerals. London: Food Standards Agency pp: 100-153.
54. Burkitt MJ (2001) A critical overview of the chemistry of copper-dependent low density lipoproteinoxidation: roles of lipid hydroperoxides, alpha-tocopherol, thiols, and ceruloplasmin. Arch Biochem Biophys 394: 117-135.
55. Miller ER, Pastor-Barriuso R, Dalal D, Riemersma RA, Appel LJ, et al. (2005) Meta-analysis: high-dosage vitamin E supplementation may increase all-cause mortality. Ann Intern Med 142: 37-46.
56. Valko M, Leibfritz D, Moncol J, Cronin MT, Mazur M, et al. (2007) Free radicals and antioxidants in normal physiological functions and human disease. Int J Biochem Cell Biol 39: 44-84.
57. Benzie IF (2003) Evolution of dietary antioxidants. Comp Biochem Physiol A Mol Integr Physiol 136: 113-126.
58. Jacob RA (1999) Vitamin C. In: Shils ME, Olson JA, Shike M, Ross AC (eds.) Modern nutrition in health and disease. Baltimore: Williams & Wilkins pp: 467-482.
59. Padayatty SJ, Katz A, Wang Y, Eck P, Kwon O, et al. (2003) Vitamin C as an antioxidant: evaluation of its role in disease prevention. J Am Coll Nutr 22: 18-35.
60. Hamilton IM, Gilmore WS, Benzie IF, Mulholland CW, Strain JJ (2000) Interactions between vitamins C and E in human subjects. Br J Nutr 84: 261-267.
61. Weeks BS, Perez PP (2007) A novel vitamin C preparation enhances neurite formation and fibroblast adhesion and reduces xenobiotic-induced T-cell hyperactivation. Med Sci Monit 13: 51-58.
62. García-Casal MN, Layrisse M, Solano L, Barón MA, Arguello F, et al. (1998) Vitamin A and beta-carotene can improve nonheme iron absorption from rice, wheat and corn by humans. J Nutr 128: 646-650.
63. Alija AJ, Bresgen N, Sommerburg O, Langhans CD, Siems W, et al. (2005) Cyto-and genotoxic potential of beta-carotene and cleavage products under oxidative stress. Biofactors 24: 159-163.
64. Alija AJ, Bresgen N, Bojaxhi E, Vogl C, Siems W, et al. (2010) Cytotoxicity of ß-carotene cleavage products and its prevention by antioxidants. Acta Biochim Pol 57: 217-221.
65. Siems W, Wiswedel I, Salerno C, Crifò C, Augustin W, et al. (2005) Beta-carotene breakdown products may impair mitochondrial functions potential side effects of high-dose beta-carotene supplementation. J Nutr Biochem 16: 385-397.
66. Siems W, Salerno C, Crifò C, Sommerburg O, Wiswedel I (2009) Beta-carotene degradation products-formation, toxicity and prevention of toxicity. Forum Nutr 61: 75-86.
67. Hallberg L, Brune M, Rossander L (1989) The role of vitamin C in iron absorption. Int J Vitam Nutr Res Suppl 30: 103-108.
68. Thankachan P, Walczyk T, Muthayya S, Kurpad AV, Hurrell RF (2008) Iron absorption in young Indian women: the interaction of iron status with the influence of tea and ascorbic acid. Am J Clin Nutr 87: 881-886.
69. Cook JD, Lipschitz DA, Miles LE, Finch CA (1974) Serum ferritin as a measure of iron stores in normal subjects. Am J Clin Nutr 27: 681-687.
70. Bezwoda WR, Bothwell TH, Torrance JD (1979) The relationship between marrow iron stores, plasma ferritin concentrations and iron absorption. Scand J Haematol 22: 113-120.
71. Taylor P, Martinez-Torres C, Leets I, Ramirez J, Garcia-Casal MN, et al. (1988) Relationships among iron absorption, percent saturation of plasma transferrin and serum ferritin concentration in humans. J Nutr 118: 1110-1115.
72. Hunt JR, Roughead ZK (2000) Adaptation of iron absorption in men consuming diets with high or low iron bioavailability. Am J Clin Nutr 71: 94-102.
73. Nemeth E, Ganz T (2006) Regulation of iron metabolism by hepcidin. Annu Rev Nutr 26: 323-342.
74. Brown EG, Dubach R, Moore CV (1958) Studies on iron transportation and metabolism. IX. Critical analysis of mucosal block by large doses of iron in human subjects. J Lab Clin Med 52: 335-355.
75. Viteri FE, Xunian L, Tolomei K (1995) True absorption and retention of supplementation iron is more efficient when iron is administered every three days rather than daily to iron-normal and iron-deficient rats. J Nutr 125: 82-91.
76. Jaleel A, Siddiqui IA, Rahman MA (2003) Do we need daily iron supplementation? Comments and controversies. J Pak Med Assoc 53: 162-165.
77. Thomas C, Mackey MM, Diaz AA, Cox DP (2009) Hydroxyl radical is produced via the Fenton reaction in submitochondrial particles under oxidative stress: implications for diseases associated with iron accumulation. Redox Rep 14: 102-108.
78. Roughead ZK, Zito CA, Hunt JR (2005) Inhibitory effects of dietary calcium on the initial uptake and subsequent retention of heme and nonheme iron in humans: comparisons using an intestinal lavage method. Am J Clin Nutr 82: 589-597.
79. Heaney RP (2001) Factors influencing the measurement of bioavailability, taking calcium as a model. J Nutr 131: 1344S-1348S.

80. Solomons N, Slavin JL (2001) What impact does stage of physiological development and/or physiological state have on the bioavailability of dietary supplements? Summary of workshop discussion. J Nutr 131: 1392S-1395S.
81. Wang L, Li Q, Duan XL, Chang YZ (2005) Effects of extracellular iron concentration on calcium absorption and relationship between Ca2+ and cell apoptosis in Caco-2 cells. World J Gastroenterol 11: 2916-2921.
82. Seligman PA, Caskey JH, Frazier JL, Zucker RM, Podell ER, et al. (1983) Measurements of iron absorption from prenatal multivitamin-mineral supplements. Obstet Gynecol 61: 356-362.
83. Gregory JF (2001) Case study: Folate bioavailability. J Nutr 131: 1376S-1382S.
84. Meydani M (2002) Antioxidants in the prevention of chronic diseases. Nutr Clin Care 5: 47-49.
85. Rajput RJ (2008) Cyclical medicine for hair loss management and improving results in hair transplant. Hair Transplant Forum International 18: 208
86. Rajput RJ (2010) Is there a role for adjuvants in the management of male pattern hair loss? Journal of Cutaneous and Aesthetic Surgery.
87. Rajput R (2015) Understanding hair loss due to air pollution & the approach to management. Hair Ther Transplant.
88. Rajput RS (2016) Benefit from vitamin therapy in smoker's hair. Hair Ther Transplant 6: 141.
89. Rajput R (2016) Improvement in hair loss and better hair quality with vitamin therapy in Monilethrix. J Cosmo Trichol 2: 113.
90. Rajput R (2016) Hair loss due to electromagnetic radiation from overuse of cell phone. J Cosmo Trichol 2: 114.
91. Rajendrasingh JR (2017) Role of non-androgenic factors in hair loss and hair regrowth. J Cosmo Trichol 3: 118.
92. Assunção Guimarães C, Linden R (2004) Programmed cell deaths. Apoptosis and alternative deathstyles. Eur J Biochem 271: 1638-1650.
93. Yoshimori T (2004) Autophagy: a regulated bulk degradation process inside cells. Biochem Biophys Res Commun 313: 453-458.
94. Bender AE (1976) Subclinical and covert malnutrition. Bull Schweiz Akad Med Wiss 31: 279-290.
95. Bailey RL, West KP, Black RE (2015) The epidemiology of global micronutrient deficiencies. Ann Nutr Metab 66 Suppl 2: 22-33.
96. Baart AM, van Noord PA, Vergouwe Y, Moons KG, Swinkels DW, et al. (2013) High prevalence of subclinical iron deficiency in whole blood donors not deferred for low hemoglobin. Transfusion 53: 1670-1677.
97. El-Eshmawy MM, Arafa MM, Elzehery RR, Elhelaly RM, Elrakhawy MM, et al. (2016) Relationship between vitamin A deficiency and the thyroid axis in clinically stable patients with liver cirrhosis related to hepatitis C virus. Appl Physiol Nutr Metab 41: 985-991.
98. Yilmaz H, Cakmak M, Darcin T, Inan O, Gurel OM, et al. (2015) Subclinical hypothyroidism in combination with vitamin D deficiency increases the risk of impaired left ventricular diastolic function. Docr Regul 49: 84-90.
99. Chanoine JP (2003) Selenium and thyroid function in infants, children and adolescents. Biofactors 19: 137-143.
100. Ravanbod M, Asadipooya K, Kalantarhormozi M, Nabipour I, Omrani GR (2013) Treatment of iron-deficiency anemia in patients with subclinical hypothyroidism. Am J Med 126: 420-424.
101. Zimmermann MB (2007) Interactions of vitamin A and iodine deficiencies: effects on the pituitary-thyroid axis. Int J Vitam Nutr Res 77: 236-240.
102. Beals KA, Manore MM (1998) Nutritional status of female athletes with subclinical eating disorders. J Am Diet Assoc 98: 419-425.

Effect of Different Corn Processing Techniques in the Nutritional Composition of Nixtamalized Corn Tortillas

Josefina Consuelo Morales* **and Rodrigo A Garcia Zepeda**

Department of Food Science and Technology, National Institute of Medical Sciences and Nutrition Salvador Zubirán, México

***Corresponding author:** Morales JC, Department of Food Science and Technology, National Institute of Medical Sciences and Nutrition Salvador Zubirán, México E-mail: josefina.moralesg@incmnsz.mx

Abstract

Maize in the form of tortilla plays an important role in the diet of Mexican population, with a per cápita consumption of 157 g/day. The two main methods for tortilla are the traditional method, which uses maize dough or masa made in the ancient manner; and the industrial method, which uses industrially-processed maize flour. Both methods are based on the alkaline-processing of maize known as nixtamalization. Chemical profiles of maize tortillas were analyzed. Samples were collected between 2012 and 2013 in three lots, one every six months, from four retail shops at 16 municipalities of Mexico City; tortillas made of maize flour were obtained from two supermarkets of four municipalities. Composition changed according to raw materials and production method. Samples made with nixtamal dough showed lower contents of moisture, of about 5%, and absence of thiamine and riboflavin than nixtamal flour. Differences in carbohydrates and iron, 0.5% more in case of iron, may be caused by maize phenotype; while differences in crude fat 1% more, dietary fiber 0.5% more, thiamine, and riboflavin are due to additives added by manufacturers; however, concentration of vitamins and minerals in the final product were below theoretical values. In case of calcium, 100% more in maize dough tortillas is due to lime amount added on each method or amount of broken grain processed. Regarding on effect of sampling, contents of protein and crude fat remained constant on dough tortillas regardless of sample collection and these were consistently higher than maize flour tortillas over time, 0.3% and 1%, respectively, which is due to maize phenotype. On flour-made tortillas, fat and dietary fibers were also constant since maize flour manufacturers add additives and nutrients to obtain certain rheological characteristics and nutritional content on maize flour tortillas.

Keywords: Maize; Nixtamal; Tortilla; Nixtamal flour; Nixtamal dough; Chemical composition

Abbreviations:

MD: Maize Dough Tortillas; MF: Maize Flour Tortillas; MD/MF: Maize Dough and Flour Tortillas; TM: Traditional Method; IM: Industrial Method; OMS: Official Mexican Standard; TS: Tortilla Shop

Introduction

Maize tortillas play an important role in diet of Mexicans, with a per capita consumption of 157 g/day [1]. Tortilla industry comprises nixtamal mills, Tortilla Shops (TS) (a shop that produces and sells tortillas), and nixtamal flour factories, which represent the main form in which maize is industrially processed in Mexico.

The methods for tortilla production based on the alkaline-processing known as nixtamalization are: Traditional Method (TM), which uses Maize Dough (MD) and Industrial Method (IM), which uses industrially-processed Maize Flour (MF).

Nixtamalization produces changes in maize such as easy pericarp removal [2], partial gelatinization of starches [3], protein solubility [4], and niacin release [5]. Furthermore, lime increase calcium content of tortilla, up to 400% as compared to unprocessed maize [3].

The nixtamalization has been previously studied, and information is available on effects of: different cooking times and temperatures, lime concentration, number of rinsing after cooking and extra soaking before cooking. The differences on the former variables affect quality of tortillas [3-10].

The Official Mexican Standard (OMS) NOM-187 [11] establishes sanitary and commercial specifications for tortillas and other nixtamal-derived products. Other OMS such as NMX-FF-034 [12] and NMX-F-046 [13] define specifications for white maize to be used in production of MD, and those for MF, respectively. However, there is still no an OMS that establishes chemical specifications for tortillas.

Given the above, the aim of this study was to systematically evaluate nutritional composition of tortillas obtained by TM and IM obtained from nixtamal corn dough and using pre-processed flour, respectively. A second purpose was to evaluate variability of composition among tortillas by raw material and point of sale, as well as variability of sampling on same groups.

Material and Methods

Collection of samples

Tortillas were obtained between 2012 and 2013, from the 16 municipalities of Mexico City. Four TS were selected randomly from each municipality, and batches of 2 kg were bought. At the same time, two supermarkets that produce their own tortillas were selected in four municipalities and 2 kg were obtained at each point of sale. In these same stores, pre-packed tortillas produced in a factory elsewhere were also purchased. All kinds were collected three times, once every six months.

Sample treatment

Moisture (AOAC 925.09) was determined on freshly samples; then were dehydrated at 67°C/14 h in an Apex Ltd. drier and grounded in a Thomas Wiley knife mill, with a 1 mm mesh.

Storage of samples

Dehydrated ground tortilla was divided into four 200 g aliquots. Two were analyzed and two were stored in hermetic plastic containers and then into boxes at room temperature (23 ± 2°C).

Analytical methods

Proximate composition, vitamins and minerals were analyzed by duplicate according to the AOAC techniques: moisture (925.09), nitrogen (977.14) using a 6.25 factor to obtain content of crude protein, fat (920.39 and 963.15), ash (923.03) and total dietary fiber (985.29) [14].

Energy content was calculated according to OMS NOM-184 appendix C, clause 1 [15] which are based on At-water factors.

Ca, Fe and Zn were analyzed with an AOAC atomic adsorption-spectrophotometric techniques: 977.29, 944.02 and 986.15, respectively. While, thiamine and riboflavin with AOAC spectroscopy-fluorometric techniques: 924.23 and 970.65 [14].

Statistical analysis

Nutrients and confidence interval at 95% are reported by mean ± SD per 100 g of fresh weight. Descriptive statistic was calculated as described in Table 1; significances by point of sale and raw material were determined by Kruskal-Wallis, followed by U of Mann-Whitney tests, and differences among collections were determined by Friedman test. All statistical evaluations were carried out with SPSS v12.0 System.

To determine the similarity in chemical composition between the groups a cluster analysis was performed.

Groups	Description
Point of sale	Tortilla shop
	Supermarkets
Raw material	Maize Flour (MF)
	Maize Dough (MD)
	Maize Flour/Maize Dough mix (MF/MD)

Table 1: Description of the study groups.

Results and Discussion

At TS was common to mix MF with MD to make tortillas. Therefore, such mix was considered as another raw material (Table 1). 192 samples were obtained from TS, 24 from supermarkets and 45 samples were commercially-branded fully industrialized tortillas.

Chemical composition of tortillas by raw material and point of sale

Proximate composition, minerals and vitamins in tortillas are shown in Tables 2 and 3. MF tortillas had consistently the highest moisture as compared to MD; this difference agrees with other reports that mention a 5 g/100 g difference in moisture [6] due to addition of CMC, gums or unsaturated fatty acids to retain water [7,16]. Other authors consider that this difference is caused by MF processing conditions, which results in higher gelatinization-index and higher water-holding capacity [5].

Protein Content (PC) varies between MD and MF tortillas. It is known that MF industry prefers hard endosperm maize, as opposed to TM that favours white landraces [17]. Previous studies report PC, on dry basis, for MD tortillas of 7.58-15.63 g/100 g [10,18-21]. These reports have different maize descriptions, suggesting phenotypes were different; but also is known PC varies according to endosperm hardness [17]. However, on dry basis, results between MD and MF, were similar ($p>0.05$) and differences, per 100 g of fresh weight, are due to losses that take place during cooking, pericarp removal and wet milling of nixtamal in TM [5,21].

Energy Content (EC) of tortillas correlated with moisture with a coefficient $r=-0.997$. MD tortillas and MD/MF did not show difference; while MF tortillas had significantly lower EC due to their higher moisture levels.

Crude Fat (CF) contents show differences by raw material or point of sale, Table 2; this may be due to maize germ losses, which has up to 90% of lipids. Germ losses can reach 30% during nixtamalization and 17% during TM nixtamal rinsing [7]. The industry prefers high endosperm maize varieties, which results in low maize germ, but also in lower protein quality [6]. Maize phenotype may also affect fat content; however, it is noteworthy that MF sometimes is added with non-polar fatty acids that work as softeners at a concentration of approximately 1% [22,23]. Such fatty acids affect the content of crude fat in the final product.

Ash contents were different ($p<0.05$) by raw material and point of sale, Tables 2 and 3. These may be due to different extent of lime removal on TM because around of 0.5% differences were reported between MD tortillas made on different maize varieties that were soaked for 12-16 h in a solution of lime 0.6-2% g/kg of grain [10,19-21]; although, some authors report that differences are due to pericarp removal [24], suggesting there is no direct relationship between amount of lime used in the process and ash content.

Dietary Fiber (DF) was lower in MF tortillas ($p<0.05$) as compared to MD and the mix (Table 2); which may be due to: 1) Differences in soaking time and cooking temperature, since soluble carbohydrates increase as a function of these variables [25], 2) Partial or null pericarp removal, which increase insoluble fibrous elements of cell wall [26]. A pericarp excess affects colour of tortillas, possibly because of that, MF tortillas were whiter than MD tortillas; 3) Presence of resistant starch which is related to a harder endosperm and requires longer cooking times to let water enter the grain and solubilize starch [3]; tortilla producers are not able to control this and do not adjust the process accordingly. MF had low content even when: 1) Is added with gums such as CMC, and 2) Starch having a higher gelatinization as caused by the industrial MF method. It is important to mention that on dry basis differences were maintained.

Nutrient	Unit	Raw Material			P value
		MFA	MDB	MF/MDC	
		(n=111)	(n=78)	(n=105)	
Moisture	g	48.98 ± 4.94[a]	43.05 ± 2.87[b]	42.87 ± 2.44[b]	0
	g*	48.02-49.94	42.51-43.59	42.32-43.42	
Protein	g	4.64 ± 0.56[a]	5.17 ± 0.32[b]	5.22 ± 0.28[b]	0
	g*	4.53-4.74	5.11-5.23	5.16-5.29	
Energy	kJ	201.02 ± 19.87[a]	223.16 ± 11.71[b]	223.87 ± 9.64[b]	0
	kJ*	197.17-204.86	220.96-225.37	221.70-226.04	
Crude fat	g	0.95 ± 0.20[a]	1.24 ± 0.26[b]	1.28 ± 0.23[b]	0
	g*	0.91-0.99	1.19-1.29	1.23-1.34	
Ash	g	1.05 ± 0.26[a]	1.14 ± 0.18[b]	1.18 ± 0.16[b]	0
	g*	1.00-1.10	1.11-1.17	1.14-1.21	
Dietary fiber	g	8.01 ± 1.22[a]	8.50 ± 1.06[b]	8.63 ± 1.25[b]	0
	g*	7.78-8.25	8.30-8.70	8.35-8.91	
Calcium (Ca)	mg	122.88 ± 70.53[a]	207.72 ± 64.67[b]	197.99 ± 69.60[b]	0
	mg*	109.23-136.53	195.56-219.88	182.30-213.68	
Iron (Fe)	mg	1.47 ± 0.97a	1.82 ± 0.62[b]	2.02 ± 1.23[b]	0
	mg*	1.28-1.66	1.71-1.94	1.74-2.29	
Zinc (Zn)	mg	1.16 ± 0.30	1.18 ± 0.19	1.14 ± 0.17	0.157
	mg*	1.10-1.21	1.14-1.21	1.10-1.17	
Riboflavin (B2)	mg	0.08 ± 0.07[a]	0.04 ± 0.03[b]	0.03 ± 0.02[b]	0
	mg*	0.07-0.10	0.03-0.05	0.03-0.04	
Thiamine (B1)	mg	0.12 ± 0.11[a]	0.04 ± 0.04[b]	0.05 ± 0.05[b]	0
	mg*	0.10-0.15	0.03-0.05	0.03-0.06	

**All nutrients are per 100 g fresh weight of edible food *Confidence interval 95% Same letters by row indicate no significant difference ($p>0.05$) [a]Maize flour, [b]Maize dough, [c]Maize flour/Maize dough

Table 2: Nutrients in maize tortillas by raw material** from 16 municipalities of Mexico City.

Calcium and Iron were significantly different between MF and MD. The latter was similar to MD/MF tortillas (Table 2). Calcium increased as a function of: 1) Maize phenotype, 2) Fractured grain percentage, and 3) Soaking time [8,27]. The higher calcium in MD tortillas may be due to: 1) longer nixtamalization and holding times, 12-18 h, even though lime amount added in each process varies considerably, TM using up to 1.2% and IM 5 to 6%; 2) Is possible that the grain used has a high % of broken grain that favours calcium diffusion, the affinity being pericarp>germ>endosperm [28]; or 3) Is caused by the lime addition to MD during kneading, before pressing it in a tortilla machine. This last practice was observed in tortilla shops and it is made with the aim of whitening and softening the product, as well as to help stop spoilage. On the other hand, calcium concentration affects tortilla moisture: at higher concentrations water absorption into starch is reduced [29]. This may explain the lower moisture in MD tortillas.

Iron in MD tortillas is of 1.5-1.7 mg [30]. In this study, MD tortillas (Tables 2 and 3) showed contents of about 2.0 mg. It's known iron is related to maize phenotype, since white maize has higher content as compared to yellow varieties and losses smaller amounts along process [9]. Therefore, longer holding time of nixtamal modifies it [8]. These considerations suggest that white maize is used in TM, while MF industry prefers yellow types [31].

Zinc contents among tortillas were not statistically different (Tables 2 and 3) between tortillas by raw material or point of sale. It's been reported that longer holding time of nixtamal has strongest effect on zinc because up to 11% of zinc may be lost as compared to initial content of grain [8]. Therefore, it's been observed that zinc in tortillas is related to maize phenotypes [32].

Nutrient	Unit	Point of sale		P value
		Tortilla shop	Supermarket	
		(n=192)	(n=102)	
Moisture	g	43.05 ± 2.74	49.01 ± 5.01	0
	g*	42.66-43.44	48.03-49.99	
Protein	g	5.19 ± 0.31	4.63 ± 0.56	0
	g*	5.14-5.23	4.52-4.74	
Energy	kJ	223.14 ± 11.08	200.94 ± 20.15	0
	kJ*	221.57-224.72	196.99-204.90	
Crude fat	g	1.25 ± 0.25	0.95 ± 0.20	0
	g*	1.22-1.29	0.92-0.99	
Ash	g	1.15 ± 0.17	1.05 ± 0.26	0.001
	g*	1.13-1.18	1.00-1.10	
Dietary fiber	g	8.54 ± 1.15	8.03 ± 1.21	0
	g*	8.38-8.71	7.79-8.26	
Calcium (Ca)	mg	201.99 ± 67.63	123.73 ± 71.33	0
	mg*	192.37-211.62	109.72-137.74	
Iron (Fe)	mg	1.90 ± 0.92	1.46 ± 0.98	0
	mg*	1.77-2.03	1.27-1.65	
Zinc (Zn)	mg	1.16 ± 0.19	1.16 ± 0.30	0.217
	mg*	1.13-1.19	1.10-1.22	
Riboflavin (B2)	mg	0.03 ± 0.03	0.08 ± 0.07	0
	mg*	0.03-0.04	0.07-0.10	
Thiamine (B1)	mg	0.04 ± 0.04	0.13 ± 0.11	0
	mg*	0.04-0.05	0.10-0.15	
**All nutrients are per 100 g fresh weight of edible food *Confidence interval 95%. Same letters by row indicate no significant difference (p>0.05)				

Table 3: Nutrients in maize tortillas by point of sale** from 16 municipalities of Mexico City.

Riboflavin and thiamine contents decreases by alkaline cooking, with losses close to 50% and 70% for riboflavin and thiamine, respectively [31]. In present study, content depend on the manufacturing process or raw material. MF tortillas showed a 100% higher content of riboflavin, as well as 200% higher for thiamine than MD tortillas, it could be due to the OMS NOM-187, which establishes that MF shall be added with 0.3 and 0.5 mg/100 g of riboflavin and thiamine, respectively [33]. It is noteworthy that these two vitamins are absent in MD tortillas.

Variation of chemical composition of tortillas along the systematic sampling

Moisture in tortillas varied along sampling by raw material and point of sale (Tables 4 and 5). This may be due, in case of MD, to the lack control during manufacturing process. It is known that TM employs subjective techniques to evaluate final products [34]; which is confirmed by the variation observed in MD tortillas by point of sale. On the other hand, addition of MF to MD seems to stabilize moisture, although samples from different collections were statistically different, but p value was close to significance; what is clear is the higher moisture content of MF tortillas.

Nutrient / Sampling	Unit	MFA 1 (n=35)	MFA 2 (n=35)	MFA 3 (n=35)	P value	MDB 1 (n =37)	MDB 2 (n=37)	MDB 3 (n=37)	P value	MF/MDC 1 (n=26)	MF/MDC 2 (n=26)	MF/MDC 3 (n=26)	P value
Moisture	g	47.30 ± 4.03^{a}	49.93 ± 7.05^{b}	49.71 ± 2.10^{b}	0.003	44.49 ± 3.66^{a}	42.67 ± 1.83^{b}	42.00 ± 2.24^{b}	0.001	43.20 ± 2.68^{a}	43.50 ± 2.55^{a}	41.92 ± 1.79^{b}	0.049
Protein	g	4.92 ± 0.51^{a}	4.67 ± 0.65^{a}	4.32 ± 0.27^{b}	0	5.15 ± 0.42	5.23 ± 0.23	5.13 ± 0.30	0.315	5.28 ± 0.30	5.22 ± 0.28	5.16 ± 0.27	0.292
Energy	kJ	207.62 ± 16.40^{a}	197.42 ± 27.99^{b}	198.00 ± 9.34^{b}	0.009	217.13 ± 15.05^{a}	224.91 ± 7.23^{b}	227.46 ± 8.96^{b}	0.001	222.91 ± 10.27	221.46 ± 10.20	227.25 ± 7.58	0.132
Crude fat	g	0.98 ± 0.23	0.95 ± 0.23	0.93 ± 0.12	0.723	1.21 ± 0.34	1.26 ± 0.20	1.26 ± 0.21	0.769	1.38 ± 0.15^{a}	1.27 ± 0.27^{a}	1.21 ± 0.23^{c}	0.038
Ash	g	1.15 ± 0.25^{a}	1.03 ± 0.28^{a,b}	0.96 ± 0.19^{b}	0.007	1.09 ± 0.18^{a}	1.17 ± 0.19^{a,b}	1.17 ± 0.14^{b}	0.037	1.17 ± 0.16	1.17 ± 0.14	1.19 ± 0.18	0.964
Dietary fiber	g	8.25 ± 0.97	7.95 ± 1.33	7.84 ± 1.32	0.707	8.01 ± 1.07^{a}	8.65 ± 0.99^{b}	8.85 ± 0.97^{b}	0.002	8.06 ± 1.08^{a}	8.93 ± 1.51^{b}	8.91 ± 0.91^{b}	0.016
Calcium (Ca)	mg	126.96 ± 68.46	114.79 ± 56.94	126.91 ± 64.77	0.905	190.04 ± 69.60^{a}	209.66 ± 72.45^{a,b}	223.46 ± 45.86^{b}	0.018	164.00 ± 53.05^{a}	214.63 ± 86.10^{b}	215.34 ± 53.74^{b}	0.002
Iron (Fe)	mg	1.58 ± 0.46	1.42 ± 0.61	1.40 ± 0.61	0.481	2.03 ± 0.53^{a}	1.74 ± 0.75^{b}	1.70 ± 0.53^{b}	0.009	2.00 ± 0.57	2.20 ± 0.88	1.85 ± 0.84	0.343
Zinc (Zn)	mg	1.16 ± 0.34	1.16 ± 0.31	1.15 ± 0.24	0.579	1.05 ± 0.17^{a}	1.26 ± 0.17^{b}	1.22 ± 0.16^{b}	0	1.07 ± 0.10^{a}	1.13 ± 0.22^{a,b}	1.20 ± 0.16^{b}	0.011
Riboflavin (B2)	mg	0.09 ± 0.07	0.07 ± 0.07	0.09 ± 0.07	0.057	0.03 ± 0.02^{a}	0.03 ± 0.02^{a,b}	0.05 ± 0.03^{b}	0	0.02 ± 0.03^{a}	0.04 ± 0.02^{b}	0.04 ± 0.02^{b}	0.041
Thiamine (B1)	mg	0.13 ± 0.11	0.13 ± 0.10	0.12 ± 0.11	0.851	0.04 ± 0.04	0.04 ± 0.04	0.04 ± 0.04	0.617	0.05 ± 0.05	0.04 ± 0.04	0.05 ± 0.05	0.787

*All nutrients are per 100 g fresh weight of edible food, a Maize flour, b Maize dough, C Maize flour/Maize dough. Same letters by row and section indicate no significant difference (p>0.05)

Table 4: Variability in nutrients of maize tortillas by raw material* from 16 municipalities of Mexico City.

Protein Content (PC) of MD and MD/MF tortillas, both collected from TS, did not show significant differences along sampling (Tables 4 and 5). Addition of MF did not affect PC at any time. MD tortillas have higher PC and differences in manufacturing conditions between traditional establishments do not seem to affect PC. The results obtained may suggest that MF tortillas have lower protein contents and this may confirm that milling of alkaline-processed grain at low moisture, in IM, has an effect on protein.

Energy Content (EC) of tortillas was different along sampling, but only those of MD/MF did not show differences (p>0.05), which may be due to % of MF added. It's been reported that 30% of MF only improves texture characteristics of MD [34]; therefore we may say that addition percentages ≥ 30% could modify the EC of MD/MF tortillas.

Crude Fat (CF) content in tortillas by raw material was not different at sampling, except for MD/MF samples. In MD tortillas, even though processing conditions vary between establishments; and in MF tortillas, since it is common, containing additives to obtain particular characteristics in final product. The consistently lower CF in all MF samples may confirm that a different phenotype is used by MF industry.

Ash content varied along sampling for both MD and MF tortillas. Variation of ash could be attributed to differences in pericarp removal or to amount of lime added during maize nixtamalization. As shown by the results, tortillas obtained by TM contain more ashes as given by process itself; or by manufacturer's addition when trying to achieve higher yields. However, this hasn't been corroborated yet.

Dietary Fiber (DF) in MF tortilla samples did not vary along time. This is explained by addition of hydrocolloids polymers or gums in order to control their functional properties. Industry includes these additives according to maize characteristics to be processed. On the other hand, DF variations of MD samples may be due to cooking temperature and longer holding times, which increases resistant starch content [35]. Cooking temperatures of tortillas on hot plates or machines may also be a factor, since it causes starch pyro-dextrinization and production of free polysaccharides, which increases non-digestible carbohydrates [36].

Calcium, Iron and Zinc contents in MF samples did not show variations along sampling. It is noteworthy that stirring, cooking time and holding time are factors that determine the degree of calcium incorporation into the grain [37]. Therefore, differences in MD tortillas indicate that amount of calcium hydroxide or magnitude of parameters mentioned above may vary considerably between establishments.

Nutrient		Tortilla shop				Supermarket			
Sampling	Unit	1	2	3	P value	1	2	3	P value
		(n=64)	(n=64)	(n=64)		(n=34)	(n=34)	(n =34)	
Moisture	g	43.99 ± 3.31^{a}	43.09 ± 2.24^{a}	42.08 ± 2.22^{b}	0	47.32 ± 4.09^{a}	49.99 ± 7.15^{b}	42.00 ± 2.13^{b}	0.003
Protein	g	5.20 ± 0.37	5.22 ± 0.25	5.14 ± 0.29	0.173	4.91 ± 0.52^{a}	4.66 ± 0.66^{a}	4.31 ± 0.26^{b}	0
Energy	kJ	219.33 ± 13.48^{a}	223.16 ± 8.98^{a}	226.94 ± 8.99^{b}	0.001	207.62 ± 16.64^{a}	197.26 ± 28.39^{b}	197.96 ± 9.48^{b}	0.012
Crude fat	g	1.27 ± 0.30	1.26 ± 0.23	1.24 ± 0.22	0.54	0.99 ± 0.23	0.95 ± 0.23	0.93 ± 0.12	0.511
Ash	g	1.12 ± 0.18	1.17 ± 0.17	1.18 ± 0.16	0.109	1.15 ± 0.26^{a}	1.03 ± 0.29^{a,b}	0.96 ± 0.20^{b}	0.007
Dietary fiber	g	7.99 ± 1.09^{a}	8.78 ± 1.22^{b}	8.86 ± 0.94^{b}	0	8.32 ± 0.88	7.91 ± 1.33	7.84 ± 1.34	0.468
Calcium (Ca)	mg	177.57 ± 65.11^{a}	210.16 ± 78.11^{b}	218.26 ± 50.83^{b}	0	128.66 ± 68.73	114.86 ± 57.79	127.66 ± 85.93	0.845
Iron (Fe)	mg	2.01 ± 0.54^{a}	1.93 ± 1.33^{b}	1.76 ± 0.67^{b}	0.005	1.57 ± 1.48	1.40 ± 0.61	1.40 ± 0.62	0.463
Zinc (Zn)	mg	1.06 ± 0.15^{a}	1.20 ± 0.20^{b}	1.21 ± 0.16^{b}	0	1.15 ± 0.34	1.17 ± 0.31	1.15 ± 0.24	0.403
Riboflavin (B2)	mg	0.03 ± 0.03^{a}	0.03 ± 0.02^{a}	0.05 ± 0.03^{b}	0	0.09 ± 0.07^{a}	0.08 ± 0.07^{a}	0.09 ± 0.07^{b}	0.049
Thiamine (B1)	mg	0.04 ± 0.04	0.04 ± 0.04	0.04 ± 0.04	0.855	0.13 ± 0.12	0.13 ± 0.10	0.12 ± 0.11	0.89

*All nutrients are per 100 g fresh weight of edible food. Same letters by row and section indicate no significant difference ($p>0.05$)

Table 5: Variability in nutrient composition of maize tortillas by point of sale* from 16 municipalities of Mexico City.

Iron and zinc are added in amounts of 40 mg/kg of MF, and per 100 g of tortillas the expected amount is of 1.62 mg of each, and these do not take into account mineral contents naturally present in maize; concentrations of these minerals in MF tortillas were lower; this may be due to a decrease during storage, iron decreases around 10%, and zinc remains constant after two months [38]. Given the above, losses seem to be around ≥15% for iron, and ≥30% for zinc.

Riboflavin and thiamine in MF tortillas were not statistically different along collections. This is due to fortification of MF, as mentioned, that is of 3 and 5 mg/kg of MF, of vitamins B2 and B1, which results in 0.12 and 0.20 mg/100 g of tortillas, respectively. However, concentrations of B1, B2 in tortillas were lower; this may be due to a decrease in vitamin content during storage, which is between 18 to 37%. When tortillas are prepared, vitamins decrease 37% further [38]. Given the above, losses seem to be around 40% for vitamins.

In MD tortillas, only thiamine did not show differences along collection period; however it was found in low concentrations that indicate a probable total loss. The addition of MF to MD, In MD/MF tortillas, seems to compensate the variation in vitamins contents.

Conclusion

Statistical differences observed in chemical composition of tortillas by raw material, particularly those found for crude fat and iron are due to maize phenotype, while those observed for dietary fiber are due to pericarp removal addition of additives. Significant difference in protein and ash contents, are due to losses during nixtamalization. Regarding ash, amount of lime added didn't seem to cause a difference, as opposed to variations in pericarp removal.

Differences in composition along sampling in MD tortillas may be due to variations in time and cooking temperature, as well as in holding time given by each establishment. However, protein and crude fat wasn't affected in final product.

Not having found variations along time in crude fat, crude fiber, calcium, iron, zinc, thiamine and riboflavin in MF tortillas are due to additives added whose purpose is to improve rheological characteristics of tortillas, as well as to fortify the product.

References

1. Secretary of Economy, General Directorate of Basic Industries (2012) Analysis of the corn-tortilla value chain: current situation and local competition factors pp: 30-31.
2. Garcia-Lopez S, Wyatt CJ (1982) Effect of fiber in corn tortillas and cooked beans on iron availability. J Agric Food Chem 30: 724-727.
3. Salinas-Moreno Y, Herrera-Corredor JA, Castillo-Merino J, Pérez-Herrera P (2003) Physicochemical changes of the starch during the nixtamalization of maize in varieties with different grain hardness. Arch Latinoam Nutr 53: 188-193.
4. Urizar Hernández AL, Bressani R (1997) The effect of lime cooking of corn on phytic acid, calcium, total and ionizable iron content. Arch Latinoam Nutr 47: 217-223.
5. Bello-Pérez L, Osorio-Díaz P, Agama-Acevedo E, Solorza-Feria J, Toro-Vázquez JF, et al. (2003) Chemical and physicochemical properties of dried wet masa and dry masa flour. J Sci Food Agric 83: 408-412.
6. Billeb de Sinibaldi AC, Bressani R (2001) Nixtamalization cooking characteristics of 11 maize varieties. Arch Latinoam Nutr 51: 86-94.
7. Arámbula-Villa G, Barrón-Ávila L, González-Hernández J (2001) Effect of nixtamalized maize grain (*Zea mayz L.*) on the physicochemical, rheological, structural and textural characteristics of the grain, dough and corn tortillas. Arch Latinoam Nutr 51: 184-194.

8. Bressani R, Turcios JC, Colmenares de Ruiz AS, de Palomo PP (2004) Effect of processing conditions on phytic acid, calcium, iron, and zinc contents of lime-cooked maize. J Agric Food Chem 52:1157-1162.

9. Bressani R, Pazy Paz R, Scrimshaw NS (1958) Chemical Changes in Corn during Preparation of Tortillas. Agric Food Chem 6: 770-774.

10. Figueroa Cárdenas JD, Acero Godinez MG, Vasco Méndez NL, Lozano Guzmán A, Flores Acosta LM, et al. (2001) Fortification and evaluation of the nixtamal tortillas. Arch Latinoam Nutr 51: 293-302.

11. DGN (2011) Official Mexican Standard NOM-187-SSA1/SCFI-2002, Products and services. Dough, tortillas, toasts and flour prepared for processing and establishments where processed. Sanitary specifications. Commercial information. Test methods. D. of the Fed.

12. Normas DG (2002) Norma Mexicana NMX-FF-034/1-SCFI-2002 Non-industrialized food products for human consumption- cereals-Part I: White corn for alkaline process for corn tortillas and nixtamalized corn products-Specifications and test methods. D of the Fed.

13. Normas DG (1980) Mexican Standard NMX-F-046-S-1980, Nixtamalized corn flour. D. of. The Fed.

14. Association of Official Agricultural Chemists (AOAC) (2012) Official Methods of Analysis of the association of Analytical Chemists International (AOAC) (19th edn.).

15. Normas DG (2002) Official Mexican Standard NOM-184-SSA1-2002, Products and services. Milk, milk formula and combined dairy product. Sanitary specifications. D. of. The Fed.

16. Vittadini E, Clubbs E, Shellhammer TH, Vodovotz Y (2004) Effect of high pressure processing and addition of glycerol and salt on the properties of water in corn tortillas. J Cereal Sci 39: 109-117.

17. Pereira RC, Davide LC, Pedrozo CA, Carneiro NP, Souza IRP, et al. (2008) Relationship between structural and biochemical characteristics and texture of corn grains. Genet Mol Res 7: 498-508.

18. Martínez-Flores HE, Figueroa JDC, Martínez-Bustos F, Gonzalez-Hernandez J, Rodríguez García ME, et al. (2002) Physical properties and composition of femurs of rat fed with diets based on corn tortillas made from different processes. Int J Food Sci Nutr 53: 155-162.

19. Gómez-Aldapa C, Martínez-Bustos, CJD Figueroa, Ordorica FCA (1999) A comparison of the quality of whole corn tortillas made from instant corn flours by traditional or extrusion processing. Int J Food Sci Technol 34: 391-399.

20. Bressani R, Benavides V, Acevedo E, Ortiz MA (1990) Changes in Selected Nutrient Contents and in Protein Quality of Common and Quality-Protein Maize During Rural Tortilla Preparation. Cereal Chem 67: 515-518.

21. Rendon-Villalobos R, Bello-Pérez LA, Osorio-Díaz P, Tovar J, Paredes-López O (2002) Effect of Storage Time on In Vitro Digestibility and Resistant Starch Content of Nixtamal, Masa, and Tortilla. Cereal Chem 79: 340-344.

22. Flores-Farías R, Martínez-Bustos F, Salinas-Moreno Y (2002) Characterization of commercial flours of nixtamalized maize. Agrociencia 36: 557-567.

23. Arámbula-Villa G, Gutiérrez-Árias E, Moreno-Martínez E (2007) Thermal properties of maize masa and tortillas with different components from maize grains, and additives. J Food Eng 80: 55-60.

24. Núñez-Santiago M, Santoyo E, Bello-Pérez L, Santoyo-Gutiérrez S (2003) Rheological evaluation of non-Newtonian Mexican nixtamalised maize and dry processed masa flours. J Food Eng 60: 55-66.

25. Bello-Pérez L, Osorio-Díaz P, Agama-Acevedo E, Núñez-Santiago C, Paredes-López YO (2002) Chemical, physicochemical and rheological properties of masses and flours of nixtamalized maize. Agrociencia 36: 319-328.

26. Dreher ML (2001) Handbook of Dietary Fiber.

27. Zazueta C, Ramos G, Fernández-Muñoz JL, Rodríguez ME, Acevedo-Hernández G, et al. (2002) A Radioisotopic Study of the Entry of Calcium Ion into the Maize Kernel During Nixtamalization. Cereal Chem 79: 500-503.

28. Gonzalez R, Reguera E, Figueroa JM, Sánchez-Sinencio F (2005) On the nature of the Ca binding to the hull of nixtamalized corn grains. LWT-Food Sci Technol 38: 119-124.

29. Sánchez-Madrigal MÁ, Meléndez-Pizarro CO, Martínez-Bustos F, Ruiz-Gutiérrez MG, Quintero-Ramos A, et al. (2014) Structural, functional, thermal and rheological properties of nixtamalised and extruded blue maize (*Zea mays L*) flour with different calcium sources. Int J Food Sci Technol 49: 578-586.

30. Krause VM, Tucker KL, Kuhnlein HV, LopezPalacios CY, Ruz M, et al. (1992) Rural-urban variation in limed maize use and tortilla consumption by women in Guatemala. Ecol Food Nutr 28: 279-288.

31. Bressani R, Rooney L, Quintero X, Serna Saldivar S (1997) Fortification of Corn Masa Flour with Iron and/or Other Nutrients? A Literature and Industry Experience Review. SUSTAIN, Washington DC, USA.

32. Dickerson G (1992) Nutritional analysis of New Mexico blue corn and dent corn kernels. pp: 1-2.

33. Normas DG (2008) Official Mexican Standard NOM-247-SSA1-2008, Products and services. Cereals and their products. Cereals, cereal flour, meal or semolina. Food based on: cereals, edible seeds, flour, semolina or semolina or their mixtures. products of. D. of. the Fed.

34. Gasca-Mancera JC, Casas-Alencáster NB (2007) Addition of nixtamalized maize flour to fresh mass of nixtamalized maize. Effect on textural properties of dough and tortilla. Rev Mex 6: 317-328.

35. Bello-Perez LA, Flores-Silva PC, Agama-Acevedo E, Figueroa-Cardenas JD, Lopez-Valenzuela JA, et al. (2014) Effect of the nixtamalization with calcium carbonate on the indigestible carbohydrate content and starch digestibility of corn tortilla. J Cereal Sci 60: 421-425.

36. Laurentin A, Cárdenas M, Ruales J, Pérez E, Tovar J (2003) Preparation of indigestible pyrodextrins from different starch sources. J Agric Food Chem 51: 5510-5515.

37. Ruiz-Gutiérrez MG, Quintero-Ramos A, Meléndez-Pizarro CO, Lardizábal-Gutiérrez D, Barnard J, et al. (2010) Changes in mass transfer, thermal and physicochemical properties during nixtamalization of corn with and without agitation at different temperatures. J Food Eng 98: 76-83.

38. Rosado JL, Cassís L, Solano L, Duarte-Vázquez MA (2005) Nutrient addition to corn masa flour: effect on corn flour stability, nutrient loss, and acceptability of fortified corn tortillas. Food Nutr Bull 26: 266-272.

Nutritional Value of Coffee Made from a Mixture of Coffee Leaf and Spices used in Ethiopia

Yitayal AA[1*] **and Tilahun RD**[2]

[1]*Kotebe Metropolitan University, Addis Ababa, Ethiopia*

[2]*Wolkite University, Gubrei, Wabe Bridge, Ethiopia*

[*]**Corresponding author:** Yitayal AA, Kotebe Metropolitan University, Addis Ababa, Ethiopia, E-mail: yituaddis@gmail.com

Abstract

In the south western part of the Southern Nations, Nationalities and Peoples Region (SNNPR) in Ethiopia, coffee is prepared not only from coffee bean but also from a mixture of coffee leaf and spices; commonly practiced in Kaffa, Sheka and Bench-Maji zones. The purpose of this study was to determine the proximate and mineral compositions of the coffee and evaluate its nutritional and energy values. The American Public Health Association (APHA) methods were employed for the determination of pH, crude fat and minerals. The phenol sulphuric acid and the Kjeldahl procedures were used for the determination of total carbohydrate and protein, respectively. The amount of energy that could be obtained from the drink was estimated by taking the sum of the proportions of fat, carbohydrate and protein. The percent values were: carbohydrate 0.92 ± 0.21-2.04 ± 0.16, protein 0.19 ± 0.01-0.44 ± 0.02 and fat 2.43 ± 0.49-4.17 ± 0.30. Energy content was 96.05 ± 13.72-434.53 ± 18.33 kcal. Considerable amounts of K (619.29–1910.67), Na (2654.19–3671.61), Fe (4.70–8.57), Mg (33.98-97.45), Ca (24.99–59.58), Mn (0.91–1.58), Cu (0.09–0.24), Zn (0.42–0.78), N (286.48–710.00) and P (24.47–59.10) mg/L were obtained. The Na:K and Ca:P ratios are found to be 1.92–4.27 and 0.62–1.02, respectively. There exist significant differences in almost all the nutrients among the roasted and other types of coffee made from a mixture of coffee leaf and spices ($P<0.05$). Generally, the drink contains significant nutrients vital for energy and health. It could be used as a supplement to satisfy human nutrition needs (food additive) so that it would partially curb nutrition insecurity problems in and out of the region and the country, especially for coffee growing countries.

Keywords: Coffee leaf; Energy; Health; Minerals; Spices

Introduction

Ethiopia is considered to be the birthplace of the coffee plant and of coffee culture. Today, over 15 million people in Ethiopia are involved in the cultivation and picking of coffee, and it remains a central part of Ethiopian culture [1].

In addition to the cultural and social value, coffee is often consumed for its stimulatory effects as caffeine is the most prominent in its composition [2]. It is reported that 70% of caffeine comes from coffee while soft drinks and tea contribute 16 and 12%, respectively [2].

Moreover, coffee contains essential substances for energy and health. For example, a nutritional analysis study on coffee bean showed the carbohydrate (cellulose and hemicelluloses which are 8.6 and 36.7 g/100 g sample respectively); proteins 13.6 g/100 g and minerals: potassium, phosphorus, magnesium, calcium, aluminum, iron, manganese, copper, zinc with contents of 3549, 1475.1, 1293.3, 777.4, 279.3, 118.7, 40.1, 32.3, 15.1 mg/kg of sample, respectively [3].

On the other hand, spices are used for different purposes such as food additives, preservatives and digestive stimulant action [4,5]. They are composed of an impressive list of phyto-nutrients, essential oils, antioxidants, minerals and vitamins; anti-inflammatory, antiviral and anti-cancer properties which increase blood circulation and reduce the risk of heart problems [6]. According to these literatures, addition of some amount of spices could be important for its nutritional and medicinal values.

A socio-cultural practice survey in the south western part of SNNPR in Ethiopia reported that coffee is prepared not only from coffee bean but also from a mixture of coffee leaf and spices. It is also indicated that about 50% of the proportion (on weight basis) is coffee leaf and the other 50%, excluding water, is the sum of all the spices: *Ocimum basilicum, Mentha piperita, Ruta chalepensis, Coriandrum sativum, Lippia javanica, Allium sativum, Anethum foeniculum, Zingiber officinale, Capsicum frutescens, Aframomum corrorima, Allium cepa* and salt (sodium chloride) added as ingredients [7].

It is also reported that in the specified part of the country coffee made from mixture of coffee leaf and spices (here after referred as CCLS) can be prepared in three different processes, and the primary purpose of drinking CCLS in the culture is to obtain considerable energy along with its socio-cultural, medicinal, economical values and stimulatory effect [7]. However, the nutritional and energy value of CCLS is not scientifically tested and reported.

This study was, therefore, intended to investigate the proximate and mineral compositions of CCLS prepared through the three different processes commonly used in Kaffa, Sheka and Bench-Maji zones in Ethiopia, and evaluate its nutritional and food security values in the region and the country.

Materials and Methods

Sample collection and preparation

The ingredients, proportions and processes for sample preparation were employed following the indigenous people practice [7]. The ingredients were collected from the gardens of the local people and the market, if not available in the garden, in Sheka, Kaffa and Bench-Maji zones. One litre samples of each of CCLS types were prepared in the laboratory by the researchers together with three selected indigenous individuals who represent the three types of CCLS, differing only in process of preparation as follows

Type one (Roasted CCLS)

The coffee leaf that is used for one round preparation was cut from the tip of the coffee plant, then roasted on a baking pan and crushed. One litre of water was added into the CCLS pot and boiled. The prepared coffee leaf was mixed with the boiling water (at 100°C) and further boiled for 10 min. Thereafter, all other ingredients *(Ocimum basilicum, Mentha piperita, Ruta chalepensis, Coriandrum sativum, Lippia javanica, Allium sativum, Anethum foeniculum, Zingiber officinale, Capsicum frutescens, Aframomum corrorima, Allium cepa* and sodium chloride) were added and the resulting mixture was boiled for 15 min. Preparation of CCLS is completed at this stage and CCLS is made ready for analysis after filtration.

Type two (Raw CCLS)

This is the same as type one. However, the leaf was not roasted but simply heated over a fire for a short period of time (5 min) and was crushed with its moisture.

Type three (Mejengir CCLS)

The third process is typical to the Mejengir community in Sheka zone of SNNPR in Ethiopia. In this type, the coffee leaf used was the same as type one, but the coffee leaf, Capsicum frutescens, and other needed spices, enumerated in type one, were boiled separately in different pots [7]. The filtrate of coffee leaf was filtered to the spices pot after the boiling stage had been completed. Finally, 30 ml of Capsicum frutescens was added to the mixture.

Determination of proximate composition

Crude fat and pH were determined according to the method described by APHA 2540D, 2540C, 5520B and 4500-H+ B, respectively [8]. The total carbohydrate was determined by following the procedures in Phenol-sulphuric Acid method as reported by Hedge and Hofreiter [9], and the protein content of CCLS samples was determined by the Kjeldahl method following the procedures enumerated in Pearson [10].

Estimation of energy content

The CCLS samples calorific value was estimated (in Kcal) by multiplying the percentage crude protein, crude lipid and carbohydrate by the recommended energy conversion factors [2.44, 8.37 and 3.57], respectively [11].

Determination of minerals

The American Public Health Association (APHA) 3500-K B and APHA 3500-Na B aqua-regia digestion flame photometric (Elico CL-378 flame photometer) method were used for the determination of potassium and sodium, respectively; and APHA 3111 B aqua-regia digestion direct air acetylene flame (PG-990 Atomic Absorption Spectrophotometer (AAS) method was used for the determination of calcium, magnesium, manganese, copper, iron and zinc. For phosphorus determination, APHA 4500-P C, aqua-regia digestion vanado-molybdo-phosphoric acid colorimetric (T-80 UV/Vis Spectrophotometer) method was applied [8].

Data analysis

The proximate and mineral composition values obtained from the three processes of CCLS preparation were compared by performing Analysis of Variance (ANOVA) using SPSS statistical programme version 20. Significant differences among the means were determined using Least Significant Difference (LSD) multiple comparison test and results were considered statistically significant at $p<0.05$. The results were presented as mean ± SD.

Results and Discussion

Proximate composition of CCLS types

The results in Tables 1 and 2 shows that the Roasted type of CCLS contains relatively high composition of nutrients. The pH of CCLS for the three types of samples showed that the drink is quite acidic with a pH range of 4.46-4.57. CCLS was found to contain carbohydrate, protein and fat in the ranges of 0.92-2.04, 0.19-0.44 and 2.43-4.17%, respectively. The results of this study showed that the Roasted type was found to contain the highest amounts of the three macro-nutrients followed by the Mejengir type.

Parameter	Roasted Type	Raw Type	Mejengir Type
pH	4.55 ± 0.11	4.57 ± 0.04	4.46 ± 0.13
Carbohydratea	2.04 ± 0.16	0.92 ± 0.21	1.78 ± 0.23
Crude Proteina	0.44 ± 0.02	0.19 ± 0.01	0.38 ± 0.07
Crude Fata	4.17 ± 0.30	2.43 ± 0.49	3.19 ± 0.46
Energyb	434.53 ± 18.33	96.05 ± 13.72	135.29 ± 15.82
a and b indicates units in %, and Kcal, respectively. Results are presented as mean ± SD			

Table 1: Proximate composition of CCLS types.

The pH value of CCLS was comparable to 4.4-4.6 reported for malt drinks in Nigeria [12], but was significantly lower than non-alcoholic beverages (pH=7.00) spiced with *Zingiber officinale* [13]. The pH was in the range of values recommended for table wine [12]. The difference in pH among the three types of CCLS was statistically not significant ($p>0.05$).

The difference in protein content among the three types, the carbohydrate contents between Roasted and Mejengir type, and the fat contents of Raw and Mejengir types were statistically not significant ($p>0.05$). The value of protein in this study was lower than the 2.2%

reported for a local drink made from Baobab fruit [14]. The fat and carbohydrate values of CCLS were lower than and the protein is almost comparable to most of the Nigerian food supplements [15], which indicates that CCLS could be used as a food supplement in Ethiopia and other coffee growing countries to partly satisfy human nutritional needs. The recommended dietary allowances of carbohydrates are 60-95, 130, 175 and 210 g/day for infants, children, adults and pregnant and lactating women, respectively [16]. Consequently, consumption of a litre of the roasted type of CCLS could provide an average of 20.40 g/day which is 30%, 16.20%, 12% and 10% of the requirements for each of the above groups, respectively. For protein it is recommended to consume 9.1, 13-19, 34-56 and 71 g/day for infants, children, other age groups, and pregnant and lactating women, respectively. Coffee made from mixture of coffee leaf and spices could provide 1.9-4.4 g protein/day if a litre is consumed per day. The recommended value for fat is achieved for infants only, which is 30-31 g/day. However, this amount could be obtained totally from other sources as the infants consume little CCLS in the culture.

Generally, these macro-nutrients provide an average total energy of 96.05, 135.29 and 434.53 Kcal per liter of CCLS consumed for the Raw; Mejengir and roasted types, respectively. These values were lower than the energy value of cinnamon [17]. The energy content of the Roasted CCLS was significantly highest ($p<0.05$), which implies that this type is a better source of energy. This could justify the indigenous people's practice of using CCLS as an energy source.

Mineral content of CCLS

Table 2 also shows that potassium (K) content was 1910.67 ± 31.15, 619.29 ± 52.05 and 619.29 ± 52.05 and that of sodium (Na) was 3671.61 ± 125.15, 2654.19 ± 171.35 and 3590.76 ± 140.78 for the Roasted, Raw and Mejengir types, respectively. The Ca and P contents ranged from 24.99-59.58 and 24.47-59.10 ppm, respectively. The roasted type contained the highest value in both nutrients. The result also showed that CCLS contained a mean of Mg (33.98 - 97.45), Mn (0.91 - 1.58), Fe (4.70 to 8.57), Zn (0.42 to 0.78) and Cu (0.09 to 0.24) ppm.

Parameter	Roasted Type	Raw Type	Mejengir Type
Potassium	1910.67 ± 31.15	619.29 ± 52.05	619.29 ± 52.05
Sodium	3671.61 ± 125.15	2654.19 ± 171.35	3590.76 ± 140.78
Magnesium	97.45 ± 9.35	33.98 ± 5.72	56.59 ± 2.74
Calcium	59.58 ± 4.81	24.99 ± 2.46	32.35 ± 3.51
Iron	8.57 ± 0.11	4.70 ± 0.15	6.47 ± 0.98
Manganese	1.58 ± 0.06	0.91 ± 0.20	1.19 ± 0.16
Copper	0.24 ± 0.09	0.09 ± 0.03	0.18 ± 0.10
Zinc	0.71 ± 0.06	0.42 ± 0.09	0.78 ± 0.17
Nitrogen	710.00 ± 22.40	286.48 ± 28.01	577.84 ± 106.19
Phosphorus	59.10 ± 4.61	24.47 ± 2.97	31.14 ± 4.80
Na:K Ratio	1.92 ± 0.10	4.27 ± 0.13	4.00 ± 0.18
Ca:P Ratio	1.01 ± 0.01	1.02 ± 0.02	0.62 ± 0.10
Results are presented as mean ± SD			

Table 2: Mineral content of CCLS types (in mg/L).

The difference among the K values of CCLS types is statistically significant ($p<0.05$), hence for better K, consumption of the Roasted type could be important. For Na the Roasted and the Mejengir types could be vital as the differences between the two are not significant ($p>0.05$). The values of Na are higher than the values obtained for malt drinks (12.92-38.00 ppm) [9], and higher than K and Na values (130 and 5.6 ppm, respectively) of a local African drink made from Baobab fruit (Adansonia digitata) pulp as reported by Adedayo et al. [14]. The population (>14 years) in the study area consumes a minimum of a litre per day (children consume less than this) of CCLS which contributes part of the Na and K consumption as the recommended acceptable intakes (AI) of K for infants, children and others is 0.4-0.7, 3.0-3.8 and 4.5-4.7, respectively; and that of Na is 0.12-0.37, 1.0-1.2 and 1.2-1.5 g/day, respectively. The K intake can be maximized up to 5.1 g/day for lactating women [16]. Potassium works with Na to maintain the body's normal blood pressure. Increasing dietary K may provide a protective effect against hypertension (high blood pressure) by increasing the amount of Na excreted from the body and reduce risk of death due to cardiovascular disease [18,19]. However, during the preparation of CCLS, salt (sodium chloride) is added which could increase the Na content and makes the Na: K ratio 1.92, 4.27 and 4.00 for the Roasted, Raw and Mejengir types, respectively (Table 2).

Relative to the other types, the ratio of the Roasted type is preferable as Na:K ratio gets minimized which should further decrease below one though it is significantly the lowest ($p<0.05$). A reduction in Na intake of about 0.03 g/day or an increase in K intake of 0.05 g/day is associated with an average 2 to 4 mmHg decrease in blood pressure

[20]. For such a reduction, either the sodium chloride added in CCLS should be minimized or potassium chloride should be used instead so that the Na:K ratio could be minimized. For those people who usually consume K rich food items like vegetables (especially tomatoes), fruits (banana, orange and avocado) and yogurt, CCLS could be important to balance the Na:K ratio [19]. This effect could be the reason why the community uses CCLS as a traditional medicine for hypertension [7]. In general, the Roasted type of CCLS could be preferable as it contains relatively the highest K, Na and lowest Na:K ratio.

Phosphorus (P) and calcium (Ca) are essential minerals for bone development and are needed for optimal bone health throughout life [21]. Statistically, the differences in Ca content of the Roasted type with the other two, and in P of the Raw type with the other two were significant ($p<0.05$). The Ca value of CCLS is significantly higher than the values reported by Adedeyo [12]; Oluwalana and Adedeji [13], but significantly lowers than that of human milk (300 mg/L) and cow milk (1230 mg/L) [22]. For P, the CCLS value is significantly lower than the values of 150 and 960 mg/L reported for human and cow milks, respectively [22]. The recommended dietary allowances of Ca is 200-260, 700-1000 and 1000-1300 mg/day, and that of P is 100-275, 460-500 and 700-1250 mg/day for infants, children and other age groups in both sexes, respectively [17]. This shows that CCLS could be one source of Ca but extra Ca and P sources would be required. The Ca:P ratios in CCLS were 0.62, 1.01 and 1.02 (Table 2) for the Mejengir type, the Roasted type and Raw type, respectively. The latter two almost agree with the optimal dietary calcium-to-phosphorus weight ratio (Ca:P) of 1.3 and cow milk (1.3), but lower than human milk [22,23]. Coffee made from a mixture of coffee leaf and spices could serve as a source of balanced Ca and P during the process of bone hardening or aging, as the Ca:P ratio gradually undergoes increases from 1:1 to 1.67 (above optimum) in this process. In conclusion, for the sake of better Ca, P and Ca:P ratio content consumption of the Roasted type of CCLS could be advisable.

For Mg content, the roasted type contains the highest amount and the difference among the three types of CCLS was significant ($p<0.05$). Daily consumption of a litre of Roasted type of CCLS could satisfy about 100% and 23-40.8% of the daily requirements of children and other age groups, respectively as the recommended dietary allowances of magnesium are 30-75, 80-130 and 240-420 mg/day for infants, children and other age groups of both sexes, respectively [17]. Therefore, consumption of CCLS (especially the Roasted type) could reduce the risk of cardiovascular diseases and atherogenesis such as increasing oxidative stress, cytokine synthesis, nitrogen oxides and mediators of inflammation, and adhesion molecules on microvascular endothelial cells which otherwise would occur due to Mg deficiency in the body [24,25].

Manganese (Mn) is an essential trace element, necessary for development and growth of organisms. The adequate content of this element in the body determines proper metabolism of amino acids, cholesterol and carbohydrates, and influences the activity of several enzymes involved in metabolic and redox processes [26]. The results of Mn content (Table 2) show that CCLS could be used as a good source to obtain adequate amounts of Mn reported to be 0.003-0.6, 1.2-1.5 and 1.6-2.6 mg/day for infants, children and other age groups, respectively [16]. This means that consuming a litre of CCLS could be enough to satisfy the Mn requirement of the human body (except for pregnant and lactating women) if consumed daily. The Mn value of CCLS is higher than the 0.01 ± 0.02 ppm for malt drinks in Nigeria [13], human milk (3-10 μg/L), cow formula (30-50 μg/L) and soy formula (200-300 μg/L) [27], but lower than the result of 13 ppm obtained for a local African drink made from Baobab fruit (Adansonia digitata) pulp [14]. The highest value of Mn was obtained from the Roasted type, and the statistical difference between this type of CCLS and the other two types was significant. Thus, the Roasted type of CCLS is important for consumption.

The Fe content of CCLS was found to be an average of 4.7-8.57 ppm, where the Roasted type contained the highest value and the difference among the three types was significant ($p<0.05$). The dietary allowances for Fe reported for infants, children and other age groups is 0.27-11, 7-10 and 8-18 mg/day, respectively, and it may reach up to 27 mg/day for pregnant women [16]. Thus, consumption of a litre of CCLS (especially the Roasted one) per day could be enough to satisfy the Fe requirement of children and almost all men. For adult women (14-50 years), an additional source of Fe or more CCLS could be needed as Fe is discharged out during regular bleeding (menstruation cycle) [28]. The Fe value of CCLS is higher than the values 0.11-0.28 ppm, 0.4-0.53 ppm and 3 ppm reported for malt drinks in Nigeria, non-alcoholic beverages spiced with *Zingiber officinale* and a local African drink made from Baobab fruit (*Adansonia digitata*) pulp, respectively [12-14]. Generally, using CCLS, specifically the Roasted type, could be important to supplement the Fe requirements of the body.

The value of Zn is almost comparable with 0.25-0.31 ppm, but higher than 0.05-0.10 [9,10]. The Mejengir type contains the highest amount of Zn though the difference is insignificant ($p>0.05$) with the Roasted type. Like the other nutrients, using CCLS (preferably the Mejengir type) also contributes to Zn requirement of the human body.

The Roasted type contains the highest value of Cu which was significantly different ($p<0.05$) with the Raw type. From the dietary reference data, the recommended dietary allowances for Cu for infants, children and other age groups is 200-300, 340-440 and 700-1000 μg/day, respectively and 1300 μg/day for lactating women [16]. Therefore, about 62 and 25% of the daily requirements of Cu for children and adults could be obtained by consuming a litre of the Roasted type of CCLS daily as Cu plays an important role in metabolism, largely because it allows many critical enzymes to function properly, and can act both as an antioxidant and a pro-oxidant [29].

Conclusion

The results of both the proximate and mineral compositions of CCLS are comparable to other energy and mineral drinks studied by other researchers. Together with carbohydrate, protein, fat and minerals, CCLS contains almost optimum K:Na and Ca:P ratios responsible for maintaining the body's normal blood pressure and processing bone hardening, respectively. In addition, it contains Fe which could be useful to supplement the Fe requirement of the body especially for adult women. In general, CCLS is found to contain significant nutritional values vital for energy and health thus plays a part in alleviating nutritional problems in the area.

Acknowledgement

This manuscript is based on the work supported by Mizan-Tepi University. The authors would like to acknowledge this institution and JJ Labo Glass along with contributions of the following individuals: Tibka Demissie, Jemayinesh Teka, Abel Mandefro, Emebet Abere, Zelalem Kibret, Sefowdin Berta and Yimam Getinet.

References

1. Heran SB (2010) Coffee, culture and intellectual property. Lessons for Africa from the Ethiopian fine coffee initiative: The pardee papers no. 11. Boston University, Boston, pp: 1-37.
2. Butt MS, Sultan MT (2011) Coffee and its consumption: benefits and risks critical. Crit Rev Food Sci Nutr 51: 363-373.
3. Mussatto SI, Carneiro LM, Silva JP, Roberto IC, Teixeira JA (2011) A study on chemical constituents and sugars extraction from spent coffee grounds. Journal of Carbohydrate Polymers 83: 368-374.
4. Platel K, Srinivasan K (2004) Digestive stimulant action of spices: A myth or reality? Indian J Med Res 119: 167-179.
5. Kassahun M (2013) Sources of milk products, milk and milk products handling, preservation and spices added to the milk products in Ada'a Woreda, Ethiopia. Int J Agric 3: 6-12.
6. Blescing U (2008) Spicy healing, the medicinal use of spices.
7. Yitayal AA, Achame HA (2014) Socio-cultural practice on coffee made from mixture of coffee leaf and spices. Int Multidiscp E-J 3: 36-45.
8. The American Public Health Association (APHA) (1999) Standard methods for the examination of water and waste water (20th edn.). Washington, DC, USA.
9. Hedge JE, Hofreiter BT (1962) Carbohydrate chemistry (17th edn.). In: Whistler RL and Be Miller JN (eds.) Academic Press, NY, USA.
10. Pearson D (1976) Chemical analysis of food (7th edn.), Church Hill Livingstone, London, UK, pp: 72-73, 138-143, 488-496.
11. Caunii A, Cuciureanu R, Zakar A, Tonea E, Giuchici C (2010) Chemical composition of common leafy vegetables. Vasile Goldis University Press 20: 45-48
12. Obuzor GU, Ajaezi NE (2010) Nutritional content of popular malt drinks produced in Nigeria. Afr J Food Sci 4: 585-590.
13. Oluwalana IB, Adedeji TO (2013) Nutritional composition of a non-alcoholic beverage spiced with Zingiber officinale extract produced from sorghum bicolor stem sheath. Int J Food Sci Nutr Eng 3: 21-27.
14. Adedayo MR, Olayemi FF, Bamishaiye EI (2011) Proximate and mineral composition of a local drink made from baobab fruit *(Adansonia digitata)* Pulp. Adv Biores 2: 82-85.
15. Okolo SC, Olajide OO, Idowu O, Doyinsola I, Adebiyi AB, et al. (2012) A Comparative proximate studies on some Nigerian food supplements. Ann Biol Res 3: 773-779.
16. DRIs (2005) Recommended dietary allowances and adequate intakes: Elements, Food and Nutrition Board, Institute of Medicine. National Academy of Sciences.
17. Gul S, Safdar M (2009) Proximate composition and mineral analysis of cinnamon. Pak J Nutr 8: 1456-1460.
18. IFICF (2011) Potassium & heart health fact sheet, Washington DC, USA.
19. Bellows L, Moore R (2013) Potassium and the Diet. Food and Nutrition Series|Health. Colorado State University. USA 2013: 1-4.
20. Khaw KT, Connor EB (1988) The association between blood pressure, age, and dietary sodium and potassium: a population study. Circulation 77: 53-61.
21. Kemi V (2010) Effects of dietary phosphorus and calcium-to phosphorus ratio on calcium and bone metabolism in healthy 20- to 43-year-old Finnish women: A dissertation in the Department of Food and Environmental Sciences University of Helsinki, Helsinki, 2010: 19-21.
22. International Federation of Accountants (IFA) (2013) Phosphorus is essential to life and bone health.
23. National Nutrition Council (2005) Finnish Nutrition Recommendations: Diet and physical activity in balance. Helsinki.
24. Stevanovicl S, Nikolic M, Stankovic A (2011) Dietary magnesium intake and coronary heart disease risk: A study from Serbia. Med Glas Ljek komore Zenicko-doboj kantona 8: 203-208.
25. Bernardini D, Nasulewic A, Mazur A, Majer JA (2005) Magnesium and microvascular endothelial cells: a role in inflammation and angiogenesis. Front Bioscience 10: 1177-1182.
26. Slowinska KZ, Grajeta H (2012) The role of manganese in etiopathogenesis and prevention of selected diseases. Postepy Hig Med Dosw 66: 549-553.
27. Aschner JL, Aschner M (2005) Nutritional aspects of manganese homeostasis. Molecular Aspects of Medicine 26: 353-362.
28. Anderson J, Fitzgerald C (2010) Iron: An Essential Nutrient. Food and Nutrition Series Health. Colorado State University, USA 2010: 1-3.
29. The Food and Agriculture Organization (FAO) (2011) United Nations Food and Agriculture Organization. Learning about carbohydrates , protein and fats.

Neuroscience of Reward: Implications for Food Addiction and Nutrition Policy

Thomas Horman and Francesco Leri*

Department of Psychology and Neuroscience, University of Guelph, Ontario, Canada

***Corresponding author:** Francesco Leri, Professor and Chair, Department of Psychology and Neuroscience, University of Guelph, Ontario, Canada
E-mail: fleri@uoguelph.ca

Abstract

According to the World Health Organization, unhealthy diet is one key contributor to the development of non-communicable diseases. The global response to this problem has primarily involved the implementation of nutritional policies intended on raising public awareness, and providing information through nutritional guidelines and product labels. However, there is experimental evidence suggesting that certain foods may promote addictive processes and consequent unhealthy dietary choices. This review discusses neurobiological mechanisms of reward involved in the consumption of refined sugars and fats, and the aforementioned indicators of their addictive characteristics. By acknowledging that these foods can act on brain reward systems to promote excessive or addictive consumption, policy makers may need to address issues of unhealthy diets by considering approaches that target availability, regulations within the food industry, taxation and advertising.

Keywords: Reward; Dopamine; Addiction; Sugar; Conditioning

Introduction

Non-communicable diseases (NCD) are the leading cause of global mortality, accounting for 63% of deaths world-wide in 2008 alone [1]. Of these diseases, the top four causes are preventable lifestyle choices including: alcohol abuse, tobacco use, inactivity, and unhealthy diets [2]. The current review focuses specifically on the overconsumption of refined sugars and fats [3], because of links to diabetes, obesity, and other metabolic diseases [2].

The global response to this problem has primarily involved implementing nutritional policies intended on raising awareness, and providing consumers information through nutritional guidelines and product labels. However, a growing body of research suggests that these regulatory strategies may not be completely effective.

Indeed, there is evidence that certain components of processed food may activate addictive processes. For example, there are a number of neurobiological similarities between behaviours reinforced by these foods and those reinforced by addictive drugs in laboratory animals [4-6]. Moreover, in clinical studies, the Yale Food Addiction Scale (YFAS) identified common neural correlates of food and substance dependence [7,8]. Finally, conditioning has been found to play a central role in excessive seeking and taking of food and drugs in both humans and animals [6,9]. This said, the "food addiction" hypothesis is often criticized for the lack of a clear definition and generally inconsistent findings [10]. Critics also suggest that food addiction may not add significant diagnostic capability beyond conditions like Binge Eating Disorder (BED) or Bulimia, nor does it adequately explain obesity. On the basis of these arguments, it can be concluded that the evidence is not convincing enough to supersede the adverse social and economic impacts of considering food addiction as a diagnosable condition.

But, rather than dismissing this relatively young field of study, examining the validity of the constructs on which it has been proposed may be beneficial. Perhaps, food addiction does not adequately explain obesity or BED, but associated health risks are not confined to these demographics either [4]. In particular, emphasis on the overweight and obese demographics has led to the misconception that perhaps addictive-like feeding behaviour leads to obesity, but this is not a universal truth [11]. Another important consideration involves employing criteria from established models of substance dependence to examine food addiction. Significant variability in diagnostic terminology, neurobiological mechanisms, and individual vulnerability exists among drugs with known abuse potential [10,12]. These issues further complicate the discussion of the addictive potential of food.

Nevertheless, it is important to recognize that for some people, in some environments, certain foods can activate addictive processes and promote unhealthy dietary choices. Acknowledging this may help policy makers learn from other addictive substances, such as alcohol and tobacco, which have transitioned from readily available to restricted through implementation of effective policies such as limiting the prevalence of associated cues, increase taxation, and/or subsidizing on particular products, or regulating availability [13]. It is anticipated that, if applied to refined sugars, these strategies will give people a better chance to follow sound nutritional advice already being promoted.

Society and Food

Unhealthy diet is a leading risk factor for developing NCDs, but what constitutes an unhealthy diet? Highly processed and refined ingredients found in fast food and ready-made to eat food are notable examples. Processing food involves the extraction or refinement of whole foods, which then generally become energy dense and nutrient deficient [14]. As a result, these foods tend to be high in fat, sugar and salt [15].

It is clear that not all fats are bad; guidelines recommend dietary levels of omega 3 and 6 fatty acids of 1-2% daily caloric intake to avoid serious deficiency [16]. Unfortunately, processed food is essentially devoid of these essential fatty acids, while retaining high levels of saturated fats and cholesterol [15]. Various health agencies, including the United States Department of Agriculture and American Heart Association, recommend that total fat intake should be 30% or less of total caloric intake, saturated fat less than 10% and cholesterol less than 300 mg/day [16], as these fats have been linked to hypertension and cardiovascular disease [2].

As well, high-fructose corn syrup, a refined sugar produced by chemical processing of corn, is one of the most commonly used food additives today. Although it is employed in many processed foods, its use in soft drinks has been suggested to have the biggest impact on health [17]. There is a significant relationship between increased consumption of sugar-sweetened beverages and weight gain [18,19], metabolic syndrome, and hypertension [20]. As illustrated below, current trends in consumption patterns make a compelling argument for the risks associated with excessive consumption of these foods.

Consumption trends and health implications

Over the past 50 years, there has been a significant global increased consumption of processed food accompanied by a decrease in the use of raw/ unprocessed culinary ingredients. Using six separate household food budget surveys, Moubarac and colleagues documented consumption trends in Canada by examining the caloric contribution of various foods (unprocessed or minimally processed foods, processed culinary ingredients, and ready-to-serve processed or ultra-processed foods) to the total dietary energy availability (kcal per capita) [15]. Their results appear staggering. Between 1938 and 2011, the proportion contributed by unprocessed or minimally processed foods dropped from 37% to 13%, while ultra-processed ready-to-serve food increased from 29% to 62%. A report by Popkin indicated that this transition is in fact a global issue and suggests that fast food and soft drink industries as primary contributors to this phenomenon [17].

Consumption rates of refined sugar are also cause for concern. The WHO has recently lowered the recommended limit of added sugar from 10% to 5% of daily caloric intake [21]. But, a report by Langlois and Garriguet revealed that Canadians are eating four times this amount, consuming enough sugar to account for 21% of daily energy intake [22]. A major contributor in this regard is the soft drink industry. Per capita consumption of soft drinks in the US has increased by 500% in the past 50 years according to the USDA [23].

Overall, the relationship between recent dietary and health trends supports the consequences of unhealthy eating behaviour. Both adult and childhood obesity have been increasing worldwide. The Center for Disease Control reported that prevalence of obesity prior to 1990 did not exceed 15% in any state, but by 2010 over a dozen states exceed 30% with several others reaching 25% [24]. This has drawn considerable attention due to the myriad of health risks exacerbated by obesity [25]. Thus, prevalence of type 2 diabetes has been rising in the general population [26], as well as in children, a condition that was relatively uncommon in youth until the early 1990's [27]. Moreover, according to the public health agency of Canada, between 1998 and 2008 the prevalence of diabetes rose from 3.3% to 5.6 % [28]. Overall, healthcare costs associated with obesity have risen by almost $60 billion between 1998 and 2008 [29]. These numbers prompted the prediction of an unprecedented decline in life expectancy in the US over the 21st century [30].

Current policy targets

Current trends of poor diet related health consequences have gained significant attention on the global stage and steps have been taken to address the issue. Examples of current strategies include: the global strategy on diet, physical activity and health (2004) and the population-based prevention strategies for childhood obesity (2009), among others. These initiatives raise awareness and mandate that producers to provide nutritional information required for people to make informed dietary decisions. Most notable are those promoting dietary guidelines and nutritional labelling, which informs the public about the contents of food and what constitutes a healthy diet.

There is some evidence that these policies are successfully raising awareness. Over the past 25 years, more shoppers reported their purchases were strongly influenced by health concerns [31]. As well, market research reported a 57% increase of annual spending from 1996 to 2006 on weight-loss programs and related products in the US [32]. Unfortunately, public awareness does not ensure that people will make healthy choices. Current nutritional policies rely on the individual's ability to self-regulate their intake of processed food but fail to consider biological and environmental influences that may compromise self-control.

Dangerous Combination

Industry response to nutrition policy

One fundamental difficulty lies with the apparent variability of industry response to nutrition policies. Private food companies probably face government pressure to transition to healthier options, and they may therefore implement policies of self-regulation such as reducing marketing to children, reducing unhealthy products in schools, and implementing responsible package labelling [33]. But, it cannot be overlooked that food has become a commodity, which means the industry must be profitable [14]. Therefore, private companies continue the sale of highly processed foods and simply offer healthier options [14]. These companies claim that there is nothing inherently wrong with the sale of processed foods in moderate quantities [14]. The core of this argument thus places the responsibility on each individual to be mindful of nutritional advices and limit consumption of unhealthy food through self-control.

While the onus rests firmly on the individual, it appears that major corporations continue to generate profit by promoting unhealthy products. Coca Cola sponsored the 5th International Congress on Physical Activity and Public Health, and they are also the official drink of the Olympics [34]. Another prominent example is McDonalds, who also sponsors the Olympics. McDonalds has started offering healthier options, such as salads and veggie wraps; however, a survey conducted by Dumanovsky et al. reported that the most popular meal purchased at McDonalds in the US is a Big Mac, fries and a medium regular soda, which contains 95 g of sugar and 1360 calories [27,35]. Other companies that are attempting a transition to healthy products are experiencing some difficulties. For example, a report on vendors in public recreation facilities in British Columbia found that those selling healthier foods were losing customers to vendors selling more palatable foods [36].

Food addiction: classic substance dependence?

Promoting nutrition awareness and relying on individual self-control may not be adequate strategies for addressing unhealthy eating behaviour [13,37]. This is because there are striking behavioural and neurobiological similarities between chronic exposure to components of processed food and to drugs of abuse, staging the suggestion that some of these foods may be addictive [3-5]. A common characteristic of addictive substances is their ability to promote consumption despite known negative consequences [12]. As such, the intent of current nutrition policy is likely to fall short of addressing health trends discussed above.

A review of the current understanding of substance dependence is beneficial before examining the validity of the food addiction hypothesis. Koob and Volkow describe substance dependence as compulsive seeking and taking of a substance leading to disruption of functional living and health [12]. Addiction is often characterized by a recurrent pattern of compulsive drug seeking, loss of control during drug intake (binging), and intense drug craving [38]. These behaviours have been categorized into 11 diagnostic criteria for substance-use disorders (SUD) in the DSM-V, and have also been adapted to animal models for the investigation of underlying biological mechanisms of addiction [12].

Addictive behaviours involve drug-induced neurobiological changes in neural systems that naturally control responses to rewards [39]. More specifically, addiction has been conceived as a learning and memory disorder, and brain reward systems adapt to repeated drug exposure and the organism develops habitual responses to environmental stimuli predictive of drugs [9]. This said, excessive intake of drugs also affects neural systems involved in executive functions and reactivity to stressful stimuli. Compromised inhibitory function and excessive reactivity to stress interact to promote the transition from drug use to addiction and dependence [12,40,41]. Although several neurochemical systems are involved in these processes [12,42], the mesolimbic (ventral tegmental area to nucleus accumbens) and mesocortical (ventral tegmental area to various cortical regions) dopamine systems are considered central [41]. Dopamine activity is involved in reward learning [43], reward sensitivity [41], as well as sensitization to drug effects [44], and cue learning by which drug predictors become salient [45].

Food is a nutritional reward required for life and, therefore, not inherently harmful. However, hyper-processing creates energy dense foods which act on dopaminergic systems producing effects similar to drugs of abuse [3]. Four lines of evidence from studies in laboratory animals support the hypothesis that food, and more specifically sugars and fats, activate addictive processes. First, there is evidence of cross-sensitization between sugar and drugs of abuse. In an elegant set of studies, Avena and Hoebel demonstrated the bi-directionality of this effect using sucrose and amphetamine [46,47]: both motor hyperactivity and hyper-consummatory behaviours were observed upon exposure to an otherwise ineffective dose of the novel substance (sucrose or amphetamine) after pre-exposure to the other. Interestingly, Foley and colleagues revealed a role of dopamine in this effect, as rats exhibited motor hyperactivity to quinpirole (a dopamine D2/D3 receptor agonist) after pre-exposure to sucrose [48].

Second, binging and withdrawal have been reported during and after prolonged sugar consumption. Thus, given intermittent daily access to glucose and food for 30 days, rats develop binging along with increased dopamine D1 receptor binding in the nucleus accumbens and decreased D2 receptor binding in the dorsal striatum [49,50]. Furthermore, somatic (tremors, chattering teeth and head shakes) [51], and emotional signs of withdrawal [51,52], as well as increased consumption upon re-exposure to sucrose [53], have also been reported. Whether withdrawal from sugar is identical to withdrawal from drugs, however, is not completely clear because it is very difficult to equate sugar to drug exposure, and it may not be ecologically valid to employ levels of sugar exposure that are necessary to observe a withdrawal response.

Third, animals that self-administer sucrose or high-fructose corn syrup in operant chambers respond in ways that closely resemble the self-administration of cocaine, and display alterations of mu-opioid and D2 dopamine receptors in the striatum that are also observed in cocaine-exposed rats [54-56]. Finally, there is evidence that unlimited exposure to palatable food can promote compulsive seeking and excessive consummatory behaviour. Teegarden and Bale reported that rats trained to consume a diet high in fat and sugars were more willing to endure an aversive environment in order to regain access to their preferred diet [57]. Johnson and Kenny explored a highly palatable, calorie dense cafeteria diet, and found that over time rats consistently preferred the cafeteria diet over the standard chow, became obese, and persisted consumption of the palatable diet despite the risk of an aversive stimulus [58]. Importantly, these behaviours were accompanied by increased brain reward threshold and a reduction of striatal dopamine receptors [58].

The YFAS scale [7,8] was developed to assess whether an individual's eating behaviour would meet the DSM criteria for substance dependence. Although scores on the YFAS do not correlate with body mass index [59], the use of this scale in overweight or obese subjects has generated interesting findings. For example, Bégin compared a sample of obese individuals seeking help controlling their eating behaviour to individuals with other substance use disorders [60]. It was found that obese individuals who scored high on the YFAS better matched individuals with other SUDs on measures of impulsivity. As well, high YFAS scores predicted the frequency of snacking, emotional eating, and associated comorbid disorders such as BED, depression, and attention deficit hyperactive disorder in childhood [59]. Interestingly, several neural correlates of addictive eating have been identified using the YFAS. In a study by Gearhardt and colleagues, fasted obese and lean subjects were shown cues of palatable food followed by the delivery of a palatable solution [61]. They found that individuals who scored higher on the YFAS demonstrated increased activation in areas of the brain involved in encoding the incentive-salience of food cues (dorso-lateral prefrontal cortex, medial orbito-frontal cortex [62], and caudate nucleus [63]). Also, high scores were associated with reduced activity in the lateral orbito-frontal cortex, a region involved in behavioural inhibition during consumption of rewards [64]. Interestingly, these brain regions are a part of the mesocortical dopamine system, which plays a key role in SUDs, as discussed above.

Another interesting finding relevant to the current discussion is evidence of cue reactivity in the context of addictive-like eating behaviour. In fact, people who struggle with substance use disorders are very familiar with the physiological responses experienced when presented with cues associated with their drug of choice [65]. Cue reactivity is well documented in animals and humans in the context of many substances including cocaine, tobacco, heroin and alcohol [65]. Meule and colleagues documented a similar effect in adults meeting criteria for food addiction using the YFAS [66]. They found that participants fitting four or more criteria demonstrated significantly greater reactivity to food cues than those fitting one or no criteria.

Because it is known that only a small fraction of individuals who use drugs eventually progress to dependence [12,41], it is expected that only vulnerable individuals will be predisposed to addictive-like eating behaviours [67]. Indeed, a genetic profile involving several alleles has been implicated in mediating reward-responsive overeating [68]. Of particular interest is the Taq1 A1 allele, which is associated with increased reward sensitivity [69], palatable food preference [70], diminished striatal dopamine activity [71], and it is expressed in many individuals with SUDs and eating disorders [72]. It has been hypothesized that individuals expressing the Taq1 A1 allele are more susceptible to seek and consume palatable food as a form of compensatory behaviour [71]. Individual vulnerabilities have also been observed in rodents: the motivation to consume palatable food is more pronounced in obesity-prone rats [73], and rats more sensitive to the incentive properties of palatable food are significantly more sensitive to the reinforcing effect of cocaine [74].

Finally, similarly to drug addiction, there is significant evidence that childhood exposure to stress and a family history of substance use can increase the risk of developing eating disorders and obesity later in life. For example, a longitudinal study found that childhood maltreatment is linked to an increased risk of developing eating disorders [75]. Interestingly, a family history of alcohol abuse is also associated with an inherent preference for sweet tastes [76] and predicts the risk of obesity in young individuals [77]. Similarly, children of mothers who smoke during pregnancy are higher risk for developing eating disorders and weight problems [78].

Implications

Given the neurobiological and behavioural evidence reviewed above, could the food industry take advantage of the addictive potential of sugars and fats to create an environment that promotes the consumption of their products? Because food is commodity, it is in companies' best interest to bombard consumers with logos and advertisements to ensure maximum profitability [14]. These can act as conditioned stimuli, much the same way a picture of a cigarette pack can act as a cue for smokers [9], hindering attempts to alter lifestyle choices and consume healthier food. Overall, the weight of the evidence above suggests that regulating marketing strategies may be effective in curbing consumption of unhealthy foods.

Adjusting the Current Mind Set

Food addiction did not appear in the recently updated DSM-V because of inconsistencies in the literature and lack of clear definition [10]. It is possible to argue that the evidence is not convincing enough to supersede potential adverse social and economic impacts of considering food addiction as a diagnosable condition. For example, it can be argued that framing food and drugs of abuse within a similar model of mental health disease can impede motivation required to make appropriate lifestyle adjustments necessary for good health such as exercise. Moreover, it has been suggested that food addiction does not adequately explain existing conditions, such as binge eating disorder, and that its inclusion in the DSM would not add significant diagnostic capability for treating these conditions. Although these are valid arguments, the food addiction hypothesis is still relatively new and rather than discarding it all together, it is more useful to examine the validity of the constructs on which it has been proposed.

One potential issue has been the focus on the obese population. Weight gain results from the overconsumption of food and consequent imbalance of energy intake, and this has led to the suggestion that addictive-like feeding behaviour is the cause of obesity. This, however, is not necessarily the case [11] because obesity is an exceptionally multifaceted issue with a complex etiology that makes it impossible to understand using a framework focused on one cause. In addition, it is possible to over consume processed food, not become overweight, and still be at an increased risk of heart disease and diabetes. There is also reasonable indication that one does not need to be obese to be addicted to food either [27]. Thus, although obesity is an important demographic variable to investigate the neurobiology of overconsumption of food, it should not be used as the prototype for food addiction [79].

Another consideration is the use of other addictive substances to model food addiction. While this approach is informative, there is a very important fundamental difference that must be taken into consideration. Food is ubiquitous throughout society and a necessity for life, which makes defining exactly when food is being abused difficult. In this regard, it is critical for research in this field to determine specifically what makes some food addictive and what sets these foods aside from those which we are required to eat [37]. Also, considerable variability exists among addictive substances regarding the underlying mechanism that initially promotes consumption. Opiate dependence is driven by a pattern of withdrawal and negative affect, psychomotor stimulants users follow a pattern of binging and intoxication, and smokers of nicotine and cannabis exhibit a preoccupation and anticipation pattern [12].

As such, there are problems with using the DSM criteria for substance dependence to define food addiction because of inappropriate terminology. This is especially evident when examining withdrawal, tolerance, and seeking characteristics. With regard to withdrawal, are the symptoms expressed while experiencing abstinence from these foods an effect of withdrawal or simply energy deficits? A recent study in laboratory animals indicated that although naltrexone precipitates robust signs of affective withdrawal in heroin pre-treated animals, the effect in animals pre-treated with high fructose corn syrup are much less pronounced [52]. In the description of tolerance, the DSM-IV highlights "intoxication," which is a term that may not be suitable for consumption of food. The DSM-V added "desired effect" but this is also ambiguous and could be difficult to interpret in the context of food consumption. Ultimately, the initial motivation to consume food is nutrition, which is not comparable to intoxication [79]. Seeking criteria are also ambiguous in the context of food consumption for two reasons: first, food seeking is a basic biological necessity; and second, food is legal, unlike many drugs, and harmful effects are not as readily apparent [10]. Essentially, you cannot go to jail for eating or overdose on food. Thus, determining when healthy food seeking becomes harmful can be difficult.

Limitations aside, the latest edition of the DSM has employed an updated framework to describe addictions that may be useful to accommodate foods. The understanding of substance dependence continues to develop and influence the diagnostic framework of SUDs. The DSM-IV used a strict categorical method, applying an indiscriminate seven item list to all substances with an all-or-nothing approach, where meeting three or more criteria indicated substance dependence. In contrast, the DSM-V employs a dimensional approach with distinct diagnostic criteria for several classes of substances, and a separate set of criteria for behavioural addictions such as gambling

[11]. Whether food addiction would best fit within substance or behavioural addictions remains unclear.

Policy Implications

If one assumes that the food addiction hypothesis is viable, then it becomes questionable whether the self-regulation approach currently employed by industry is sufficient to address the adverse health trends discussed above [37]. But, if regulatory policies were to be implemented, what would they look like? Also, there are significant hurdles to overcome in order to implement effective policy changes. For example, one would expect that regulations could have damaging implications to corporations such as McDonald's or Coca-Cola, which have billions of dollars at stake [13]. Perhaps, considering legislative progress involved in regulating other addictive substances such as alcohol and tobacco, may offer some insight for effective policy approaches regarding unhealthy foods [37].

Several addictive substances have undergone notable transitions from freely available to restricted. Examples include opium, cocaine (formerly a primary ingredient in Coca-Cola), and most recently tobacco [80]. Tobacco has become more difficult to obtain due to a series of restrictions implemented over the past 40 years [37]. Of particular relevance to the current discussion is the elimination of public advertisement and restrictions on the displays of cigarette packaging in stores. A survey conducted in Norway, found that eliminating tobacco displays in point-of-sale settings was perceived as particularly beneficial and significantly reduced the temptation to purchase cigarettes by youth [81]. Should the advertisement of products high in sugars and fats be similarly restricted?

Ultimately, policy makers should employ a substance-focused approach to strengthen current nutrition policy [13,37]. This could include restricting advertisements that promote processed food, removing sweets from point-of-sale settings, subsidizing the production of whole foods, and taxing products containing added sugar. These policies would provide incentive for the food industry to endorse a bona fide transition toward healthier food, promote an environment that supports healthy lifestyle choices, and reinforce sound nutritional advice already being promoted. Interestingly, a few of these approaches are already being implemented. For example, several countries, including Great Brittan, Mexico, Hungary, and Finland have implemented a sugar tax [82], and PepsiCo has recently announced that they will cut all sugar content from their drinks by 2025 [83]. It is important to continue monitoring the impact of these approaches to determine their effectiveness over time.

Conclusion

It appears that current regulatory strategies inadequately address the prevalence of unhealthy diets and the related health consequences. Effective government intervention must implement nutrition policies that consider both the biological and environmental influences on negative eating behaviours presented throughout this review. The global response currently addressing this issue is effectively increasing public concern; however, unhealthy food remains a popular choice and adverse health trends continue to present difficulties for public health.

Current nutrition policy allows companies to continue the sale of unhealthy food under industry-derived self-regulation policies that place the onus entirely on the public to practice self-control. Evidence presented in this review indicates that prevalent food cues combined with addictive potential of certain foods creates an environment that ultimately compromises this strategy. Therefore, introducing policies that limit the use of refined sugar or restrict advertisement on products containing sugar may be an effective and pragmatic first step in reducing the prevalence of unhealthy diets.

Finally, the study of food addiction is in its infancy and there is much to discover. Indeed, only a small proportion of obesity is linked to food addiction; but, individual vulnerability to the health consequences and addictive processes associated with the consumption of processed food are not confined to this demographic. Ultimately, the long-term consequences of the effect of sugar on the brain are not yet known. Is it possible that excessive exposure to sugar in children may predispose them to reward related pathologies in adulthood? How can neuroscience address this question and how would this impact nutrition policies?

Author Contributions

T.H. and F.L. contributed to the conception and designed of this review; T.H. and F.L. wrote the paper.

Acknowledgments

This research was conducted with the support of the Ontario Brain Institute, an independent non-profit corporation, funded partially by the Ontario government. The opinions, results and conclusions are those of the authors and no endorsement by the Ontario Brain Institute is intended or should be inferred.

References

1. Alwan A (ed.) (2010) Global Status Report on Non-communicable Diseases 2010. World Health Organization: Geneva, Switzerland.
2. World Health Organization (2003) Diet, Nutrition and the Prevention of Chronic Diseases. World Health Organization; report of joint WHO/FAO expert consultation. Geneva, Switzerland.
3. Ifland JR, Preuss HG, Marcus MT, Rourke KM, Taylor WC, et al. (2009) Refined food addiction: a classic substance use disorder. Med Hypotheses 72: 518-526.
4. Parylak SL, Koob GF, Zorrilla EP (2011) The dark side of food addiction. Physiol Behav 104: 149-156.
5. Avena NM, Rada P, Hoebel BG (2008) Evidence for sugar addiction: behavioral and neurochemical effects of intermittent, excessive sugar intake. Neurosci Biobehav Rev 32: 20-39.
6. Murray S, Tulloch A, Gold MS, Avena NM (2014) Hormonal and neural mechanisms of food reward, eating behaviour and obesity. Nat Rev Endocrinol 10: 540-552.
7. Gearhardt AN, Corbin WR, Brownell KD (2009) Preliminary validation of the Yale Food Addiction Scale. Appetite 52: 430-436.
8. Gearhardt AN, Corbin WR, Brownell KD (2016) Development of the Yale Food Addiction Scale Version 2.0. Psychol Addict Behav 30: 113-121.
9. Hyman SE (2005) Addiction: a disease of learning and memory. Am J Psychiatry 162: 1414-1422.
10. Ziauddeen H, Fletcher PC (2013) Is food addiction a valid and useful concept? Obes Rev 14: 19-28.
11. Meule A, Gearhardt AN (2014) Food addiction in the light of DSM-5. Nutrients 6: 3653-3671.
12. Koob GF, Volkow ND (2010) Neurocircuitry of addiction. Neuropsychopharmacology 35: 217-238.
13. Gearhardt AN, Brownell KD (2013) Can food and addiction change the game? Biol Psychiatry 73: 802-803.
14. Moodie R, Stuckler D, Monteiro C, Sheron N, Neal B, et al. (2013) Profits and pandemics: prevention of harmful effects of tobacco, alcohol, and ultra-processed food and drink industries. Lancet 381: 670-679.

15. Moubarac JC, Batal M, Martins AP, Claro R, Levy RB, et al. (2014) Processed and ultra-processed food products: consumption trends in Canada from 1938 to 2011. Can J Diet Pract Res 75: 15-21.
16. Lichtenstein AH, Kennedy E, Barrier P, Danford D, Ernst ND, et al. (1998) Dietary fat consumption and health. Nutr Rev 56: S3-S19.
17. Popkin BM (2006) Global nutrition dynamics: the world is shifting rapidly toward a diet linked with non-communicable diseases. Am J Clin Nutr 84: 289-298.
18. Bray GA, Nielsen SJ, Popkin BM (2004) Consumption of high-fructose corn syrup in beverages may play a role in the epidemic of obesity. Am J Clin Nutr 79: 537-543.
19. Malik VS, Schulze MB, Hu FB (2006) Intake of sugar-sweetened beverages and weight gain: a systematic review. Am J Clin Nutr 84: 274-288.
20. Khitan Z, Kim DH (2013) Fructose: a key factor in the development of metabolic syndrome and hypertension. J Nutr Metab 2013: 12.
21. Owens B (2014) Storm brewing over WHO sugar proposal. Nature 507: 150.
22. Langlois K, Garriguet D (2011) Sugar consumption among Canadians of all ages. Health Rep 22: 23-27.
23. Morris MJ, Beilharz JE, Maniam J, Reichelt AC, Westbrook RF (2014) Why is obesity such a problem in the 21st century? The intersection of palatable food, cues and reward pathways, stress, and cognition. Neurosci Biobehav Rev.
24. Center for Disease Control and Prevention (2010) Obesity Trends Among U. S. Adults Between 1985 and 2010.
25. Thow AM, Armstrong T, Candeias V, Randby S, Xuereb G (2010) Population-Based Prevention Strategies for Childhood Obesity: Report of a WHO forum and techincal meeting. World Health Organization, Geneva, Switzerland.
26. Danaei G, Finucane MM, Lu Y, Singh GM, Cowan MJ, et al. (2011) National, regional, and global trends in fasting plasma glucose and diabetes prevalence since 1980: systematic analysis of health examination surveys and epidemiological studies with 370 country-years and 2·7 million participants. Lancet 378: 31-40.
27. Lustig RH (2013) Fat Chance: Beating the Odds against Sugar, Processed Food, Obesity, and Disease. New York, Penguin Publishing Group, New York.
28. Pelletier C, Dai S, Roberts KC, Bienek A, Onysko J, et al. (2012) Report summary. Diabetes in Canada: facts and figures from a public health perspective. Chronic Dis Inj Can 33: 53-54.
29. Finkelstein EA, Trogdon JG, Cohen JW, Dietz W (2009) Annual medical spending attributable to obesity: payer-and service-specific estimates. Health Aff (Millwood) 28: w822-w831.
30. Olshansky SJ, Passaro DJ, Hershow RC, Layden J, Carnes BA, et al. (2005) A potential decline in life expectancy in the United States in the 21st century. N Engl J Med 352: 1138-1145.
31. Mancino L, Kinsey J (2008) Is dietary knowledge enough? Hunger, stress, and other roadblocks to healthy eating. U.S. Department of Agriculture, Economic Research Service.
32. Baradel LA, Gillespie C, kicklighter JR, Doucette MM, Penumetcha M, et al. (2009) Temporal changes in trying to lose weight and recommended weight-loss strategies among overweight and obese Americans, 1996-2003. Prev Med 49: 158-164.
33. Sharma LL, Teret SP, Brownell KD (2010) The food industry and self-regulation: Standards to promote success and to avoid public health failures. Am J Public Health 100: 240-246.
34. de Sá TH (2014) Can Coca Cola promote physical activity? Lancet 383: 2041.
35. Dumanovsky T, Nonas CA, Huang CY, Silver LD, Bassett MT (2009) What people buy from fast-food restaurants: caloric content and menu item selection, New York City 2007. Obesity (Silver Spring) 17: 1369-1374.
36. Vander Wekken S, Sørensen S, Meldrum J, Naylor PJ (2012) Exploring industry perspectives on implementation of a provincial policy for food and beverage sales in publicly funded recreation facilities. Health Policy 104: 279-287.
37. Gearhardt AN, Grilo CM, DiLeone RJ, Brownell KD, Potenza MN (2011) Can food be addictive? Public health and policy implications. Addiction 106: 1208-1212.
38. Koob GF, Le Moal M (2008) Neurobiological mechanisms for opponent motivational processes in addiction. Philos Trans R Soc Lond B Biol Sci 363: 3113-3123.
39. Berridge KC, Robinson TE (1998) What is the role of dopamine in reward: hedonic impact, reward learning, or incentive salience? Brain Res Brain Res Rev 28: 309-369.
40. Robinson TE, Berridge KC (2008) Review. The incentive sensitization theory of addiction: some current issues. Philos Trans R Soc Lond B Biol Sci 363: 3137-3146.
41. Volkow ND, Wang GJ, Fowler JS, Tomasi D (2012) Addiction circuitry in the human brain. Annu Rev Pharmacol Toxicol 52: 321-336.
42. Wang GJ, Volkow ND, Thanos PK, Fowler JS (2004) Similarity between obesity and drug addiction as assessed by neurofunctional imaging: a concept review. J Addict Dis 23: 39-53.
43. Schultz W (2010) Dopamine signals for reward value and risk: basic and recent data. Behav Brain Funct 6: 24.
44. Robinson TE, Berridge KC (2000) The psychology and neurobiology of addiction: an incentive-sensitization view. Addiction 2: S91-S117.
45. Berridge KC, Kringelbach ML (2008) Affective neuroscience of pleasure: reward in humans and animals. Psychopharmacology (Berl) 199: 457-480.
46. Avena NM, Hoebel BG (2003) Amphetamine-sensitized rats show sugar-induced hyperactivity (cross-sensitization) and sugar hyperphagia. Pharmacol Biochem Behav 74: 635-639.
47. Avena NM, Hoebel BG (2003) A diet promoting sugar dependency causes behavioral cross-sensitization to a low dose of amphetamine. Neuroscience 122: 17-20.
48. Foley KA, Fudge MA, Kavaliers M, Ossenkopp KP (2006) Quinpirole-induced behavioral sensitization is enhanced by prior scheduled exposure to sucrose: A multi-variable examination of locomotor activity. Behav Brain Res 167: 49-56.
49. Colantuoni C, Schwenker J, McCarthy J, Rada P, Ladenheim B, et al. (2001) Excessive sugar intake alters binding to dopamine and mu-opioid receptors in the brain. Neuro report 12: 3549-3552.
50. Avena NM (2007) Examining the addictive-like properties of binge eating using an animal model of sugar dependence. Exp Clin Psychopharmacol 15: 481-491.
51. Colantuoni C, Rada P, McCarthy J, Patten C, Avena NM, et al. (2002) Evidence that intermittent, excessive sugar intake causes endogenous opioid dependence. Obes Res 10: 478-488.
52. Daniels S, Marshall P, Leri F (2016) Alterations of naltrexone-induced conditioned place avoidance by pre-exposure to high fructose corn syrup or heroin in Sprague-Dawley rats. Psychopharmacology (Berl) 233: 425-433.
53. Wideman CH, Nadzam GR, Murphy HM (2005) Implications of an animal model of sugar addiction, withdrawal and relapse for human health. Nutr Neurosci 8: 269-276.
54. Levy A, Marshall P, Zhou Y, Kreek MJ, Kent K, et al. (2015) Fructose:glucose ratios-A study of sugar self-administration and associated neural and physiological responses in the rat. Nutrients 7: 3869-3890.
55. Leri F, Zhou Y, Goddard B, Levy A, Jacklin D, et al. (2009) Steady-state methadone blocks cocaine seeking and cocaine-induced gene expression alterations in the rat brain. Eur Neuropsychopharmacol 19: 238-249.
56. Leri F, Zhou Y, Carmichael B, Cummins E, Kreek MJ (2012) Treatment-like steady-state methadone in rats interferes with incubation of cocaine sensitization and associated alterations in gene expression. Eur Neuropsychopharmacol 22: 143-152.
57. Teegarden SL, Bale TL (2007) Decreases in dietary preference produce increased emotionality and risk for dietary relapse. Biol Psychiatry 61:

1021-1029.

58. Johnson PM, Kenny PJ (2010) Dopamine D2 receptors in addiction-like reward dysfunction and compulsive eating in obese rats. Nat Neurosci 13: 635-641.

59. Davis C, Curtis C, Levitan RD, Carter JC, Kaplan AS, et al. (2011) Evidence that 'food addiction' is a valid phenotype of obesity. Appetite 57: 711-717.

60. Bégin C (2012) Does food addiction distinguish a specific subgroup of overweight/obese overeating women? Health 4: 1492-1499.

61. Gearhardt AN, Yokum S, Orr PT, Stice E, Corbin WR, et al. (2011) Neural correlates of food addiction. Arch Gen Psychiatry 68: 808-816.

62. Wilson SJ, Sayette MA, Fiez JA (2004) Prefrontal responses to drug cues: a neurocognitive analysis. Nat Neurosci 7: 211-214.

63. Delgado MR, Stenger VA, Fiez JA (2004) Motivation-dependent responses in the human caudate nucleus. Cereb Cortex 14: 1022-1030.

64. Elliott R, Dolan RJ, Frith CD (2000) Dissociable functions in the medial and lateral orbitofrontal cortex: evidence from human neuroimaging studies. Cereb Cortex 10: 308-317.

65. Carter BL, Tiffany ST (1999) Meta-analysis of cue-reactivity in addiction research. Addiction 94: 327-340.

66. Meule A, Lutz A, Vögele C, Kübler A (2012) Women with elevated food addiction symptoms show accelerated reactions, but no impaired inhibitory control, in response to pictures of high-calorie food-cues. Eat Behav 13: 423-428.

67. Volkow ND, Wise RA (2005) How can drug addiction help us understand obesity? Nat Neurosci 8: 555-560.

68. Davis C, Loxton NJ, Levitan RD, Kaplan AS, Carter JC, et al. (2013) 'Food addiction' and its association with a dopaminergic multilocus genetic profile. Physiol Behav 118: 63-69.

69. Davis C, Levitan RD, Kaplan AS, Carter J, Reid C, et al. (2008) Reward sensitivity and the D2 dopamine receptor gene: a case-control study of binge eating disorder. Prog Neuro-Psychopharmacology Biol Psychiatry 32: 620-628.

70. Epstein LH, Temple JL, Neaderhiser BJ, Salis RJ, Erbe RW, et al. (2007) Food reinforcement, the dopamine D2 receptor genotype, and energy intake in obese and nonobese humans. Behav Neurosci 121: 877-886.

71. Stice E, Spoor S, Bohon C, Small DM (2008) Relation between obesity and blunted striatal response to food is moderated by TaqIA A1 allele. Science 322: 449-452.

72. Carlier N, Marshe VS, Cmorejova J, Davis C, Müller DJ, et al. (2015) Genetic similarities between compulsive overeating and addiction phenotypes: a case for "food addiction"? Curr Psychiatry Rep 17: 96.

73. Pickering C, Alsiö J, Hulting AL, Schiöth HB (2009) Withdrawal from free-choice high-fat high-sugar diet induces craving only in obesity-prone animals. Psychopharmacology 204: 431-443.

74. Levy A, Salamon A, Tucci M, Limebeer CL, Parker LA, et al. (2013) Co-sensitivity to the incentive properties of palatable food and cocaine in rats; implications for co-morbid addictions. Addict Biol 18: 763-773.

75. Johnson JG, Cohen P, Kasen S, Brook JS (2002) Childhood adversities associated with risk for eating disorders or weight problems during adolescence or early adulthood. Am J Psychiatry 159: 394-400.

76. Fortuna JL (2010) Sweet preference, sugar addiction and the familial history of alcohol dependence: shared neural pathways and genes. J Psychoactive Drugs 42: 147-151.

77. Grucza RA, Krueger RF, Racette SB, Norberg KE, Hipp PR, et al. (2010) The emerging link between alcoholism risk and obesity in the United States. Arch Gen Psychiatry 67: 1301-1308.

78. Oken E, Levitan EB, Gillman MW (2008) Maternal smoking during pregnancy and child overweight: systematic review and meta-analysis. Int J Obes (Lond) 32: 201-210.

79. Ziauddeen H, Farooqi IS, Fletcher PC (2012) Obesity and the brain: how convincing is the addiction model? Nat Rev Neurosci 13: 279-286.

80. Austin GA (1978) Perspetives on the history of psychoactive substance use. National Institue on Drug Abuse, Rockville, Maryland.

81. Scheffels J, Lavik R (2013) Out of sight, out of mind? Removal of point-of-sale tobacco displays in Norway. Tob Control 22: e37-e42.

82. Briggs A (2016) Sugar tax could sweeten a market failure. Nature 531: 551.

83. Aubrey A (2016) PepsiCo pledges to guc sugar as big soda comes under scrutiny. National Public Radio.

Natural Ingredient Edible Coatings on Italian Millet: Effect on Functional and Cooking Characteristics

Ranjitha and Neena Joshi*

Department of Food Science and Nutrition, GKVK, University of Agricultural Sciences, Bengalore, India

***Corresponding author:** Neena Joshi, Department of Food Science and Nutrition, GKVK, University of Agricultural Sciences, Bengalore, India
E-mail: nj_pande@yahoo.com

Abstract

Edible coatings are generally defined as continuous matrices that can be prepared from edible materials. Italian millet contains appreciable amounts of PUFA concentrated on the top layer of the milled grains that are involved in the development of rancidity on storage. Due to their high antioxidant activity Bangalore blue grapes, green tea and tulsi were selected as edible coating material for Italian millet. Dehusked grains were coated with edible material and dried. These were then analysed for functional properties and cooking characteristics. The bulk density was in the range of 0.69-0.82. There was no significant difference between solubility, swelling power, water and oil absorption capacity. Cooking time ranged from 13.16-15.20 min. Water uptake ratio ranged from 17-24. Coatings resulted in lighter product with a slightly reduced cooking time and higher water absorption than the non-coated grains. Coatings resulted in a lighter cooked sample, slight reduction in cooking time and higher water absorption capacity. However, the cooking and functional characteristic of the grain was acceptable.

Keywords: Italian millet; Natural ingredient; Edible coatings; Functional properties; Cooking characteristics

Introduction

Millets are minor cereals and form the staple food for a large segment of the population. Millet contains 9-14% protein, 70-80% carbohydrates and is rich source of dietary fibre [1]. It is a starchy food with a 25:75 amylose to amylopectin ratio and it is a fairly good source of lipids (3-6%) with about 50% of the lipids in the form of polyunsaturated fatty acids. Even though the nutritional qualities of millet have been well [2,3], its utilization for food is confined to the traditional consumers in tribal populations, mainly due to non-availability of consumer friendly, ready-to-use or ready-to-eat products as are found for rice and wheat. One of the reasons for this is attributed to the fact that Italian millet contains appreciable amounts of PUFA concentrated on the top layer of the milled grains which are involved in the development of rancidity on storage.

Italian millet (*Setariaitalica*) is one of the important food crops in parts of the Indian subcontinent. It is also known as foxtail, German, Hungarian or Siberian millet. Simple processing methods like dehulling, soaking and cooking are reported to result in significant decreases in antinutrients and improved bioavailability of minerals like iron and zinc and also protein digestibility [4]. Italian millet is highly nutritious, non-glutinous, and like buckwheat and quinoa, is not an acid forming food so it is soothing and easy to digest. It is considered to be one of the least allergenic and most digestible grains available [5].

Foxtail millet is largely utilized in the form of millet rice which is obtained after the millet is dehusked and polished. Dehusking strips a significant quantity of antioxidants and fatty acids from the surface of the grain. However, during this process it exposes the fat which is principally PUFA to the atmospheric oxygen causing rapid onset of rancidity. Millet rice thus has a short shelf life.

Edible coatings are generally defined as continuous matrices that can be prepared from edible materials. They can be used as thin wraps or formed as coatings on food or between food components. In fact, edible coatings have been used for centuries to prevent moisture migration, improve food appearance and increase shelf-life. However, in recent years edible coatings have been recognized for more innovative uses. One major advantage of coatings is that several active ingredients can be incorporated into the polymer matrix and consumed with the food, thus enhancing safety or even nutritional and sensory attributes [6].

Incorporation of coated millets in food formulations have shown to improve their keeping quality. The question whether incorporation of natural antioxidants rich coatings on Italian millet brings about any change to its functional or cooking quality needs to be answered. Thus, the effect of these on functional and cooking characteristics of edible coated Italian millet was examined.

Materials and Methods

The variety of Italian millet used for the study was Prasad (SiA 326). The samples were procured from All India Coordinate Research Project on Millets, UAS, GKVK, Bangalore. Tulsi was obtained from plants maintained in Dept. of Horticulture UAS Bangalore. Other ingredients were procured from the local market in Bangalore.

Preparation and selection of coating

Most of the coating solutions/paste were prepared by slowly mixing a known amount of coating material into 75-100 ml distilled water with continuous stirring until the coating materials were suspended in the solution. The consistency of solution was such that it could be mixed by a hand. The weight of the coating substance was therefore dependent on the desirable consistency. The coating material was rubbed into the grains and mixed thoroughly till the material was uniformly distributed. This was assured by closely examining the grain visually. The procedure was standardized to ensure that there were no excess lumps of the coating material in the sample.

The weight of the coating material was recorded and respective quantity of coating material used throughout the study for treating the Italian millet grain. The quantity of the paste/solution was also recorded. This information is given in the following paragraphs for the three treatments.

Bangalore blue grapes (*Vitisvinifera* L.), green tea (*Camellia sinensis*) and tulsi (*Ocimum sanctum linn*) were selected as coating material due to their high antioxidant activity [7].

Grapes: Slurry of Bangalore blue grapes (seed, pulp and skin) which were freshly procured from the market was used. For 100 g of grains 6.25 g of grape paste was applied. The paste was rubbed into the dehusked grains manually.

Green tea: Green tea (Sencha Japanese green tea) was purchased from the market and stored in refrigerator (4°C) till use. Green tea infusion was used for coating the grains. Green tea infusion (extract) was prepared according to procedure described by Manay and Shadakshari [8]. Hundred ml of water was heated at 85°C in a steel container. Then 10 g of green tea was added to it. The container was covered and tea was allowed to steep for period of 3 min. The decoction was then strained and cooled. This decoction was rubbed in manually into the dehusked grains. For 100 g of grains 10 ml of green tea decoction was used.

Tulsi: Fresh leaves of tulsi were harvested from the plants maintained in Dept. of Horticulture UAS Bangalore. The leaves were dried in microwave oven for a minute. Dried leaves were powdered. 5 g of powdered tulsi was mixed with 20 ml of water. For 100 g of grains 6.25 g of tulsi paste was used. The paste was rubbed into the dehusked grains manually.

Drying of coated grains

Coated grains were dried under shade and constant stream of circulating air at room temperature (26°C ± 2°C, RH 40%). The grains dried within 5 h. The treated grains were stored in HDPE pouches at room temperature for storage and shelf life study and at -10°C until analysis. A view of the samples after drying process was complete is shown in Figure 1.

Functional properties

Bulk density (g/ml): A calibrated centrifuge tube was weighed and flour samples were filled to 10 ml mark by constant tapping, until there was no further change in volume. The content was weighed and from the difference in weight, the bulk density of the sample was calculated and the results are expressed as g/ml [9].

Water and oil absorption capacity: One-gram sample was mixed with 10 ml of either distilled water or in 15 ml oil for 30 min. The contents were allowed to stand at 30°C in a water bath for 30 min and then centrifuged at 3000-5000 rpm for 20-30 min. After centrifuging the volume of the supernatant was recorded and used for determination of water and oil absorption and the results were expressed as g/g sample [10].

Solubility and swelling power: Two hundred and fifty mg finely ground sample was thoroughly mixed with 15 ml of distilled water and heated to 65°C (being the initial temperature at which gelatinization of starch granules begins). The content was then cooled to room temperature and centrifuged at 5000 rpm for 10 min. The soluble solids content was calculated as percentage of sample soluble in water. At the same time, this was used to calculate the swelling power, since the sample has been heated at 65°C for 30 min, the residue was weighed and the increase in weight was calculated as the swelling power of the sample at that particular temperature [11].

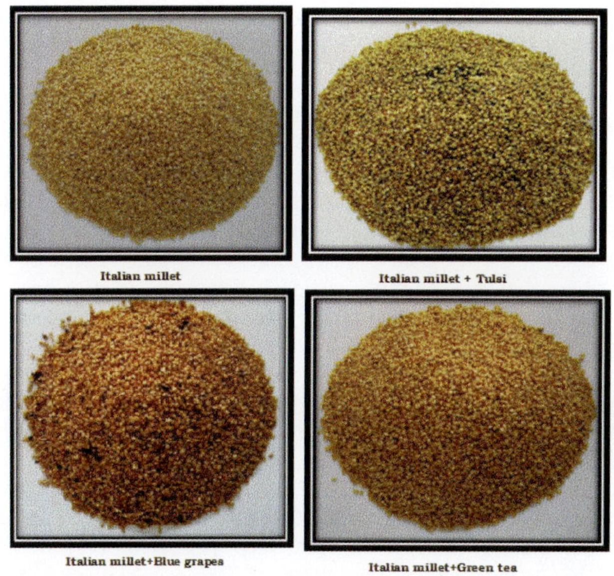

Figure 1: A view of Italian millet coated with antioxidant rich ingredients.

Cooking characteristics

The methods suggested by Bhattacharjee and Kulkarni [12] were followed to evaluate the cooking quality. Weighed sample (2 g) was placed in test tubes containing boiling water (20 ml) and heated on boiling water bath.

Cooking time: Optimum cooking time was determined by pressing few grains between two slides frequently taken from the cooking tube and noting the time when opaque core has just disappeared.

Percentage increase in weight (g): The increase in weight of the Italian millet was determined by weighing the Italian millet before and after cooking and finding the difference between the two as shown below.

$$Per\ cent\ increase\ in\ weight = \frac{Weight\ of\ cooked\ foxtail\ millet - Weight\ of\ raw\ foxtail\ millet}{Amount\ of\ foxtail\ millet} \times 100$$

Percentage increase in volume (ml): Volume of water in a volumetric cylinder containing 100 ml of water before and after the samples cooked was measured. Increase in volume was calculated as follows:

$$Per\ cent\ increase\ in\ volume = \frac{Weight\ of\ cooked\ foxtail\ millet - Volume\ of\ raw\ foxtail\ millet}{Amount\ of\ foxtail\ millet} \times 100$$

Water uptake ratio: The water uptake ratio was obtained by dividing the apparent water uptake at 80°C by the apparent water uptake at 90°C and the value was expressed in percentage (W2-W1) × 100.

Dispersed solids: Solids leached out into the cooking water was determined as follows. The water drained out after cooking the rice was taken in a Petri dish and dried in a hot air oven and weighed.

Weight of the Petri dish=W1

Weight of Petri dish+leached out solid after drying=W2

Therefore, total leached out solids=W2-W1

Results and Discussion

The functional properties of coated Italian millet are presented in Table 1. Bulk density of the samples ranged from 0.69-0.82 g/ml. Highest bulk density was found in uncoated Italian millet (0.82 g/ml) followed by green tea coated Italian millet (0.78 g/ml). The least bulk density was found in the tulsi coated Italian millet (0.69 g/ml). The bulk density of Italian millet variety Prasad was 0.82 g/ml which was heavier than values reported for millets. The bulk density of millet grain by Ocheme et al. [13] was 0.67 g/cm^3. The values of bulk density for coated grains ranged between 0.69 g/ml and 0.78 g/ml. Thus, coating with different antioxidant rich ingredients resulted in lighter product. Significant differences were found in bulk density among the treatments ($P \leq 0.05$). Lightness of the coated Italian millet can be attributed to larger air spaces between the particles when compared to uncoated Italian millet. The solubility per cent ranged from 0.74-0.76%. There was no significant difference observed between coated and uncoated samples ($P \leq 0.05$). This quality has implications in product development to improve the quality traits. Water absorption capacity of coated and uncoated Italian millet ranged from 1.1-1.2 g/ml. Ocheme and Chinma [14] reported that water absorption capacity in millet flour was 1.31 g/g. Dietary fiber is known to bind water. Thus, presence of fiber in the samples contributed to its water uptake. Oil absorption capacity ranged from 0.80-1.15 g/ml. There were no significant differences in water and oil absorption capacity among different Italian millet samples ($P \leq 0.05$). The coating with different ingredients did not change the characteristic of either water or oil uptake, suggesting that coated grains may be suitable for preparation of the traditional products from Italian millet.

Cooking characteristics of coated Italian millet samples were compared with uncoated de husked Italian millet are presented in Table 2. The cooking characteristics studied were cooking time, per cent increase in weight, per cent increase in volume, water uptake ratio and gelatinisation temperature. Least cooking time (13.16 min) was recorded in tulsi coated Italian millet. The type of coating influenced the cooking time in the order; green tea (15.16 min) > grapes (14.16 min) > tulsi (13.16 min). Yareshimi [15] reported that cooking time of some rice varieties ranged from 16-20 min. Thus, when compared to rice, Italian millet samples had lower cooking time. This could be attributed to its smaller size and therefore a larger surface area. The coating treatment further reduced the cooking time; this could be due to some alterations in the absorptive surface of the grain. Tulsi coated Italian millet recorded significantly higher per cent increase in weight (149%) followed by grapes (137%) and green tea (131%) coated Italian millet samples; while, it was lowest (125%) in uncoated Italian millet. Maximum per cent increase in volume (250%) was observed in tulsi coated Italian millet, followed by grapes (248%) and green tea (241%) coated Italian millet while lowest (240%) was in uncoated Italian millet. These may be due to the higher water absorption capacity of tulsi coated Italian millet during cooking as discussed in above paragraph on water absorption capacity. Pavithra [16] in her study on cooking quality of rice found that water absorption capacity was influenced by moisture content of the raw grains. This also may have contributed to the differences in values in the present study.

Treatments	Bulk density (g/ml)	Solubility (%)	Swelling power (%)	Water absorption (g/ml)	Oil absorption (g/ml)
Italian millet	0.82	0.74	4.03	1.12	1
Italian millet +Grapes	0.75	0.75	3.99	1.18	0.92
Italian millet+Green tea	0.78	0.75	3.96	1.1	0.8
Italian millet+Tulsi	0.69	0.76	4.1	1.2	1.15
F value	*	NS	NS	NS	NS
SEm ± (0.05)	0.0058	0.0128	0.0501	0.0501	0.151
CD (0.05)	0.0188	-	-	-	-

*Significant ($p \leq 0.05$); NS: Non significant

Table 1: Functional properties of Italian millet treated with different antioxidant rich ingredients.

Italian millet coated with tulsi, grapes, green tea and uncoated Italian millet had water uptake ratio of 24, 19, 18 and 17 respectively. The order of dispersed solids was tulsi coated (3.4%) > grapes coated (3.2%) > green tea coated (2.6%) > uncoated Italian millet (2.4%). There were significant difference between the coated samples in water uptake ratio and dispersed solids ($P \leq 0.05$). Yareshimi [15] reported that water uptake ratio and dispersed solids of some rice varieties ranged from 29.80-40.29 and 2.60-5.00% respectively. Thus, when compared to rice, Italian millet samples have lower water uptake ratio and dispersed solids. This could be attributed to amylose content. This might be also as a result of high moisture content. The coating treatment further increased the water uptake ratio and dispersed solids; this could be due to some alterations in the moisture level and absorptive surface of the grain after coating. Rice contains more moisture percentage than the Italian millet. There is relationship between amylose content and moisture to the water uptake ratio and dispersed solids [17]. The amylose content of Italian millet was reported as 17.5 per cent [18]. Gelatinisation temperature of the treated and untreated Italian millet samples ranged between 71.06°C and 73.00°C. Increase in starch-lipid complex formations decreases the extent of hydration in the amorphous areas, thus, resulting in an increased amount of thermal energy required for melting [15]. On cooking, the gelatinized starch tends to return from the soluble, dispersed and amorphous state to an insoluble crystalline state. It is enhanced with low gelatinization temperature and high concentration of starch [19]. The differences between Yareshmi's values and those observed in the present study might be explained by the fact that Italian millet has a higher fat content compared to rice. The higher onset temperature for uncooked flour indicated that more energy is required to initiate starch gelatinisation from uncooked flour when compared to hydrated flour. Generally, the completion temperature increases with the protein content and melting enthalpy of starch-lipid complexes [20]. However, the values are in the same range as those reported by some other workers for millet and other cereals. Jideani and Scott [21] reported gelatinisation temperature of pearl millet (51.3-86.9) which was similar to the Italian millet. For cereal grains, the value is usually around 65-70°C [22].

Treatments	Cooking time (min)	Percent increase in weight (%)	Percent increase in volume (%)	Water uptake ratio	Dispersed solids (%)	Gelatinization temperature (°C)
Italian millet	15.2	125	240	17	2.4	72.1
Italian millet+Grapes	14.16	137.33	248	19	3.2	73
Italian millet+Green tea	15.16	131.25	240.16	18	2.6	72.16
Italian millet+Tulsi	13.16	149	250.33	24	3.4	71.06
F value	*	*	*	*	*	NS
SEm ± (0.05)	0.15	0.54	0.67	0.57	0.05	0.58
CD (0.05)	0.5	1.78	2.19	1.88	0.18	-

*Significant ($p \leq 0.05$); NS: Non significant

Table 2: Cooking characteristics of Italian millet treated with different antioxidant rich ingredients.

Conclusion

Italian millet has unique cooking as well as functional characteristics that lends itself to many conventional and modern ways of product preparation. Using edible coating in this study was a novel approach to incorporate antioxidant rich ingredients. As incorporation of these coatings did not bring about any undesirable changes in its functional and cooking characteristics it may be concluded that this approach may be acceptable for enhancing antioxidant content of Italian millet without affecting its cooking quality.

References

1. Hadimani A, Malleshi NG (1993) Studies on milling, physic chemical properties, nutrient composition and dietary fiber content of millets. J Food Sci and Technol 30: 17-20.
2. Saleh ASM, Zhang Q, Chen J, Shen Q (2013) Millet Grains: Nutritional Quality, Processing, and Potential Health Benefit. Compr Rev Food Sci Food Saf 12: 281-295.
3. Hulse JH, Laing EM, Pearson OE (1980) Sorghum and millets: Their composition and nutritive Value. Academic Press, London.
4. Pawar VD, Machewad GM (2006) Processing of foxtail millet for Improved nutrient availability. J Food Process Preser 30: 269-279.
5. Kamara MT, Ming ZH, Kexue Z (2009) Extraction, characterization andnutritional properties of two varieties of defatted foxtail millet flour (*Setaria italica* L.) grown in China. Asian J Biochem 4: 88-98.
6. Paviath AE, Orts W (2009) Edible Films and Coatings: Why, What, and How? In: Edible Films and Coatings for Food applications, Embuscado ME, Huber KC (eds.) Springer Science and Business Media, LLC.
7. Ramamoorthy KP, Bono A (2007) Antioxidant activity, total phenolic and flavonoid content of Morinda citrifolia fruit extracts from various extraction processes. J Engg Sci Technol 2: 70- 80.
8. Manay NS, Shadaksharswamy M (2001) Food facts and principles. New Age International Publishers (P) Ltd., New Delhi, India.
9. Narayana K, Rao NMS (1982) Functional properties of raw and processed winged bean flour. J Food Sci 47: 137-140.
10. Rosario RD, Flores DM (1981) Functional properties of flour types on mung bean flours. J Sci Food Agric 32: 172-180.
11. Iyer I, Singh V (1997) Functional properties of wheat and chickpea composite flours. Food Australia 49: 27-31.
12. Bhattacharjee P, Kulkarni PR (2000) A comparative study on the physical characteristics and cooking quality parameters of commercial brands of Basmati rice. Int J Food Sci Nutr 51: 295-299.
13. Ocheme OB, Olundamilola O, Gladys ME (2010) Effect of lime soaking and cooking (nixtamalization) on the proximate, functional and some anti-nutritional properties of millet flour. Aus J Technol 14: 131-138.
14. Ocheme OB, Chinma CE (2008) Effects of soaking and germination on some physicochemical properties of millet flour for porridge production. J Food Technol 6: 185-188.
15. Yareshimi S (2011) Processing and nutritional qualities of biofortified (iron and zinc) aerobic rice varieties. M.Sc. Thesis, Univ Agri Sci, Bangalore.
16. Pavithra V (2007) Physiological and biochemical changes in rice varieties grown under aerobic and anaerobic condition. M.Sc. Thesis, Univ Agri Sci, Bangalore.
17. Oko AO, Ubi BE, Dambaba N (2012) Rice cooking quality and physicochemical characteristics: a comparative analysis of selected local and newly introduced rice varieties in Ebony state, Nigeria. J Food and Public Health 2: 43-49.
18. Lorenz K, Hinze C (1976) Functional characteristics of starches from proso and foxtail millets. J Agric Food Chem 24: 911-914.
19. Tomita Y, Sugimot Y, Sakamoto S, Fuwa H (1981) Some properties of starches of grain amaranth and several millets. J Nutri Sci Vitaminol 27: 471-484.
20. Liu QZ, Donner E, Tetlow L, Emes M (2007) Investigation of digestibility in vitro and physicochemical properties of A and B type starch from soft and hard wheat flour. Cereal Chem 84: 15-21.
21. Jideani VA, Scott DJ (2012) Hydrothermal characteristics of pearl millet (Pennisetum glaucum) flour during cooking into fura. African J Agric Res 7: 2751-2756.
22. Sozer N, Dalgic AC, Kaya A (2007) Thermal, textural and cooking properties of spaghetti enriched with instant starch. J Food Engg 81: 476-484.

Under Nutrition and Associated Factors among Adolescent Pregnant Women in Shashemenne District, West Arsi Zone, Ethiopia

Belete Y[1,*], Negga B[2] and Firehiwot M[3]

[1]*College of Medicine and Health Sciences, Debre Markos University, P.O. Box269, Debre Markos, Ethiopia*

[2]*College of Health and Medical Sciences, Haramaya University, P.O. Box 235, Harar, Ethiopia*

[3]*College of Health and Medical Sciences, Haramaya University, P.O. Box 235, Harar, Ethiopia*

[*]**Corresponding author:** Belete Yimer, College of Medicine and Health Sciences, Debre Markos University, PO Box 269, Debre Markos, Ethiopia
E-mail: byimer04@gmail.com

Abstract

Background: Pregnancy places adolescent females who, in general, are at risk for nutritional problems at even greater risk. This study aimed to determine prevalence of under nutrition and identifying associated factors among adolescent pregnant women in Shashemenne district, West Arsi Zone, Ethiopia from March 10/2015-March 31/2015.

Methods: A cross-sectional, community based study was conducted on 424 adolescent pregnant women existing in ten randomly selected rural and urban kebeles (kebele is the smallest administrative unit in Ethiopia). Data were collected using a pre-tested, structured questionnaire and anthropometric measurement in their own respective homes. MUAC of <22 cm defined under nutrition. Data were analyses by SPSS version 21. A multivariable logistic regression was used to identify the predictors of under nutrition.

Results: In this study, the mean MUAC (± SD) of the study participants was 22.0cm (± 2.8) and 34.0%, 95%CI: 29.5%, 38.4% of the women were undernourished. Women married before 15 years [AOR=7.3, 95%CI (9.5-23.7)] were sixteen times more likely undernourished than those married between 18-19 years. Whereas; Literate women [AOR=0.3, 95%CI (0.2-0.8)], No ANC visits [AOR=6.0, 95%CI (1.2-30.1)], Less than three pregnancies [AOR=0.1, 95%CI (0.03-0.3)], having support [AOR=0.4, 95%CI (0.2-0.8)] and Workload [AOR=13.6, 95%CI (6.3-28.8)]. Conclusion: The level of under nutrition was high. Thus, pregnant teenager's targeted efforts should be made by al concerned bodies to improve the health and nutritional conditions of teenage mothers and their offspring.

Keywords: Under nutrition; Antenatal care; Demographic survey; Health

Abbreviations

ANC: Antenatal care

BMI: Body Mass Index AOR: Adjusted odds ratio

CI: Confidence Interval

EDHS: Ethiopian Health and Demographic Survey

MUAC: Mid Upper Arm Circumference

WHO: World Health Organization Conflict of Interests

Background

Adolescence refers to the developmental period between childhood and adulthood. The World health organization (WHO) defines adolescents as individuals between the ages of 10-19 years [1,2]. Adolescence is a time of rapid physical growth with nutritional requirements increasing significantly to support growth and development. A combination of the energy demands of the adolescent growth spurt and inadequate diet has contributed a lot to the poor nutritional status of adolescents. The additional energy and nutrient demands of pregnancy place adolescents at nutritional risk [3-10].

Due to the high rate of adolescent marriage in some developing countries, pregnancy during adolescence is still common. The magnitude of teenage pregnancy differs across countries of the developing world. According to EDHS 2005, despite a minimum legal marriage of 18 years in Ethiopia, early marriage remains common, with a median age at first marriage 16.1 years. Almost all pregnancies in Ethiopia occur within marriage, and the median age at first birth is about 17 years. Levels of contraceptive use are low, at 15% among married women of reproductive age.

Teenagers had lower contraceptive prevalence and used family planning methods sporadically compared with young adults age 20-24 and about 40% of women had begun childbearing by age 19, and many as early as age 15 or 16 [11]. In developing countries, many adolescents are undernourished and still growing when they enter pregnancy. Due to chronic malnutrition, age at menarche is delayed by about 3 years and growth continues until age 20. In cases in which a woman has not completed her physical, psychological, and social development, the pregnancy period affects the mother and infant negatively [12-14].

Adolescent pregnant women encounter challenges in addition to those encountered by all women who are pregnant. They are at greater risk for certain health conditions, such as pregnancy induced hypertension, pre-eclampsia, intra-uterine growth retardation, preterm delivery, low birth weight, and inadequate weight gain, related to their age and developmental stage, and have limited knowledge of their bodies, reproduction, pregnancy, and birth. Also adolescent pregnant women have been found to be at higher risk when compared to pregnant adults for certain social problems, such as discontinuation of education, unemployment, and social isolation [15-19]. Factors at individual, household and community level, or a combination of these factors, may contribute to poor nutrition and health status. Previous studies have shown that family income, education, MUAC and pregnancy body mass index (BMI) were associated with nutrient inadequacy [20,21]. Adolescents in populations with minimal access to contraception are likely to have many closely spaced pregnancies over their childbearing years. In such adolescents, changes in nutritional status during pregnancy may be predictive of long term reproductive nutritional depletion [22-24].

Nutritional deficiencies are far reaching consequences in adolescent pregnant women. Pregnancy among those who themselves are children can result in pregnancy complications. If their nutritional needs are not met, they are likely to give birth to undernourished children, thus transmitting under nutrition to future generations [3,4,12,13]. Addressing the nutritional needs of adolescent pregnant women could be an important step towards breaking the vicious cycle of intergenerational malnutrition. The vicious cycle of under nutrition, if not broken, will go on resulting in more and more severe cob nsequences. One way to break the intergenerational cycle of under nutrition is to improve the nutrition of adolescent girls prior to conception in general and during pregnancy in particular [25].

Despite the fact that adolescence in general and adolescent pregnancy in particular is one of windows of opportunity in the life cycle nutritional interventions, a few studies have reported the nutritional status of pregnant adolescents. Nutritional requirements during adolescent pregnancy are greater than during adult pregnancy. If an adolescent is well nourished during pregnancy, she will have adequate fat and other nutrient reserves that can be used to compensate partially for her additional requirements and her foetus. Because of this, and the importance of nutrition in the course and outcome of pregnancy, all adolescent pregnant women should have a formal assessment of their nutritional status at the beginning of their prenatal care, with ongoing surveillance throughout the pregnancy. So, information on nutritional status and associated factors of the adolescent pregnant women is urgently needed for prioritizing, designing and initiating intervention programs aimed at improving maternal nutrition. The process of priority setting should start with the assessment and analysis of the situation that adolescent pregnant women face in their environment. In Ethiopia where marriage is universal and occurs at younger ages; the nutritional status and associated factors of pregnant adolescents is of prime public health importance. To the best of principal investigator's knowledge, there is no research based information regarding pregnant adolescent's nutritional status and associated factors from the study communities. Thus, the objective of this study was to assess the level of undernutrition and associated factors among adolescent pregnant women in Shashemene district.

Methods

Study setting, design and period

A community-based cross-sectional study was conducted in Shashamane district, West Arsi Zone, Oromia National Regional State, Ethiopia from March 10/2015-March 31/2015 among adolescent pregnant women. The district is one of 13 districts in West Arsi zone and its population is divided into rural and urban dwellers. Shashemenne is its capital city (the capital city of West Arsi zone); it is located 206 Kms from Adama (the capital city of Oromia Regional State) and 251 Kms from Addis-Ababa (the capital city of Ethiopia). According to Shashemenne district health office report, the total population of the district, in the year 2014, was estimated to be 328,035 (156, 237 males and 171,798 females) and 24% [78,729] of the population are women of reproductive age group and about a quarter(19,682) of those women are teenagers. The total numbers of adolescent pregnant women, which were the source population, in the district were 2,007. The district is constituted by 47 kebeles (10 urban and 37 rural kebeles). The district has two hospitals, 14 health centers, 47 health posts, 3 small, 5 medium and 6 higher private clinics, one private hospital and 12 private drug vendors. The potential health service coverage in the district is 98% [26].

Study population, sample size and sampling

Adolescent pregnant women between the ages of 10-19 years in the randomly selected kebeles of the district were the study population. Pregnant women were identified by self-report, from the report of health extension workers in the kebeles. A sample size of 434 adolescent pregnant women was calculated using a single population proportion formula with a 95% confidence level, 5% margin of error, and 15.1% estimated prevalence of chronic wasting (MUAC<22 cm) in the study area [27] and by considering a non-response rate of 10%. This study was based on the random sample of ten kebeles of the forty seven kebeles existing in the district. The total kebeles in the district were initially stratified into rural and urban (10 urban and 37 rural) areas. Then, ten (three from urban and seven from rural) were selected randomly based on Probability Proportional to Size (PPS) sampling technique and then the determined sample size was distributed proportional to total adolescent pregnant women of each stratum. After that, simple random sampling was used to select the required number of adolescent pregnant women.

Data collection methods and procedures

Data was collected by four grade twelve complete female data collectors and supervised by one BSc nurse and principal investigator who were able to speak and write local languages. Data was collected using a pre-tested, structured questionnaire adapted from related studies and anthropometric measurement. The adapted questionnaire was modified, contextualized to the local situation and the research objectives. Information on socio-demographic, psychosocial, eating habits and maternal health variables of the identified eligible respondents' were assessed using a structured face-to-face interview administered questionnaire in their own respective homes.

Anthropometric measurement

The nutritional status of pregnant women is often measured using mid upper arm circumference (MUAC). MUAC is independent of pregnancy or lactation status and therefore can be used as an effective indicator of women's nutritional status throughout the reproductive years. MUAC is more useful than weight during pregnancy, as it varies little during pregnancy and has been associated with maternal BMI and weight, maternal and infant mortality, prematurity and other poor foetal outcomes [28]. Because of MUAC instrument is simple and the training is straightforward, MUAC measurement was taken by the grade twelve complete data collectors. MUAC is the circumference of the left upper arm measured in centimeters using a non-stretchable MUAC tape. The point is between the tip of the shoulder and the elbow. Wasting in pregnant women can be defined as a mid- upper arm circumference (MUAC) <22 cm [29].

Statistical analysis

Data was double entered and cleaned in EPI data software version 3.1. The entered data were exported and analyses with SPSS version 21. Descriptive tests like proportions mean and standard deviation was used to describe the data. Bivariate and multivariate logistic regression analyses with an odds ratio along with the 95% confidence interval were used to ascertain the association between covariates and under nutrition among adolescent pregnant women. Hosmer- Lomeshow goodness-of-fit is used to test model fitness. Only covariates that have (P<0.2) at the bivariate level were included in the multivariate logistic regression to control for all possible confounders. For all statistical tests P-value ≤ 0.05 was considered for level of statistical significance.

Ethical consideration

Officially written approval letter from Haramaya University institutional research ethics and review committee (IRERC) was obtained prior to the study. Then, informed consent was obtained, privacy and confidentiality was maintained for the participants. For adolescent pregnant women below 18 years, the interview was conducted after informed consent from their husband/male partner or parents/legal guardians. Verbal assent was also obtained from the adolescent pregnant women under 18 years. The purposes, the data collection procedures, the risks, and the benefits of the research were explained to the eligible respondents before obtaining their informed consent.

Results

Socio-demographic characteristics of the respondents

A total of 424 adolescent pregnant women were interviewed making a response rate of 97.5%. The median (±SD) age of mothers was 18.0 (±1.2) years. The majority of participants were Oromo (67.2%) and Muslim (66.5%), (Table 1).

Variable	Category	Number	Percentage (%)
Age	15-17	146	34.4
	18-19	278	65.6
Age at first marriage	Never married	48	11.3
	<15	35	8.3
	15-17	306	72.1
	18-19	35	8.3
Occupation	House wife	191	45.1
	Merchant	98	23.2
	Gov't employee	56	13.2
	Others	79	18.7
Educational status	Illiterate	151	35.5
	Literate	273	64.5
Current marital relationship	Never married	48	11.3
	Married	303	71.5
	Other	73	17.2
Marriage type	Never married	48	11.3
	Arranged marriage	207	48.8
	Love marriage	169	39.9
Residence	Urban	65	15.3
	Rural	359	84.7

Table 1: Characteristics of pregnant women in Shashemene, southern Ethiopia April, 2015.

Under nutrition and associated factors

The mean MUAC (± SD) of the study participants was 22.0cm (± 2.8). Among 424 women interviewed, 144 (34.0%, 95%CI: 29.5%, 38.4%) were undernourished (MUAC<22 cm) (Figure 1).

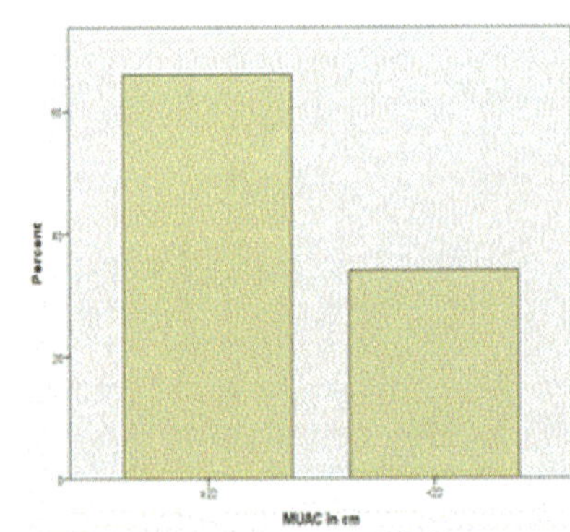

Figure 1: MUAC measurement of adolescent pregnant women in shashemene, Ethiopia April 2015.

In the bivariate analysis; literate women were nine times less likely to be undernourished than those illiterate women. Women married before 15 years were sixteen times more likely to be undernourished than those married between 18-19 years and women who had exposure to mass media and live in urban were eight and five times less likely to be undernourished than their counterparts respectively. Women who get pregnant less than three times were nine times less likely to be undernourished than their counterparts. Women who desired their current pregnancy were eight times protected from under nutrition than women who did not desire their current pregnancy. Respondents those who avoid any foods during their pregnancy time were three times more likely to be undernourished than their counterparts. Women having literate partner and desired pregnancy by partner were less likely to be under nourished and respectively. In multivariate analysis, Compared to respondants married between 18-19 years, those married before 15 years were about seven times more likely to be undernourished. On the other hand, literate women were protected from under nutrition. The odds of under nutrition were 70% lower for the literate adolescent pregnant women` than the illiterate women. Aadolescent pregnant women who didn't visit ANC were six times more likely to be undernourished when compared to respondents who attended ANC greater or equal to four times. Adolescent pregnant women who get pregnant less than three times were less likely to be under nourished than those who had more pregnancy. Moreover, adolescent pregnant women having partner, peer or family support were protected from being under nourished. Adolescent pregnant women having daily heavy workload were thirteen times more likely to be undernourished as compared to their counterparts (Table 2).

Variable	**Under nutrition**		**COR**	**AOR**	**P-value**
	Yes	**No**	**(95% CIs)**	**(95%CI)**	
Age(years)					
15-17	74(50.7%)	72(49.3%)	3.1(2.0-4.7)*	1.4(0.6-3.7)	0.448
18-19	70(25.2%)	208(74.8%)	1		
Marital status					
Never married	9(23.7%)	39(76.3%)	1.3(0.5-3.4)	5.2(0.03-9.9)	0.539
Married	124(40.9%)	179(59.1%)	3.9(2.0-7.7)*	1.5(0.4-5.8)	0.55
Other	11(15.1%)	62(84.9%)	1		
Age at 1st Marriage					
Never married	9(23.7%)	39(76.3%)	2.6(0.9-7.4)	1	
<15	14(39.5%)	21(60.5%)	16.0(6.5-39.4)*	7.3(9.5-23.7)*	0.022
15-17	118(38.6%)	188(61.4%)	7.0(3.1-16.2)*	0.5(0.1-2.3)	0.353
18-19	3(8.2%)	32(91.8%)	1	1	
Marriage type					
Never married	9(23.7%)	39(76.3%)	2.9(1.2-6.9)*	1	
Arranged	120(58.3%)	86(41.7%)	15.4(8.4-28.5)*	0.8(0.2-2.4)	0.641
Love	14(8.3%)	155(91.7%)	1	1	
Educational status					
Literate	49(17.9%)	224(82.1%)	0.1(0.1-0.2)*	0.4(0.2-0.8)*	0.043
Illiterate	95(62.9%)	56(37.1%)	1	1	
Occupation					
House wife	103(53.9%)	88(46.1%)	1.2(0.7-2.0)	1.1(0.3-3.7)	0.854
Merchant	16(16.3%)	82(83.7%)	0.3(0.1-0.5)*	1.2(0.3-4.4)	0.762
Gov't employee	11(19.6%)	45(80.4%)	0.2(0.1-0.4)*	0.5(0.1-4.3)	0.54
Other	55(69.6%)	24(30.4%)	1	1	
Numbers of pregnancy					
<3	91(23.3%)	268(74.7%)	0.1(0.04-0.2)*	0.1(0.03-0.3)*	0.0001
≥3	53(81.5%)	12(18.5%)	1	1	
ANC visits					
No ANC	114(55.3%)	92(44.7%)	11.4(6.3-20.5)*	6.0(1.2-30.1)*	0.031

<4 visits	27(27.8%)	70(72.2%)	4.6(2.4-8.8)*	1.2(0.2-6.5)	0.834
≥4 visits	3(2.5%)	118(97.5%)	1	1	
Number of meals/day					
<3meal	28(71.8%)	11(28.2%)	3.4(1.7-7.1)*	1.1(0.3-3.4)	0.897
≥3meal	116(30.1%)	269(69.9%)	1	1	
Meal pattern					
Regular	51(19.7%)	208(80.3%)	0.2(0.2-0.4)*	1.2(0.6-2.5)	0.63
Irregular	93(56.4%)	72(43.6)	1	1	
Change in food intake					
No change	112(50.2%)	111(49.2%)	6.0(3.5-11.7)*	0.5(0.2-1.5)	0.199
Frequency	15(26.3%)	42(73.7%)	2.0(1.0-4.0)*	0.7(0.2-2.4)	0.624
Amount	7(16.3%)	36(83.7%)	2.0(1.0-4.5)*	0.6(0.2-2.6)	0.543
Freq. & amt.	10(9.9%)	91(90.1%)	1	1	
Workload					
Yes	119(72.6%)	45(27.4%)	7.3(4.7-11.3)*	13.6(6.3-28.8)*	0.0001
No	25(9.6%)	235(90.4%)	1	1	
Support					
Yes	53(18.1%)	240(81.9%)	0.2(0.1-0.3)*	0.4(0.2-0.8) *	0.007
No	91(69.5%)	40(30.5%)	1	1	

Table 2: Key: COR=crude odds ratio, AOR=Adjusted odds ratio, CI=confidence interval, *=P-value ≤ 0.05 for statistical significance.

Discussion

The study showed a high prevalence of under nutrition. Age at first marriage, educational status, ANC visits, and numbers of pregnancy, work load and support during pregnancy remained the main significant factors associated with under nutrition. The result of the study was almost consistent with findings on the level of under nutrition in some parts of the country; the prevalence of wasting among adolescent pregnant women of the Tigray region and Southern region was (37.5%) and (37%) respectively [30]. This result is also consistent with study from Philippines where the prevalence of wasting was 33.1% [31]. But more than two times finding from Aletawondo, Southern region of Ethiopia which is 15.1% [27] and finding from South Africa (13%), [32]. The level of under nutrition in this study also much higher than findings from other different countries, i.e., 6.4% in Uganda [33], 18.1% in Thailand [34], 25% in Bangladesh [35] and 20% in Nigeria [36]. The probable reason for the above variation in rates could be little interventions on adolescents' health, nutrition, early marriage, family planning and other adolescent women empowering programs by the government as well as other non-governmental organizations in the study area which in turn resulted in chronic energy deficiency, inadequate weight gain during pregnancy and poor nutritional status of adolescent pregnant women. This finding evidenced that, those married before 15 years were more likely undernourished. This was in line with other studies [37]. The practices of early marriage, which was a case in the study area (The median age at first marriage was 16.0(±1.3) years which was almost similar with the national figure which is 16.1 [11], limit the education and development of girls which in turn trigger the occurrence of under nutrition. Compared to illiterate women, literate women were protected from under nutrition. This is consistent with other studies [38]. This may be due to educated adolescent pregnant women have adequate knowledge about their own health, development and nutritional needs and also education affects fertility through delay in age at marriage, improving knowledge and access to effective family planning methods and ability on decision making on number of children needed.

Compared to respondents who visits ANC greater or equal to four times (which is recommended), those who did not visit ANC were more likely under nourished. The risk is higher than the study finding from Aletawondo where the odds of under nutrition (MUAC<22 cm) during pregnancy among women who did not visit ANC were 2.9 compared with other women [27]. This might be because those who frequently visit the health institutions were getting health and nutrition educations as well as advice from the respective health professionals. Similarly, compared to respondents who get pregnant greater or equal to three times, those who get pregnant less than three times were less likely under nourished. This is in line with other study [27]. This may be due to the average age of marriage for women have a significant effect on the teenage birth rate. So, adolescents in populations where early marriage is common together with minimal access to contraception are likely to have many closely spaced pregnancies.

In this study, adolescent pregnant women having daily heavy workload were more likely undernourished as compared to their counterparts. This was in line with study from Aletawondo [27]. The practices of arranged marriage, which is a case in the study area, may limits the love, attention and care given by the partner which in turn make pregnant adolescents work largely on the families' jobs. Adolescent pregnant women having adequate partner, peer or family support were protected from being undernourished. This is in line with study from South Africa [32,39]. It should be noted that; woman who has not completed her physical, psychological, and social development needs support to protect the health and nutritional conditions of the growing mother and her foetus.

Contrary to the general perception, age of respondents, occupation, exposure to mass media, avoid eating any food during pregnancy, meal pattern and desiredness of pregnancy was found to have no significant association with under nutrition in our study. The finding of a lack of association could reflect effect modification on the basis of settings or cultural contexts. Major strengths of this study were the community based approach and random selection of the study households or kebeles. This may made generalization possible to the study communities as an attempt was made to identify randomized households and adolescent pregnant women from the study communities. The study couldn't establish firm causal links though association was observed due to its cross-sectional design. This study also used only MUAC measurement for nutritional assessment which is indirect measure of nutrition and status. As study was based on the women's self-reported pregnancy, there was the cultural unacceptability and fear of disclosing the issue and this may have resulted in under reporting.

Conclusion

There was high level of under nutrition among the Adolescent pregnant women in the study area. Age at first marriage, respondent's educational status, and number of pregnancy, ANC visits, workload and support during pregnancy were found to be the main significant factors associated with under nutrition. Thus, adolescent pregnant women in the study area are at higher risk of under nutrition which may affect the health of the growing mother and their foetus negatively. Therefore, there should be the community awareness in the setting to respect a Federal family guidance (delay marriage until after 19 years of age) and incentives for girls to stay in school. There is need to identify and target post-menarcheal married nulligravid and unmarried adolescents who are undernourished for food supplementation programs and family planning programs which should preferentially target adolescent married girls through incentives to delay their first pregnancy and to increase birth intervals. The intervention should also focus on nutritional screening for adolescent pregnant women and close monitoring of pregnancy weight gain especially during ANC visits and to deal with the special needs of adolescents in a friendly manner and health education to pregnant teenagers and their families like avoiding work load and adequate support during pregnancy.

Conflicts of Interest

The authors did not receive payments, funding, or salary from any organization in relation to the work and publication of this paper in the past five years and there will also be no financial support to be received in the future. There is not any organization affected positively or negatively by the publication of this paper. There are not any competing interests related with patents of the content of the paper. The authors also declare that there are not any other financial or nonfinancial competing interests.

Authors' Contribution

All authors, Belete Yimer, Negga Baraki, and Firehiwot Mesfin, conceptualized the research question, monitored and managed fieldwork, analyzed and interpreted the findings, and written the paper.

Acknowledgment

Haramaya University provided financial and other supports for this research project. The authors are grateful to the pregnant women who sacrificed their time. The authors also thank the HEWs working in the selected kebeles of the district for their necessary support and the data collectors for their responsible data collection. The authors got enabling cooperation from Haramaya District Administration, District Health Office, and the Administrations of the Selected Kebeles during the fieldwork.

References

1. World Health Organization (WHO) (2007) Adolescent pregnancy-unmet needs and undone deeds: a review of the literature and programmes. Geneva, Switzerland: WHO Press.
2. UNICEF (2005) State of the world's Children. House, 3 UN plazas, New York, NY 10017, USA.
3. Harrison KA, Fleming AF, Briggs ND, Rossiter CE (2005) Growth during pregnancy in Nigerian primigravidae. Br J Obstet Gynaecol 92: 32-39.
4. Naeya RL (2001) Teenaged and pre-teenaged pregnancies: consequences of the fetal maternal competition for nutrients. Paediatrics 67: 146-150.
5. Spear BA (2002) Adolescent growth and development. J Am Diet Assoc 102: S23-S29.
6. Nwokocha ARC (2009) Adolescence and associated problems. In Paediatrics and child health in a tropical region. Azubuike JC, Nkanginieme KEO (eds) Services, PO Box 1691 and 2 Dengramite Avenue, Owerri, Nigeria: Nigeria African Educational Services; 97-109.
7. Heald FP, Gong EJ (2005) Diet, nutrition and adolescence. Modern nutrition in health and disease. Ninthth edition. Shils ME, Ross AC (eds) Maryland, USA: Williams and Wilkins.
8. Rees JM, Nuumark SD, Kohn M, Jocobson M (2007) Improving the nutritional health of adolescents- position statement- society for adolescent medicine. J Adolesc Health 24: 461-462.
9. Chauliac M, Raimbault AM (2012) Adolescent pregnancy. Dev Sante, 98: 23-25.
10. Story M, Alton I (2005) Nutrition issues and adolescent pregnancy. Nutr Today 30: 142-151.
11. Wubegzier MA (2013) Differentials of Early Teenage Pregnancy in Ethiopia, 2000 and 2005. DHS working papers, No. 90.
12. Riley AP, Huffman SL, Chowdhury AK (2009) Age at menarche and postmenarcheal growth in rural Bangladeshi females. Ann Hum Biol 16: 347-359.
13. Scholl TO, Hediger ML, Cronk CE, Schall JI (2013) Maternal growth during pregnancy and lactation. Horm Res 39: 59-67.
14. Leenstra T, Petersen LT, Kariuki SK (2005) Prevalence and severity of malnutrition and age at menarche; cross-sectional studies in pregnant adolescent in Western Kenya. Eur J Clin Nutr 59: 41-48.
15. Koniak GD, Turner PC (2001) Health risks and psychosocial outcomes of early childbearing: a review of the literature. J Perinat Neonatal Nurs 15: 1-17.
16. Abu HA, Ali AM, Al DS (2002) Obstetrics and perinatal outcome of adolescent nulliparous pregnant women. Gynecol Obstet Invest 53: 90-92.

17. Klima CS (2003) Centering pregnancy: a model for adolescent pregnant women. J Midwifery Women's Health 48: 220-225.
18. Dubois S, Coulombe C, Pencharz P, Pinsonneault O, Duquette MP (2007) Ability of the Higgins Nutritional Intervention Program to improve adolescent pregnancy outcome. J Am Diet Assoc 97: 871-878.
19. Semiha TA, Elçin B, Osman G (2010) Comparison of life quality of adolescent pregnant women with that of pregnant adults in Turkey. Upsala Journal of Medical Sciences 115: 275-281.
20. Orvos H, Nyirati I, Hajdu J, Pál A, Nyári T, et al. (2009) Is adolescent pregnancy associated with adverse perinatal outcome? J Perinat Med 27: 199-203.
21. Asha K, Salil S (2010) Nutrient Intake of pregnant adolescent mothers from rural areas and urban areas. Indian J Soc Res 39: 2.
22. Begum F, Buckshe K, Pande JN (2003) Risk factors associated with preterm labor. Bangladesh Med Res Counc Bull 29: 59-66.
23. Christian P, Katz J, Wu L, Kimbrough-Pradhan E, Khatry SKet al. (2008) Risk factors for pregnancy-related mortality: a prospective study in rural Nepal. Public Health 122: 161-172.
24. Liljestrand J, Bergström S (2011) Antenatal nutritional assessment: the value of upper arm circumference. Gynecol Obstet Invest 32: 81-83.
25. Nega T (2010) Dietary Adequacy and Nutritional Practice of adolescent women. MSc thesis. Hawassa, Oromia Regional State: Hawassa University, College of Agriculture, Institute of Nutrition, Food Science and Technology, Shashemene district health office report; 2014; Shashemene, Ethiopia.
26. Mukhopadhyay A, Bhadra M, Bose K (2010) Anthropometric assessment of nutritional status of adolescent pregnant women of Aletawondo district, Southern region of Ethiopia. J Hum Ecol 18: 213-216.
27. Maso MJ, Gong EJ, Jacobson MS, Bross DS, Heald FP (2008) Anthropometric predictors of low birth weight outcome in teenage pregnancy. Adolesc Health Care 9: 188-193.
28. WHO collaborative study (WHO) (2011) Monitoring of pregnancy weight gain in outpatient clinics. Bull World Health Orga 73: 1-98.
29. Central Statistical Agency (CSA) [Ethiopia] and ORC Macro (2006) Ethiopia Demographic and Health Survey 2005. Addis Ababa, Ethiopia: Central Statistical Agency and ORC Macro.
30. Madriaga JR, Cheong RL, Perlas LA (2004) Anthropometric assessment of adolescent pregnant women, Philipines. Food and Nutrition Research Institute FNRI. 5th National nutrition survey results 150-8925.
31. Kesa H, Oldewage-Theron W (2011) Anthropometric indications and nutritional intake of women in the Vaal Triangle, South Africa. Public Health 119: 294-300.
32. Lynn A, Florence M, Annika J, Edward KK, Elisabeth F (2012) Evaluaton of nutritional status of adolescent pregnant women-in Wakiso district, Uganda; African Health Sciences 5: 304-3098.
33. Phnom S, Tippawan L, Virasakdi C, Praneed S, Vosasit S, et al. (2010) Inadequacy of nutrients intake among pregnant women in the Deep South of Thailand. BMC Public Health 10: 572, 1471-2458.
34. Ahmed F, Zareen M, Khan MR, Banu CP, Haq MN, et al. (2008) Dietary pattern, nutrient intake and growth of adolescent women in urban Bangladesh. Public Health Nutr 1: 83-92.
35. Alabi A (2009) The relationship between basal blood pressure and body mass index in apparently healthy Nigerian adolescents. Dissertation submitted to West African college of physicians. Lagos State: West African College of Physicians.
36. Teller H, Yimer G (2000) Level and determinants of malnutrition in pregnant adolescent and adult women in Southern Ethiopia. Ethiop J Health Dev 4: 57-66.
37. Abdullah M, Wheeler EF (2005) Seasonal variations, and the intra-household distribution of food in a Bangladeshi village. Am J Clin Nutr 41: 1305-1313.
38. Ronsmans C, Collin S, Filippi V (2008) Maternal Mortality in Developing Countries: Nutrition and Health in Developing Countries (2ndedn). 999 Riverview Drive, Suite 208, Totowa, NJ 07512, Humana Press, USA.
39. Soriano G (2005) Malnutrition in children of adolescent mothers. Arch Domin Pediatr 27: 5-8.

Changes in Polyphenol Content of Newly Released Varieties of Wheat during Different Processing Methods

Neera Parmar[1], Saroj Dahiya[1] and Sanjay Kumar[2*]

[1]Department of Foods and Nutrition, Chaudhary Charan Singh Haryana Agricultural University, India

[2]Department of Biochemistry, Central University of Haryana, India

[*]**Corresponding author:** Sanjay Kumar, Assistant Professor, Department of Biochemistry, Central University of Haryana, India, E-mail: sanjaykumar@cuh.ac.in

Abstract

Background: Wheat *(Triticum aestivum)* is the most important food crop in India and most important cereal grain. It is widely consumed in northern India. It is the leading source of all the macronutrients like proteins (especially vegetable protein), energy and carbohydrates and micronutrients like minerals (iron, calcium, zinc, potassium etc.) and B vitamins. It is currently second to rice in terms of total production (tonnes) as the main human food crop. The wheat flour besides various nutrients also contains anti-nutrients like phytates, oxalates, polyphenols, tannins etc. Polyphenol are the phytochemicals i.e., compounds which are found abundantly in natural plant food sources that have antioxidant properties. These phytochemicals are found in many types of plant foods, such as grains like wheat, pearl millet, maize etc., legumes like peanuts and soybeans, nuts, and seeds. There are various factors which affect the polyphenol content of plants and these include environmental factors, degree of ripeness at the time of harvesting, processing and storage. Polyphenolic content of the foods are greatly affected by environmental factors as well as edaphic factors like soil type, sun exposure, rainfall etc.

Methods: The treatments like soaking, roasting, sprouting and malting reduce the polyphenolic content in wheat varieties. Two newly released varieties of wheat (WH-1080 and WH-1025) and one conventional wheat variety C-306 were collected from the Department of Genetics and Plant Breeding, College of Agriculture, CCS HAU, Hisar in a single lot.

All the three wheat varieties obtained were cleaned, washed well under running tap water to get rid of all the dust, soil particles and foreign matter adhered to the grains, dried and ground to flour using conventional flour mill and processed in three different ways roasting, sprouting and malting and then used for nutritional evaluation of raw and processed wheat varieties and interpretation.

Results: Polyphenol content in wheat varieties which were unprocessed ranged from 234.15-338.4 mg/100 g (on dry weight basis) and in processed wheat varieties from 218.98-338.4 mg/100 g. Processing treatments showed significant decrease in the polyphenol levels. Lowest polyphenol content was found in sprouted WH-1080 variety 218.98 mg/100 g. Sprouting significantly ($P<0.05$) reduced the polyphenol content as compared to malting and roasting.

Conclusion: Sprouting treatment was found to be most advantageous in reducing the polyphenol content in all the wheat varieties when compared to other treatments like roasting and malting.

Keywords: Anti-nutrients; Polyphenols; Malting; Sprouting; Roasting; Phytochemicals

Introduction

Wheat (*Triticum aestivum*) is the most important staple form of food crop which is rich in macronutrients and micronutrients. It is especially rich in proteins especially vegetable proteins, energy, carbohydrates, and vitamins and minerals like calcium, phosphorus, magnesium, zinc, iron etc., thus making it a wholesome crop. India is the fourth largest producer of wheat in the world after Russia, the USA and China and accounts for 8.7% of the world's total wheat production. Uttar Pradesh, Punjab and Haryana are the three prominent wheat producing states. These states account for about 60% of the wheat area and produce about three-fourths of the total wheat production in India

Wheat is one of the least expensive cereal grains available amongst rice, pearl millet, maize flour etc., in fabricated form which rich in nutrition as it contains a variety of minerals like iron, calcium, phosphorous, zinc, potassium, magnesium etc. [1,2], vitamins like thiamine [3], and fatty acids like stearic acid, myristic acid, palmitic acid etc. The nutritional content of wheat on an average are energy 320-350 kcal, protein 10-13%, carbohydrate 74-78%, lipids 1-3% and considerable amounts of vitamins i.e., thiamine 0.3-0.5 mg and riboflavin 0.2-0.45 mg and minerals mg, iron 2.8-3.5 mg, zinc 2.0-3.43 and magnesium 110-130 mg/100 g, on dry weight basis. The wheat flour has various anti-nutrients like phytates, oxalates, polyphenols, tannins etc. [4,5]. The most important anti-nutrients found out of these are phytic acid and polyphenols. Polyphenol are the phytochemicals meaning compound found abundantly in natural plant food sources that have antioxidant properties. These are found in many types of plant foods, such as grains (wheat, maize, pearl millet etc.), legumes (including peanuts and soybeans), nuts, and seeds. There are various factors which affect the polyphenol content of plants and these include environmental factors, degree of ripeness at the time of harvesting, processing and storage. Polyphenolic content of the foods are greatly affected by environmental factors as well as edaphic factors like soil type, sun exposure, rainfall etc.

These anti-nutrients like phytates, polyphenols, tannins, oxalates are reduced by some cooking treatments which are boiling, sprouting, fermentation, roasting, malting etc. [6,7]. The above mentioned antinutrients are reduced considerably and thus the products which are consumed have low levels of these anti-nutrients as the flour has been processed to make the products organoleptically acceptable.

Review of Literatures

Hooda [8] analysed the anti-nutritional factors in wheat and found that the polyphenol concentration as 355.11 mg/100 g (dry weight basis) in wheat flour samples. Sangwan and Dahiya [9] also evaluated the wheat grains for polyphenol content in and found that the polyphenol concentration is 320.4 mg/100 g (dry weight basis). Varsha [10] also evaluated polyphenol content in wheat flour samples and found that it was 465 mg/100 g. Sikandra [1] in 2005 also evaluated the polyphenolic content in wheat flour samples and the result obtained was 275-342 mg/100 g concentration of polyphenol. Ragee and Kiefer [11] studied the phenolic composition of cereals for food use and found that Mg content in refined flours, Polyphenols was found to be 562 μg/g in hard wheat flour (bread flour) which was more than soft wheat flour about 501 μg/g. Manu [12] in 2006 also evaluated the polyphenol content in whole wheat flour and compared it to the composite wheat flour with supplementation and found that it was 299.20 mg/100 g of polyphenol in whole wheat flour. Singh [13] in the year 2006 also evaluated the polyphenols levels and the result showed that the polyphenol content was 298.39 mg/100 g of wheat flour. Nikita and the group in 2008 analyzed the proximate composition of five wheat varieties which were grown under both organic and inorganic farming conditions and found that on average, the polyphenol content of inorganic wheat was significantly higher than that of organic wheat varieties Among the five varieties a significant variation (275-342 mg) in polyphenol contents was observed; the C-306 and WH-711 varieties had the maximum amount of polyphenols. Rakhi and Punia [14,15] in 2013 while evaluating polyphenol content in wheat varieties found that polyphenol content of unprocessed wheat varieties ranged from 487.16 mg/100 g and 502.33 mg/100 g which decreased to 335.14-385.51 mg/100 g after germination.

Materials and Methods

The investigation or the experiment was conducted in the Department of Foods and Nutrition, I.C. College of Home Science, CCS Haryana Agricultural University, and Hisar. Two newly released varieties of wheat (WH-1080 and WH-1025) and one conventional variety of wheat C-306 were procured from the Department of Genetics and Plant Breeding, College of Agriculture, CCS HAU, Hisar in a single lot.

This section of materials and the methods will provide relevant information related to the research design and the methodologies used for the present investigation. All the research procedures have been clearly described below under the following headings and subheadings: 1) Procurement of material from the store; 2) Processing of raw wheat varieties: Roasting, Sprouting, and Malting; 3) Estimation of polyphenol content in the raw & processed wheat varieties.

Procurement of material from the store

Both the newly released wheat varieties (WH 1025, WH 1080) and one conventional variety C-306 was obtained from the Department of Genetics & Plant Breeding, CCS Haryana Agricultural University, and Hisar in a single lot. All the wheat varieties were first cleaned, washed thoroughly under running tap water so as to get rid of all the dust, soil particles and foreign matter adhered to the grains and then dried & ground to flour using flour mill which was available in the departmental laboratory and then the flour was used for nutritional evaluation of raw and processed wheat varieties and inference.

Processing of raw wheat varieties

Roasting: The wheat grains of all the three varieties which were procured were washed to remove dust and other foreign particles and then were dried under sun to remove excess water and then again dried in hot air oven at the temperature of 50°C for 24 hrs.

Sprouting: Wheat grains of all the varieties after washing and cleaning remove soil and dust were soaked for 12 hrs and after that they were kept in petri dishes or containers which were lined with wet filter paper to promote germination/sprouting and then kept in an incubator at 30°C for 48 hrs. All the grains were kept moist by sprinkling distilled water frequently. After 48 hrs sprouting occurs and the sprouts can be seen emerging out.

Malting: Malting process was done by the standard and approved method of Chaturvedi and Sarojini [16]. There were altogether four major stages involved. These were:

- **Steeping:** This process involves soaking of wheat grains in excess water for rehydration and to facilitate germination in the grains. All the three wheat varieties were soaked in germinating dish by using double the amount of 0.1% formaldehyde solution (to avoid microbial degradation). The mouth of the dish was covered with a cloth preferably muslin cloth by using rubber band and then the grains were allowed to soak for 6 hr at 25-30°C in an incubator. The un-imbibed water left was drained off without removing the cloth.
- **Aeration:** After steeping aeration was done by removing cloth for a period of 3 hrs in a well-ventilated room to enhance the enzyme activity. During aeration process, grains were rotated by glass rod occasionally. After aeration, grains were subjected to steeping with fresh formaldehyde solution for a period of 16 hrs and then the mouth of the dish was again covered. At the end of steeping period, extra water was drained off from the container and cloth was removed and the sample was air rested for a period of 2 hrs.
- **Germination:** The seeds which were soaked were sprayed with 25 ml of 0.1% formaldehyde solution to prevent the mold growth and then were allowed to germinate in an incubator at 25-30°C. The germinated grains were roasted twice daily. A constant humid atmosphere was maintained inside the incubator by means of keeping a pan of water. After 48 hrs and 72 hrs grain samples were removed from the incubator.
- **Kilning:** The grains which were germinated were dried in hot air oven at a temperature of 50°C for 24 hrs. Then the kilned grains were de vegetated by abrasive action. After kilning, grains which had characteristic malt aroma were obtained.

Polyphenol estimation

Total Polyphenols were extracted by the method of Singh and Jambunathan [17].

Defatted sample (500 mg) was refluxed with 50 ml methanol containing 1% HCL for four hours. The extract was concentrated by evaporating on a hot water bath and brought its volume to 25 ml with methanolic–HCL. The amount of polyphenolic compounds was estimated as tannic acid equivalent according to Folin-Davis procedure.

Reagents required

Folin-denis reagent preparation: To 750 ml water, 100 g sodium tungstate, 20 g phosphomolybdic acid and 50 ml phosphoric acid were added and heated and then refluxed for two hours.

Tannic acid (Stock solution): 100 mg of tannic acid was weighed and then dissolved in distilled water and the volume was made up to one liter. In order to use a working standard solution, 20 ml stock solution was diluted to 100 ml with water and the aliquot was made.

Saturated aqueous sodium carbonate solution: Sodium carbonate of amount 350 g was dissolved in one litre of hot distilled water at the temperature of 70-80°C, cooled and filtered through glass wool.

Procedure: In a graduated test tube add 1.5 ml of test solution/sample and 8.5 ml of distilled water. After thorough mixing, add Folin–Denis reagent and the tubes were well shaken. Exactly after 3 minutes, one ml of saturated sodium carbonate solution was added and the tubes were thoroughly shaken again. After an hour, the absorbance was read at 725 nm on UV-VIS Spectrophotometer -118 using a suitable blank. If the solution was cloudy or precipitates appeared, it was centrifuged before readings were taken. A standard curve was plotted by taking 0.5-4 ml working tannic acid standard solution containing 10-80 μg tannic acid.

Where,

M: Concentration of extract elute obtained from graph;

V: Volume made of Extract (ml);

W: Weight (g) of sample;

V1: Volume of extract aliquot taken (ml).

Results

The analysis was conducted with the objective of assessing the nutrient composition of the two newly released wheat varieties viz. WH-1080 & WH-1025 and one conventional variety i.e., C-306.

Various treatments like roasting, sprouting & malting were used to check the levels of polyphenol. The results obtained during the analysis or experiment was subjected to suitable statistical analysis, tabulated and have been presented systematically in the Table 1.

The polyphenol content of all the three wheat varieties ranged from 307.56-338.4 mg/100 g. The newly released varieties WH-1080 and WH-1025 did not differ significantly (P<0.05) among themselves and thus have similar polyphenol content (307.56 mg/100 g and 311.4 mg/100 g respectively).

The variety C-306 had significantly (P<0.05) higher polyphenol content (338.4 mg/100 g) as compared to the newly released varieties.

Varieties	Polyphenols
WH-1080	307.56+1.8
WH 1025	311.4+1.7
C 306	338.4+2.3
C.D (P<0.05)	4.03
Values represented are mean ± SE of three independent observations.	

Table 1: Polyphenol content of varieties of wheat (mg/100 g, on dry weight basis).

Variety Treatment	WH-1080	WH 1025	C-306	Mean of varieties
Unprocessed (Control)	307.56+1.8	311.4+1.7	338.4+2.3	304.84+0.23
Roasted	267.12+0.15	263.11+1.1	275.85+0.5	249.56 +11.89
Sprouted	218.98+1.1	241.42+2.3	229.51+1.7	294.58 +4.53
Malted	251.48+2.3	245.67+2.3	242.82+1.1	284.64 +4.64
Treatment Mean	261.28+0.21	267.15 +0.16	271.64 +0.29	-
CD(P<0.05)	Variety: 2.77 Treatment: 2.58 Interaction: 5.13			
Values represented are mean ± SE of three independent observations.				

Table 2: Effect of processing methods on polyphenol content of varieties of wheat (mg/100 g, as on dry weight basis).

Polyphenol content in wheat varieties which were not processed ranged from 307.56-338.4 mg/100 g and in processed wheat varieties from 218.98-275.85 mg/100 g. The processing methods resulted in significant decrease in polyphenol content. Highest reduction was observed in sprouting method (22.47-32.17%) and the decrease was significantly (P<0.05) higher than the other two treatments like roasting (13.14-18.48%) and malting (18.23-28.24%). Lowest polyphenol content was observed in sprouted WH-1080 variety (218.98 mg/100 g) (Table 2).

Discussion

The experiment was conducted to evaluate two newly released varieties of wheat namely WH-1080, WH-1025 and one conventional (already checked) wheat variety C-306 for their physico-chemical properties and nutritional composition. All the three wheat varieties were procured from the Department of Genetics and Plant Breeding, College of Agriculture, CCS HAU, Hisar in a single lot. The next step was cleaning of the wheat varieties and it was done manually to remove broken seeds, dust and other foreign matter and then washed under running water which was then dried & ground to flour using flour mill. All the three wheat varieties were processed using treatments like roasting, sprouting and malting using the standard procedures. The variety WH-1080 was found to have the lowest polyphenol content (307.56 mg/100 g) and variety C-306 had highest polyphenol content (338.4 mg/100 g). Many factors such as genetics, type of soils, environmental fluctuations, and year and fertilizer application influence the anti-nutrient composition of cereal grains as shown by the evidences [18].

Sprouting treatment significantly decreased polyphenol content among all the three wheat varieties when compared to the other two processing methods like roasting and malting. A significant difference in all the varieties was found to exist. Rakhi and Punia [15] found that there was reduction of polyphenol content after germination/sprouting and heat treatment. As polyphenols are present in the periphery of the seed there is possibility of their passing out into soaking water through seed coat. The reduction of polyphenolic compounds (tannins) after heat treatment (blanching) may be due to fact that these compounds, in addition to their predominance in seed coats are water soluble and consequently leach into the liquid medium [19]. This decrease could also be associated to that fact that these anti-nutrients are not heat stable and usually degrade upon heat treatment [20].

Summary and Conclusions

The varietyWH-1080 had lowest polyphenol content (307.56 mg/100 g) and variety C-306 had highest polyphenol content (338.4 mg/100 g). There existed significant difference in all the varieties. Sprouting significantly ($P<0.05$) reduced the anti-nutrient as compared to malting and roasting. A reduction of 22.47-32.17% of polyphenols levels during sprouting was observed. Thus method that was found to be most advantageous in reducing anti-nutrient (polyphenol) of all the processing methods in all the wheat varieties is sprouting.

References

1. Sikandra (2005) Development of value added products from sorghum and their nutritional and sensory evaluation. CCSHAU, Hisar, India
2. Hussain MA, Choudhary A, Howladar MA, Kabir KA (2010) Biochemical and functional properties of some newly released wheat varieties of Bangladesh. J Agric Res 24: 211-218.
3. Yadav S, Kumar P, Yadava RK, Gollen B, Kumar S, et al. (2011) Nutritional Contents and Medicinal Properties of Wheat. Life Sci Med Res 22: 1-10.
4. Qazi IM, Wahab S, Shad AA, Zeb A, Ayub M (2003) Effect of different fermentation time and baking on phytic acid content of whole wheat flour bread. Asian J Plant Sci 2B: 597-601.
5. Mallick SA, Kousar A, Gupta M, Sharma V, Sinha BK (2013) Characterization of grain nutritional quality in wheat. Ind J Plant Physiol 18 :183-186
6. Hemlatha M, Manu B, Bhagwat S, Leelawathi, Rao U (2007) Protein characteristics and peroxidase activities of different Indian Wheat varieties and their relationship to chapatti making quality. Europ Food Res Technol 225: 463-471.
7. Priyanka K, Sehgal S (2011) Nutritional evaluation of raw and processed chickpea varieties and its utilization for product development. CCSHAU, Hisar, India.
8. Hooda S (2002) Nutritional evaluation of fenugreek supplemented wheat products. Unpublished M.Sc. Thesis, CCS HAU, Hisar, India.
9. Sangwan V, Dahiya S (2002) Development and nutritional evaluation of wheat, sorghum, soybean composite flours biscuits. CCSHAU, Hisar, India
10. Varsha S (2003) Nutritional evaluation of utilization of selected cereals and pulses for value addition of wheat based products. CCSHAU, Hisar, India.
11. Ragee K (2006) Nutritional analysis of Cereals for food use. Int J Plant Physiol 88: 111-116.
12. Manu (2006) Development and nutritional evaluation of traditional food products incorporating calcium rich underutilized grains and leaves. CCS Haryana Agricultural University, Hisar, India.
13. Singh M, Sharma N, Khatkar BS (2006) End use quality of Indian wheat's: Milling properties and composition. J Food Sci Technol 43: 322-324.
14. Nikita, Punia D, Khetarpaul N (2008) Physico-chemical characteristics, nutrient composition and consumer acceptability of wheat varieties grown under organic and inorganic farming conditions. Int J Food Sci Nutr 59: 224-245.
15. Rakhi S, Punia D (2013) Nutritional evaluation and development of products from wheat. CCSHAU, Hisar, India.
16. Chaturvedi A, Sarojini G (1996) Malting of pearl millet (*Pennisetum typhoideum).* Its effect on starch and protein digestibility. J Food Sci Technol 33: 342-344.
17. Singh U, Jambunathan R (1981) Studies on desi and kabuli chickpea (*Cicer arietinum*) cultivars, Level of protease inhibitors, levels of polyphenolic compounds and *in vitro* protein digestibility. J Food Sci 46: 1364-1367.
18. Muahamad N, Faqir MA, Rai MA, Moazzam RK, Shahzad H, et al. (2010) An overview of anti-nutritional factors in cereal grains with special reference to wheat-A review. Pak J Food Sci 20: 54-61.
19. Reddy NR, Pierson MD, Sathe SK, Salunkhe DK (1989) Occupance Distribution Content and Dietary Intake of phytate in Cereal and Legumes. Thomson Science, London, pp: 39-56.
20. Rakic S, Petrovic S, Kukic J, Jadranin M, Tesevic V, et al. (2007) Influence of thermal treatment on phenolic compounds and antioxidant properties of oak acorns from Serbia. J Food Chem 104: 830-834.

Hypolipidemic Effect of Purslane (*Portulaca oleracea* L.) in Rats Fed on High Cholesterol Diet

Niharika Shanker and Sukumar Debnath*

Department of Traditional Food and Sensory Science, CSIR-Central Food Technological Research Institute, Mysore-570020, India

***Corresponding author:** Sukumar Debnath, Department of Traditional Food and Sensory Science, CSIR-Central Food Technological Research Institute, Mysore-570020, India, E-mail: debnath@cftri.res.in

Abstract

Purslane is a vegetarian source of n-3 PUFA (α-linolenic acid). The objective of the present work was to explore purslane as n-3 source to mitigate hyperlipidemia in rat model. Group of rats (n=48) were fed on high cholesterol diet to induce hyperlipidemia. Group 1,2,3,4 and 5 (n=6/group) were fed on aqueous extract of purslane (AEP) and lovastanin diet while group 6 and 7 were treated as hyperlipidemic and normal control. The results revealed a significant ($p<0.05$) reduction in serum TC, LDL-C, VLDL-C, TAG, increase in serum HDL-C level observed in AEP fed rats as compared to cholesterol induced hyperlipidemic control group. Groups treated with AEP and lovastatin also demonstrated considerable decrease in LDL-C: HDL-C ratios, levels of SGOT, SGPT, ALP activities and body weight in comparison to control group. Therefore, administration of AEP concluded that 150 mg/kg body weight AEP is a potent cardio-protective agent having preventive and curative effect against hyperlipidemia.

Keywords: Purslane; Hypolipidemia; Drying; PUFA; Cardio-protective agent

Introduction

The current lifestyle with high fat diet and less physical activity notably contribute to hypercholesterolemia and cardiovascular diseases [1]. Oxidative stress caused by reactive oxygen species (ROS) also plays main role in the etiology of numerous diseases including atherosclerosis and coronary heart disease [2]. Hyperlipidemia is one of the risk factors for coronary heart diseases. Epidemiological evidence supports that polyphenolic compounds found in fruit, vegetables and other plant material reduce coronary heart disease complications. Studies indicate that plant phenolics, flavonoids, flavonolignans and phenolic acids act at a molecular level as antioxidants and exhibits health-promoting properties. Furthermore, there are data suggesting the capability of phenolics to modulate and positively affect lipoprotein metabolism. Clinical trials also suggest that plant-based phenolics play a beneficial role in the prevention of coronary heart disease. Hence for herbal based cures is general practice. Hence nutraceuticals which can able to reduce hyperlipidemia induced complication or to control serum cholesterol and triacylglycerol levels has gained significant importance over the years, studied hypolipidemic and hepato-protective effect of n-3 and n-6 fatty acids rich flax and pumpkin seed lipids in hypercholesterolemic rats [3]. Although plant extracts compose potential candidates like phenolics they often have complexed with other molecules including antioxidants and pro-oxidant properties [4]. Owing to this reason in the present extract of purslane was investigated for its hypolipidemic potential. Reduction of the level of cholesterol in plasma is an efficient way to treat atherosclerosis. There are chemical drugs available (fibrates and statins) which has lipid-lowering potential. However, they fail to meet the demands for treatment further, patients prepare natural treatment rather synthetic drug due to their adverse effects and great drug dependence [5]. Hence, plant materials and their extracts became popular in treating hyperlipidemia with no adverse effects. Purslane, a member of Portulacaceae family, is well-known weed and has been ranked the eight mainly common plants in the world [6]. It has been reported to be the richest plant source of omega-3 fatty acids [FA] yet examined. Subsequent reports have confirmed the high levels of n-3 fatty acids and traces of EPA (C22: 5) and DHA (22: 6) [7] whose concentration is the highest in the leaves among leafy vegetables. Glutathione, glutamic acid and aspartic acid were also found in purslane. It is reported as the super food of the future due to its high nutritive and anti-oxidant properties [8]. It is considered as vegetable for long life in China and sold in theshops of United Arab Emirates and Oman. It is used as a traditional Chinese herbal medicine for skin [9]. A wide range of other pharmacological effects of purslane, such as antibacterial, analgesic, anti-inflammatory, wound-healing activities present in purslane. Anti-diabetic effect of extracts from purslane as alternate in streptozotocin induced diabetic rat model has also been reported [10]. Hypercholesterolemia has been reported to induce oxidative stress in various organs like liver, heart and kidney [11]. It has been shown that plants bio-actives antioxidants are better and random potential role in protecting people from numerous illnesses such as cardiovascular diseases. Purslane has also been reported to have a multiplicity of biological effects including hypoxia, hepato-protective properties and anti-hypertension effect, however, scientific validation on its efficacy is scarce in the literature. Clinical studies proposed that dyslipidaemiais one of the most important risk factors for coronary disease. It was reported from the preclinical studies that hypercholesterolemia promotes accumulation of low-density lipoprotein in the arterial wall, endothelial cell dysfunction and expansion of atherosclerosis [12]. It is evident from the literature there is no systematic similar studies available, hence based on the available information, it is hypothesized that extract of purslane may ameliorate hypercholesterolemic condition by affecting on various biochemical markers responsible for hypercholesterolemia in a rat model. Therefore, this study attempts to appraise the hypocholesteromic effect of purslane extract. The outcome of the study will have implications for improving hypercholesteromic condition and purslane serve as partial replacement of anti-hyperlipidemic drug which causes side effects.

Materials and Methods

Plant material and preparation of purslane leaf extracts

Fresh purslane was procured from super market Mysore India. The leaves were collected and surface sterilized after washing thoroughly in tap water to remove adhering dust and mud particles, followed by rinsed in distilled water and the excess water was drained off. The dried leaves were stored at room temperature in a dry place prior to use. Oven-dried (50-60°C) [13] leaves of the plant were divided into three parts weighing 25 g each. Then they were finely powdered and extracted by maceration with (3×250 mL) of water at ambient temperature for 12 h with continuous stirring. The process was repeated thrice. The aqueous extracts were filtrated with No. 1 Whatman filter paper and concentrated to dryness with a rotary evaporator at 50 ± 1°C to give solid residues. The yield was calculated to be 16.71 ± 0.7%. The dried extracts were kept in the dark at 4°C prior analysis.

Drugs and chemicals

Statin was purchased from Mysore, Solvents like methanol, chloroform, petroleumether, acetone, di-ethyl ether were of analytical grade (Rankem, Bangalore, India). Serum Cholesterol kit, Serum Triglyceride kit, Serum HDL Cholesterol kit, Serum LDL-Cholesterol kit, SGOT, SGPT, ALP were purchased from Aggape (Kumar diagnostic, Mysore). Standard mixtures of fatty acid methyl esters (C8-C24) were procured from Supelco-Sigma Aldrich, Bangalore, India.

Total phenolic contents

Total phenol content was determined using [14] method. One and a half millilitre of Folin–Ciocalteu's reagent (diluted 10 times) and 1.2 mL of Na_2CO_3 (7.5% w/v) solution were added to 300 mL of plant extract. Solution was shaken and kept to stand at room temperature (25 ± 2°C) for 30 min prior to measuring absorbance at 765 nm with a spectrophotometer (Anthelie Advanced 5 Secoman, France). The total phenol content (TPC) was expressed as gallic acid equivalent in mg/100 g fresh plant material.

Determination of antioxidant activity

The capability of a compound to donate a hydrogen atom was assessed on the basis of the scavenging activity of the DPPH (1,1-diphenyl-2-picrylhydrazyl) radical according to Miliauskas et al. [15] with slight modifications. Two millilitres of 0.15 mm DPPH was added to 1 mL of extracts in different dilutions. A control was prepared by adding 2 mL of DPPH to 1 mL of methanol. The contents of the tubes were mixed, allowed to stand for 30 min and absorbance was measured at 517 nm. Triplicate tubes were prepared for each extract. The results were expressed as % radical scavenging activity, which is:

$$\frac{\text{Controlabsorbance-sampleabsorbance}}{\text{Controlabsorbance}} \times 100 \text{ (Equation 1)}$$

Determination of phenolics by HPLC procedure

The HPLC–MS system was composed of Shimadzu LC20AD HPLC system, ShimadzuSPD20AV UV–vis detector, and Shimadzu 2010EV mass spectrometer fitted with an electrospray interface (Shimadzu, Kyoto, Japan). The column was an Alltech PrevailC18 (Alltech, Deerfield, IL), 150 mm to 4.6 mm. The mobile phase was 0.05% (v/v) aqueous acetic acid (phase A) and 0.05% acetic acid in 80% acetonitrile +20% methanol (phase B) at a flow rate of 0.8 mL/min. The linear gradient of phase B was 5%for the first 2 min, increased from 5% to 40% from 2 min to 48 min, maintained at 40% from 48 min to 57 min, and decreased from 40% to 5% from 57 min to 57.1 min. Finally, isocratic elution with 5% phase B was maintained until 65 min. UV–vis detector wavelength was set at 280 nm. Mass spectra were acquired in negative ion mode. Ion was scanned from m/z 150–600 with scan speed 1000 amu/s. Nebulizing gas flow was 1.5 L/min. Drying gas pressure was 0.1 MPa.

Lipid extraction and analysis of fatty acids

Total lipids were extracted by the method of Bligh and Dyer [16] with minor modifications. In brief, 0.5 g of dehydrated leaf sample was homogenized with chloroform–methanol (2:1 v/v) solution. To the homogenate, 1% KCl (w/v) was added and the content was filtered through filter paper (Whatman no 1). The filtrate was allowed to separate into two phases and the lower (chloroform) phase was collected into previously weighted test tube, dried under the stream of N_2 vapour and total lipid content was determined gravimetrically. To find out fatty acid profile of lipid, fatty acid methyl esters (FAME) were prepared using BF_3 in methanol method [17]. Peak identification of fatty acids was performed by comparison of the retention time with respective reference standards.

Analysis of FAME by GC-MS

FAMEs were analysed by GC-MS (Perkin Elmer, Turbomass Gold, Mass spectrometer) equipped with FID using fused silica Rtx-2330 column (Restek made, 30 m×0.32 mm ID and 0.20 μm film thickness]. Injector port and the detector were set up at 230 and 250°C respectively. N_2 was used as a carrier gas. Initially, column temperature was maintained at 120°C, followed by increasing to 220°C in 20 min, and hold at 220°C for 10 min. The fatty acids were identified by comparing their fragmentation pattern and retention time with authentic standards and also the NIST library.

Animals grouping

Male Wistar rats (OUTB-Wistar) weighing 150 g ± 10 g were grouped by random distribution n=6. They were placed in individual cagesin an approved animal house facility at CSIR-Central Food Technological Research Institute, Mysore, India. Institutional animal ethical committee approved the experimental protocol. Animals were given fresh diet daily and left over dietswere weighed and discarded. The Gain in body weight of animal was monitored at regular intervals. The animals had free access to food and water throughout the study. They were maintained under standard laboratory conditions (temperature 20 ± 3°C; 12 h light–dark cycle).

Induction of hypercholesterolemia with high cholesterol diet

The rats were fed ad libitum AIN-93 [18] supplemented (control group), and other groups were fed ad libitum AIN-93 diet containing with 1% cholesterol (experimental group). The feeding experiment was conducted over aperiod of 60 days. The experimental procedures was carried out according to the National Institute of Health Guidelines for Animal Care and approved by the Ethics Committee of our Institution.

In the present study, four doses of the AEP extract were selected as 50 mg, 100 mg, 150 mg and 200 mg/kg bw.

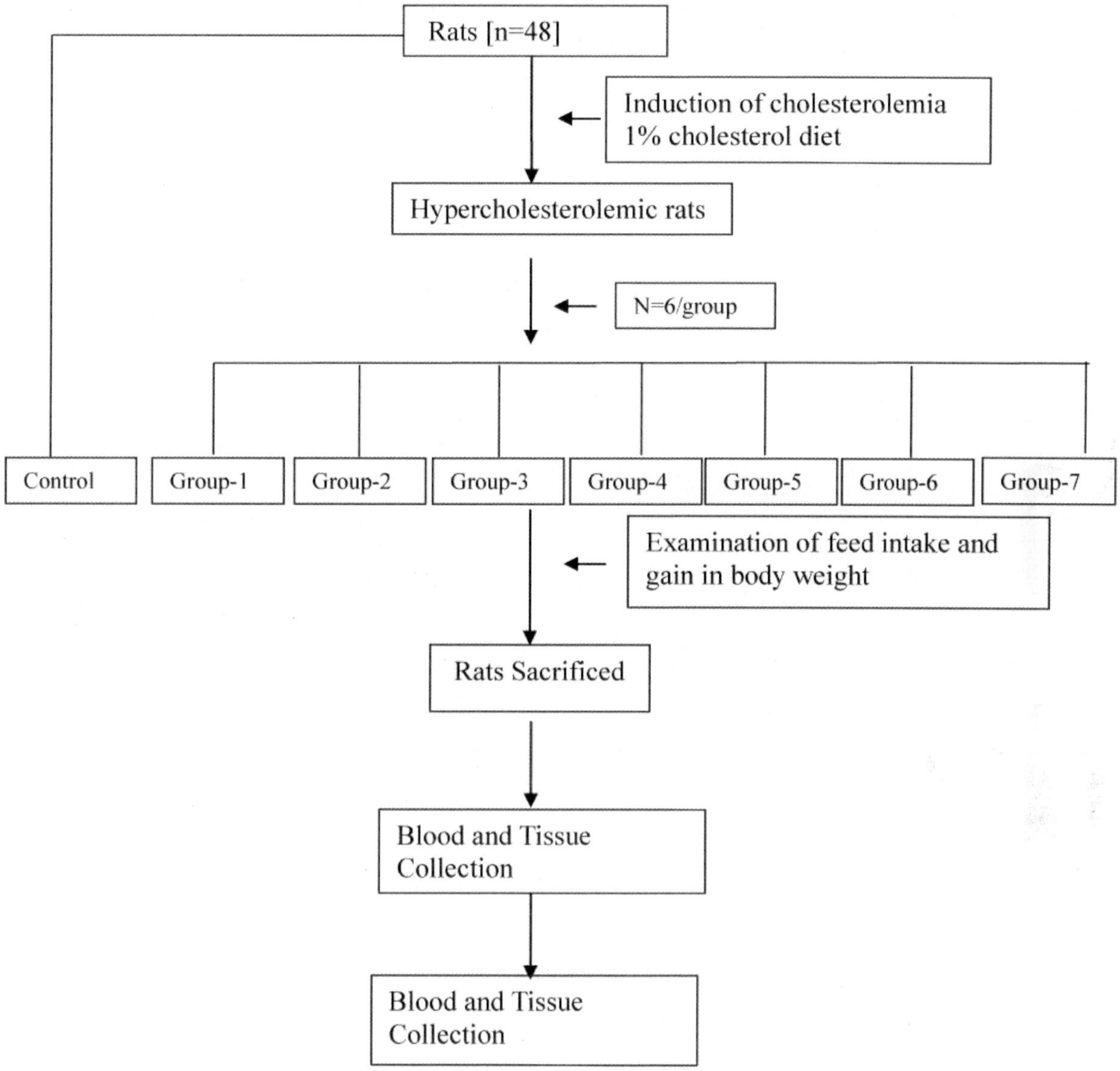

Figure 1: Experimental design.

The rats were randomly divided into seven groups of six each (Figure 1).

Group (Control): The Normal group in which the rats were daily given AIN-93 diet.

Group II: Hyperlipidemic group in which the rats were daily administered with 1% cholesterol in diet.

Group III: Test group in which the rats were daily administered with aqueous extract of purslane (50 mg/kg/day) along with 1% cholesterol in the diet.

Group IV: Test group in which the rats were daily administered with aqueous extract of purslane (100 mg/kg/day) along with 1% cholesterol in diet.

Group V: Test group in which the rats were daily administered with aqueous extract of purslane (150 mg/kg/day) along with 1% cholesterol in the diet.

Group VI: Test group in which the rats were daily administered with aqueous extract of purslane (200 mg/kg/day) along with 1% cholesterol in the diet.

Group VII: Standard group in which the rats were daily administered with Atorvastatin (20 mg/kg/day) along with 1% cholesterol in the diet.

Body weight

The body weight (in g) was recorded on day one and then weekly consecutively for 59 days using a laboratory animal weighing balance.

Biochemical analysis

All the animals were sacrificed on the 60th day of the experiment by cervical dislocation. The blood samples were collected by cardiac puncture and separately sterilized into dry centrifugation tubes and allowed to stand for 30 min at 20-25°C.

The clear serum was separated at 3000 rpm for 10 min using a centrifuge. Levels of serum glucose, total TC, HDL-C, TG, LDL-C, SGOT, SGPT and ALP were determined to analyze using auto-analyzer (semi-autoanalyzer Erba), with commercial kits (Kumar diagnostics Pvt Ltd.). The Friedewald formula was used to calculate VLDL (=total cholesterol-HDL-LDL) and atherogenic index (=(TCHDL-C)/HDL-C)).

In-vivo antioxidant activity: preparation of liver homogenate

The liver samples stored were thawed and used for analysis of antioxidant enzyme. Liver samples were homogenized in ice-cold 0.1 M phosphate buffered saline of pH 7.4 (10% homogenate) followed by centrifugation at 10,000 rpm for 10 min. The supernatant was used to prepare aliquots of homogenates to carry out the superoxide dismutase (SOD) and catalase assays.

Estimation of super oxide dismutase (SOD)

An indirect method of inhibiting auto-oxidation of epinephrine to its adrenochrome was used to analyze SOD activities in blood serum. About 0.5 mL of blood serum was diluted with 0.5 mL of distilled water, to this 0.25 mL of ethanol; 0.5 mL of chloroform (all chilled reagents) was added. The mixture was allowed to vortex for 1 min and centrifuge at 2000 rpm for 20 min.

The SOD activity in the supernatant was determined by the addition of 0.05 mL of carbonate buffer (0.05 M pH 10.2) and 0.5 mL of EDTA. The reaction was initiated by addition of 0.4 mL of epinephrine and read the O.D using spectrophotometer at 480 nm. The SOD activity was expressed as Units/mg protein transformed in optical density/mm. About 50% inhibition of epinephrine to adrenochrome transition by the enzyme is taken [19].

Estimation of catalase (CAT)

The activity of catalase (CAT) in liver homogenate was measured by the decrease in absorption at 240 nm using spectrophotometer. Reaction mixture consists of 995 microliter phosphate buffer (0.1 nm, ph-7), 5 mL of sample and 50 mL of (8.8 nM). One CAT activity is defined as the amount of enzyme required to decompose I milt of H_2O_2/min liver homogenate [20].

Statistical analysis

Results were presented as mean ± S.D. The significance of variation among the groups was observed using one way analysis of variance (ANOVA). All the experiments were repeated thrice.

Results and Discussion

Hyperlipidemia continues to be a main health problem in India and other developing countries, which lead to vital risk factors like atherosclerosis, stroke etc.

Hyperlipidemia evokes the damages in various tissues, which in turn, deregulates the cellular functions foremost to various pathological conditions. It is known that nutrition plays an important role in the etiology of hyperlipidemia and atherosclerosis [21].

Phytochemical analysis

The results of the preliminary phytochemical screening of aqueous extract of purslane leaves (AEP) showed the presence of total polyphenol, antiradical activity (Table 1a) and flavonoids (Table 1b).

Total Polyphenol content (mg GAE/100DW)	283.17 ± 0.6
Antiradical activity (%)	86.79 ± 0.14
Values are expressed as mean ± standard deviation	

Table 1a: Total polyphenol content and antiradical activity of aqueous extract of dried purslane.

Sample	Phenolic acids (mg/100 g dry wt.)		Flavonoids content (mg/100 g dry wt.)		
	Rosmarinic acid	Ferulic acid	Kaempferol	Quercetin	Coumaric acid
Aqueous extract of Purslane	0.55 ± 0.02	4.85 ± 0.06	0.41 ± 0.08	0.92 ± 0.03	0.34 ± 0.02
Values are expressed as mean ± standard deviation					

Table 1b: Phenolic acids and flavonoids content of aqueous extract of dried purslane.

Fatty acid profile of purslane

The Tables 2a and 2b showed that the presence of PUFA and α-linolenic acid (ALA) was observed in the dried purslane to an extent of 52.65% and 60.97% respectively.

Capric acid (C10:0)	Lauric acid (C12:0)	Myristic acid (C14:0)	Palmitic acid (C16:0)	Stearic acid (C18:0)	Oleicacid (C18:1)	Linoleic acid (C18:2)	α-Linolenic acid (C18:3)
	-	-					-
1.4 ± 0.2	0.75 ± 0.1	0.8 ± 0.3	19.7 ± 0.1	7.1 ± 0.3	9.5 ± 0.2	12.1 ± 0.1	48.6 ± 0.3

Table 2a: Fatty acid (% relative area).

SFA	MUFA	PUFA	ALA
29.75 ± 0.2	9.5 ± 0.1	60.7 ± 0.2	48.6 ± 0.3
Where, S: Saturated; MU: Monounsaturated; PU: Polyunsaturated; FA: Fatty acids; ALA: α-Linolenic acid			

Table 2b: Distribution of SFA, MUFA and PUFA content of dried purslane.

Effects of high-fat diet and AEP on body and organ weight

There was no difference among the treatment groups at the commencement. However upon animals fed with cholesterol diet showed significant increase in body weight compared to those feed with control diet (p<0.01) (Table 3). The untreated hyperlipidemic group showed significantly higher organ weight (liver) in comparison with HCD group (p<0.05). However, no significant difference was found in the weight of kidney and heart between high-fat diet and control group.

Initial weeks	Control (g)	Untreated (g)	Drug Treated (g)	50 concentration (mg/kg bw)	100 concentration (mg/kg bw)	150 concentration (mg/kg bw)	200 concentration (mg/kg bw)
Initial bw (g)	193.4 ± 1.3	180 ± 2.1	198 ± 0.9	195.75 ± 1.4	201.25 ± 2.3	195 ± 1.4	200.5 ± 1.3
2nd	224.0 ± 0.7	231.0 ± 2	233.0 ± 0.7	235.0 ± 0.8	213.0 ± 1.4	230.0 ± 0.8	239.1 ± 2.6
3rd	230.0 ± 0.9	247.0 ± 1	240.0 ± 0.8	244.0 ± 0.6	225.0 ± 1.7	235.0 ± 2.5	226.0 ± 1.9
4th	250.0 ± 0.6	288.0 ± 1	261.7 ± 1.3	259.7 ± 1.5	254.5 ± 1	260.0 ± 1.6	252.2 ± 0.9
5th	262.5 ± 1.4	316.0 ± 2	271.2 ± 0.8	271.2 ± 1.7	266.0 ± 0.6	278.5 ± 1.3	268.7 ± 0.5
6th	269.2 ± 0.9	330.0 ± 0.6	278.0 ± 2.4	281.2 ± 1.2	272.4 ± 1	285.2 ± 0.7	285.2 ± 1.4
7th	278.5 ± 2.4	341.0 ± 2	296.6 ± 1.7	289.7 ± 1.8	281.2 ± 1.3	296.2 ± 0.5	289.2 ± 2.3
Final bw	265.0 ± 1.6	333.7 ± 0.5	285.0 ± 1.4	273.5 ± 1.4	267.0 ± 0.8	288.0 ± 1.6	280.0 ± 1.2
Liver weight	7.75 ± 0.3	9.8 ± 0.6	7.8 ± 0.5	7.95 ± 0.4	7.46 ± 0.3	7.65 ± 0.6	7.47 ± 0.7
Heart weight	0.8 ± 0.5	0.8 ± 0.4	0.8 ± 0.3	0.80 ± 0.7	0.75 ± 0.2	0.75 ± 0.4	0.53 ± 0.3
Kidney weight (g)	1.32 ± 0.9	1.8 ± 0.7	1.63 ± 0.4	1.5 ± 0.6	1.34 ± 0.7	1.57 ± 0.7	1.65 ± 0.6
Where, bw: Body weight of animals							

Table 3: Variation in body weight of rats fed a 1% cholesterol diet and treated with AEP extracts for 7 weeks.

Effect of administration of AEP on biochemical parameters of high cholesterol diet induced hyperlipidemia

The effect of AEP on lipid levels of serum in treated rats is shown in Figure 2. The results showed that the levels of TG, TC, LDL-C and VLDL-C in the HCD treated group were significantly higher ($p<0.05$), while the level of HDL-C was significantly lower ($p<0.01$), when compared to normal and other treated groups. The results on serum lipid profile of HCD groups with doses of AEP (150 mg/kg), showed significant ($p<0.01$) decrease in serum parameters TG, TC, LDL, VLDL and significantly ($p<0.05$) increase in HDL, whereas atorvastatin showed significantly ($p<0.05$) decrease in TG, TC, LDL, VLDL and increase ($p<0.01$) in HDL when compare with that of high cholesterol diet group. The effect of AEP as a feed supplement at four doses, i.e., 50, 100, 150 and 200 mg/kg bw, resulted in a dose-dependent reduction in lipid profiles.

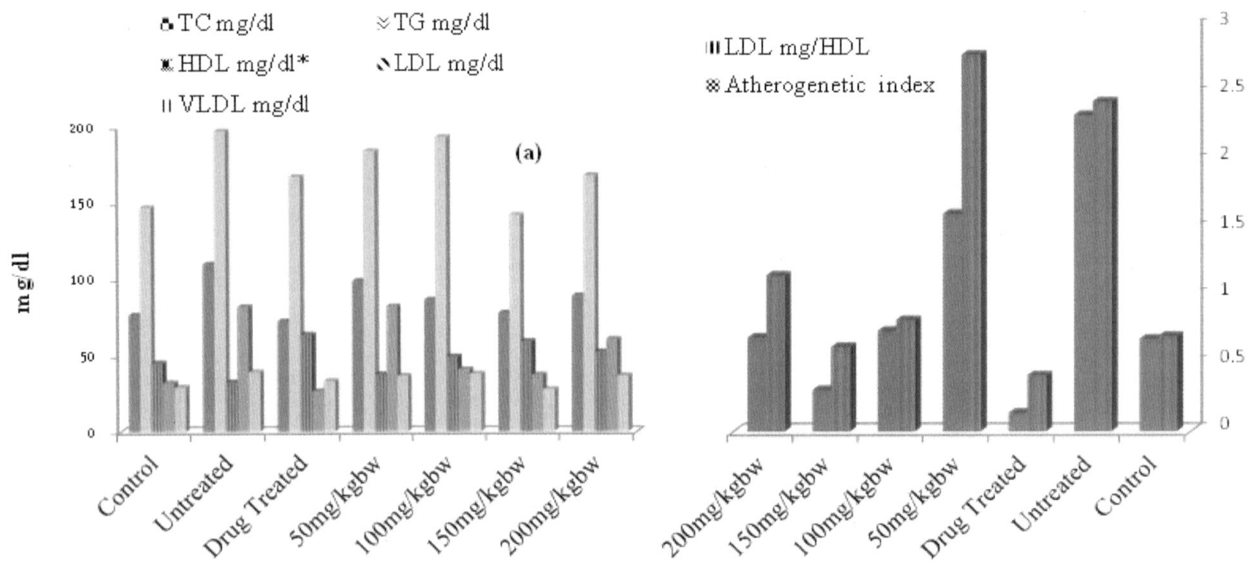

Figure 2: Serum lipid profile of adult male albino wistar rats fed on 1% cholesterol diet with the AEP (Values are expressed as mean SEM, n=6. Comparison made between normal control to hyperlipidemic control and drug treated groups ($p<0.05$, $^*p<0.01$)).

Excessive amounts of PUFA (omega6 fatty acids) and a very high omega6 fatty acids/omega3 fatty acids ratio, as is found in today's Western diets, promote the pathogenesis of many diseases, including cardiovascular disease, cancer, inflammatory and autoimmune diseases, whereas increased levels of omega3 fatty acids (a lower omega-6 fatty acids/omega3 fatty acids ratio), exert suppressive effects. In the secondary prevention of cardiovascular disease, a ratio of 4/1 was associated with a 70% decrease in total mortality. In our study also we found that 200 mg/kg wt group rats were having some toxic effect.

Effects of AEP on LDL/HDL and Atherogenic index

As seen from Figure 2 the leaves of LDL/HDL and Atherogenic index are higher in the HCD treated groups compared to normal and other treated groups.

Effect of AEP extract on liver enzymes

As shown in Table 4a, treatment with AEP extracts exhibit a hepatoprotective effect, indicated by decreased levels of SGOT, SGPT, and ALP. The increased liver enzyme levels and the formation of hepatic steatosis (fatty liver) in the high cholesterol diet-fed groups are allied with a significant increase of liver weight. The administration of the extract resulted in the prevention of hepatic fatty deposition in hepatocytes.

The superoxide dismutase (SOD) activity in the hyperlipidemic control group has shown (Table 4b) considerable decline as compared to the normal group. The treatment with standard drug Atorvastatin as well as the four doses of the AEP led to the significant ($p<0.05$) increase in SOD activity levels thus demonstrating the antioxidant activity of the extract. The Atorvastatin treated group showed the highest increase in SOD activity, followed by the 200 mg/kg body weight. As it is seen from Table 4b, the catalase activity has also showed a considerable decrease in the hyperlipidemic control group. Treatment by the standard drug Atorvastatin and the two doses of the AEP led to a significant ($p<0.05$) increase in catalase activity. The Atorvastatin treated group showed the highest increase in catalase activity, followed by the 150 mg/kg body weight doses of the AEP. The cholesterol lowering effect of purslane may be attributed to the combined effect of omega-3 fatty acids, phenolics compound and pectin [22]. As shown in the present study, while elevating plasma HDL-c levels, AEP lowered to plasma total cholesterol and LDL-c levels dose dependently. There is a positive correlation exists among the risk of developing ischemic heart disease and raised plasma total cholesterol and LDL-c concentrations [23]. The weight losing effect of AEP observed in this study could either be as a result of its lipid lowering or appetite inhibiting of binding affinity of pectin with dietary lipids that is not available for absorption [24]. The protective role of glutathione, as an antioxidant and detoxifying agent, has been demonstrated in various clinical studies [25]. It is a ubiquitous compound that is synthesized rapidly in the liver, kidney and other tissues, including the gastrointestinal tract. In animal cells, glutathione acts as a substrate for glutathione peroxidase, which reduces lipid peroxides that are formed from polyunsaturated fatty acids (PUFA) in the diet and as a substrate for glutathione S-transferase, which conjugates electrophilic compounds. Many evidences showed that glutathione obtained from the diet is directly absorbed by the gastrointestinal tract and thus dietary glutathione can readily increase the antioxidant status in humans [26]. The antioxidant enzymes such as GPx, GR, SODand GST, take part in maintaining GSH homeostasis in tissues [27]. Also, increased levels of GPx, GR, GST, CAT and SOD, were all found to correlate with elevated glutathione level and depressed MDA and NO in rats, showing the antioxidant activity of purslane. In conclusion, purslane leaf is beneficial for hepatic and cardio-protective activities as it has an antioxidant properties and nutritive value.

	Control	Untreated	Drug Treated	50 concentration (mg/kg bw)	100 concentration (mg/kg bw)	150 concentration (mg/kg bw)	200 concentration (mg/kg bw)
SGOT U/dL	40.14 ± 0.4	56.71 ± 1.2	38.83 ± 0.9	58.02 ± 1.4	41.88 ± 0.6	47.99 ± 1.1	46.05 ± 0.8
SGPT U/dL	56.78 ± 0.3	78.17 ± 1.4	54.15 ± 0.9	58.75 ± 1.5	64.56 ± 0.7	40.57 ± 1.4	57.94 ± 1.6
ALP U/dL	152 ± 0.7	256 ± 1.1	157 ± 0.8	280 ± 1.4	211 ± 1.6	172.4 ± 0.8	225 ± 1.8
Values are expressed as mean ± SE of animals, p values <0.05							

Table 4a: Effect of AEP on liver enzyme activity in normal and hypercholesterolemic rats.

Dosage Groups	SOD	Catalase
	(Units/min/mg protein)	(µmoles of H_2O_2/min/mg)
Control	12.33 ± 0.5	222.5 ± 2.8
High Cholesterol Die (HCD)	5.31 ± 0.2	110.3 ± 2.6
HCD+AEP 50 mg/kg	6.18 ± 0.2	132.7 ± 1.1
HCD+AEP 100 mg/kg	8.12 ± 0.4	149.8 ± 3.2
HCD+AAEE 150 mg/kg	10.22 ± 0.4	192.8 ± 2.2
HCD+AEP 200 mg/kg	9.12 ± 0.3	205.8 ± 1.4
HCD+STD (Atorvastatin)	11.08 ± 0.8	237.5 ± 3.6
Values are expressed as Mean ± SEM, (=6). Significant difference compared to control; significant difference compared to HFD, <0.05		

Table 4b: Effect of AEP on antioxidant activity of SOD and catalase in hyperlipidemic rats.

Conclusion

Purslane is used traditionally in medicine to manage, control, and/or treat diabetes mellitus and hypertension. The present study demonstrate the aqueous extract (50-200 mg/kg bw) of leaves fed to hyperglycaemic rats indicate that the leaf aqueous extract of purslane possesses hypolipidemic properties, and thus purslane can be used in the management or control of hyperlipidemia. However, dietary studies are needed to further confirm the impact of purslane on lipid metabolism. Further purslane can be used as an easily accessible source of natural antioxidants.

Acknowledgement

The authors thank Professor Ram Rajasekharan, Director, CSIR-CFTRI, Mysore, for providing infrastructure, constant encouragement and support. The authors also thank the Head, Department of Animal House, CSIR-CFTRI, Mysore, for providing all the facilities and suggestions during animal study. The first author gratefully acknowledges U.G.C for providing the financial assistance to carry out the present investigation. The help of Dr V Baskaran, Senior Principal Scientist, Department of Biochemistry, CSIR-CFTRI, Mysore, is highly acknowledged.

References

1. Donahue RP, Abbott RD, Bloom E, Reed DM, Yano K (1987) Central obesity and coronary heart disease in men. Lancet 1: 821-824.
2. Tribble DL (1999) Antioxidant consumption and risk of coronary heart disease: emphasis on vitamin C, vitamin E, and ß-carotene: A statement for healthcare professionals from the American Heart Association. Circulation 99: 591-595.
3. Makni M, Fetoui H, Gargouri NK, Garoui el M, Jaber H, et al. (2008) Hypolipidemic and hepatoprotective effects of flax and pumpkin seed mixture rich in omega-3 and omega-6 fatty acids in hypercholesterolemic rats. Food Chem Toxicol 46: 3714-3720.

4. Parejo I, Viladomat F, Bastida J, Rosas-Romero A, Flerlage N, et al. (2002) Comparison between the radical scavenging activity and antioxidant activity of six distilled and nondistilled Mediterranean herbs and aromatic plants. J Agri Food Chem 50: 6882-6890.
5. Alsheikh-Ali AA, Kuvin JT, Karas RH (2004) Risk of adverse events with fibrates. Am J Cardiol 94: 935-938.
6. Osman SM, Hussein MA (2015) Purslane Seeds Fixed Oil as a Functional Food in Treatment of Obesity Induced by High Fat Diet in Obese Diabetic Mice. J Nutr Food Sci 5: 1.
7. Ezekwe MO, Omara-Alwala TR, Membrahtu T (1999) Nutritive characterization of purslane accessions as influenced by planting date. Plant Foods Hum Nutr 54: 183-191.
8. Al-Howiriny T (2008) Protective effect of purslane on rat liver injury induced by carbon tetrachloride. Saudi Pharm J 16: 239-244.
9. Hu LF, Xu XY, Wang BQ (2003) Research and utilization situation of *Portulaca oleracea* L. in China. Prac. J Med Pharm 20: 315-316.
10. Singh V, Kori ML (2014) Antidiabetic effect of hydroalchololic combined plant extract of *portulaca oleracea* and caralluma attenuate in streptozotocin induced diabetic rats. Indo Am J Pharm Res 4: 03.
11. Vijayakumar RS, Surya D, Nalini N (2004) Antioxidant efficacy of black pepper (Piper nigrum L.) and piperine in rats with high fat diet induced oxidative stress. Redox Rep 9: 105-110.
12. Takahashi Y, Zhu H, Yoshimoto T (2005) Essential roles of lipoxygenases in LDL oxidation and development of atherosclerosis. Antioxid Redox Signal 7: 425-431.
13. Niharika S, Sukumar D (2015) Impact of dehydration of purslane on retention of bioactive molecules and antioxidant activity. J Food Sci Technol 52: 6631-6638.
14. Singleton VL, Rossi JA (1965) Colorunetry of total phenolics with phosphomolybdic-phosphotungstic acid reagents. Am J Enol Viticul 16: 144-158.
15. Miliauskas G, Venskutonis PR, Van Beek TA (2004) Screening of radical scavenging activity of some medicinal and aromatic plant extracts. Food Chem 2: 231-237.
16. Bligh EG, Dyer WJ (1959) A rapid method of total lipid extraction and purification. Can J Biochem Physiol 37: 911-917.
17. O'Fallon JV1, Busboom JR, Nelson ML, Gaskins CT (2007) A direct method for fatty acid methyl ester synthesis: application to wet meat tissues, oils, and feedstuffs. J Anim Sci 85: 1511-1521.
18. Reaves GP, Nielsen HF, Fohey CG (1993) AIN- 93 purified diets for laboratory rodents: Final report of the American Institute of Nutrition. Ad hoc writing committee on the reformulation of the AIN- 76A rodent diet. J Nutr 123.
19. Misra HP, Fridovich I (1976) The oxidation of phenylhydrazine: superoxide and mechanism. Biochemistry 15: 681-687.
20. Aebi H, Bergmeyer HV (1974) Methods in enzymatic analysis, New York: Academic press 2: 674-684.
21. Dhulasavant V, Shinde S, Naikwade MPNS (2010) Antihyperlipidemic activity of Cinnamomum tamala Nees on high cholesterol diet induced. Int J Pharm Tech Res 2: 2517-2521.
22. Car NM, Go I, Larraur JA, Alonso AG, Calixto FS (1999) Reduction in serum total and LDL cholesterol concentrations by a dietary fiber and polyphenol-rich grape product in hypercholesterolemic rats. Nutr Res 19: 1371-1381.
23. Oladele SB, Ayo JO, Adaudi AO (1995) Medicinal and physiological properties of flavonoids, coumarin derivatives and anthraquinones of plant origin. West African J Pharmacol Drug Res 11: 134-144.
24. Liya LI, Xu J, Mu Y, Han L, Liu R, et al. (2015) Chemical characterization and anti-hyperglycaemic effects of polyphenol enriched longan (Dimocarpus longan Lour) pericarp extracts. J Func Foods 13: 314-332.
25. Simopoulos AP (2004) Omega-3 fatty acids and antioxidants in edible wild plants. Biol Res 37: 263-277.
26. Jones DP, Hagen TM, Weber R, Wierzbicka GT, Bonkovsky HL (1989) Oral administration of glutathione (GSH) increases plasma GSHconcentrations in humans. FASEB J 3: A1250.
27. Abdel-Moneim AE, Dkhil MA, Al-Quraishy S (2011) The redox status in rats treated with flaxseed oil and lead-induced hepatotoxicity. Biol Trace Elem Res 143: 457-467.

Effect of Storage on Physicochemical Properties of Spiced Fish Sauce

Dagadkhair AC[1*], Pakhare KN[2] and Gadhave RK[3]

[1]Department of Food Chemistry and Nutrition, Vasantrao Naik Marathwada Krishi Vidyapith, Parbhani, MH, India

[2]Department of Technology, Food Technology Division, Shivaji University, Kolhapur, MH, India

[3]Department of Food Engineering and Technology, SLIET, Sangrur, Punjab, India

[*]**Corresponding author:** Dagadkhair AC, Department of Food Chemistry and Nutrition, College of Food Technology, Vasantrao Naik Marathwada Krishi Vidyapith, Parbhani, MH, India, E-mail: amoldagadkhair007@gmail.com

Abstract

The study encompasses the influence of storage on physicochemical properties of spiced sauce at ambient temperature on 15 days interval up to 60 days. The results pertaining to physicochemical properties studied on fresh day and 60 days demonstrate that the moisture content of sauce was gradually increased from (65.81 g/100 g) to (66.20 g/100 g), fat was slightly decreased from (6.20 g/100 g) to (6.08 g/100 g), protein was increased from (5.72 g/100 g) to (6.25 g/100 g), carbohydrate steadily decreased during storage time from (16.15 g/100 g) to (15.10 g/100 g), total ash was constantly between 2.88 g/100 g to 2.90 g/100 g during whole study, Salt found 3.20 g/100 g to 3.18 g/ 100 g during storage, the pH was (5.62) to (4.87), the total organic acidity was 1.05 to 1.23, TSS of sauce was slightly increased during storage was increased from fresh (21° Bx) to 60th days (23° Bx) simultaneously. And the viscosity of sauce drastically decreases with storage during study as from fresh (282.0 cP) to 60th day (260.4 cP). The results obtained reveals that change in the physicochemical properties of spiced fish sauce was due to lactic acid fermentation during storage. The dominant flora was counted on same day of chemical analysis simultaneously and the results revealed gradual increase in growth from fresh day 2.9×10^3 to 4.1×10^3 at 60th day.

Keywords: Spiced ish sauce; Storage; LAB's fermentation; Physicochemical properties

Introduction

India is the second largest producer of marine water fish and the second largest producer of fresh water fish in the world. Fish production has increased from 41.57 lakh tonnes (24.47 lakh tonnes for marine and 17.10 lakh tonnes for inland fisheries) in 1991-92 to 86.66 lakh tonnes (33.71 lakh tonnes for marine and 52.95 lakh tonnes for inland fisheries) in 2011-2012 [1].

Fish is a rich source of animal protein and its culture is an efficient protein food production system from aquatic environment. The main role of fish culture is its contribution in improving the nutritional standards of the people. Fish and fishery products represent a valuable source of nutrients of fundamental importance for diversified and healthy diets. Fish provides not only high-value protein, but also a wide range of essential micronutrients, including various vitamins (D, A and B), minerals (including calcium, iodine, zinc, iron and selenium) and polyunsaturated omega-3 fatty acids (docosahexaenoic acid and eicosapentaenoic acid) [2,3]. The nutritive value of fish proteins is comparatively high because of the favorable essential amino acid pattern. Fish proteins are rich in all the essential amino acids (particularly methionine and lysine), in contrast with most proteins from plant sources, which lack adequate amounts of one or more essential amino acids. As compared with red meat, fish proteins are considered nutritionally equivalent or slightly superior [4].

Fermentation is one of the oldest techniques in food preservation as it not only extends the shelf-life but also enhances the flavour and nutritional quality of the product [5]. In Southeast Asia, fish sauce is made from various types of fish, from both freshwater and marine fish species, by various methods. Each has its unique taste and characteristic. Fish sauce is known as '*nampla*' in Thailand, '*patis*' in Philippines, '*kecapikan*' in Indonesia, '*budu*' in Malaysia, '*nuocnam*' in Vietnam, '*toeuk trey*' in Cambodia and '*nganpyaye*' in Myanmar [6-9].

Fish sauce is a translucent amber liquid with a unique aroma and flavour and is rich in amino acids. Fish sauce is basically a protein hydrolysate that results from a natural fermentation of fish and salt [9]. Protein hydrolysis is induced by endogenous proteinases in fish muscle and digestive tract as well as proteinases produced by halophilic bacteria [10,11]. Degradation of fish protein to free amino acids is primarily responsible for the delicious taste of fish sauce [12]. Various volatile compounds, including acids, carbonyls, nitrogen-containing compounds, and sulfur-containing compounds, are formed during fermentation and believed to be responsible for the distinct aroma of fish sauce [13,14]. Fish sauce has been used as a condiment and an important ingredient in Southeast Asia cooking. In addition, fish sauce is also a rich source of essential amino acids especially lysine. Many vitamins and mineral were also found in fish sauce. Fish sauce is a very good source of vitamin B12 and many minerals such as sodium (Na), calcium (Ca), magnesium (Mg), iron (Fe), manganese (Mn) and phosphorus (P) [15]. Fish sauces contain about 20 g/l of nitrogen, of which 80% is in the form of amino acids; thus they may be considered an important sources of protein [16].

Spices and herbs have been used for thousands of centuries by many cultures to enhance the flavor and aroma of foods. Early cultures also recognized the value of using spices and herbs in preserving foods and for their medicinal value [17].

In the view of the importance of freshwater fish like Catla, to reduce the post-harvest losses and to increase the production of processed fish products in country, the sincere effort were taken to carry the mentioned study in laboratory. Hence the results are narrated here.

Materials and Methods

Preparation of plain and spiced fish sauce

The plain fish sauce was prepared by using sweet water fish variety i.e., Catla (Indian major carp). Firstly the fish was washed and eviscerated then clean by water to remove blood clots and other unwanted parts. The fish was cut into small strips of required size and shape then mixed with salt in 3:1 proportion and mixed well. The mixture was kept in glass chamber and the lid was closed tightly, to avoid air contamination. The mixture was allowed to ferment for 2 months, after fermentation clear amber liquid i.e., plain fish sauce was extracted from fermented mass and used for further study. The spiced fish sauce was prepared by using plain fish sauce 1 kg, Wheat 1.5 kg, Cumin seeds 500 g, coriander 1 kg, mustard 1 kg, fennel seed 750 g, black pepper 100 g and water 8 litre [18]. All spices were roasted, ground and then mixed thoroughly with plain fish sauce.

The spiced sauces were prepared by using three recipes made i.e., T1, T2 and T3 and the spice mix was prepared according to standard recipe adopted from [18]. The recipe was standardized by using 10 g of plain fish sauce and 80 ml water with 30, 40 and 50 g spice mix in T1, T2 and T3 respectively. The panel of semi-trained judges consisting of 25 members was given the spiced fish sauce samples for evaluation of organoleptic characteristics viz. colour, taste, flavour and overall acceptability. After organoleptic assessment of spiced fish sauce, the spiced sauce containing 40 g spice mix having a best sensory acceptability than remaining other two samples.

Physicochemical analysis of spiced fish sauce

Chemical constituents like moisture, fat, protein, carbohydrate, total ash, salt, TSS, TS and total organic content and pH were determined by AOAC (for salt only) [19,20] and Ranganna [21].

Determination of moisture: Moisture was estimated by accurately weighing the 5 g sample, it was ground and subjected to oven drying at 105°C for 4 hr. It was again weighed after cooling in desiccators until constant weight. The resultant loss in weight was calculated as moisture content [19].

Determination of fat: 5 g ground de-moisturised sample was weighed accurately in thimble and defatted with petroleum ether in Soxhlet apparatus for 6-8 hrs. at 60°C. The resultant ether extract was evaporated and lipid content was calculated [19].

Determination of protein: Protein was determined by micro-Kjeldahl method using 0.2 g of sample by digesting the same with concentrated sulfuric acid (H_2SO_4) containing catalyst mixture for 3-4 hrs at 70°C. Then it was distilled with 40 per cent NaOH and liberated ammonia was trapped in 2 per cent boric acid containing methyl red indicator and then it was titrated with 0.01 N H_2SO_4. The per cent nitrogen was calculated and protein percentage was estimated in the sample by multiplying with appropriate factor. To calculate protein content %N was determined by given formula [19].

Determination of carbohydrate: Total carbohydrate content of foods has, for many years, been calculated by difference, rather than analysed directly. Under this approach, the other constituents in the food (protein, fat, water, alcohol, ash) are determined individually, summed and subtracted from the total weight of the food. This is referred to as total carbohydrate by difference and is calculated by the following formula:

100-(Weight in grams [protein+fat+water+ash+other constituent] in 100 g of food)

It should be clear that carbohydrate estimated in this fashion includes fibre, as well as some components that are not strictly speaking carbohydrate, e.g. organic acids [22].

Determination of ash: 5 g sample was weighed into silica crucible and heated at low flame till all the material was completely charred and cooled. Then it was kept in muffle furnace for about 4 hr at 600°C. It was again cooled in desiccator and weighed and repeated until two consecutive weights were constant. The per cent ash was calculated by knowing the difference between the initial and final weight [19].

Determination of total organic acidity: A total acidity was determined as a total organic acidity Take 25-40 ml of the sauce, (previously filtered to remove suspended matter if any) in a 200 ml flask, add 25-50 ml water if desired and titrate against standard Sodium hydroxide solution using phenolphthalein as indicator till a faint pink color persists for 15 seconds. Calculate acidity by using a standard formula [23].

Determination of salt: Weigh 10 g sample was taken into 250 ml Erlenmeyer flask. Add 20 ml of the standardized 0.1 N $AgNO_3$ or more than enough to precipitate all Cl as AgCl. Add 20 ml of HNO_3. It was boiled gently on a hot plate until all solids except AgCl solids dissolve (usually 15 min). Cooled, then 50 ml H_2O and 50 ml indicator was added and titrated with 0.1 N NH_4SCN solution until solution becomes permanent light brown. Subtracted the ml 0.1 N NH_4SCN used from ml 0.1 N $AgNO_3$ added and calculate difference as NaCl. With 10 g sample each ml 0.1 N $AgNO_3$ = 0.058% NaCl [20].

Determination of total soluble solids: Total soluble solids were measured by using hand refractometer (Erma Japan) and reported as °Bx. The TSS of sauce was affected by the concentration of salt, protein, fat and minerals in the sauce.

Determination of viscosity: Viscosity was determined to check the flowing nature and thickness or viscosity (resistance to flow) of sauce which is one of the quality criteria of fish sauce, determined by using the Brookfield viscometer DV-E at different speed and at constant temperature 25°C with a spindle number S-62 and it were expressed in terms of centipoises (cP).

Result and Discution

Effect of storage (ambient temperature) on physicochemical properties of spiced fish sauce

The storage of spiced sauce at ambient temperature affects the physicochemical properties of fish sauce. The study involves the effect of storage on physicochemical properties of spiced sauce and the results were noted on 15 days period intervals up to 60th day.

The moisture content of spiced fish sauce indicates the prime quality parameter and it drastically affects the shelf life of product and also other components of food. The results revealed the moisture content of spiced was gradually increased and the values narrate to moisture was from fresh day (65.81 g/100 g) to 60th day (66.20 g/100 g). The increase in moisture content of spiced sauce may be the effect of degradation and hydrolysis of protein and carbohydrate during storage by fermentation of lactic acid bacteria's. The fat percentage was slightly decreased during storage period from fresh (6.20 g/100 g) to 60th day (6.08 g/100 g). The similar results pertaining to fat changes during storage were observed by Magdi. The protein content of spiced sauce in the Table 1 demonstrates that the protein content was drastically increased during storage. The data exists to protein shows that it was increased from fresh (5.72 g/100 g) to 60th day (6.25 g/100 g). The steady increase in protein concentration of spiced fish sauce was the effect of increase in bulk concentration of microbes in the sauce. The similar findings were quoted in Nicole. scientific literature. The data pertaining to carbohydrates in the Table 1 prove that the carbohydrate steadily decreased during storage from fresh (16.15 g/100 g) to 60th day (15.10 g/100 g). The ultimate results states that carbohydrate content was decreased during storage and this may the effect of utilization of carbohydrate by microbes in the sauce. The similar results were noted by Magdi. The total ash content of sauce indicates the concentration of minerals in the sauce. It could be observed from the Table 1 that the ash content of sauce was found between 2.88 g/100 g to 2.90 g/ 100 g while during study. The salt content of spiced sauce was not much affected during storage. And it was constantly between 3.20 g/100 g to 3.18 g/ 100 g.

No.	Characteristics	Values in g/100 g					Mean	SE ±
		Fresh	15 days	30 days	45 days	60 days		
1	Moisture	65.81	65.85	65.89	65.95	66.2	65.94	0.0191
2	Fat	6.2	6.16	6.15	6.12	6.08	6.142	0.0103
3	Protein	5.72	5.79	5.84	5.97	6.25	5.914	0.0129
4	Carbohydrates	16.15	15.87	15.7	15.57	15.1	15.678	0.0214
5	Salt	3.2	3.2	3.19	3.18	3.18	3.19	0.0115
6	Total Ash	2.9	2.9	2.89	2.88	2.88	2.89	0.0096
7	pH	5.62	5.45	5.32	5.1	4.87	5.272	0.0187
8	Total organic acidity	1.05	1.08	1.12	1.17	1.23	1.13	0.032
9	Total soluble solids	21	22	22	23	23	22.2	1.0645
10	LAB's	$2.9{\times}10^3$	$3.1{\times}10^3$	$3.4{\times}10^3$	$3.6{\times}10^3$	$4.1{\times}10^3$	-	-

Table 1: Effect of storage (ambient temperature) on physicochemical properties of spiced fish sauce (*Each value represents the mean of three determinations).

The pH of spiced sauce was gradually decreased during storage and it affected the quality of sauce, the pH declined drastically affected the micro flora of sauce. The pH of sauce during storage was noted from fresh (5.62) to 60th day (4.87). The results reveals that fall in pH was due to increase in acidity of sauce and this may be the effect of lactic acid fermentation during storage. Also decline in pH was indications of increase in LAB's and decrease in other pH dependent micro flora. The total organic acidity of fish sauce refers to the lactic acid dominantly and the results were noted on first day 1.05 and 60th day 1.23 of study.

The total soluble solids content shows the amount of soluble fraction of food components in the product. The data related to total soluble solids from Table 1 expresses that TSS of sauce was fairly decreased during storage from fresh (21° Bx) to 60th day (23° Bx). The increase in TSS of sauce may be due to degradation and hydrolysis of carbohydrate and fat during storage by microbes.

The crucial factor for the changes occurred in physicochemical properties of spiced fish sauce during storage was ongoing fermentation. The halophilic LAB's was found dominant at the final stage of fermentation, coinciding with a period when color, aroma and flavor are fully developed. This has led to an assumption that halophilic LAB's could play a significant role in the distinct characteristics of fish sauce [10]. According to Jedah et al. [18] the addition of spices can act as stimulants for the growth of LAB's. Also LAB's are able to improve the shelf life of several food products. Result concerning to the LAB's count during storage has noted in the above Table 1 revealed that the LAB's count was progressively increased during storage right from the fresh day ($2.9{\times}10^3$ cfu/ml) to 60th day ($4.1{\times}10^3$ cfu/ml). Similar interpretations were found in the work (Figure 1) [18].

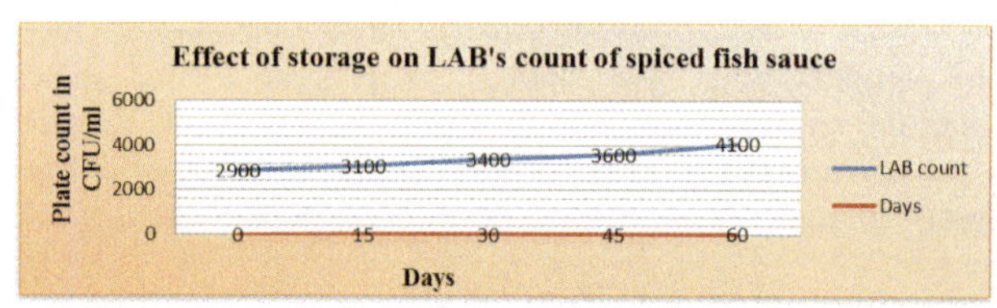

Figure 1: Effect of storage on LAB count of spiced fish sauce.

The viscosity of sauce (other viscous products also) is a major physical quality parameter in respect to consumer acceptance. Therefore, reliable and accurate rheological data are necessary for designing and optimization of various foods processing equipment. The viscosity of sauce was initially increased by addition of wheat flour. The various parameters affect the viscosity of food viz. temperature, chemical composition, storage and etc., during the study the effect of storage was carefully considered on fresh to 60th day by 15 days intervals regularly.

It could be observe from Table 2 that the viscosity was constantly decreased during storage. The results obtained from the table shows that the viscosity was gradually decreased from fresh (282.0 cP) to 60th day (260.4 cP). The change in viscosity during storage may be the effect of fermentation and hydrolysis of food components. Similar results were expressed by Beal et al. (Figure 2) [24].

No.	Days	Viscosity in Centipoise (cP)
1	Fresh	282.0
2	15	278.2
3	30	275.3
4	45	268.6
5	60	260.4
6	Mean	272.9
7	SE ±	3.1166

Table 2: Effect of storage (ambient temperature) on Viscosity of spiced fish sauce (*Each value represents the mean of three determinations).

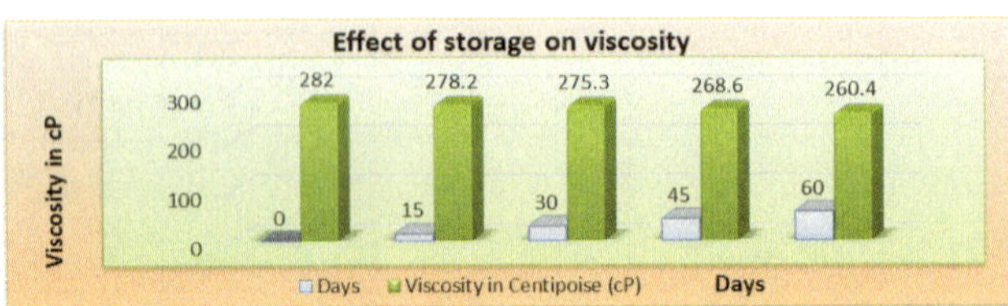

Figure 2: Effect of storage (ambient temperature) on viscosity of spiced fish sauce.

Conclusion

A good quality spiced fish sauce can prepare by using given formulation and mature for valid time which carries various changes during storage or alteration of physicochemical properties of sauce due to the fermentation. The change in properties was effect of fermentation and degradation of chemical components of sauce during storage by fermentation. Also it causes loss of viscosity of product at the end of study.

References

1. Anonymous (2013) Annual Report 2012-13, Department Of Animal Husbandry, Dairying and Fisheries Ministry of Agriculture, Government of India, New Delhi.
2. FAO (2012) State of World Fisheries and Aquaculture. Food and Agricultural Organization of the United Nations, Rome.
3. Jitender KJ, Pal AK, Devivaraprasad AR, Sahu NP, Venkateshwarlu G, et al. (2012) Fatty acids composition of some selected Indian fishes. African Journal of Basic and Applied Sciences 4: 155-160.
4. Venugopal V (2006) Seafood processing adding value through quick freezing, retortable packaging, and cook-chilling. Taylor and Francis group, LLC, Boca Raton London.
5. Visessanguan W, Benjakul S, Riebroy S, Thepkasikul P (2004) Changes in composition and functional properties of proteins and their contributions to Nham characteristics. Food Chemistry 66: 579-588.
6. Ismail MS (1977) Accelerated fermentation of fish soy paste and fish soy-sauce by using Aspergillus oryzae NRRL 1989. Symposium on Indigenous Fermented Foods, Bangkok, Thailand.
7. Putro S (1993) Fish Fermentation Technology in Indonesia. In: Lee CH, Steinkraus KH and Alan Reilly PJ (eds.), In fish fermentation technology. United Nations University Press, Tokyo, Japan.
8. Phithakpol B, Varanyanond W, Reungmaneepaitoon S, Wood H (1995) The traditional fermented foods of Thailand. ASEAN Food Handling Bureau.
9. Tran TD (2002) Country Report-Vietnam. In: Third Regional Workshop on the application of HACCP in the fish processing industry in Southeast Asia.
10. Saisithi P (1994) Traditional fermented fish: Fish sauce production. In: Martin AM (ed.), Fisheries processing biotechnological application. London: Chapman and Hall.
11. Gildberg A, Thongthai C (2001) The effect of reduced salt content and addition of halophilic lactic acid bacteria on quality and composition of fish sauce made from sprat. Journal of Aqua Food Production 10: 77-88.
12. Chayovan S, Rao RM, Liuzzo JA, Khan MA (1983) Chemical characterization and sensory evaluation of a dietary sodium-potassium fish sauce. Journal of Agriculture Food Chemistry 31: 859-863.
13. Shimoda M, Peralta RR, Osajima Y (1996) Headspace gas analysis of fish sauce. Journal of Agriculture and Food Chemistry 44: 3601-3605.
14. Fukami K, Ishiyama S, Yaguramaki H, Masuzawa T, Nabeta Y (2002) Identification of distinctive volatile compounds in fish sauce. Journal of Agriculture Food Chemistry 50: 5406-5412.
15. Wilaipan P (1990) Halophilic bacteria producing lipase in fish sauce. MS thesis, Chulalongkorn University, Bangkok.
16. Mizutani T, Kimizuka A, Ruddle K, Ishige N (1992) Chemical components of fermented fish products. Journal Food Composition Analysis 5: 152-159.
17. Erturk O (2006) Antibacterial and antifungal activity of ethanolic extracts from eleven spice plants. Section Cellular and Molecular Biology 61: 275-278.
18. Al-Jedah JH, Alib MZ, Robinson RK (2000) The inhibitory action of spices against pathogens that might be capable of growth in a fish sauce (mehiawah) from the Middle East. International Journal of Food Microbiology 57: 129-133.
19. AOAC (1990) Official method of analysis Volume II, Association of Official Analytical Chemists, Washington.
20. AOAC (2005) Official Methods of Analysis of the AOAC International (18th edn.), Association of Official Analytical Chemists, Gaithersburg, MD.
21. Ranganna S (2007) Handbook of analysis and quality control for fruit and vegetable products. II Ed. Tata Macgraw-Hill Publishing Company Ltd, New Delhi.
22. Merrill AL, Watt BK (1973) Energy value of foods: basis and derivation. Agriculture Handbook No. 74. Washington, DC, ARS United States Department of Agriculture.
23. Food Safety and Standards Authority of India (2015) Manual of methods of analysis of foods, meat and meat products and fish and fish products. Lab Manual 6.
24. Beal C, Skokanova J, Latrille E, Martin N, Corrieu G (1999) Combined Effects of Culture Conditions and Storage Time on Acidification and Viscosity of Stirred Yogurt. Journal of Diary Science 82: 673-681.

Permissions

All chapters in this book were first published in JN&FS, by OMICS International; hereby published with permission under the Creative Commons Attribution License or equivalent. Every chapter published in this book has been scrutinized by our experts. Their significance has been extensively debated. The topics covered herein carry significant findings which will fuel the growth of the discipline. They may even be implemented as practical applications or may be referred to as a beginning point for another development.

The contributors of this book come from diverse backgrounds, making this book a truly international effort. This book will bring forth new frontiers with its revolutionizing research information and detailed analysis of the nascent developments around the world.

We would like to thank all the contributing authors for lending their expertise to make the book truly unique. They have played a crucial role in the development of this book. Without their invaluable contributions this book wouldn't have been possible. They have made vital efforts to compile up to date information on the varied aspects of this subject to make this book a valuable addition to the collection of many professionals and students.

This book was conceptualized with the vision of imparting up-to-date information and advanced data in this field. To ensure the same, a matchless editorial board was set up. Every individual on the board went through rigorous rounds of assessment to prove their worth. After which they invested a large part of their time researching and compiling the most relevant data for our readers.

The editorial board has been involved in producing this book since its inception. They have spent rigorous hours researching and exploring the diverse topics which have resulted in the successful publishing of this book. They have passed on their knowledge of decades through this book. To expedite this challenging task, the publisher supported the team at every step. A small team of assistant editors was also appointed to further simplify the editing procedure and attain best results for the readers.

Apart from the editorial board, the designing team has also invested a significant amount of their time in understanding the subject and creating the most relevant covers. They scrutinized every image to scout for the most suitable representation of the subject and create an appropriate cover for the book.

The publishing team has been an ardent support to the editorial, designing and production team. Their endless efforts to recruit the best for this project, has resulted in the accomplishment of this book. They are a veteran in the field of academics and their pool of knowledge is as vast as their experience in printing. Their expertise and guidance has proved useful at every step. Their uncompromising quality standards have made this book an exceptional effort. Their encouragement from time to time has been an inspiration for everyone.

The publisher and the editorial board hope that this book will prove to be a valuable piece of knowledge for researchers, students, practitioners and scholars across the globe.

List of Contributors

Aina A T
Department of Microbiology, University of Ibadan, Ibadan, Nigeria

Adel A A Ismail
Consultant in Clinical Biochemistry and Chemical Endocrinology (RTD), Pinderfiels and Leeds Teaching Hospitals, West Yorkshire, England

Nour A Ismail
Pinderfiels and Leeds Teaching Hospitals, West Yorkshire, England

Dworzanski T and Celinski K
Chair and Department of Gastroenterology, Medical University of Lublin, Poland

Dworzanska E
Department of Pediatric Neurology, Medical University of Lublin, Poland

Lach T
Medical University of Lublin, Poland

Gordillo-Bastidas E
Department of Endocrinology and Nutrition, Hospital Clínic, Barcelona, Spain

Roura E and Massanés T
Fundació Alícia, Barcelona, Spain

Díaz-Rizzolo DA
Diabetes and Obesity Research Laboratory, IDIBAPS, Barcelona, Spain

Gomis R
Department of Endocrinology and Nutrition, Hospital Clínic, Barcelona, Spain
Diabetes and Obesity Research Laboratory, IDIBAPS, Barcelona, Spain
University of Barcelona, Barcelona, Spain

Ibok O and Ellis W O
Food Science and Technology Department, College of Science, Kwame Nkrumah University of Science and Technology, Kumasi, Ghana

Mensah E O
Food Science and Technology Department, College of Science, Kwame Nkrumah University of Science and Technology, Kumasi, Ghana
International Potato Centre (CIP), c/o CSIR-CRI, Kumasi, Ghana

Carey E E
International Potato Centre (CIP), c/o CSIR-CRI, Kumasi, Ghana

Rohmah Z and Fitria L
Faculty of Biology, Universitas Gadjah Mada, Yogyakarta 55281, Indonesia

Kang S J, Kim J S and Choi B D
Department of Seafood and Aquaculture Science, The Institute of Marine Industry, Gyeongsang National University, Tongyeong 53064, Korea

Lee J J
Department of Food and Nutrition, Chosun University, Gwangju 61452, Korea

Ha Y L
Antiaging Institute, HK Biotech Co. Ltd., Jinju 52840, Korea

Rintu Das, Silpak Biswas and Ena Ray Banerjee
Department of Zoology, University of Calcutta, India

Garcia J S, Palacios V and Roldán A
Department of Chemical Engineering and Food Technology, University of Cádiz, PB 40, Poligono Rio San Pedro, Puerto Real 11510, Cádiz, Spain

Jentzsch N S, Silveira FJF and Wainstein APDL
Faculty of Medical Sciences of Minas Gerais, Belo Horizonte/MG, Brazil

Cruz L L
School of Nutrition, Federal University of Ouro Preto, Ouro Preto/MG, Brazil

Previato HDRA
Department of Food and Nutrition, School of Food Engineering, University of Campinas, Campinas/SP, Brazil

Jiri O and Mafongoya P
School of Agricultural, Earth and Environmental Sciences, University of KwaZulu-Natal, Private Bag X01, Scottsville, Pietermaritzburg, 3209, South Africa

Rates SPM, Capanema F D, Albuquerque S R, Cordeiro M L and Laguardia S
College of Health and Human Ecology (FASEH), Alterosa Garden, Vespasian-MG, Brazil

Rocha D S
Federal University of Bahia, Campus Teixeira, Candeias, Victory of the Conquest, BA, Brazil

Lamounier J A
School of Medicine, Federal University of Minas Gerais, Santa Efigenia, Belo Horizonte-MG, Brazil

Nguyen Thi Nhu Quynh and Tran Chi Hai
Ho Chi Minh City University of Food Industry, Ho Chi Minh City, Vietnam

Phan Van Man
Faculty of Chemical and Food Technology, Ba Ria Vung Tau University, Vietnam

Le Thanh Thanh
Thu Dau Mot University, Bình Dương, Vietnam

Roba K T, Abdo M and Wakayo T
College of Health and Medical Sciences, Haramaya University, Eastern Ethiopia, Harar, East Harargie 0000, Ethiopia

Imai E, Nakade M, Kasaoka Tsuboyama and Takimoto H
Department of Nutritional Epidemiology, National Institutes of Biomedical Innovation, Health and Nutrition, Tokyo, Japan

Wenpeng You
Biological Anthropology and Comparative Anatomy Unit, The University of Adelaide, Adelaide, SA, Australia

Maciej Henneberg
Institute of Evolutionary Medicine, University of Zurich, Switzerland

Ibegbulem C O, Ene A C and Igwe C U
Department of Biochemistry, Federal University of Technology, Owerri, Nigeria

Nwanpka P and Chikezie P C
Department of Biochemistry, Imo State University, Owerri, Nigeria

Ting Liu, Zhentian Li, Tengfei Wang and Xiaoyan Zhu
College of Animal Science and Veterinary Medicine, Henan Agricultural University, Zhengzhou, PR China

Bayomy H M and Rozan M A
Department of Food Science and Technology, Damanhour University, Egypt

Mohammed G M
Department of Nutrition and food Science, Tabuk University, KSA

Debnath M and Agrawal S
Sports Authority of India, Netaji Subash Eastern Centre, Salt Lake, Kolkata, India
Department of Food and Nutrition, Bajbaj College, Kolkata, India

Osilesi O and Onajobi F D
Department of Biochemistry, Babcock University, Ilishan-Remo, Ogun State, Nigeria

Adebawo O O
Department of Biochemistry, Olabisi Onabanjo University, Ikenne, Ogun State, Nigeria

Karigidi K O
Department of Chemical Sciences, Ondo State University of Science and Technology, Okitipupa, Nigeria

Ibrahim H O
Department of Biochemistry, Babcock University, Ilishan-Remo, Ogun State, Nigeria
Department of Science Laboratory Technology, Federal Polytechnic, Offa, Kwara State, Nigeria

Muhammad L B
Department of Science Laboratory Technology, Federal Polytechnic, Offa, Kwara State, Nigeria

Emana Megersa
Department of Animal Science, Gambella Agricultural, Technical and Vocational Training College, Ethiopia

Ashenafi Mengistu
Department of Tropical Animal Production and Health, College of Veterinary Medicine and Agriculture, Addis Ababa University, Ethiopia

Getahun Asebe
Department of Animal Science, College of Agriculture and Natural Resource, Gambella University, Ethiopia

Karina Huber, Priscila Brigide, Eloá Bolis Bretas and Solange Guidolin Canniatti-Brazaca
Food and Nutrition Department, Luiz de Queiroz College of Agriculture, University of São Paulo, Brazil

Rajendrasingh Rajput
Hair Transplant Surgeon, Member ISHRS, IAT, and AHRS, India

Josefina Consuelo Morales and Rodrigo A Garcia Zepeda
Department of Food Science and Technology, National Institute of Medical Sciences and Nutrition Salvador Zubirán, México

Yitayal A A
Kotebe Metropolitan University, Addis Ababa, Ethiopia

Tilahun R D
Wolkite University, Gubrei, Wabe Bridge, Ethiopia

Thomas Horman and Francesco Leri
Department of Psychology and Neuroscience, University of Guelph, Ontario, Canada

Ranjitha and Neena Joshi
Department of Food Science and Nutrition, GKVK, University of Agricultural Sciences, Bengalore, India

Belete Y
College of Medicine and Health Sciences, Debre Markos University, Debre Markos, Ethiopia

Negga B
College of Health and Medical Sciences, Haramaya University, Harar, Ethiopia

Firehiwot M
College of Health and Medical Sciences, Haramaya University, Harar, Ethiopia

Neera Parmar and Saroj Dahiya
Department of Foods and Nutrition, Chaudhary Charan Singh Haryana Agricultural University, India

Sanjay Kumar
Department of Biochemistry, Central University of Haryana, India

Niharika Shanker and Sukumar Debnath
Department of Traditional Food and Sensory Science, CSIR-Central Food Technological Research Institute, Mysore-570020, India

Dagadkhair A C
Department of Food Chemistry and Nutrition, Vasantrao Naik Marathwada Krishi Vidyapith, Parbhani, MH, India

Pakhare K N
Department of Technology, Food Technology Division, Shivaji University, Kolhapur, MH, India

Gadhave R K
Department of Food Engineering and Technology, SLIET, Sangrur, Punjab, India

Index